EXERCISE

AND THE

HEART

EXERCISE
AND THE
HEART

FIFTH EDITION

Victor F. Froelicher, M.D.
Professor of Medicine
Director ECG/Exercise Laboratory
VA Palo Alto Health Care System
Stanford University
Palo Alto, California

Jonathan Myers, Ph.D.
Clinical Associate Professor of Medicine
VA Palo Alto Health Care System
Stanford University
Palo Alto, California

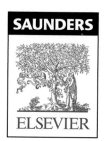

SAUNDERS

ELSEVIER

SAUNDERS
ELSEVIER

1600 John F. Kennedy Blvd.
Ste 1800
Philadelphia, PA 19103-2899

EXERCISE AND THE HEART, Fifth Edition

ISBN-13: 978-1-4160-0311-3
ISBN-10: 1-4160-0311-8

Copyright © 2006, Elsevier Inc.

Notice

Knowledge and best practice in this field are constantly changing. As new research and experience broaden our knowledge, changes in practice, treatment and drug therapy may become necessary or appropriate. Readers are advised to check the most current information provided (i) on procedures featured or (ii) by the manufacturer of each product to be administered, to verify the recommended dose or formula, the method and duration of administration, and contraindications. It is the responsibility of the practitioners, relying on their own experience and knowledge of the patient, to make diagnoses, to determine dosages and the best treatment for each individual patient, and to take all appropriate safety precautions. To the fullest extent of the law, neither the publisher nor the authors assume any liability for any injury and/or damage to persons or property arising out of or related to any use of the material contained in this book.

The Publisher

Library of Congress Cataloging-in-Publication Data

Froelicher, Victor F.
    Exercise and the heart/Victor F. Froelicher, Jonathan Myers.—5th ed.
       p.;cm
    Includes bibliographical references and index.
    ISBN 1-4160-0311-8
       1. Exercise tests. 2. Heart function tests. 3. Heart—Diseases—Diagnosis. I. Myers, Jonathan, 1957- II. Title.
       [DNLM: 1. Heart Diseases—rehabilitation. 2. Exercise Test—methods. 3. Exercise Therapy—methods. 4. Exertion. WG 141.5.F9 F926e 2006]
    RC683.E.E94F76 2006
    616.1′20754—dc22

2005051641

Editor: Susan F. Pioli
Senior Editorial Assistant: Joan Ryan
Publishing Services Manager: Joan Sinclair
Project Manager: Mary Stermel
Design Direction: Gene Harris
Marketing Manager: Dana Butler

Printed in the United States of America

Last digit is the print number: 10   9   8   7   6   5   4   3   2   1

Working together to grow
libraries in developing countries

www.elsevier.com | www.bookaid.org | www.sabre.org

ELSEVIER   BOOK AID International   Sabre Foundation

To Susan, my wife and best friend.

VFF

To my two older brothers,
Chris and Tim, who are no longer with us.
Their intellect eluded me but was always and
continues to be a source of motivation and inspiration.

JM

Welcome to the fifth edition of *Exercise and the Heart*. Since the fourth edition, there have been numerous important documents published, including an update of the American Heart Association (AHA)/American College of Cardiology (ACC) guidelines on exercise testing, the American Thoracic Society/American College of Chest Physicians Statement on Cardiopulmonary Exercise Testing, an AHA Scientific Statement on Exercise and Heart Failure, an AHA Scientific Statement on Physical Activity in the Prevention of Cardiovascular Disease, new editions of the American Association of Cardiovascular and Pulmonary Rehabilitation Guidelines, and the American College of Sports Medicine Guidelines on Exercise Testing and Prescription. Relevant information from these updated documents has been incorporated into this fifth edition. The necessity of practicing evidence-based medicine makes it critical that all of us defer to the panels of experts who write these guidelines. In rare cases in which the guidelines are inconsistent or we offer an opinion or recommendation that differs from the guidelines, we alert the reader.

As the field of cardiology has continued to evolve, it is important to note some of the new or changed acronyms in medicine.

HF has been recommended as the acronym to replace CHF, because CHF has confusingly represented either chronic or congestive (acute) heart failure.

PCI (percutaneous coronary intervention) has replaced PTCA, because currently many techniques in addition to balloon angioplasty are performed by interventionalists.

AED (automated external defibrillator) and ICD (implantable cardiac defibrillator) are used for the new biphasic defibrillator products.

CRT (cardiac resynchronization therapy) is an implantable pacemaker for improving cardiac function that is often combined with an ICD.

ACS (acute coronary syndrome) is the term now widely used to describe the spectrum of conditions associated with acute myocardial ischemia, including unstable angina pectoris and non-Q wave MIs.

In this edition, we've tried to incorporate the influence of the remarkable advances in cardiology in the subject matter. These advances are listed below (not in order of impact), because each by themselves has strongly influenced exercise testing, exercise training, and clinical exercise physiology.

1. Designation of ACSs
2. Biomarkers for ischemia and volume overload/left ventricular dysfunction at point of contact (troponin and brain natriuretic peptide [BNP])
3. Advances in percutaneous coronary interventions (PCI) culminating in drug-eluting stents that have greatly reduced stent failure
4. Evidence-based recommendations that PCI is better than thrombolysis for acute myocardial infarction
5. Medications that convincingly improve survival in patients with heart disease

6. Pacemakers for CRT
7. Further advances in exercise training for patients with heart failure and other groups previously excluded from rehabilitation
8. The basic role of endothelial function in maintaining cardiovascular health and how it is affected by exercise training
9. Human genomics studies related to sudden death (LQT1) and training (ACE)
10. Advances in cardiac defibrillators (implantable and portable units)

These advances have actually interacted with one another, so it is best to address them in groupings that impact health care in a similar fashion. We address those that impact the *diagnostic use of exercise testing* first. Many patients who required diagnostic exercise testing after the first appearance of symptoms now have the diagnosis made based on an elevation of troponin. They frequently go straight to cardiac catheterization. Many cardiologists believe that advances in PCI make the noninvasive diagnosis of ischemic chest pain moot, because angiography can be used to make the diagnosis and treat the problem by averting all steps in between. The lowered restenosis rate associated with drug-eluting stents has removed, in their minds, all the reasons not to diagnose and fix the problem all in one relatively low-risk procedure. However, it is important to keep in mind that health care costs continue to rise and fewer people are insured or able to afford this invasive approach. As clinicians continue to deal with the problems of cost-efficacy, we contend that the exercise test remains the most logical gatekeeper to more expensive and/or invasive diagnostic tests. When a biomarker that can be measured at point of contact becomes validated as a way to increase the sensitivity of the test along with multivariate scores, reasonable clinicians apply the exercise test first. Although some would disagree, we contend that the "art" of medical decision making and the use of noninvasive tests are currently more important than ever.

Next, let us consider the advances in health care that affect the prognostic use of exercise testing. PCI for acute myocardial infarction has been shown to be better for improving prognosis and lessening myocardial damage than thrombolysis. The reason this is so is that it is more effective than thrombolytic drugs in opening coronary arteries blocked by thrombosis. Improved patency rates mean that follow-up exercise testing is less likely to be needed routinely after MI to determine who needs coronary angiography. However, when the

patient and physician want or need individualized prognostic information, there is no test more valuable than the standard exercise test. Several recent studies have confirmed that exercise capacity alone has independent and significant prognostic power regardless of the patient's clinical history.

Surprisingly, the next two items, which relate to patients with HF, have resulted in new ideas regarding cardiovascular physiology. First, HF results in major metabolic and cellular changes that can be improved by an exercise program. These alterations have provided interesting insights into the exercise response, because changes in endothelial function appear to be a major contributor to these improvements. Second, implanted synchronous pacemakers have been shown to improve both ventricular function and exercise capacity. This is somewhat surprising, because previously it was thought that myocyte damage was the primary event leading to LV dysfunction and that conduction disturbances were a result of this. However, improvement in function resulting from correction of dysynchrony suggests that damage to the conduction system can be the cause of LV dysfunction and impair exercise capacity.

There are two important bench findings that are impacting our understanding of cardiac pathophysiology. First, regular exercise can have a powerful effect on endothelial dysfunction, and now this mechanism is proposed as one of the major beneficial actions that exercise has on health. Second, we are only on the threshold of using human genomics to understand exercise and the heart. Congenital diseases that cause exercise-related sudden death have been localized to specific genes (for instance, LQT1). The ACE gene appears to be an important determinant of the response to exercise training.

Finally, advances in defibrillators have had an important impact on exercise for the public. Biphasic units resulting in lower energy needs for defibrillation, long-life lithium batteries, and smart arrhythmia algorithms are the basis for these advances. Cardiopulmonary resuscitation (CPR) has been improved by AEDs, and they are now widely used by the public, resulting in better outcomes following arrhythmic events. These devices are now ubiquitous and are mandatory at gyms and sporting events; importantly, the AHA has developed guidelines for their use in health clubs. However, studies on the number of sudden cardiac deaths (50,000/year in the United States; approximately one fifth of the number estimated initially and used as the impetus for AEDs) and their location (most sudden deaths occur at home and not in public places) have led to some reassessment of their use. Randomized trials have demonstrated a survival benefit for ICDs in most patients with LV dysfunction. Now patients with these devices must be dealt with in the context of cardiac rehabilitation and exercise laboratory settings.

The following is our strongest variance from the guidelines: Exercise testing should be used for screening healthy, asymptomatic individuals along with risk factor assessment. We plan to lobby with our colleagues on this point for the following reasons:

- A number of contemporary studies have demonstrated remarkable risk ratios for the combination of the standard exercise test responses and traditional risk factors.

- Other modalities without the favorable test characteristics of the exercise test are being promoted for screening.

- Physical inactivity has reached epidemic proportions, and the exercise test provides an ideal way to make patients conscious of their deconditioning and to make physical activity recommendations.

- Adjusting for age and other risk factors, each MET increase in exercise capacity equates to a 10% to 25% improvement in survival.

With this fifth edition, we once again have assumed the writing by ourselves. Though it is obvious which one of us was the main author for the various chapters, we collaborated on all of them and take both blame and credit. With the volume of studies on exercise testing and training now all available on the world wide web, it is no longer practical to review in detail as many individual studies, however important they are. Although we have been careful to update our citations, we felt it necessary to keep the classic studies related to particular issues. Wherever possible, we have tried to summarize the major studies in tables, followed by a comment and then our overall view or recommendation on a given issue.

Once again we feel it is important to provide the following precepts in the preface regarding methodology even though the details are in the chapters:

- The treadmill protocol should be adjusted to the patient; one protocol is not appropriate for all patients.

- Exercise capacity should be reported in METs, not minutes of exercise.

- Hyperventilation before testing is not indicated but can be used at another time if a false-positive test is suspected.

- ST measurements should be made at ST0 (J-junction), and ST depression should be considered abnormal only if horizontal or downsloping; most clinically important ST depression occurs in V5, particularly in patients with a normal resting ECG.

- Patients should be placed supine as soon as possible post exercise without a cool-down walk in order for the test to have its greatest diagnostic value.

- The 2- to 4-minute recovery period is critical to include in analysis of the ST response.

- Measurement of systolic blood pressure during exercise is extremely important, and exertional hypotension is ominous; at this point, only manual blood pressure measurement techniques are valid.

- Age-predicted heart rate targets are largely useless because of the wide scatter for any age; a relatively low heart rate can be maximal for a given patient and submaximal for another.

- The Duke Treadmill Score should be calculated automatically on every test except for the elderly.

- Other predictive equations and heart rate recovery should be considered a standard part of the treadmill report.

To ensure the safety of exercise testing and reassure the noncardiologist performing the test, the following list of the most dangerous circumstances in the exercise testing lab should be considered:

- Testing patients with aortic valvular disease or obstructive hypertrophic cardiomyopathy (ASH or IHSS) should be done with great care. Aortic stenosis can cause cardiovascular collapse, and these patients may be difficult to resuscitate because of the outflow obstruction; IHSS can become unstable due to arrhythmia. Because of these conditions, a physical exam including assessment of systolic murmurs should be done before all exercise tests. If a significant murmur is heard, an echocardiogram should be considered before performing the test.

- When patients without diagnostic Q-waves on their resting ECG exhibit exercise-induced

ST segment elevation (i.e., transmural ischemia), the test should be stopped; this can be associated with dangerous arrhythmias and infarction. This occurs in about 1 of 1000 clinical tests.

■ A cool-down walk is advisable in the following instances:

1. When a patient with an ischemic cardiomyopathy exhibits significant chest pain due to ischemia, because the ischemia can worsen in recovery
2. When a patient develops exertional hypotension accompanied by ischemia (angina or ST depression) or when it occurs in a patient with a history of HF, cardiomyopathy, or recent MI
3. When a patient with a history of sudden death or collapse during exercise develops PVCs that become frequent

Appreciation of these circumstances can help avoid any complications in the exercise lab.

As in previous editions, there are many premedical and medical students, graduate students, residents, fellows, visiting professors, and international medical graduates who have contributed to the studies discussed in this book. They are too numerous to mention individually, but their work is cited extensively in this edition. One of the most gratifying things about what we do is to have the opportunity to host these individuals and gain the friendships that result through the inevitable battles that occur in trying to answer a research question. Because of this, we have maintained a wide range of contacts around the world, and many of them continue to collaborate with us. A few individuals in particular warrant mentioning here, because their contributions to this edition are significant. They include Paul Dubach from Switzerland, Euan Angus Ashley from Scotland (now a Stanford cardiology fellow), and Kari Saunamaki from Denmark. Takuya Yamazaki was our most recent research fellow from Japan (of a list of many), and his desk is currently occupied by Tan Swee Yaw from Singapore. Notable PhDs who keep a close eye on our science are Barry Franklin, Paul Ribisl, and Bill Herbert. We have profited both personally and professionally by our association with all of these individuals and treasure the friendships that began through research collaboration.

Given this background, we are targeting this book as a reference for the clinical aspects of exercise testing and training. It is meant for the serious student, academic, or health care provider who wants to have available much of the knowledge in this field summarized in one source. Hopefully it will find an appropriate niche on the shelves in many exercise labs, cardiac rehabilitation departments, and educational training programs. We have tried to incorporate the latest available guidelines, position statements, and meta-analyses. Our love of the subject has led to the incorporation of details that some could consider minutia yet we might have missed some work considered important by our colleagues. We hope you enjoy this book and that it is helpful to you.

Victor F. Froelicher
Jonathan Myers

contents

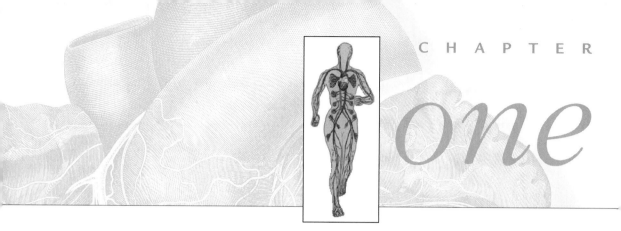

CHAPTER one

Basic Exercise Physiology

Exercise physiology is the study of the physiologic responses and adaptations that occur as a result of acute or chronic exercise. Exercise is the body's most common physiologic stress, and it places major demands on the cardiopulmonary system. For this reason, exercise can be considered the most practical test of cardiac perfusion and function. Exercise testing is a noninvasive tool to evaluate the cardiovascular system's response to exercise under carefully controlled conditions. The adaptations that occur during an exercise test allow the body to increase its resting metabolic rate up to 20 times, during which time cardiac output may increase as much as six times. The magnitude of these adjustments is dependent upon age, gender, body size, type of exercise, fitness, and the presence or absence of heart disease. Although major adaptations are also required of the endocrine, neuromotor, and thermoregulatory systems, the major focus of this chapter is on the cardiovascular response and adaptations of the heart to acute exercise. Cardiovascular adaptations to chronic training in humans and animals are reviewed in Chapter 12.

It is important to understand two basic principles of exercise physiology with regard to exercise testing. The first is a physiologic principle: total body oxygen uptake and myocardial oxygen uptake are distinct in their determinants and in the way they are measured or estimated (Table 1-1). Total body or ventilatory oxygen uptake (VO_2) is the amount of oxygen that is extracted from inspired air as the body performs work. Conversely, myocardial oxygen uptake is

the amount of oxygen consumed by the heart muscle. Accurate measurement of myocardial oxygen consumption requires the placement of catheters in a coronary artery and in the coronary venous sinus to measure oxygen content. The determinants of myocardial oxygen uptake include intramyocardial wall tension (left ventricular pressure × end-diastolic volume), contractility, and heart rate. It has been shown that myocardial oxygen uptake can be reasonably estimated by the product of heart rate and systolic blood pressure (double product). This information is valuable clinically because exercise-induced angina often occurs at the same myocardial oxygen demand (double product) and thus is a useful physiologic variable when evaluating therapy. When it is not the case, the influence of other factors should be suspected, such as a recent meal, abnormal ambient temperature, or coronary artery spasm.

The second principle of exercise physiology is one of pathophysiology: considerable interaction takes place between the exercise test manifestations of abnormalities in myocardial perfusion and function. The electrocardiographic response to exercise and angina are closely related to myocardial ischemia (coronary artery disease), whereas exercise capacity, systolic blood pressure, and heart rate responses to exercise can be determined by the presence of myocardial ischemia, myocardial dysfunction, or responses in the periphery. Exercise-induced ischemia can cause cardiac dysfunction that results in exercise impairment and an abnormal systolic blood pressure response. Often it is difficult to separate the impact of

1

TABLE 1-1. Two basic principles of exercise physiology

Myocardial oxygen consumption	≈ Heart rate × systolic blood pressure (determinants include wall tension ≅ left ventricular pressure × volume; contractility; and heart rate)
Ventilatory oxygen consumption (VO_2)	≈ External work performed, or cardiac output × a-VO_2 difference*

*The arteriovenous O_2 difference is approximately 15 to 17 vol% at maximal exercise in most individuals; therefore, VO_2 max generally reflects the extent to which cardiac output increases.

ischemia from the impact of left ventricular dysfunction on exercise responses. An interaction exists that complicates the interpretation of the exercise test findings. The variables affected by both myocardial ischemia and ventricular dysfunction (i.e., exercise capacity, maximal heart rate, and systolic blood pressure) have the greatest prognostic value.

The severity of ischemia or the amount of myocardium in jeopardy is known clinically to be inversely related to the heart rate, blood pressure, and exercise level achieved. However, neither resting nor exercise ejection fraction nor a change in ejection fraction during exercise correlates well with measured or estimated maximal oxygen uptake, even in patients without signs or symptoms of ischemia.[1,2] Moreover, exercise-induced markers of ischemia do not correlate well with one another. Silent ischemia (i.e., markers of ischemia presenting without angina) does not appear to affect exercise capacity in patients with coronary heart disease. Although not conclusive, radionuclide studies support this position.[3] Cardiac output is generally considered the most important determinant of exercise capacity, but studies suggest that in some patients with heart disease, the periphery plays an important role in limiting exercise capacity.[1,4]

Concepts of Work. Because exercise testing fundamentally involves the measurement of work, there are several concepts regarding work that are important to understand. *Work* is defined as force moving through a given distance ($W = F \times D$). If muscle contraction results in mechanical movement, then work has been accomplished. Force is equal to mass times acceleration ($F = M \times A$). Any weight, for example, is a force that is undergoing the resistance provided by gravity. A great deal of any work that is performed involves overcoming the resistance provided by gravity.

The basic unit of force is the newton (N). It is the force that, when applied to a 1-kg mass, gives it an acceleration of 1 m multiplied by sec^{-2}. Since work is equal to force (in newtons) times distance (in meters), another unit for work is the newton meter (Nm). One Nm is equal to one joule (J), which is another common expression of work. Because work is nearly always expressed per unit of time (i.e., as a rate), an additional unit that becomes important is *power*, the rate at which work is performed. The body's metabolic equivalent (MET) of power is *energy*. Therefore, it is easy to think of work as anything with weight moving at some rate across time (which is often analogous to distance). The common biologic measure of total body work is the oxygen uptake, which is usually expressed as a rate (making it a measure of power) in liters per minute. MET is a term commonly used clinically to express the oxygen requirement of the work rate during an exercise test on a treadmill or cycle ergometer. One MET is equated with the resting metabolic rate (≈3.5 mL of O_2/kg/min), and a MET value achieved from an exercise test is a multiple of the resting metabolic rate, either measured directly (as oxygen uptake) or estimated from the maximal workload achieved using standardized equations.[5]

Energy and Muscular Contraction. Muscular contraction is a complex mechanism involving the interaction of the contractile proteins actin and myosin in the presence of calcium. The British scientist A.F. Huxley proposed that the myosin and actin filaments in the muscle slid past one another as the muscle fibers shortened during contraction. Huxley won the Nobel Prize for this concept, which is still generally considered correct. The source of energy for this contraction is supplied by adenosine triphosphate (ATP), which is produced in the mitochondria. ATP is stored as two products, adenosine diphosphate and phosphate, at specific binding sites on the myosin heads.

The sequence of events that occurs when a muscle contracts has three other major players: calcium and two inhibitory proteins, troponin and tropomyosin. Voluntary muscle contraction begins with the arrival of electrical impulses at the myoneural junction, initiating the release of calcium ions. Calcium is released into the sarcoplasmic reticulum that surrounds the muscle filaments. The calcium binds to a special protein, troponin-C, which is attached to tropomyosin (another protein that inhibits the binding of actin and myosin), and actin. When calcium binds to troponin-C, the tropomyosin molecule is removed from its blocking position between actin and myosin. The myosin head then attaches to actin, and muscular contraction occurs.

The main source of energy for muscular contraction, ATP, is produced by oxidative phosphorylation. The major fuels for this process are carbohydrates (glycogen and glucose) and free fatty acids. At rest, roughly equal amounts of energy are derived from carbohydrates and fats. Free fatty acids contribute greatly to the energy supply during low levels of exercise, but greater amounts of energy are derived from carbohydrates as exercise progresses. Maximal work relies virtually entirely on carbohydrates. Because endurance performance is directly related to the rate at which carbohydrate stores are depleted, major advantages exist for both: (1) having greater glycogen stores in the muscle and (2) deriving a relatively greater proportion of energy from fat during prolonged exercise. Both of these benefits are conferred with training.

Oxidative phosphorylation initially involves a series of events that take place in the cytoplasm. Glycogen and glucose are metabolized to pyruvate through glycolysis. If oxygen is available, pyruvate enters the mitochondria from the sarcoplasm and is oxidized to a compound known as acetyl CoA, which then enters a cyclical series of reactions known as the Krebs cycle. By-products of the Krebs cycle are CO_2 and hydrogen. Electrons from hydrogen enter the electron transport chain, yielding energy for the binding of phosphate (phosphorylation) from adenosine diphosphate to ATP. This process, oxidative phosphorylation, is the greatest source of ATP for muscle contraction. A total of 36 ATP molecules per glucose molecule are formed in the mitochondria during this process.

The mitochondria can produce ATP for muscle contraction only if oxygen is present. However, at higher levels of exercise, total body oxygen demand may exceed the capacity of the cardiovascular system to deliver oxygen. Historically, "anaerobic" (without oxygen) glycolysis has been the term used to describe the synthesis of ATP from glucose under these conditions. Many researchers have superseded this term with more functional descriptions, such as "oxygen independent," "nonoxidative," or "rapid" glycolysis, because "anaerobic" incorrectly implies that glycolysis occurs only when there is an inadequate

oxygen supply. Under such conditions, glycolysis progresses in the cytoplasm much the same way as aerobic metabolism until pyruvate is formed. However, electrons released during glycolysis are taken up by pyruvate to form lactic acid. Rapid diffusion of lactate from the cell inhibits any further steps in glycolysis. Thus, oxygen-independent glycolysis is inefficient; two ATP molecules per glucose molecule is the total yield from this process.

The fact that lactate accumulates in the blood during rapid glycolysis is an important concept in exercise science. The relative exercise intensity in which lactate accumulation occurs is an important determinant of endurance performance. The degree to which lactate accumulates in the blood is related to exercise intensity and the extent to which fast-twitch (type IIB) fibers are recruited. This subject is discussed further in Chapter 3.

Although lactate can contribute to fatigue by increasing ventilation and inhibiting other enzymes of glycolysis, it can also serve as an important energy source in muscles other than those in which it was formed, and it serves as an important precursor for liver glycogen during exercise.[6-8]

Muscle Fiber Types. The body's muscle fiber types are classified on the basis of the speed with which they contract, their color, and their mitochondrial content. Type I, or slow-twitch fibers, are red in color and contain high concentrations of mitochondria. Type II, or fast-twitch fibers, are white in color and have low concentrations of mitochondria. Fiber color is related to the degree of myoglobin, which is a protein that both stores oxygen in the muscle and carries oxygen in the blood to the mitochondria. Not surprisingly, slow-twitch fibers with their high myoglobin content are more resistant to fatigue; thus, a muscle with a high percentage of slow-twitch fibers is well suited for endurance exercise. However, slow-twitch fibers tend to be smaller and produce less overall force than fast-twitch fibers. Fast-twitch fibers are generally larger and tend to produce more force, although they fatigue more easily. Research suggests that the speed of contraction for each fiber type is based largely on the activity of the enzyme myosin ATPase, which sits in the myosin head and to which ATP combines.

It is important to note that although the two fiber types can be separated by distinct characteristics, both fibers function effectively for virtually all physical activities. Evidence also suggests that slow-twitch and fast-twitch fibers are not as dichotomous as previously thought.

Myosin ATPase activity and speed of contraction of some slow-twitch fibers approximate those of fast-twitch fibers. Moreover, type II (fast-twitch) fibers have been further divided into three sub-categories: type IIA, type IIB, and type IIC. The type IIA fiber mimics the type I fiber in that it has a high capacity for oxidative metabolism. It has been suggested that the type IIA fiber actually is a type II fiber that has been adapted for endurance exercise, and endurance athletes are known to have a relatively large number of these fibers.[9] The type IIB fiber is a "true" type II fiber in that it contains few mitochondria and is better adapted for short bursts of activity. The type IIC fiber is poorly understood; it may represent an "uncommitted" fiber, capable of adapting into one of the other fiber types. Historically, it has been thought that endurance athletes were obliged to be genetically endowed with larger percentages of type I fibers, and that the opposite was true of sprinters or jumpers. Numerous cross-sectional studies have confirmed these differences in fiber types between endurance and sprint-type athletes since the advent of the muscle biopsy technique. However, fiber types may in fact represent a continuum, with some capable of adapting toward the characteristics of another fiber.

ACUTE CARDIOPULMONARY RESPONSE TO EXERCISE

The cardiovascular system responds to acute exercise with a series of adjustments that assure (1) active muscles receive blood supply appropriate to their metabolic needs, (2) heat generated by the muscles is dissipated, and (3) blood supply to the brain and heart is maintained. This response requires a major redistribution of cardiac output along with a number of local metabolic changes.

The usual measure of the capacity of the body to deliver and utilize oxygen is the maximal oxygen uptake (VO_2 max). Thus, the limits of the cardiopulmonary system are historically defined by VO_2 max, which can be expressed by the Fick principle:

$$VO_2 \text{ max} = \text{maximal cardiac output} \times \text{maximal arteriovenous oxygen difference}$$

Cardiac output must closely match ventilation in the lung in order to deliver oxygen to the working muscle. VO_2 max is determined by the maximal amount of ventilation (VE) moving into

and out of the lung and by the fraction of this ventilation that is extracted by the tissues:

$$VO_2 = VE \times (FiO_2 - FeO_2)$$

where VE is minute ventilation, and FiO_2 and FeO_2 are the fractional amounts of oxygen in the inspired and expired air, respectively. (For the moment, this equation is oversimplified, as the measurement of VO_2 also requires a determination of expired CO_2, as detailed in Chapter 3.)

Therefore, the cardiopulmonary limits (VO_2 max) are defined by (1) a central component (cardiac output) that describes the capacity of the heart to function as a pump and (2) peripheral factors (arteriovenous oxygen difference) that describe the capacity of the lung to oxygenate the blood delivered to it and the capacity of the working muscle to extract this oxygen from the blood. Figures 1-1 and 1-2 outline the many factors affecting cardiac output and arteriovenous oxygen difference. An abnormality in one or more of these components often characterizes the presence and extent of some form of cardiovascular or pulmonary disease. In the following, these models are reviewed in the context of the cardiovascular response to exercise.

Central Factors

Figure 1-1 shows the central determinants of maximal oxygen uptake.

Heart Rate

Sympathetic and parasympathetic nervous system influences underlie the cardiovascular system's first response to exercise, an increase in heart rate. Sympathetic outflow to the heart and systemic blood vessels increases and vagal outflow decreases. Of the two major components of cardiac output, heart rate and stroke volume, heart rate is responsible for most of the increase in cardiac output during exercise, particularly at higher levels. Heart rate increases linearly with workload and oxygen uptake. Increases in heart rate occur primarily at the expense of diastolic, not systolic time. Thus, at very high heart rates, diastolic time may be so short as to preclude adequate ventricular filling.

The heart rate response to exercise is influenced by several factors, including age, type of activity, body position, fitness, the presence of heart disease, medications, blood volume,

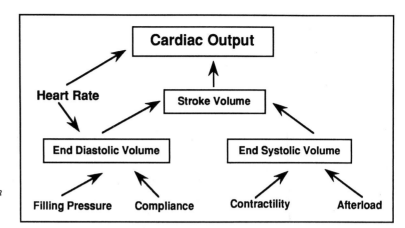

FIGURE 1-1

Central determinants of maximal oxygen uptake. *(From Myers J, Froelicher VF: Hemodynamic determinants of exercise capacity in chronic heart failure. Ann Intern Med 1991;115:377-386.)*

and environment. Of these, the most important factor is age; a decline in maximal heart rate occurs with increasing age.[10] This decline appears to be due to intrinsic cardiac changes rather than to neural influences. It should be noted that there is a great deal of variability around the regression line between maximal heart rate and age; thus, age-related maximal heart rate is a relatively poor index of maximal effort (see Chapter 5). Maximal heart rate is unchanged or may be slightly reduced after a program of training. Resting heart rate is frequently reduced after training as a result of enhanced parasympathetic tone.

Stroke Volume. The product of stroke volume (the volume of blood ejected per heartbeat) and heart rate determines cardiac output. Stroke volume is equal to the difference between end-diastolic and end-systolic volume. Thus, a greater diastolic filling (preload) will normally increase stroke volume. Alternatively, factors that increase arterial

blood pressure will resist ventricular outflow (afterload) and result in a reduced stroke volume. During exercise, stroke volume increases up to approximately 50% to 60% of maximal capacity, after which increases in cardiac output are due to further increases in heart rate. The extent to which increases in stroke volume during exercise reflect an increase in end-diastolic volume or a decrease in end-systolic volume, or both, is not entirely clear but appears to depend upon ventricular function, body position, and intensity of exercise. In healthy subjects, stroke volume increases at rest and during exercise after a period of exercise training. Although the mechanisms have been debated, evidence suggests that this adaptation is due more to increases in preload—and possibly local adaptations that reduce peripheral vascular resistance—than to increases in myocardial contractility.

In addition to heart rate, end-diastolic volume is determined by two other factors: filling pressure and ventricular compliance.

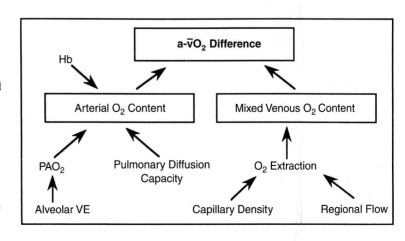

FIGURE 1-2

Peripheral determinants of maximal oxygen uptake. The a-$\bar{V}O_2$ difference is the difference between arterial and venous oxygen. Hb, hemoglobin; PAO_2, partial pressure of alveolar oxygen; VE, minute ventilation. *(From Myers J, Froelicher VF: Hemodynamic determinants of exercise capacity in chronic heart failure. Ann Intern Med 1991;115:377-386.)*

Filling Pressure. The most important determinant of ventricular filling is venous pressure. The degree of venous pressure is a direct consequence of the amount of venous return. The Frank-Starling mechanism dictates that, within limits, all the blood returned to the heart will be ejected during systole. As the tissues demand greater oxygen during exercise, venous return increases, which in turn increases end-diastolic fiber length (preload), resulting in a more forceful contraction. Venous pressure increases as exercise intensity increases. Over the course of a few beats, cardiac output will equal venous return.

A number of other factors affect venous pressure, and therefore filling pressure, during exercise. These factors include blood volume, body position, and the pumping action of the respiratory and skeletal muscles. A greater blood volume increases venous pressure and therefore end-diastolic volume by making more blood available to the heart. Because the effects of gravity are negated, filling pressure is greatest in the supine position. In fact, stroke volume generally does not increase from rest to maximal exercise in the supine position. The intermittent mechanical constriction and relaxation in the skeletal muscles during exercise also enhance venous return. Finally, changes in intrathoracic pressure that occur with breathing during exercise facilitate the return of blood to the heart.

Ventricular Compliance. Compliance is a measure of the capacity of the ventricle to stretch in response to a given volume of blood. Specifically, compliance is defined as the ratio of the change in volume to the change in pressure. The diastolic pressure/volume relation is curvilinear; that is, at low end-diastolic pressures, large changes in volume are accompanied by small changes in pressure, and vice versa. At the upper limits of end-diastolic pressure, ventricular compliance declines; that is, the chamber stiffness increases as it fills. Because of the difficulty in measuring end-diastolic pressure during exercise, few data are available concerning ventricular compliance during exercise in humans.

End-systolic volume is a function of two factors: contractility and afterload.

Contractility. Contractility describes the forcefulness of the heart's contraction. Increasing contractility reduces end-systolic volume, which results in a greater stroke volume and thus greater cardiac output. This process is precisely what occurs with exercise in the normal individual; the percentage of blood in the ventricle that is ejected with each beat increases, owing to an altered cross-bridge formation. Contractility is commonly quantified by the ejection fraction, the percentage of blood ejected from the ventricle during systole using radionuclide, echocardiographic, or angiographic techniques. Despite its wide application as an index of myocardial contractility, ejection fraction has been repeatedly shown to correlate poorly with exercise capacity.

Afterload. Afterload is a measure of the force resisting the ejection of blood by the heart. Increased afterload (or aortic pressure, as is observed with chronic hypertension) results in a reduced ejection fraction and increased end-diastolic and end-systolic volumes. During dynamic exercise, the force resisting ejection in the periphery (total peripheral resistance) is reduced by vasodilation, owing to the effect of local metabolites on the skeletal muscle vasculature. Thus, despite even a fivefold increase in cardiac output among normal subjects during exercise, mean arterial pressure increases only moderately.

Volume Response to Exercise. Results of studies evaluating the volume response to exercise have varied greatly. Although the advent of radionuclide techniques in the 1970s offered promise for the noninvasive assessment of ventricular volumes during exercise, the results have been disappointing. Because of technical limitations, most of these studies have been performed in the supine position. Early studies employing radionuclide or echocardiographic techniques during supine exercise among normal subjects reported that end-diastolic volume remained constant or diminished slightly,[11-14] increased in the order of 27%,[15] or varied greatly depending on the subject.[16-18] Among patients with coronary artery disease exercised in the supine position, increases in end-diastolic volume were observed among patients with exercise-induced angina, whereas end-diastolic volume did not change in patients who were asymptomatic. Sharma et al[19] and Jones et al[20] reported increases in both end-diastolic and end-systolic volumes in patients who developed angina during exercise. Slutsky et al[11] reported that end-diastolic volume remained unchanged in patients with coronary artery disease whether or not they developed angina. Manyeri and Kostuk[21] reported large increases in both end-systolic and end-diastolic volumes during supine exercise among 20 patients with coronary artery disease, 13 of whom developed angina during exercise.

The ventricular volume response to upright exercise also varies greatly, even in similar populations. The results of some of the major studies in this area are listed in Table 1-2. Among normal subjects, end-diastolic volume has been reported to increase greatly,[15,21,22] increase moderately,[23-27] or decrease slightly during upright exercise.[28-31] End-diastolic volume has been reported to increase in the range of 8% to 56% among patients with coronary artery disease, and end-systolic volume has been shown to increase in the range of 16% to 94% in response to upright exercise.[21,23,32-37] Among normal subjects, end-systolic volume has generally been reported to decrease in response to maximal upright exercise (range 4% to 79%).[21,23-33,38] Higginbotham et al,[22] however, observed a 48% increase in end-systolic volume among normal subjects; others have reported lesser increases. Less is known about the ventricular response to upright exercise in patients with chronic heart failure. Sullivan et al,[39] Tomai et al,[31] and Delahaye et al[40] all observed increases in both end-systolic and end-diastolic volumes from rest to peak exercise ranging between 10% and 20% in patients with left ventricular dysfunction.

The inconsistent results concerning the ventricular volume response to both supine and upright exercise have led investigators to raise questions concerning the validity of radionuclide techniques for assessing ventricular function. For example, Jensen et al[41] studied the individual variability of radionuclide ventriculography in patients with coronary artery disease with repeat testing for more than 1 year. Although differences in end-diastolic volume measurements between initial and repeat testing were small, the standard deviations of the individual differences between tests at rest and peak exercise were large, on the order of 38 and 49 mL, respectively. Variability in the ejection fraction and end-systolic volume responses to exercise were of a similar magnitude.

In light of the apparent shortcomings of the radionuclide techniques, investigators have

TABLE 1-2. Ventricular volume response to upright exercise using radionuclide of echocardiographic techniques

Investigator	Population	Technique	Percent change EDV	Percent change ESV
Rerych et al 1978[23]	Normals (n = 30)	RN	Increase 10	Decrease 35
	CAD (n = 20)	RN	Increase 56	Increase 94
Freeman et al 1981[34]	Normals (n = 10)	RN	Increase 25	Increase 10
	CAD (n = 22)	RN	Increase 30	Increase 38
Wyns et al 1982[28]	Normals (n = 10)	RN	Decrease 8	Decrease 65
Manyeri and Kostuk 1983[21]	Normals (n = 22)	RN	Increase 31	Decrease 22
Crawford et al 1983[33]	CAD (n = 10)	Echo	Increase 8	Increase 22
	CAD (n = 20)	RN	Increase 45	Increase 48
Kalischer et al 1984[36]	CAD (n = 18)	RN	Increase 27	Increase 48
	CAD (n = 10)	RN	Increase 24	Increase 38
Hakki and Iskandrian 1985[43]	Mixed (n = 117)	RN	Increase 15	—
Shen et al 1985[35]	Normals (n = 17)	RN	Increase 22	Increase 27
	CAD (n = 14)	RN	Increase 26	Increase 29
Higginbotham et al 1986[22]	Normals (n = 24)	RN	Increase 45	Increase 48
Iskandrian and Hakki 1986[24]	Normals (n = 41)	RN	Increase 6	Decrease 35
Plotnick et al 1986[27]	Normals (n = 30)	RN	Increase 4	Decrease 50
Renlund et al 1987[29]	Normals (n = 13)	RN	Decrease 3	Decrease 79
Sullivan et al 1988[39]	CHF (n = 20)	RN	Increase 20	Increase 20
Ginzton et al 1989[38]	Normals (n = 14)	Echo	Decrease 26	Decrease 48
Younis et al 1990[25]	Normals (n = 9)	RN	Increase 17	Decrease 4
Goodman et al 1991[26]	Normals (n = 15)	RN	Increase 19	Decrease 14
Myers et al 1991[37]	CAD (n = 8)	Echo	Increase 16	Increase 16
Schairer et al 1992[30]	Normals (n = 15)	Echo	Decrease 4	Decrease 52
Tomai et al 1992[32]	Normals (n = 12)	RN	Decrease 8	Decrease 42
Tomai et al 1993[31]	Normals (n = 10)	RN	Decrease 8	Decrease 43
	CHF (n = 10)	RN	Increase 12	Increase 14
Delahaye et al 1997[40]	CHF (n = 13)	RN	Increase 15	Increase 23
Lapa-Bula et al 2002[41]	CHF (n = 10)	Echo	Increase 4	Decrease 5

CAD, coronary artery disease; CHF, chronic heart failure; Echo, echocardiography; EDV, end-diastolic volume or end-diastolic volume index; ESV, end-systolic volume or end-systolic volume index; RN, radionuclide ventriculography.

employed alternative methods for quantifying ventricular function during exercise. Crawford et al[33] evaluated the feasibility and reproducibility of two-dimensional echocardiography for assessing left ventricular function during exercise. A 9% test-retest difference in end-diastolic volume was demonstrated. End-diastolic volume was reported unchanged from rest to peak exercise in patients with coronary disease, but it increased significantly (20%) from rest to peak exercise in normal subjects. Ginzton et al[38] compared athletes with sedentary subjects during upright exercise using two-dimensional echocardiography. After a slight increase in end-diastolic volume submaximally in both groups, end-diastolic volume decreased 39% and 35% at peak exercise among athletes and sedentary subjects, respectively. Although both groups decreased end-systolic volume progressively during exercise, the reduction was greater among the athletes (70% versus 52%).

Thus, the ventricular volume response to exercise is not entirely clear, but it appears to depend upon the type of disease, method of measurement (radionuclide or echocardiographic), type of exercise (supine versus upright), and exercise intensity (submaximal versus maximal). Much of the disagreement on this issue can no doubt be attributed to differences in the exercise level at which measurements were taken. With this in mind, some rough generalizations may be made concerning changes in ventricular volume in response to upright exercise.

In normal subjects, the response from upright rest to a moderate level of exercise is an increase in both end-diastolic and end-systolic volumes of about 15% and 30%, respectively. As exercise progresses to a higher intensity, end-diastolic volume probably does not increase further,[27] but end-systolic volume decreases progressively. At peak exercise, end-diastolic volume may even decline somewhat, while stroke volume is maintained by a progressively decreasing end-systolic volume. Based on six studies that have quantified the volume response of patients with coronary artery disease in the upright position,[21,23,34-37] end-diastolic volume has been reported to increase 16% to 56% during exercise. The increase in end-systolic volume has been reported to range from 16% to 48%. An exception, however, is a study performed by Rerych et al[23] that reported a 94% increase in end-systolic volume. Sullivan et al,[39] Tomai et al,[31] and Delahaye et al[40] reported approximately 20% increases in both end-systolic and end-diastolic volumes from rest

to maximal exercise during upright exercise among patients with chronic heart failure, whereas Lapu-Bula et al[42] reported that volumes changed minimally during exercise. Few other data are available for this group in the upright position.

Peripheral Factors (a-VO$_2$ Difference)

Figure 1-2 shows the peripheral determinants of maximal oxygen uptake. Oxygen extraction by the tissues during exercise reflects the difference between the oxygen content of the arteries (generally 18 to 20 mL O_2/100 mL at rest) and oxygen content in the veins (generally 13 to 15 mL O_2/100 mL at rest, yielding a typical a-VO$_2$ difference at rest of 4 to 5 mL O_2/100 mL, $\approx$23% extraction). During exercise, this difference widens as the working tissues extract greater amounts of oxygen; venous oxygen content reaches very low levels and a-VO$_2$ difference may be as high as 16 to 18 mL O_2/100 mL with exhaustive exercise (exceeding 85% extraction of oxygen from the blood at VO$_2$ max). Some oxygenated blood always returns to the heart, however, as smaller amounts of blood continue to flow through metabolically less active tissues that do not fully extract oxygen. Generally, a-VO$_2$ difference does not explain differences in VO$_2$ max between subjects who are relatively homogenous. That is, a-VO$_2$ difference is generally considered to widen by a relatively "fixed" amount during exercise, and differences in VO$_2$ max have been historically explained by differences in cardiac output. However, some patients with cardiovascular or pulmonary disease exhibit reduced VO$_2$ max values that can be attributed to a combination of central and peripheral factors.

Determinants of Arterial Oxygen Content. Arterial oxygen content is related to the partial pressure of arterial oxygen, which is determined in the lung by alveolar ventilation and pulmonary diffusion capacity, and in the blood by hemoglobin content. In the absence of pulmonary disease, arterial oxygen content and saturation are usually normal throughout exercise, even at very high levels. This is true even for patients with severe coronary disease or chronic heart failure. However, often patients with symptomatic pulmonary disease neither ventilate the alveoli adequately nor diffuse oxygen from the lung into the bloodstream normally, and a decrease in arterial oxygen saturation during exercise is one of the hallmarks of this disorder. Arterial hemoglobin content is also usually normal throughout exercise. Naturally, a condition such as anemia would reduce the oxygen-carrying capacity of the blood, along with any condition that would shift the O_2 dissociation curve leftward, such as reduced 2, 3-diphosphoglycerate, PCO_2, or elevated temperature.

Determinants of Venous Oxygen Content. Venous oxygen content reflects the capacity to extract oxygen from the blood as it flows through the muscle. It is determined by the amount of blood directed to the muscle (regional flow) and capillary density. Muscle blood flow increases in proportion to the increase in work rate and thus the oxygen requirement. The increase in blood flow is brought about not only by the increase in cardiac output, but also by a preferential redistribution of the cardiac output to the exercising muscle. A reduction in local vascular resistance facilitates the greater skeletal muscle flow. In turn, locally produced vasodilatory mechanisms, along with neurogenic dilatation resulting from higher sympathetic activity, mediate the greater skeletal muscle blood flow. A marked increase in the number of open capillaries reduces diffusion distances, increases capillary blood volume, and increases mean transit time, facilitating oxygen delivery to the muscle.

Cross-sectionally, fit individuals have a greater skeletal muscle capillary density than sedentary subjects. In addition, fit subjects may have a greater capacity to redistribute blood flow toward the working muscle and away from nonexercising tissue. The converse is true in many patients with cardiovascular disease. For example, one of the characteristics of the patient with chronic heart failure is an "exaggeration" of the deconditioning response. These patients exhibit a reduced capacity to redistribute blood, a reduced capacity to vasodilate in response to exercise or following ischemia, and a reduced capillary-to-fiber ratio.

SUMMARY

The major cardiopulmonary adaptations that are required of acute exercise make exercise testing a very practical test of cardiac perfusion and function. The rather remarkable physiologic adaptations that occur with exercise have made exercise a valuable research medium not just for the study of cardiovascular disease, but also for studying physical performance in athletes and for studying the normal and abnormal physiology of other organ systems.

A major increase and redistribution of cardiac output underlies a series of adjustments that allow the body to increase its resting metabolic rate as much as 10 to 20 times with exercise. The capacity of the body to deliver and utilize oxygen is expressed as the maximal oxygen uptake. Maximal oxygen uptake is defined as the product of maximal cardiac output and maximal arteriovenous oxygen difference. Thus, the cardiopulmonary limits are defined by (1) a central component (cardiac output) that describes the capacity of the heart to function as a pump and (2) peripheral factors (arteriovenous oxygen difference) that describe the capacity of the lung to oxygenate the blood delivered to it and the capacity of the working muscle to extract this oxygen from the blood. Hemodynamic responses to exercise are greatly affected by the type of exercise being performed, by whether or not disease is present, and by the age, gender, and fitness of the individual.

Coronary artery disease is characterized by reduced myocardial oxygen supply, which, in the presence of an increased myocardial oxygen demand, can lead to myocardial ischemia and reduced cardiac performance. Despite years of study, a number of dilemmas remain with regard to the response to exercise clinically. Although myocardial perfusion and function are intuitively linked, it is often difficult to separate the impact of ischemia from that of left ventricular dysfunction on exercise responses. Indices of ventricular function and exercise capacity are poorly related. Cardiac output is considered the most important determinant of exercise capacity in normal subjects and in most patients with cardiovascular or pulmonary disease. However, among patients with disease, abnormalities in one or several of the links in the chain that defines oxygen uptake contribute to the determination of exercise capacity.

The transport of oxygen from the air to the mitochondria of the working muscle cell requires the coupling of blood flow and ventilation to cellular metabolism. Energy for muscular contraction is provided by three sources: stored phosphates (ATP and creatine phosphate), oxygen-independent glycolysis, and oxidative metabolism. Oxidative metabolism provides the greatest source of ATP for muscular contraction. Muscular contraction is accomplished by three fiber types that differ in their contraction speed, color, and mitochondrial content. The duration and intensity of activity determine the extent to which these fuel sources and fiber types are called upon.

REFERENCES

1. Myers J, Froelicher VF: Hemodynamic determinants of exercise capacity in chronic heart failure. Ann Intern Med 1991;115:377-386.
2. McKirnan MD, Sullivan M, Jensen D, Froelicher VF: Treadmill performance and cardiac function in selected patients with coronary heart disease. J Am Coll Cardiol 1984;3:253-261.
3. Hammond HK, Kelley TL, Froelicher VF: Noninvasive testing in the evaluation of myocardial ischemia: Agreement among tests. J Am Coll Cardiol 1985;5:59-69.
4. Clark AL, Poole-Wilson PA, Coats AJ: Exercise limitation in chronic heart failure: Central role of the periphery. J Am Coll Cardiol 1996;28:1092-1102.
5. American College of Sports Medicine: Guidelines for Exercise Testing and Prescription, 6th ed. Philadelphia, Lea & Febiger, 1999.
6. Brooks GA: Intra- and extra-cellular lactate shuttles. Med Sci Sports Exerc 2000;32:790-799.
7. Brooks GA: Lactate shuttles in nature. Biochem Soc Trans 2002;30:258-264.
8. Myers J, Ashley E: Dangerous curves: A perspective on exercise, lactate, and the anaerobic threshold. Chest 1997;111:787-795.
9. Saltin B, Henriksson J, Hugaard E, Andersen P: Fiber types and metabolic potentials of skeletal muscles in sedentary man and endurance runners. Ann NY Acad Sci 1977;301:3-29.
10. Hammond K. Froelicher VF: Normal and abnormal heart rate responses to exercise. Prog Cardiovasc Dis 1985;27:271-296.
11. Slutsky R, Karliner J, Ricci D, et al: Response of left ventricular volume to exercise in man assessed by radionuclide equilibrium angiography. Circulation 1979;60:565.
12. Cotsamire DL, Sullivan MJ, Bashore TM, Leier CV: Position as a variable for cardiovascular responses during exercise. Clin Cardiol 1987;10:137-142.
13. Stein RA, Michelli D, Fox EL, Krasnow N: Continuous ventricular dimensions in man during supine exercise and recovery. Am J Cardiol 1978;41:655-660.
14. Bevegard BS, Shepherd JT: Regulation of circulation during exercise in man. Physiol Rev 1967;47:178-213.
15. Poliner LR, Dehmer GJ, Lewis SE, et al: Left ventricular performance in normal subjects: A comparison of the responses to exercise in the upright and supine positions. Circulation 1980;62:528-534.
16. Bristow JD, Klosten FE, Farrahi C, et al: The effects of supine exercise on left ventricular volume in heart disease. Am Heart J 1966;71:319-329.
17. Adams KF, Vincent LM, McAllister SM, et al: The influence of age and gender on left ventricular response to supine exercise in asymptomatic normal subjects. Am Heart J 1987;113:732-742.
18. Granath A, Jonsson B, Strandall T: Circulation in healthy old men, studied by right heart catheterization at rest and during exercise in supine and sitting position. Acta Med Scand 1964;176:425-446.
19. Sharma B, Goodwin JF, Raphael MJ, et al: Left ventricular angiography on exercise: A new method of assessing left ventricular function in ischemic heart disease. Br Heart J 1976;38:59-70.
20. Jones R, McEwan P, Newman G, et al: Accuracy of diagnosis of coronary artery disease by radionuclide measurement of left ventricular function during rest and exercise. Circulation 1981;64:586-601.
21. Manyeri DE, Kostuk WJ: Right and left ventricular function at rest and during bicycle exercise in the supine and sitting positions in normal subjects and patients with coronary artery disease. Assessment by radionuclide ventriculography. Am J Cardiol 1983;51:36-42.
22. Higginbotham MB, Morris KG, Williams RS, et al: Regulation of stroke volume during submaximal and maximal upright exercise in normal man. Circ Res 1986;58:281-291.
23. Rerych SK, Scholz PM, Newman GE, et al: Cardiac function at rest and during exercise in normals and in patients with coronary heart disease. Evaluation by radionuclide angiography. Ann Surg 1978;187:449-464.
24. Iskandrian AS, Hakki AH: Determinants of the changes in left ventricular end-diastolic volume during upright exercise in patients with coronary artery disease. Am Heart J 1986;112:441-446.
25. Younis LT, Melin JA, Robert AR, Detry JMR: Influence of age and sex on left ventricular volumes and ejection fraction during upright exercise in normal subjects. Eur Heart J 1990;11:916-924.
26. Goodman JM, Lefkowitz CA, Liu PP, et al: Left ventricular functional response to moderate and intense exercise. Can J Sport Sci 1991;16:204-209.
27. Plotnick GD, Becker L, Fisher ML, et al: Use of the Frank–Starling mechanism during submaximal versus maximal upright exercise. Am J Physiol 1986;251:H1101-H1105.
28. Wyns W, Melin JA, Vanbutsele RJ, et al: Assessment of right and left ventricular volumes during upright exercise in normal men. Eur Heart J 1982;3:529-536.
29. Renlund DG, Lakatta EG, Fleg JL, et al: Prolonged decrease in cardiac volumes after maximal upright bicycle exercise. J Appl Physiol 1987;63:1947-1955.
30. Schairer JR, Stein PD, Keteyian S, et al: Left ventricular response to submaximal exercise in endurance-trained athletes and sedentary adults. Am J Cardiol 1992;70:930-933.
31. Tomai F, Ciavolella M, Crea F, et al: Left ventricular volumes during exercise in normal subjects and patients with dilated cardiomyopathy assessed by first-pass radionuclide angiography. Am J Cardiol 1993;72:1167-1171.
32. Tomai F, Ciavolella M, Gaspardone A, et al: Peak exercise left ventricular performance in normal subjects and in athletes assessed by first-pass radionuclide angiography. Am J Cardiol 1992;70:531-535.
33. Crawford MH, Amon KW, Vance WS: Exercise 2-dimensional echocardiography. Quantitation of left ventricular performance in patients with severe angina pectoris. Am J Cardiol 1983;51:1-6.
34. Freeman MR, Berman DS, Staniloff H, et al: Comparison of upright and supine bicycle exercise in the detection and evaluation of extent of coronary artery disease by equilibrium radionuclide ventriculography. Am Heart J 1981;102:182-189.
35. Shen WF, Roubin GS, Choong CY-P, et al: Left ventricular response to exercise in coronary artery disease: Relation to myocardial ischemia and effects of nifedipine. Eur Heart J 1985;6:1025-1031.
36. Kalisher AL, Johnson LL, Johnson YE, et al: Effects of propranolol and timolol on left ventricular volumes during exercise in patients with coronary artery disease. J Am Coll Cardiol 1984;3:210-218.
37. Myers J, Wallis J, Lehmann K, et al: Hemodynamic determinants of maximal ventilatory oxygen uptake in patients with coronary artery disease. Circulation 1991;84:II-150.
38. Ginzton LE, Conant R, Brizendine M, Laks MM: Effect of long-term high-intensity aerobic training on left ventricular volume during maximal upright exercise. J Am Coll Cardiol 1989;14:364-371.
39. Sullivan MJ, Higginbotham MB, Cobb FR: Exercise training in patients with severe left ventricular dysfunction. Hemodynamic and metabolic effects. Circulation 1988;78:506-515.
40. Delahaye N, Cohen-Solal A, Faraggi M, et al: Comparison of left ventricular responses to the six-minute walk test, stair climbing, and maximal upright bicycle exercise in patients with congestive heart failure due to idiopathic dilated cardiomyopathy. Am J Cardiol 1997;80:65-70.
41. Lapu-Bula R, Robert A, Van Craeynest D, et al: Contribution of exercise-induced mitral regurgitation to exercise stroke volume and exercise capacity in patients with left ventricular systolic dysfunction. Circulation 2002;106:1342-1348.
42. Jensen DG, Genter F, Froelicher VF, et al: Individual variability of radionuclide ventriculography in stable coronary artery disease patients over one year. Cardiology 1984;71:255-265.
43. Hakki AH, Iskandrian AS: Determinants of exercise capacity in patients with coronary artery disease: Clinical implications. J Cardiac Rehabil 1985;5:341-348.

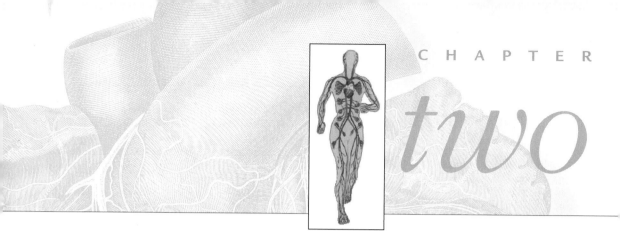

Exercise Testing Methodology

Despite the many advances in technology related to the diagnosis and treatment of cardiovascular disease, the exercise test remains an important diagnostic modality. Its numerous applications, widespread availability, and high yield of clinically useful information continue to make it an important gatekeeper for more expensive and invasive procedures. However, the many different approaches to the exercise test have been a drawback to its proper application. Excellent guidelines have been updated by organizations such as the American Heart Association, American Association of Cardiovascular and Pulmonary Rehabilitation, and American College of Sports Medicine. These guidelines are based on a multitude of research studies over the last 30 years and have led to greater uniformity in methods. Nevertheless, in many laboratories, methodology remains based on tradition, convenience, equipment, or personnel available.

New technology, while adding convenience, has also raised new questions with regard to methodology. For example, all commercially available systems today depend upon computers. Do computer-averaged exercise electrocardiograms (ECGs) improve test accuracy, and should the practitioner rely on this processed information or on the raw data? What about the many computerized exercise scores that now can so easily be calculated? Technology has changed the exercise-testing laboratory environment, and concerns such as these have arisen. Though many of these techniques are attractive, in many

instances not enough data are yet available to validate them, so they should be used judiciously. Also, what about the various ancillary tests and the nonexercise stress modalities? In this chapter, we will address basic methodology and comment on the impact these advances in technology have had. We start by listing the advantages and disadvantages of exercise ECG testing. These considerations are important because the health care provider must evaluate the suitability of the various testing modalities in each situation.

ADVANTAGES AND DISADVANTAGES OF EXERCISE ECG TESTING

ADVANTAGES OF THE STANDARD EXERCISE ECG TEST

1. Low cost
2. Availability of trained personnel
3. Exercise capacity determined
4. Patient acceptability
5. Takes less than an hour to accomplish
6. Convenience
7. Availability
8. Long history of use, validation of responses, application of multivariate scores

---

SAFETY PRECAUTIONS AND RISKS

The safety precautions outlined by the American Heart Association are very explicit in regard to the requirements for exercise testing. Everything necessary for cardiopulmonary resuscitation must be available, and regular drills should be performed to ascertain that both personnel and equipment are prepared for a cardiac emergency. The classic survey of clinical exercise facilities by Rochmis and Blackburn in 1971[1] showed exercise testing to be a safe procedure, with approximately only one death and five nonfatal complications per 10,000 tests. Perhaps because of an expanded knowledge concerning indications, contraindications, and endpoints, data suggest that maximal exercise testing is safer today than 30 years ago. In 1989, Gibbons et al[2] reported the safety of exercise testing in 71,914 tests conducted over a 16-year period. The complication rate was 0.8 per 10,000 tests. In a recent survey of 71 exercise testing laboratories throughout the Veterans Administration Health Care System including 75,828 tests, we observed an event rate of 1.2 per 10,000 tests.[3] The fact that the event rate was similar between a clinically referred population (the Veterans Administration, a higher risk group), and a generally healthier population[2] underscores the fact that the test is extremely safe. Gibbons et al[2] suggested that the low complication rate in their study was due to the inclusion of a cool-down walk, but we have observed a low rate of ventricular tachycardia,[4] and a low overall complication rate[3] despite having patients assume a supine position immediately after the test and despite exercising higher risk patients. This issue is addressed in more detail in Chapter 13, and a summary of these studies is presented in Table 13-6.

However, it is important to note that there have been reports of complications, including acute infarctions and deaths, associated with exercise testing. Although the test is remarkably safe, the population referred for this procedure usually is at high risk for coronary events. Irving and Bruce[5] have reported an association between exercise-induced hypotension and ventricular fibrillation. Shepard[6] has hypothesized the following risk levels for exercise: (1) three or four times normal in a cross-country foot race, (2) 6 to 12 times normal when patients at risk for coronary artery disease (CAD) are performing unaccustomed exercise, and (3) as high as 60 times normal when patients with existing CAD are performing exercise in a stressful environment, such as a physician's office. Cobb and Weaver[7] estimated the risk to be over 100 times in the latter situation and point out the dangers of the recovery period. The risk of exercise testing in patients with CAD cannot be disregarded even with its excellent safety record. Studies documenting the risks of exercise training are presented in more detail in Chapter 12.

Indications to stop an exercise test, in addition to the factors to consider in assessing the degree of exertion, are outlined in Table 2-1. Most problems can be avoided by having an experienced physician, nurse, or exercise physiologist standing next to the patient, measuring blood pressure, and assessing patient appearance during the test. The exercise technician should operate the recorder and treadmill, take the appropriate tracings, enter data on a form, and alert the physician to any abnormalities that may appear on the monitor scope. If the patient's appearance is worrisome, if systolic blood pressure drops or plateaus, if there are alarming ECG abnormalities, if chest pain occurs and becomes worse than the patient's usual pain, or if the patient wants to stop the test for any reason, the test should be stopped, even at a submaximal level. In most instances, a symptom-limited maximal test is preferred, but it is usually advisable to stop if 0.2 mV of additional ST-segment elevation occurs, or if 0.2 mV of flat or downsloping ST-segment depression occurs. In some patients estimated to be at high risk because of their clinical history, it may be appropriate to stop at a submaximal level, as it is not unusual for severe ST-segment depression, dysrhythmias, or both to occur in the postexercise period. If the measurement of maximal exercise capacity or other information is needed, it may be preferable to repeat the test later, once the patient has demonstrated a safe performance of a submaximal workload.

Exercise testing should be an extension of the history and physical examination. A physician obtains the most information by being present to talk with, observe, and examine the patient in

---

TABLE 2-1. Indications for terminating an exercise test and assessment of maximal effort

Absolute Reasons or Indications to Terminate
Acute myocardial infarction
Severe angina—chest pain score of 4 out of 4
Exertional hypotension—a drop in systolic blood pressure of ≥10 mmHg, or drop below the value obtained in the standing position prior to testing, particularly in patients who have heart failure, have had a prior myocardial infarction, or are exhibiting signs or symptoms of ischemia ≥1.0 mm ST elevation in leads without diagnostic Q waves
Serious arrhythmias—ventricular tachycardia, third-degree heart block
Poor perfusion as judged by skin temperature and cyanosis
Neurologic signs—confusion, lightheadedness, vertigo
Technical problems—inability to interpret the ECG pattern; any malfunction of the recording or monitoring device; inability to measure the systolic blood pressure
Patient's request to terminate

Relative Reasons or Indications to Terminate
The following indications may be superseded if done so in the context of good clinical judgment.
Increasing chest pain—chest pain score of 3 out of 4 ≥ 2.0 mm horizontal or downsloping ST depression
Pronounced fatigue or shortness of breath
Wheezing
Leg pain or claudication
Increase in systolic blood pressure to 250 mmHg or increase in diastolic blood pressure to 115 mmHg
Less serious arrhythmias than those in preceding list (frequent or mutifocal premature ventricular contractions, supraventricular tachycardia, bradyarrhythmias)
Bundle branch block or another rate-dependent intraventricular conduction defect that cannot be distinguished from ventricular tachycardia

Assessment of Maximal Effort
As no single marker of effort is usually specifically indicative of a maximal effort, it is best to consider multiple responses.
Borg scale 17-20
Signs of fatigue, profound shortness of breath, or exhaustion
Age-predicted maximal heart rate, with a population-specific regression equation
Expired gas measurements, including respiratory exchange ratio (>1.10)

---

conjunction with the test. A brief physical examination should always be performed to rule out any contraindications that exist. Accordingly, individuals who supervise exercise tests must have the cognitive and technical skills necessary to be competent to do so. The American College of Cardiology, American Heart Association, and the American College of Physicians, with broad involvement from other professional organizations involved with exercise testing, such as the American College of Sports Medicine, have outlined the cognitive skills needed to competently supervise exercise tests.[8] These skills include knowledge of appropriate indications and contraindications to testing, an understanding of risk assessment, the ability to recognize and treat complications, and knowledge of basic cardiovascular and exercise physiology, along with the ability to interpret the test in different patient populations.

The need for physician presence during exercise testing has been the subject of a great deal of discussion in the past. In many cases, exercise tests can be supervised by properly trained and competent exercise physiologists, physical therapists, nurses, physician assistants, or medical technicians who are working under the direct supervision of a physician. However, the physician must be in the immediate vicinity or on the premises or the floor and available for emergencies.[8,9] In situations where the patient is deemed to be at higher risk for an adverse event during exercise testing, the physician should be physically present in the exercise testing room to personally supervise the test. Such cases include, but are not limited to, patients with recent acute coronary syndrome or myocardial infarction (within 7 to 10 days), severe LV dysfunction, severe valvular stenosis (e.g., aortic stenosis), or known complex arrhythmias. The physician's reaction to signs or symptoms should be moderated by the information the patient gives regarding his or her usual activity. If abnormal findings occur at levels of exercise that the patient usually performs, then it may not be necessary to stop the test for them. Also, the patient's activity history should help determine appropriate work rates for testing.

CONTRAINDICATIONS

Table 2-2 lists the absolute and relative contraindications to performing an exercise test.

TABLE 2-2. Contraindications to exercise testing

Absolute
Acute myocardial infarction (within 2 days)
Unstable angina not stabilized by medical therapy
Uncontrolled cardiac arrhythmias causing symptoms or hemodynamic compromise
Symptomatic severe aortic stenosis
Uncontrolled symptomatic heart failure
Acute pulmonary embolus or pulmonary infarction
Acute myocarditis or pericarditis

Relative*
Left main coronary stenosis or its equivalent
Moderate stenotic valvular heart disease
Electrolyte abnormalities
Uncontrolled arterial hypertension†
Tachyarrhythmias or bradyarrhythmias
Hypertrophic cardiomyopathy and other forms of outflow tract obstruction
Mental or physical impairment leading to inability to exercise adequately
High-degree atrioventricular block

*Relative contraindications can be superseded if benefits outweigh risks of exercise.
†In the absence of definitive evidence, a systolic blood pressure of 200 mmHg and a diastolic blood pressure of 110 mmHg are reasonable criteria.

Good clinical judgment should be foremost in deciding the indications and contraindications for exercise testing. In selected cases with relative contraindications, testing can provide valuable information even if performed submaximally.

PATIENT PREPARATION

Preparations for exercise testing include the following:

1. The patient should be instructed not to eat or smoke at least 2 to 3 hours prior to the test and to come dressed for exercise.
2. A brief history and physical examination (particularly for patients with systolic murmurs) should be performed to rule out any contraindications to testing (see Table 2-2).
3. Specific questioning should determine which drugs are being taken, and potential electrolyte abnormalities should be considered. The labeled medication bottles should be brought along so that they can be identified and recorded. It is generally no longer considered necessary for most patients to stop taking their beta-blockers prior to testing. If it is considered necessary to do so in selected patients, they should be stopped gradually in order to avoid the "rebound" phenomenon, which can be dangerous.

The tapering of beta-blockers should be overseen by a physician.
4. If the reason for the exercise test is not apparent, the referring physician should be contacted such that this gets clarified.
5. A 12-lead ECG should be obtained in both the supine and standing positions. The latter is an important rule, particularly for patients with known heart disease, since an abnormality may prohibit testing. On rare occasions, a patient referred for an exercise test will instead be admitted to the coronary care unit.
6. The patient should receive careful explanations of why the test is being performed and of the testing procedure, including its risks and possible complications. A demonstration should be provided of how to get on and off the treadmill and how to walk on it. The patient should be told that he or she can hold on to the handrails initially but then should use the rails only for balance (discussed in the following section).

TREADMILL

The treadmill should have front and side rails for patients to steady themselves, and some patients may benefit from the helping hand of the person administering the test. The treadmill should be calibrated at least monthly. Some models can be greatly affected by the weight of the patient and will not deliver the appropriate workload to heavy patients. An emergency stop button should be readily available to the staff only. A small platform or stepping area at the level of the belt is advisable so that the patient can start the test by "pedaling" the belt with one foot prior to stepping on. After they become accustomed to the treadmill, patients should not grasp the front or side rails, as this decreases the work performed and thus the oxygen uptake, which increases exercise time, resulting in an overestimation of exercise capacity. Gripping the handrails also increases ECG muscle artifact. For patients who have difficulty letting go of the handrails, it is helpful to have them take their hands off the rails, close their fists, and extend one finger on each hand, touching the rails only with those fingers in order to maintain balance while walking. Some patients may require a few moments before they feel comfortable enough to let go of the handrails, but we strongly discourage grasping the handrails after the first minute of exercise.

LEGAL IMPLICATIONS OF EXERCISE TESTING

In any procedure with a risk of complications, it is advisable to make certain the patient understands the situation and acknowledges the risks. Some physicians feel that informing patients of the risks involved will occasionally make them overly anxious or discourage them from performing the test. Because of this, and the fact that a signed consent form does not necessarily protect a physician from legal action, there has been less insistence on consent forms. However, a great deal of case law exists suggesting that a written informed consent before the exercise test is important to protect the patient, physician, and institution.

Establishment of physician-patient communication before and after performance of the exercise test should be the first legal consideration. A test should not be performed without first obtaining the patient's informed consent, after the patient is made aware of the potential risks and benefits of the procedure. A physician may be held responsible in the event of a major untoward event, even if the test is carefully performed, in the absence of informed consent. The argument can be made that the patient would not have undergone the procedure had he or she been made aware of the risks associated with the test.

After the test, responsibility rests with the physician for prompt interpretation and consideration of the implications of the test. Communication of these results to the patient is necessary—with advice concerning adjustments in lifestyle—and this should be done immediately after the test is performed.

The second consideration should be adherence to proper standards of care during performance of the test. Exercise testing should be carried out only by persons thoroughly trained in its administration and in the prompt recognition of problems that may arise. A physician trained in exercise testing and resuscitation should be readily available during the test to make judgments concerning test termination. Resuscitative equipment should always be available. As mentioned above, an updated joint position statement from several professional organizations was published in 2000, outlining the standards for physician competence for performing exercise testing.[8]

BLOOD PRESSURE MEASUREMENT

Although numerous clever devices have been developed to automate blood pressure measurement during exercise, none can be recommended. The time-proven method of the physician holding the patient's arm with a stethoscope placed over the brachial artery remains the most reliable method to obtain the blood pressure. The patient's arm should be free of the handrails so that noise is not transmitted up the arm. It is sometimes helpful to mark the brachial artery. An anesthesiologist's auscultatory piece or an electronic microphone can be fastened to the arm. A device that inflates and deflates the cuff on the push of a button can also be helpful. If systolic blood pressure appears to be increasing sluggishly or decreasing, it should be taken again immediately. If a drop in systolic blood pressure of 10 to 20 mmHg or more occurs, or if it drops below the value obtained in the standing position prior to testing, the test should be stopped. This is particularly important in patients who have heart failure, a prior myocardial infarction, or are exhibiting signs or symptoms of ischemia. An increase in systolic blood pressure to 250 mmHg or an increase in diastolic blood pressure to 115 mmHg are also indications to stop the test. The clinical implications of abnormal blood pressure responses to the exercise test are discussed in detail in Chapter 5.

ECG RECORDING INSTRUMENTS

Many technologic advances in ECG recorders have taken place. The medical instrumentation industry has promptly complied with specifications set forth by various professional groups. Machines with high-input impedance ensure that the voltage recorded graphically is equivalent to that on the surface of the body despite the high natural impedance of the skin. There remains some concern about mismatching lead impedance, which can result in distortion. Optically isolated buffer amplifiers have ensured patient safety, and machines with a frequency response from 0 to 100 Hz are commercially available. The 0 Hz lower end is possible because DC coupling is technically feasible.

Some ECG equipment has monitoring and diagnostic modes, particularly equipment used in coronary care units. The diagnostic mode follows diagnostic instrument specifications with a frequency response from 0.05 to 100 Hz. In the monitor mode, there can be distortion of the ECG. The monitor mode is available to lessen the effects of electrical interference, motion, and respiration on the ECG and should not be used for exercise testing. The type of distortion is affected by the ECG waveform that is presented. If the ECG waveform is a tall R wave without an S wave, the ST-segment distortion can be different than if there is an R wave followed by a large S wave. In general, an inadequate low-frequency response can greatly decrease the Q- and R-wave amplitude and create S waves. Alteration of the 25 to 45 Hz frequency response is the most common cause of ST-segment distortion found in tracings with abnormal ST segments. Some of the newer filtering techniques delay the appearance of the ECG signal on the monitor screen by several seconds.

WAVEFORM AVERAGING

Digital averaging techniques have made it possible to average ECG signals to remove noise. There is a need for consumer awareness in these areas, since most manufacturers do not specify how the use of such procedures modifies the ECG. Signal averaging can actually distort the ECG signal. These techniques are attractive because they can produce a clean tracing in spite of poor skin preparation. However, the common expression used by computer scientists, "Garbage in, garbage out," has never been more applicable than to the computerized ECG. The clean-looking exercise ECG signal produced may not be a true representation of the actual waveform and in fact may be dangerously misleading. Also, the instruments that make computer ST-segment measurements cannot be totally reliable as they are based on imperfect algorithms. For instance, the algorithm that measures QRS end at 70 or 80 msec after the peak of the R wave can hardly be valid, particularly with a changing heart rate.

Because of physician insistence on having exercise tracings as clean as resting tracings, manufacturers have taken some worrisome steps with filtering and ECG presentation. One such approach is "linked medians," in which averages are connected together at the same R-R interval as raw data. Even though these tracings are appropriately labeled, and often presented with a channel of raw data as well, most physicians do not realize that they are dealing with created waveforms instead of raw data.

ECG PAPER RECORDERS

For some patients it is advantageous to have a recorder with a slow paper speed option such as 5 mm/sec. This speed makes it possible to record an entire exercise test and reduces the likelihood of missing any dysrhythmias when specifically evaluating patients with these problems. A faster paper speed of 50 mm/sec can be helpful for making accurate ST-segment slope measurements. Many different types of ECG paper can be used. Wax-treated paper is known to retain an ECG image for 20 years or longer; however, it is pressure-sensitive and easily marked. Thermochemically treated paper is sturdy and resists marking. There are many different types of thermochemically treated paper, and the life expectancy of images recorded on them is usually adequate. However, at least one instance of ECG paper losing a recorded image resulted in legal action by a hospital against a manufacturer. Ceramic-coated paper is very sturdy and comparable in price to other ECG papers. It has a hard finish with a high contrast, which makes it durable and easy to interpret. Untreated paper is the cheapest ECG paper, but the ink-jet and carbon-transfer techniques characteristically produce fuzzy images on untreated paper. The ink-jet and carbon-transfer recorders are available with six channels and are expensive, but they do have an excellent upper-frequency response for phonocardiography. The ceramic paper also requires an ink-jet rather than a heat stylus. Ink-jet recorders require more maintenance and have largely been replaced by thermal head printers. Copying can be a problem as some photographic reproduction machines poorly copy reds and blues.

Thermal head printers have nearly totally replaced all other types of printers. These recorders are remarkable in that they can use blank thermal paper and write out the grid as well as the ECG, vector loops, and alphanumerics. They can record graphs and figures as well as tables and typed reports. They are totally digitally driven and can produce very high resolution records. The paper price is comparable to that for paper used with other recorders, and these devices are themselves reasonably priced and very durable, particularly because no stylus is needed. Some exercise systems use a laser printer, but this is not suitable for the exercise environment, where recording the ECG is delayed by the 5 to 20 seconds required for the printing to occur.

Z-fold paper has the advantage over roll paper in that it is easily folded, and the study can be interpreted in a manner similar to paging through a book. Exercise ECGs can be microfilmed on rolls, cartridges, or in fiche cards for storage. They can also be stored in digital or analog format on magnetic media or optical discs. The latest technology involves recording on CD-ROM discs that are erasable and have fast access and transfer times. These devices can be easily interfaced with microcomputers and can store gigabytes of digital information.

EXERCISE TEST MODALITIES

Three types of exercise can be used to stress the cardiovascular system: isometric, dynamic, and a combination of the two. *Isometric exercise*, defined as constant muscular contraction without or with minimal external movement (such as handgrip), imposes a disproportionate pressure load on the left ventricle relative to the body's ability to supply oxygen. *Dynamic exercise* is defined as rhythmic muscular activity resulting in movement, and it initiates a more appropriate increase in cardiac output and oxygen exchange. Since a delivered workload can be accurately calibrated and the physiologic response easily measured, dynamic exercise is preferred for clinical testing. With progressive workloads of dynamic exercise, patients with CAD can be protected from rapidly increasing myocardial oxygen demand. Although bicycling is a dynamic exercise and appropriate for exercise testing, most individuals perform

slightly more work on a treadmill. This is because a greater muscle mass is involved, in addition to the fact that most subjects are more familiar with walking than cycling.

Numerous modalities have been used to provide dynamic exercise for exercise testing, including steps, escalators, and ladder mills. Today, however, the bicycle ergometer and the treadmill are the most commonly used dynamic exercise devices. The bicycle ergometer is usually cheaper, takes up less space, and makes less noise. Upper body motion is usually reduced, but care must be taken so that the arms do not perform isometric exercise. The workload administered by the simple bicycle ergometers is not well calibrated and is dependent upon pedaling speed. It can be easy for a patient to slow pedaling speed during exercise testing and decrease the administered workload. More modern electronically braked bicycle ergometers keep the workload at a specified level over a wide range of pedaling speeds. Electrically braked ergometers are particularly needed for supine exercise testing.

ARM ERGOMETRY

Alternative methods of exercise testing are necessary for patients with vascular, orthopedic, or neurologic conditions that prevent them from performing leg exercise. Arm ergometry is one such alternative. For a given submaximal workload, arm exercise is performed at a greater physiologic cost than is leg exercise. However, at maximal effort, physiologic responses are generally significantly greater in leg exercise than in arm exercise. At a given power output (expressed as kilopond meters per minute [kpm/min] or watts), heart rate, systolic and diastolic blood pressure, the product of heart rate and systolic blood pressure, minute ventilation, and blood lactate concentration are higher during arm exercise. In contrast, stroke volume and the ventilatory threshold (the latter expressed as a percentage of aerobic capacity) are lower during arm exercise than during leg exercise.[10-13] Because cardiac output is nearly the same in arm and leg exercise at a given oxygen uptake,[14] the elevated blood pressure during arm exercise is due to increased peripheral vascular resistance.

This difference in cardiopulmonary and hemodynamic responses to arm exercise as compared with leg exercise at identical workloads appears to be due to several factors. First, mechanical efficiency is lower during arm exercise than leg exercise. This lower efficiency may reflect the involvement of smaller muscle groups and the static effort by the torso muscles to stabilize the shoulder required for arm work.[15] Both factors could increase oxygen requirements yet not affect the external work performed by the arms. The higher rate-pressure product and estimated myocardial oxygen demand at a given external workload for arm work as compared to leg work may be due to increased sympathetic tone during arm exercise (owing to reduced stroke volume with compensatory tachycardia), isometric contraction of torso muscles, or vasoconstriction in the nonexercising leg muscles.[16-18]

Maximal oxygen uptake (VO_2 max) during arm ergometry in men generally varies between 64% and 80% of leg ergometry VO_2 max. Similarly, maximal cardiac output is lower during arm exercise than during leg exercise, whereas maximal heart rate, systolic blood pressure, and rate-pressure product are comparable[19] or slightly lower[20] during arm exercise. Although women have a lower arm VO_2 max than men, it appears that their aerobic capacity for arm work is not disproportionately inferior to men's. Vander et al[21] found that the relationship between arm and leg

ergometry in women, expressed as arm VO_2 max/leg VO_2 max, was 79%, compared to the mean value of 72% derived from seven separate studies on men. A summary of the studies comparing maximal heart rate responses to arm and leg exercise is presented in Table 2-3.

Fardy et al[22] reported a greater arm VO_2 max than leg VO_2 max when aerobic capacity was expressed per milliliter of limb volume. Because the arms were approximately one-third the volume of the legs, and the VO_2 max for the arms was two thirds that of the legs, VO_2 max for arm exercise was twice that of the legs. The twofold increase in oxygen use per unit of arm volume may be spurious, because arm ergometry also utilizes muscles of the back, shoulders, and chest.

Several investigators have examined the ability of leg or arm exercise testing to conversely predict performance capacity of the other extremities in able-bodied subjects. Asmussen and Hemmingsen[23] showed that it was not possible to estimate leg VO_2 max from experiments with arm work, and vice versa. Franklin et al[24] found weak correlations between maximal power output (kpm/min) or VO_2 max (metabolic equivalents;

TABLE 2-3. Comparison of the maximal heart rate (HR max) in response to arm and leg exercise in men and women

Investigator	HR max (beats/min) Arms	Legs	HR max difference Ratio legs/arms beats/min	Ratio arms/legs (%)
Men (normal)				
Astrand et al. (1968)	177	190	13	93
Stenberg et al. (1967)	178	188	10	95
Bar-Or and Zwiren (1975)	173	195	22	89
Bergh et al. (1976)	176	189	13	93
Davis et al. (1976)	184	193	9	95
Fardy et al. (1977)	174	185	11	94
Magel et al. (1978)	174	195	21	89
Bouchard et al. (1979)	183	186	3	98
De Boer et al. (1982)	167	190	23	88
Sawka et al. (1982)	169	179	10	94
Franklin et al. (1983)	172	184	12	93
Balady et al. (1986)	160	160	0	100
Men (cardiac patients)				
Schwade et al. (1977)	122	129	7	95
DeBusk et al. (1978)	142	145	3	98
Balady et al. (1985)	101	109	8	93
Women (normal)				
Vander et al. (1984)[21]	169	177	8	95
Mean Results	164	174	11	94

METs) for arm and leg exercise. Schwade et al[25] also reported a poor correlation ($r = 0.37$) between peak workloads during arm and leg exercise in patients with ischemic heart disease.

To determine the sensitivity of arm exercise in detecting CAD, Balady et al[26, 27] tested 30 patients with angina pectoris using both arm ergometry and a treadmill before coronary angiography. All patients had at least 70% diameter reduction in one or more major coronary arteries. Ischemic ST depression (≥ 0.1 mV) or angina occurred more frequently with leg exercise (86%, 26 patients) than with arm exercise (40%, 12 patients). No significant difference in peak rate-pressure product was seen between tests, although peak VO_2 was greater during leg exercise than during arm exercise (18 versus 13 mL/kg/min). For concordantly positive tests, oxygen uptake at the onset of ischemia was significantly lower during arm testing than during leg testing (12 versus 17 mL/kg/min). No significant difference in heart rate was seen between tests at the onset of ischemia. Thus, arm exercise testing is a reasonable, but not equivalent, alternative to leg exercise testing in patients who cannot perform leg exercise.

SUPINE VERSUS UPRIGHT EXERCISE TESTING

A great deal of the information available on hemodynamic responses to exercise has come from supine exercise, mostly because cardiac catheterization is required to obtain much of this information. However, there are marked differences between the body's response to acute exercise in the supine versus upright position. During supine bicycle exercise, stroke volume and end-diastolic volume do not change much from values obtained at rest, whereas in the upright position, these values increase during mild work and then plateau. Naturally, exercise capacity is markedly lower in the supine position than during upright cycling. In patients with heart disease, left ventricular filling pressure is more likely to increase during exercise in the supine position than in the upright position. When patients with angina perform identical submaximal bicycle workloads in supine and upright positions, heart rate is higher and angina will develop at a lower double product while the patient is supine. ST-segment depression is often greater in the supine position because of the greater left ventricular volume.

As with upright exercise, a linear relationship between cardiac output and oxygen uptake during supine bicycle exercise has been observed and has been used to separate heart disease patients from normal subjects. *Exercise factor*, or the increase in cardiac output for a given increase in oxygen uptake, is based on studies of normal subjects. For every 100 mL increase in oxygen consumption, cardiac output should increase by 500 mL. Left ventricular filling pressure does not increase in proportion to work in normal persons, but it often increases in patients with heart disease. Radionuclide imaging has shown that the ejection fraction usually increases in normal subjects but can decrease during exercise in patients with ischemia or left ventricular dysfunction. However, many patients with heart disease demonstrate discordance between their disease and ventricular function and can respond normally to exercise.

BICYCLE ERGOMETER VERSUS TREADMILL

In most studies comparing the upright cycle ergometer with treadmill exercise, maximal heart rate values have been demonstrated to be roughly similar, whereas maximal oxygen uptake has been shown to be 6% to 25% greater during treadmill exercise.[28-31] Early hemodynamic studies by Niederberger et al[32] concluded that bicycle exercise constitutes a greater stress on the cardiovascular system for any given oxygen uptake than does treadmill exercise. The clinical importance of these findings in relation to patients with cardiovascular disease undergoing exercise testing is that slightly higher maximal oxygen uptakes are achieved with slightly less hemodynamic stress when treadmill exercise is used. Wicks et al[33] reported similar ECG changes with treadmill testing as compared to bicycle testing in coronary patients. Rather than for any clinical reason, however, the treadmill is the most commonly used dynamic testing modality in the United States because patients are more familiar with walking than they are with bicycling. Patients are more likely to give the muscular effort necessary to adequately increase myocardial oxygen demand by walking than by cycling.

EXERCISE WITH INTRACARDIAC CATHETERS

Exercise testing with intracardiac catheters has significant advantages over alternative diagnostic methods for: (1) separation of cardiac from pulmonary dyspnea, (2) separation of LF systolic from diastolic dysfunction, and (3) quantitative evaluation of the clinical significance of valvular disease.

Cardiac versus Pulmonary Dyspnea. Patients with severe chronic obstructive pulmonary disease (COPD) have clinical findings that make the assessment of left ventricular function extremely difficult. Many patients with COPD have left-sided heart disease secondary to CAD, hypertension, or left-sided valvular disease. In patients with left-sided heart disease, the common denominator for cardiac dyspnea is elevation of left atrial pressure. This leads to elevation of the pulmonary wedge pressure, which leads to increased pulmonary interstitial fluid, decreased pulmonary compliance, and dyspnea. In contrast, significant elevation of left atrial or pulmonary wedge pressure is unusual in uncomplicated COPD cases. Measurement of rest/exercise wedge pressure allows one to distinguish the pathophysiology of COPD from left-sided heart disease. In the former case, pulmonary artery pressure may rise markedly, but pulmonary wedge pressure will remain below 20 mmHg even with maximal supine exercise. In left-sided heart disease, a pulmonary wedge pressure greater than 25 mmHg often occurs at maximal exercise.

Left Ventricular Systolic versus Diastolic Dysfunction. Left ventricular systolic dysfunction with a resultant increase in left ventricular volume leads to an increase in diastolic filling pressure. The patient with heart failure after a myocardial infarction is the classic example of systolic dysfunction. In hypertrophic cardiomyopathy, systolic or contractile function can be normal or even better than normal, but a thick, noncompliant ventricle that cannot readily fill leads to an increased pulmonary wedge pressure. Diastolic dysfunction is characterized by a normal cardiac output for a given workload, but this output comes at the expense of an elevated filling pressure. The distinction between systolic and diastolic function requires the measurement of cardiac output.

Quantitation of Valvular Disease. Patients whose symptoms seem out of proportion to their valvular disease can be assessed using these invasive techniques. In the case of significant valvular lesions, exercise leads to an increase in pulmonary wedge pressure. Forward output may be maintained until late in their course. Elevation of exercise pulmonary wedge pressure at symptom-limited exercise suggests that valve disease rather than concomitant pulmonary disease is the cause of clinical symptoms.

EXERCISE PROTOCOLS

The many different exercise protocols in use have led to some confusion regarding how physicians compare tests between patients and serial tests on the same patient. The most common protocols, their stages, and the predicted oxygen cost of each stage are illustrated in Figure 2-1. When treadmill and cycle ergometer testing were first introduced into clinical practice, practitioners adopted protocols used by major researchers such as Balke and Ware,[34] Astrand and Rodahl,[35] Bruce,[36] and Ellestad[37] and their coworkers. In 1980, Stuart and Ellestad[38] surveyed 1375 exercise laboratories in North America and reported that of those performing treadmill testing, 65.5% use the Bruce protocol for routine clinical testing. A survey published in 2001 among 71 exercise laboratories at Veterans Administration Medical Centers indicated that the percentage of exercise laboratories primarily using the Bruce protocol is similar to that 20 years earlier.[3] Thus, this protocol remains widely used. A disadvantage of the Bruce protocol is that it uses relatively large and unequal 2 to 3 MET increments in work every 3 minutes. Large and uneven work increments such as these have been shown to result in a tendency to overestimate exercise capacity.[9,30,31,39] In part for this reason, many investigators, along with exercise testing guidelines, have since recommended protocols with smaller and more equal increments.[9,30,31,39-42]

In a classic study, Redwood et al[42] performed serial testing in patients with angina and reported that work rate increments that were too rapid resulted in a reduced exercise capacity and could not be reliably used for studying the effects of therapy. When excessive work rates were used, the reduction in myocardial oxygen demand as a result of nitroglycerin administration was minor, suggesting that protocols placing heavy and abrupt demands on the patient may mask a potential salutary effect of an intervention. These investigators recommended that the protocol be individualized for each patient to elicit angina within 3 to 6 minutes. Smokler et al[43] reported that among 40 pairs of treadmill tests conducted within a 6-month period, tests that were less than 10 minutes in duration showed a much greater percentage of variation than those that were

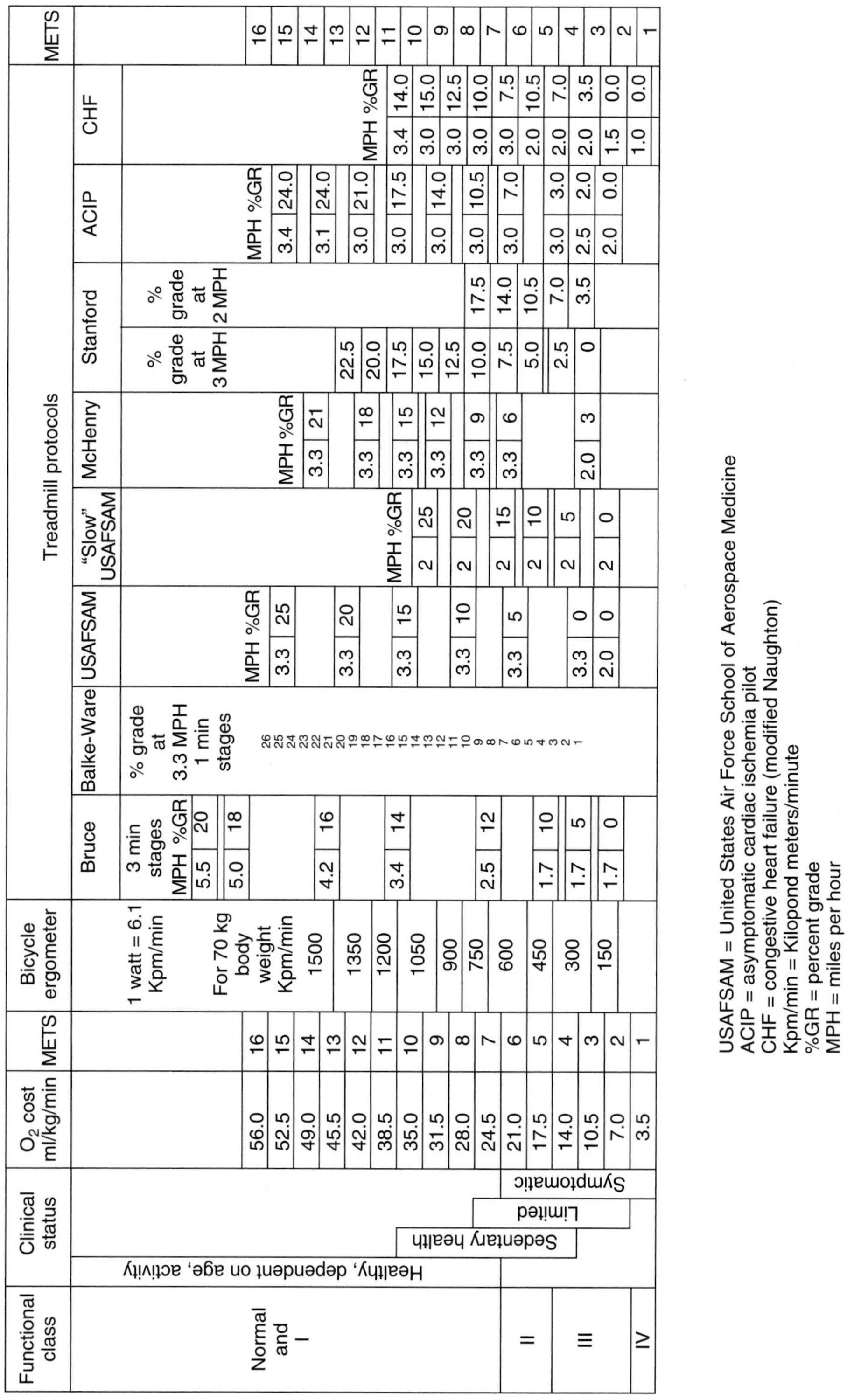

FIGURE 2-1
The oxygen cost per stage for most of the commonly used treadmill protocols.

Functional class	Clinical status	O₂ cost ml/kg/min	METS	Bicycle ergometer Kpm/min (for 70 kg body weight; 1 watt = 6.1 Kpm/min)	Bruce (3 min stages) MPH / %GR	Balke-Ware %grade at 3.3 MPH, 1 min stages	USAFSAM MPH / %GR	"Slow" USAFSAM MPH / %GR	McHenry MPH / %GR	Stanford %grade at 3 MPH	Stanford %grade at 2 MPH	ACIP MPH / %GR	CHF MPH / %GR	METS
Normal and I — Healthy, dependent on age, activity		56.0	16		5.5 / 20	26, 25								16
		52.5	15		5.0 / 18	24, 23	3.3 / 25					3.4 / 24.0		15
		49.0	14	1500		22, 21			3.3 / 21			3.1 / 24.0		14
		45.5	13		4.2 / 16	20, 19	3.3 / 20							13
		42.0	12	1350		18, 17			3.3 / 18	22.5		3.0 / 21.0		12
		38.5	11	1200	3.4 / 14	16, 15	3.3 / 15	2 / 25	3.3 / 15	20.0		3.0 / 17.5		11
		35.0	10	1050		14, 13		2 / 20	3.3 / 12	17.5		3.0 / 14.0	3.4 / 14.0	10
		31.5	9			12, 11	3.3 / 10	2 / 15	3.3 / 9	15.0		3.0 / 10.5	3.0 / 15.0	9
		28.0	8	900	2.5 / 12	10, 9		2 / 10	3.3 / 6	12.5		3.0 / 7.0	3.0 / 12.5	8
II — Sedentary healthy		24.5	7	750		8, 7	3.3 / 5			10.0	17.5	3.0 / 3.0	3.0 / 10.0	7
		21.0	6	600	1.7 / 10	6, 5		2 / 5	2.0 / 3	7.5	14.0	2.5 / 2.0	3.0 / 7.5	6
		17.5	5	450	1.7 / 5	4, 3	3.3 / 0			5.0	10.5	2.0 / 0.0	2.0 / 10.5	5
III — Limited		14.0	4	300	1.7 / 0	2, 1	2.0 / 0	2 / 0		2.5	7.0		2.0 / 7.0	4
		10.5	3							0	3.5		2.0 / 3.5	3
IV — Symptomatic		7.0	2	150									1.5 / 0.0	2
		3.5	1										1.0 / 0.0	1

USAFSAM = United States Air Force School of Aerospace Medicine
ACIP = asymptomatic cardiac ischemia pilot
CHF = congestive heart failure (modified Naughton)
Kpm/min = Kilopond meters/minute
%GR = percent grade
MPH = miles per hour

greater than 10 minutes in duration. Buchfuhrer et al[30] performed repeated maximal exercise testing in five normal subjects while varying the work rate increment. Maximal oxygen uptake varied with the increment in work; the highest values were observed when intermediate increments were used. These investigators suggested that an exercise test with work increments individualized to yield a duration of approximately 10 minutes was optimal for assessing cardiopulmonary function. Lipkin et al,[44] on the other hand, observed that among patients with chronic heart failure, small work increments yielding a long test duration (mean 31 ± 15 minutes) resulted in reduced values for maximal oxygen uptake, minute ventilation, and arterial lactate compared with tests using more standard increments. These observations have led a number of investigators to suggest that protocols should be individualized for each patient such that test duration falls within the range of 8 to 12 minutes, and this recommendation is reflected in the various exercise testing guidelines published over the last 2 decades.

RAMP TESTING

An approach to exercise testing that has gained interest is the ramp protocol, in which work increases constantly and continuously (Fig. 2-2). The popular call for "optimizing" exercise testing would appear to be facilitated by the ramp approach, because: (1) work increments are small and (2) this protocol allows for increases in work (ramp rate) to be individualized, allowing a given test duration to be targeted.

Our laboratory compared ramp treadmill and bicycle tests to protocols more commonly used clinically.[31] Ten patients with chronic heart failure, 10 with CAD who were limited by angina during exercise, 10 with CAD who were asymptomatic during exercise, and 10 age-matched normal subjects performed three bicycle tests (25 W/2-minute stage, 50 W/2-minute stage, and ramp) and three treadmill tests (Bruce, Balke, and ramp) in randomized order on different days. For the ramp tests, ramp rates on the bicycle and treadmill were individualized to yield a test duration of approximately 10 minutes for each subject. Maximal oxygen uptake was significantly higher (18%) on the treadmill protocols than on the bicycle protocols collectively, confirming previous observations. However, only minor differences in maximal oxygen uptake were observed when the treadmill protocols were compared with one another and when the cycle ergometer protocols were compared with one another.

The relationships between oxygen uptake and work rate (predicted oxygen uptake), defined as a slope for each protocol, are illustrated in Table 2-4. These relationships, which reflect the degree of change in oxygen uptake for a given increase in work (a slope of unity would suggest that the cardiopulmonary system is adapting in direct accordance with the demands of the work), were highest for the ramp tests and lowest for the protocols containing the greatest increments in work. Further, the variance about the slope

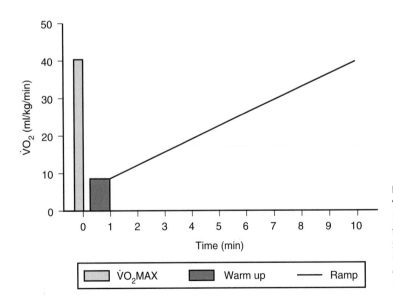

■ FIGURE 2-2

The ramp treadmill test. Following a 1-minute warmup at 2.0 mph/0% grade, the rate of change in speed and grade is individualized to yield a work rate (x axis) corresponding to an estimated exercise capacity (y axis) in approximately 10 minutes.

TABLE 2-4. Slopes in oxygen uptake versus work rate for 40 subjects performing six exercise protocols

	Treadmills			Bicycles		
	Bruce	**Balke**	**Ramp**	**25 W**	**50 W**	**Ramp**
Slope	0.62	0.79	0.80	0.69	0.59	0.78
SEE	4.0	3.4	2.5	2.3	2.8	1.7

Note: Each slope ≥ 0.78 was significantly different from each slope ≥ 0.69 (p <0.05 except Balke versus 25 W, p = 0.07). If the change in ventilatory oxygen uptake were equal to change in work rate, the slope would be 1.0. SEE, standard error of the estimate (mL O_2/kg/min); 25 W, 25 w/stage; 50 W = 50 w/stage.

(standard error of the estimate in oxygen uptake, mL/kg/min) was largest for the tests with the largest increments between stages (Bruce treadmill and 50 w/stage bicycle) and smallest for the ramp tests. These observations suggest that: (1) oxygen uptake is overestimated from tests that contain large increments in work and (2) the variability in estimating oxygen uptake from work rate is markedly greater on these tests than for an individualized ramp test.

It is also interesting how oxygen uptake kinetics were influenced by the presence of disease. The oxygen uptake slopes were generally steeper (closer to unity) among normal subjects regardless of the protocol used (Table 2-5). Patients with heart disease had reduced slopes compared with normal subjects, confirming previous investigations. However, we observed a pronounced improvement in the slope of the oxygen uptake/work rate relation in these patients when using an individualized protocol. In fact, the response of patients with heart failure was similar to that of normal subjects when both groups performed ramp treadmill tests (Fig. 2-3).

Because this approach appears to offer several advantages, we now perform all our clinical and research testing using the ramp. However, this approach is empirical and more data from other laboratories are necessary to confirm its utility.

A number of equipment manufacturers have developed treadmills that can perform ramping. The ramp appears to offer a better method of testing patients than the traditional, single-protocol approaches.

WALKING TESTS

Guyatt et al[45] point out that bike and treadmill exercise tests can be difficult for many patients with heart failure and may not reflect their capacity to undertake day-to-day activities as accurately as a walking test will. Walking tests have proven useful as measures of outcomes for patients with chronic heart failure and pulmonary disease. They can be simply done in a hospital or clinic by determining how far a patient walks in 6 minutes over a measured corridor (the "6-minute walk test"). To investigate the potential value of the 6-minute walk as an objective measure of exercise capacity in patients with chronic heart failure, the test was administered six times over 12 weeks to 18 patients with chronic heart failure and 25 patients with chronic lung disease. The subjects also underwent bike testing, and their functional status was evaluated by conventional measures. The walking test proved highly acceptable to the patients, and reproducible results were achieved after the first two walks.

TABLE 2-5. Slopes in oxygen uptake versus work rate for each patient subgroup performing each of six exercise protocols

	CAD	Angina	CHF	Normal
Slope	0.51	0.53	0.53	0.71*
SEE	2.6	3.1	2.8	4.2

*P < 0.001 versus other groups. CAD, coronary artery disease; CHF, chronic heart failure; SEE, standard error of the estimate (mL O_2/kg/min). If the change in ventilatory oxygen uptake were equal to the change in work rate, the slope would be 1.0.

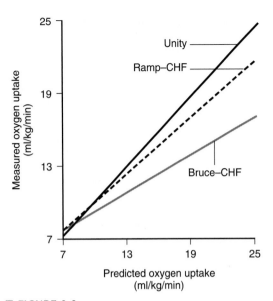

FIGURE 2-3

Relation between the change in measured and predicted oxygen uptake for the ramp and Bruce treadmill protocols among patients with chronic heart failure (CHF). The unity line is achieved when predicted oxygen uptake is equal to measured oxygen uptake. The regression equation was $y = 0.80x + 2.0$ for the ramp test and $y = 0.54x + 3.8$ ($p < 0.01$ for slope) for the Bruce test.

The results correlated with the conventional measures of functional status and exercise capacity. The "6-minute" or other walking tests are now frequently incorporated into pharmaceutical trials as an additional measure of efficacy among patients with heart disease. In patients with heart failure, the 6-minute walk test has been demonstrated by several groups to have prognostic value.[46-48] However, as pointed out in Chapter 5, we and other investigators have observed that 6-minute walk performance correlates only modestly with exercise tolerance on the treadmill (see Table 5-1).

SUBMAXIMAL EXERCISE TESTING

Submaximal exercise testing is useful clinically for predischarge post-myocardial infarction evaluations (see Chapter 9), and versions of submaximal tests are commonly used for fitness screening evaluations, such as in health clubs. Such tests are rather limited for the latter purpose as most of them use an extrapolation of the heart rate response to estimate fitness. A common submaximal cycle ergometer test is outlined by the YMCA, in which work is incremented based on the heart

rate response up to a submaximal level.[49] When used clinically, one problem with submaximal tests is that the most vulnerable patients can be stressed to a relatively greater extent, whereas the less impaired may be limited by submaximal target heart rates. A submaximal test is clinically indicated for patients in the predischarge post-myocardial infarction or post-bypass surgery period, and these tests have been shown to be important in risk stratification for such patients.[50,51] Submaximal tests in the early post-myocardial infarction or postsurgery period are also useful for making appropriate activity recommendations, for modifying the medical regimen, and for identifying the need for further interventions. A submaximal test is also an appropriate option for patients with a high probability of serious arrhythmias.

The testing endpoints for submaximal, predischarge testing have traditionally been arbitrary, but should always be based on clinical judgment. A heart rate limit of 140 beats/min and a MET level of 7 are often used for patients younger than age 40 years, and limits of 130 beats/min and a MET level of 5 are often used for patients older than 40 years. For those using beta-blockers, a Borg perceived exertion level in the range of 7 to 8 (1-to-10 scale) or 15 to 16 (6-to-20 scale) are conservative endpoints. The initial onset of symptoms, including fatigue, shortness of breath, or angina, is also an indication to stop the test. A low-level protocol should be used, that is, one that uses no more than 1-MET increments per stage. The Naughton protocol is commonly used for submaximal testing. Ramp testing is also ideal for this purpose because the ramp rate (such as 5 METs achieved over a 10-minute duration) can be individualized depending on the patient tested.

PERCEIVED EXERTION

Rather than use heart rate to clinically determine the intensity of exercise, it is preferable to use either the 6-to-20 Borg scale or the later, nonlinear 1-to-10 scale of perceived exertion.[52,53] The 6-to-20 scale was developed by noting that young men could approximate their exercise heart rate if a scale ranging from 60 to 200 was aligned with labels ranging from very, very light for 60 to very, very hard for 200. The last digit was dropped, and the scale was used for all ages. Because sensory perception of pain or exertion is nonlinear, Borg then developed the 1-to-10 scale. Since the development of the Borg scales, many studies have associated ratings of perceived exertion with physiologic responses to exercise, and these scales have been widely used to estimate effort during exercise testing.[53]

SKIN PREPARATION

Proper skin preparation is essential for the performance of an exercise test. Because noise increases with the square of resistance, it is extremely important to lower the resistance at the skin-electrode interface during exercise and thereby improve the signal-to-noise ratio. It is often difficult to ensure that technicians consistently prepare the skin properly, because doing so may cause the patient discomfort and minor skin irritation. Yet, the performance of an exercise test with an ECG signal that cannot be continuously monitored and accurately interpreted because of artifact is worthless and can even be dangerous.

The general areas for electrode placement should be cleansed with an alcohol-saturated gauze pad, then the exact areas for electrode application may be marked with a felt-tip pen. The mark serves as a guide for removal of the superficial layer of skin. The electrodes are placed using anatomic landmarks that are best found with the patient supine. Some individuals with loose skin can have a considerable shift of electrode positions when they assume an upright position. The next step is to remove the superficial layer of skin using light abrasion with fine-grain emery paper designed for this purpose. Skin resistance should be reduced to 5000 Ω or less, which can be verified prior to the exercise test with an inexpensive AC-impedance meter driven at 10 Hz. A DC meter should not be used, since it can polarize the electrodes. Each electrode can be tested against a common electrode with an ohmmeter, and when 5000 Ω or less is not achieved, the electrode must be removed and skin preparation repeated. Clever devices have been designed for this purpose. This maneuver saves time by obviating the need to interrupt a test because of noisy tracings.

ELECTRODES AND CABLES

The only suitable electrodes are constructed with a metal interface, sunken to create a column that can be filled with either an electrolyte solution or a saturated sponge. These fluid-column electrodes markedly decrease motion artifact as compared to older designs that required direct metal-to-skin contact. Many disposable electrodes have been shown to perform well for exercise testing. Silver plate or silver-silver chloride crystal pellets are the best electrode materials. Platinum is too expensive, and the frequently used German silver is actually an alloy. If electrodes of different types of metals are used together, an offset voltage can be generated that makes it impossible to record an ECG. The disposable electrodes have the advantages of quick application and no need for cleansing for reuse. They are more expensive to use than the older nondisposable electrodes, but have replaced them completely.

Developing suitable connecting cables between the electrodes and the recorder has been a problem in gathering exercise ECG data. The earliest versions of these cables were subject to wire-continuity problems, frequent failures, and motion artifact; they were improperly shielded, they used inadequate connectors, and many did not perform well in metropolitan areas or near x-ray or other high-voltage equipment. Several commercial companies have concentrated on solving these problems, and currently there are exercise cables available that are constructed to avoid these problems. Buffer amplifiers carried by the patient are no longer advantageous. Cables develop continuity problems over time with use and require replacement rather than repair. We find replacement to often be necessary after roughly 500 tests. Some systems have used analog-to-digital converters carried by the patient in the electrode junction box. Digital signals are relatively impervious to noise, so the patient cable can be unshielded and is very light. Several companies have developed systems that transmit the ECG signal in wireless format, obviating the need for cables.

LEAD SYSTEMS

Electrodes have been placed in a variety of ways using many different lead systems. This has complicated making comparisons of the ST-segment response to exercise. The four major exercise ECG lead systems are the bipolar, the Mason-Likar 12-lead,[54] a simulation of Wilson's central terminal, and the three-dimensional (either orthogonal or nonorthogonal systems).

Bipolar lead systems have been used because of the relatively short time required for placement, the relative freedom from motion artifact, and the ease with which noise problems can be located. Figure 2-4 illustrates the electrode

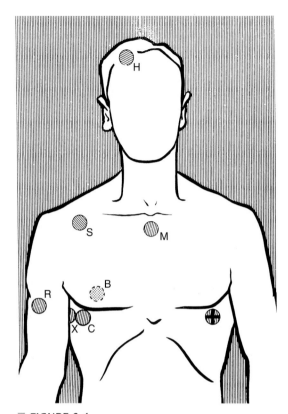

■ **FIGURE 2-4**

The common bipolar ECG leads used during exercise testing.

placements for most of the bipolar lead systems. The usual positive reference is an electrode placed the same as the positive reference for V_5. The negative reference for V_5 is Wilson's central terminal, which consists of connecting the limb electrodes—right arm (RA), left arm (LA), and left leg (LL). The only other no-table bipolar lead system is the roving bipolar lead, which was introduced by McHenry. In this system, beginning with a CC_5 placement, the electrodes are moved around to obtain the maximal R wave with a small S wave.

The problem with comparing the results of ST-segment analysis if different leads are used has been demonstrated by a computer analysis study.[55] ST-segment depression and slope measurements were made on signals gathered simultaneously from CC_5, CM_5, and V_5. A common positive reference electrode was used. CM_5 consistently had a more negative J-junction and a more positive slope than did V_5 and CC_5, whereas V_5 and CC_5 were essentially identical on the basis of standard analysis but differed statistically when computer measurements were compared.

This difference in the leads most likely explains why investigators using CM_5 have reported an inadequate ST slope to be as serious as horizontal depression. Specific ST-segment responses relative to test sensitivity and different lead systems are presented in more detail in Chapter 6.

Vector Leads

A number of three-dimensional or vectorcardiographic (VCG) lead systems can be used during exercise. The corrected Frank-lead system has the advantage that the electrical activity of the heart is orthogonally represented in the three derived signals. The relative ease of placement of its electrodes and the fact that there are only seven of them have made the Frank system the most popular orthogonal lead system. Care should be taken so that the X and Z electrodes are placed as described by Frank in his original paper, at the fifth intercostal space level and the sternum. The VCG approach makes it possible to evaluate the spatial changes of the ST-segment vector. The Frank X is a left precordial lead but is about 25% smaller in amplitude than V_5 because of the Frank network resistance, which is an attempt to electrically move the heart to the center of the chest. However, ST-segment criteria have not been adjusted for this. In both the 12-lead and Frank systems, several electrodes can be shared. V_4 and V_6 are I and A, respectively, LF can also be F, and in this way 14 electrodes can be used to obtain both systems.

The Dalhousie square is a simple way to assist with the proper and reproducible placement of the Frank electrodes and of the Wilson precordial electrodes.[56] It is a simple right-angle device that is held to the chest. Proper placement is necessary for the application of ECG/VCG interpretive criteria. Reproducible placement is essential to assess serial changes.

Mason–Likar Electrode Placement

Because a 12-lead ECG could not be obtained accurately during exercise with electrodes placed on the wrists and ankles, in 1966 Mason and Likar[54] first suggested that adhesive electrodes be placed in the base of the limbs for exercise testing. In addition to providing a noise–free exercise tracing, their modified placement apparently showed no differences in ECG configuration as compared with the standard limb lead placement.

However, others have found that the Mason–Likar placement causes amplitude changes and axis shifts when compared with standard placement, which could lead to diagnostic changes. Consequently, it has been recommended that the modified exercise electrode placement not be used for recording a resting ECG. The pre-exercise test ECG has been further complicated by the recommendation that it be obtained standing, as that is the same position maintained during exercise. This recommendation is made more difficult to follow by the common practice of moving the limb electrodes onto the chest in order to minimize motion artifact.

Figure 2-5 illustrates the Mason–Likar torso-mounted limb lead system. The conventional ankle and wrist electrodes are replaced by electrodes mounted on the torso at the base of the limbs. In this way, the artifact introduced by movement of the limbs is avoided. The standard precordial leads use Wilson's central terminal as their negative reference, which is formed by connecting the right arm, left arm, and left leg. This triangular configuration around the heart results in a zero voltage reference through the cardiac cycle. The use of Wilson's central terminal for the precordial leads (V leads) requires the

negative reference to be a combination of three additional electrodes rather than the single electrode used as the negative reference for bipolar leads. Simulation of Wilson's central terminal by other combinations of electrodes has not been validated, and therefore such alternate configurations should be avoided.

The University of California, San Diego (UCSD) Electrode Placement Study

It is clinically important to obtain an accurate pre-exercise ECG, which should be compared with previous tracings in order to determine if any changes have occurred, and because it is needed as a baseline for testing. We hypothesized that much of the confusion regarding distortion of the pre-exercise ECG was due to: (1) misplacement of limb electrodes medially on the torso and (2) obtaining the ECG in the standing position. Therefore, we compared 12-lead ECGs utilizing the standard limb placement (electrodes on wrists and ankles) against two modified exercise placements in the supine and standing positions in the same patients.[57]

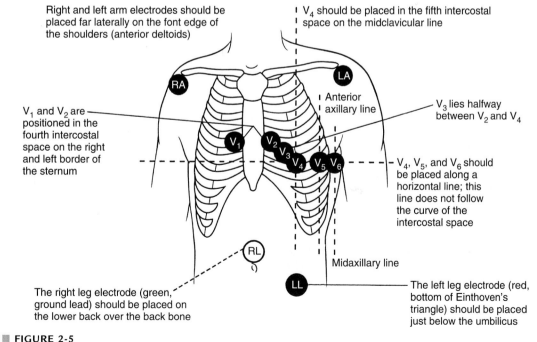

Right and left arm electrodes should be placed far laterally on the font edge of the shoulders (anterior deltoids)

V1 and V2 are positioned in the fourth intercostal space on the right and left border of the sternum

The right leg electrode (green, ground lead) should be placed on the lower back over the back bone

V4 should be placed in the fifth intercostal space on the midclavicular line

Anterior axillary line

V3 lies halfway between V2 and V4

V4, V5, and V6 should be placed along a horizontal line; this line does not follow the curve of the intercostal space

Midaxillary line

The left leg electrode (red, bottom of Einthoven's triangle) should be placed just below the umbilicus

■ **FIGURE 2-5**
The Mason–Likar-simulated standard 12-lead ECG electrode placement for exercise testing.

Prior to exercise testing, 104 male patients with stable coronary heart disease were studied. Included were 30 men with ECG criteria for an inferior myocardial infarction, 13 with an anterior myocardial infarction, five with diagnostic Q waves in multiple locations, six with right bundle branch block (three with diagnostic Q waves), 33 with other abnormalities, and 17 with normal ECGs. Just prior to a treadmill test, each patient had 12-lead ECGs recorded with lead placements as illustrated in Figure 2-6. The four electrode placements were as follows:

- Placement 1—the standard limb lead electrode placement on the wrists and ankles; supine ("standard").

- Placement 2—arm electrodes placed medially on the torso, 2 cm below the midpoint of the clavicle and leg electrodes below the umbilicus ("misplaced").

- Placement 3—the "correct" Mason–Likar placement with the arm electrodes placed at the base of the shoulders against the deltoid border 2 cm below the clavicle, and the leg electrodes the same as in placement 2 with the patient supine ("exercise supine").

- Placement 4—the same as placement 3 except that the patient is standing ("exercise standing").

In addition, the Frank X, Y, Z leads were recorded at the same time as the exercise-supine and exercise-standing ECGs.

The tracings were read by two blinded observers looking for definite diagnostic changes that might be clinically important (including "new" Q waves in aV_L or III) and other obvious changes. Q waves were considered diagnostic if they were 25% or greater of the following R-wave amplitude and 40 msec or longer in duration. Visual analyses of each of the 104 patients' four ECGs were performed independently and by consensus of two observers. The tracings were interpreted separately and then compared with the standard limb lead ECG to reveal any "serial" changes in the other three tracings.

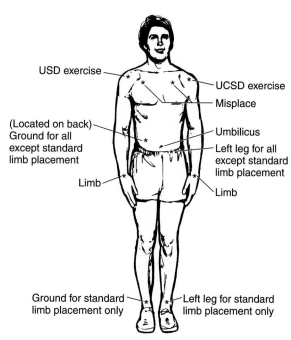

■ FIGURE 2-6

Electrode placement of the University of California, San Diego (UCSD) study of the effects of limb lead placement and standing on the routine ECG.

Differences between the standard limb lead ECG and the other ECGs were grouped into three categories: (1) diagnostic changes, (2) clinically important changes, and (3) other obvious changes (Table 2-6). The category "diagnostic changes" contained tracings with waveforms that had changed when the lead placement was altered or the patient stood in such a way that the diagnosis was different than for the supine limb lead ECG. In all cases except one, the change in diagnosis was either the loss or appearance of an inferior infarction. The one exception was a standing tracing showing that the change in position had caused an anterior infarct pattern

TABLE 2-6. Differences noted by standard visual interpretation between exercise test electrode placements and standard supine electrocardiogram

	Misplaced	Exercise-standing	Exercise-supine
Diagnostic Changes	6	12	3
Important Changes	19	12	7
Other Obvious Changes	3	6	0
Total Changes	28	30	10

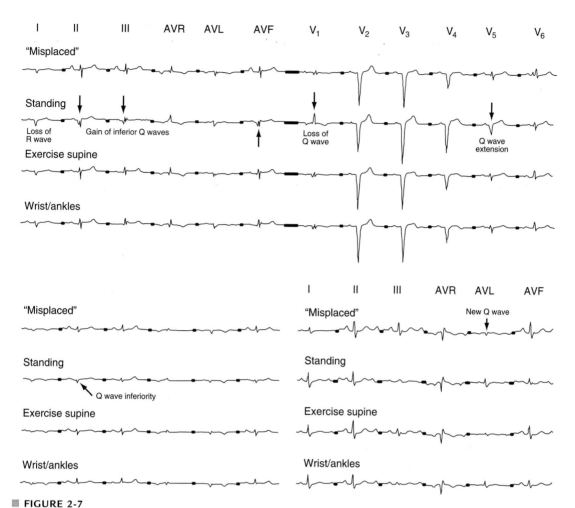

| I | II | III | AVR | AVL | AVF | V₁ | V₂ | V₃ | V₄ | V₅ | V₆ |

■ FIGURE 2-7

Examples of the artifact seen in the pre-exercise test 12-lead ECG study.

to disappear. The "exercise standing" placement had a total of 12 diagnostic changes: seven where a new diagnosis of inferior infarction was made, four where an inferior infarction diagnosis was lost, and the previously mentioned exception of losing an anterior infarction diagnosis. The "misplaced" electrode placement had six diagnostic changes: one where the criterion for an inferior infarction was reached and five where it was lost. The "exercise supine" placement had three diagnostic changes, all showing a loss of the criteria for an inferior infarction compared with the standard ECG.

The category "important changes" consisted of changes that might be clinically important but did not of themselves alter the ECG diagnosis. Such changes included significant Q waves in III or aV$_L$ alone, ST-segment and T-wave changes such as flipped or flattened T waves or ST

depression, and one instance of a Q wave appearing in V$_6$. The "misplaced" placement had various important changes: eight where a new Q wave appeared in aV$_L$; seven where a Q wave disappeared in only III; three where a Q wave appeared in III; two ST-segment or T-wave changes; and one where a Q wave appeared in aV$_L$. The "exercise supine" placement had seven important changes: four where a Q wave disappeared in III, one where it appeared, and two where a Q wave appeared in aV$_L$. Figure 2-7 illustrates the changes seen in three patients; in the bottom two tracings, changes occurred only in the limb leads.

QRS frontal axis means, standard deviations, and differences analyzed by computer for the four electrode placements are given in Table 2-7. When compared with the standard electrode placement, "misplaced" showed an average of 26 degrees of

TABLE 2-7. Computer analysis of QRS axis in frontal plane as mean values, standard deviation, mean of differences, and standard deviation of difference

	Standard	Supine-exercise	Misplaced	Standing-exercise
Mean	18	27	44	18
Standard Deviation	43	48	48	53
Mean Difference		9	26	−3
Standard Deviation of Differences		36	41	48
Significant Difference		NS	$P < 0.01$	NS

deviation to the right ($p < 0.01$), "supine exercise" showed an average of 9 degrees of rightward deviation (not significant), and "standing exercise" showed an average of 3 degrees of deviation to the left (not significant). "Standing exercise" showed the greatest amount of variability, with a standard deviation of 53 degrees.

Other Electrode Placement Studies

Kleiner et al[58] compared ECGs gathered on 75 patients using the standard wrist and ankle placement against the Mason–Likar placement. Fifty of the 75 patients had a rightward axis shift of 30 degrees or more on the modified ECG compared with the standard. In addition, 11 of these patients had a rightward shift in axis on their modified ECG that resulted in Q- and T-wave inversion in lead aV_L, without prior history of myocardial infarction by ECG. Seventeen patients had diagnostic criteria for an old inferior myocardial infarction, and seven of them (41%) had these criteria erased by the rightward axis shift on the modified placement. These investigators cautioned that the modified exercise placement of Mason and Likar should not be considered interchangeable with the standard electrode placement. However, it was not stated where the shoulder electrodes were placed or if the modified ECG was recorded supine or standing. Rautaharju et al[59] came to a similar conclusion as Kleiner et al.[58]

The pre-exercise ECG is further complicated by positional differences. Shapiro et al[60] studied the differences between supine and sitting Frank-lead VCGs in 59 adult male patients with suspected CAD. They observed that QRS spatial and R-wave amplitudes in lead Z were significantly higher and R-wave amplitudes in lead Y lower for sitting than for supine positions. They concluded that the pre-exercise ECG should be obtained with the patient in the same position as that

maintained during exercise. Other studies have also shown differences between ECGs taken supine versus sitting or standing. Sigler[61] studied 100 patients and found a tendency for the QRS axis to shift to the left for abnormal tracings and to the right for normal tracings when the patient changed from a supine to standing position. Dougherty[62] correlated changes in the frontal plane QRS axis with changes in heart position measured with a chest x-ray brought about by moving the patient from a supine to a standing position. He found that every degree of positional heart change caused a 3-degree shift in QRS frontal axis throughout the normal range in the same direction. Bruce et al[63] found a higher prevalence of false-positive polar cardiographic criteria for myocardial infarction in 72 normal men and women.

Another complicating factor is the effect of respiration on inferior Q waves. Because it has been suggested that inspiration caused Q waves in lead III to diminish or disappear in normal subjects and to persist in patients with inferior myocardial infarctions, Mimbs et al[64] studied the effect of respiration on the Q wave in lead III in normal subjects and in patients with documented inferior myocardial infarctions. They found that the Q wave in III decreased on inspiration in 82% of patients with a recent myocardial infarction and in 44% of patients with an old infarction. Among eight normal subjects with a Q wave in III, only one showed a decrease in amplitude; others showed no change. The researchers concluded that the effect of inspiration on the ECG was variable, although they did not report specific amplitude changes.

As part of a detailed study of 194 patients, Reikkinen and Rautaharju[65] analyzed the effects of respiration and sitting on the VCG. Because of the great variability of the changes, though rarely with any significant differences in the means, they reported the percentage of patients who had increases or decreases in specific values beyond an arbitrary threshold. The changes with deep inspiration were much more prominent than those with deep expiration. With inspiration, 35% of the patients had a posterior shift in the horizontal plane, whereas 8% had an anterior shift; 45% had a rightward shift in the frontal plane, whereas 3% had a leftward shift. R-wave amplitude in lead Z decreased a mean of 0.5 mV, Q-wave amplitude decreased, and the QRS-T angle increased. During sitting, R-wave amplitude increased in Z, Q-wave amplitude decreased in Y, and the mean QRS maximal spatial magnitude increased. Sitting also caused 26% of patients to have a posterior shift in the horizontal plane, whereas 10% had an anterior shift; 15% had a rightward shift in the frontal plane, whereas 10% had a leftward shift, and 36% of patients had an increase in the QRS-T angle.

The results of the UCSD lead study clarify much of the confusion regarding the pre-exercise test ECGs.[57] Misplacement of the Mason–Likar arm leads is common; published articles have even described it as the correct exercise modification. By placing the leads medially, near the midclavicular line, we found that the frontal plane axis shifts rightward an average of 26 degrees. This shift caused decreased amplitudes in the Q wave in III and of the R wave in I and aV_L, and it caused increased amplitudes in the Q wave in aV_L and the R wave in II, III, and aV_F. Of clinical importance is what these shifts did to the visual interpretation of the ECG. In five patients the ECG diagnosis of old inferior infarct was lost. In addition, seven patients lost significant Q waves in III alone. There were also instances of Q waves gained. Eight patients had no Q waves in aV_L, one had a new Q wave in III and II, one had a new Q wave in V_6, and one gained an inferior infarct diagnosis. Although these "serial" changes are merely artifacts produced by electrode misplacement, they could be very misleading. The changes, reported to be caused by misplaced electrode arrangement in the UCSD study,[57] were very similar to those reported by Kleiner et al.[58]

Standing can cause many changes in the visual interpretation of the ECG, including those that would be most alarming—that is, appearance of new Q waves (particularly inferiorly). The misplacement of the arm electrodes in the midclavicular area also causes many clinical changes, including the appearance of Q waves in aV_L and large axis shifts and amplitude changes. The correct Mason and Likar modification can likewise cause amplitude and duration changes, but they are less clinically important. The modified exercise electrode placement should not be used for routine resting ECGs. The changes caused by

the exercise electrode placement can be kept to a minimum by: (1) keeping the arm electrodes off the patient's chest and putting them on the shoulder (anterior deltoid) instead and (2) obtaining the pretest, resting ECG with the patient supine. However, the standing ECG using the modified exercise limb lead placement of Mason and Likar can serve as the reference ECG prior to an exercise test.

Relative Sensitivity of Leads

Numerous studies comparing the relative sensitivity of different ECG leads were reported in the 1970s. Robertson et al[66] compared the performance of different ECG leads among 39 patients with both an abnormal exercise test and an abnormal coronary angiogram. Eighteen percent had an abnormal response in leads other than V_5. Patients with right coronary artery lesions usually showed ST-segment depression in the inferior leads, and patients with left coronary system lesions usually showed ST-segment depression in leads I and aV_L and in the chest leads. Almost a third of the patients showed ST-segment depression in leads other than those anticipated from their angiographic anatomy. Tucker et al[67] performed 12-lead exercise tests in 100 consecutive patients who were also studied with coronary angiography. Forty-eight had abnormal tests, with 30% of the abnormal responses occurring in leads other than V_5 (17% in aV_F and 13% in other leads). Two false positives occurred in V_5 and two in aV_F, whereas 16 positives occurred in leads other than V_5 or aV_F. Of those abnormal in aV_F alone, five had lesions in the right coronary or left circumflex artery, and two had disease in the left anterior descending artery.

Chaitman et al[68] evaluated the role of multiple-lead ECG systems and clinical subsets in interpreting treadmill test results. Two hundred men with normal ECGs at rest had a maximal treadmill test using 14 ECG leads and then underwent coronary angiography. This study included standard leads plus three bipolar leads. The prevalence of significant coronary stenosis was 86% in 87 men with typical angina, 65% in 64 men with probable angina, and 28% in 49 men with nonspecific chest pain. The predictive value of ST-segment deviation in any one of 14 leads was 45% in men with nonspecific chest pain versus 70% in men with probable angina, and 55% in men with typical angina. In the latter, recording a single lead such as CM_5 was adequate. In men with typical or probable angina, a normal response in 14 leads associated with treadmill exercise time longer than 9 minutes reduced the chance of three-vessel disease to less than 10%. The likelihood of multivessel disease in a patient with an abnormal ST response and a treadmill time equal to or less than 3 minutes was approximately 90%. In patients with angina, the use of 14 leads increased sensitivity over that of V_5 alone from 52% to 75%. This value was increased even further, to 86%, by the additional consideration of bipolar leads.

Miranda et al[69] studied 178 males who had undergone both exercise testing and coronary angiography to determine the diagnostic value of ST-segment depression occurring in the inferior leads. Lead V_5 had a better sensitivity (65%) and specificity (84%) than that of lead II (sensitivity and specificity being 71% and 44%, respectively) at a single cut point. Receiver operating characteristic curve analysis demonstrated that lead V_5 (area = 0.759) was markedly superior to lead II (area = 0.582) over multiple cut points. Moreover, the area under the curve in lead II was not significantly greater than 0.50, suggesting that for the identification of CAD, ST-segment depression isolated to lead II is unreliable.

It remains to be demonstrated precisely what the specificity of leads other than V_5 is, but one has the impression that inferior leads produce more false positives and may require different criteria. This apparent lack of specificity may be due to the effect of atrial repolarization in the inferior leads, which causes depression of the ST segment. With adequate experience, atrial repolarization can be recognized as causing ST-segment depression. The end of the PR segment can be seen to be depressed in a curved fashion to the same level that the ST segment begins. Such findings also support the concept of *intercoronary artery steal* during exercise; that is, ischemic areas obtain blood flow through collaterals. This phenomenon makes it impossible for ST-segment depression with multiple-lead exercise testing to enable prediction of the location of coronary artery occlusions.

BODY SURFACE MAPPING

Studies in Normal Subjects

The normal repolarization response to exercise using large electrode arrays has been described by Mirvis et al[70] and by Miller et al.[71] Mirvis et al[70] used a 42-electrode left precordial lead system in 15 normal volunteers during supine exercise. Analyses of the exercise isopotential maps revealed a minimum amplitude during the early portions of the ST segment located below the standard V_3 and V_4 chest positions, with negative potentials involving most of the precordial region. Isopotential "difference" maps were constructed by subtracting potentials at the beginning of the ST segment from potentials later in the ST segment. These maps characterized the direction and magnitude of ST-segment slopes and revealed up-sloping ST segments over regions of negative ST potentials.

Miller et al[71] obtained total thoracic surface exercise maps in 20 normal subjects, recording from 24 electrode sites and deriving the remaining potentials at 150 locations using previously developed mathematical transformations. Isopotential maps during the early ST segment were less negative than those described by Mirvis et al[70] primarily because of Miller's "zone" reference potential. The end of the PR segment was chosen, in contrast to the use of the ST segment by Mirvis et al[70] (which shortens with heart rate increases). Exercise isopotential maps in normal subjects were characterized by a left anterior maximum during ST-T.

Studies in Patients with Coronary Artery Disease

Fox et al[72] from London used very simple exercise ECG mapping techniques to detect myocardial ischemia. Using a 16-lead precordial map and visual interpretation of the ECG data, they drew contour maps for each patient illustrating regions on the precordial surface where significant ST-segment depression was observed. The first of these studies involved 100 patients undergoing coronary angiography for evaluation of chest pain. The sensitivity of the precordial mapping technique (96%) for diagnosing coronary disease was better than the modified 12-leads (80%), using 0.1 mV horizontal ST-segment depression as the criterion for abnormal. The higher sensitivity using mapping was due to the improved recognition of single-vessel disease. Also of interest was the regional localization of the ischemic ST contours in single-vessel disease. ST-segment depression involving the uppermost horizontal row of electrodes was highly sensitive for proximal left anterior descending or left main CAD. This result was obtained without a loss in specificity (90%).

In a second study involving 200 patients undergoing coronary angiography, Fox et al[73] again compared the 12-lead ECG to a 16-lead map and found that the standard precordial leads sampled only 41% of the ST-segment depression projected to the front of the chest. However, in only 7% of patients was the ST-segment depression not apparent in the standard precordial leads. The rightmost column of electrodes never recorded ST-segment depression that was not seen in one or more of the remaining 12 electrodes on the precordial surface. The researchers concluded that these 12 precordial leads, along with the standard limb leads, would optimize the detection of ST-segment changes.

Yanowitz et al[74] at the University of Utah have reported using a 32-lead electrode array to derive torso potential distributions at 192 locations by means of a mathematical transformation. These investigators evaluated this system during exercise testing in 25 patients with documented CAD. The distribution of 80-msec ST-segment isoarea contours (ST80 isoarea maps) was plotted and compared with the standard precordial leads. It was found that in 25% of patients with ischemic ECG changes the maximal ST change was located at sites distant to the standard leads. In addition, there was some evidence of localization in patients with single-vessel disease.

Simoons and Block[75] recorded exercise body surface maps in 25 normal subjects and 25 patients with coronary disease using a system of 120 thoracic surface electrodes. Evaluation of normal subjects revealed a low-level (<90 μV) precordial minimum during early ST, followed by the development of a prominent maximum later in the ST-T wave, similar to the observations of Miller et al.[71] In the coronary patients, exercise maps frequently showed a prolonged negative area in the precordium, with varying locations of the minimum. There was no relation between the specific ST isopotential distributions and either the coronary anatomy or the location of thallium scan defects. However, the maps were more sensitive (84%) in detecting abnormal repolarization patterns in coronary patients than the 12-lead exercise ECG (60%), using an ST-segment minimum of 90 μV at 60 msec after the J-point as the criterion for an abnormal map. None of the normal subjects had negative ST potentials of this magnitude (specificity of 100%).

It is simplistic to consider ST-segment mapping data as having the ability to directly quantitate ischemic myocardium. The physiologic mechanisms responsible for ST-segment (and TQ-segment) shifts in ischemic injury are complex and depend upon the shape and location of the ischemic region in relation to the electrode sites on the body surface. Since currents of injury primarily occur at the boundaries between normal and abnormal tissue, cancellation of forces will likely distort the relationships between body surface ST-segment changes and the degree of ischemia. The subendocardial and nontransmural locations of most exercise-induced ischemia make it unreasonable to expect that body surface ECG recordings will reflect the extent, magnitude, and location of the ischemic tissues.

Experimental confirmation of these concerns has been provided by Mirvis and Ramanathan.[76] Body surface maps were obtained in dogs with previously placed amaroid constrictors around one of the three major coronary arteries. Atrial pacing induced reversible myocardial ischemia. Although the location of the ischemic repolarization abnormalities on the maps varied with the particular artery involved, significant spatial overlap was observed so as to preclude any identification of discrete ischemic zones unique to a given arterial lesion. These findings, plus consideration of the added cost of specialized recorders and more electrodes, leave mapping as a research tool without much clinical applicability.

NUMBER OF LEADS TO RECORD

In patients with normal resting ECGs, V_5 or a similar bipolar lead along the long axis of the heart usually is adequate. In patients with ECG evidence of myocardial damage or with a history suggestive of coronary spasm, additional leads are needed. As a minimal approach for these patients, it is advisable to record three leads: a V_5-type lead, an anterior V_2-type lead, and an inferior lead such as aV_F. Alternatively, the Frank X, Y, and Z leads may be used. The continuous monitoring of at least three leads is also helpful for the detection and identification of dysrhythmias. It is advisable to record a second three-lead grouping consisting of V_4, V_5, and V_6. Occasionally, abnormalities that are seen as borderline in V_5 are clearly abnormal in V_4 or V_6. This issue is less of a concern today because the medical electronics industry has made 12 leads the standard available in all machines.

POSTEXERCISE PERIOD

If maximal sensitivity is to be achieved with an exercise test, patients should be supine during the postexercise period. It is advisable to record about 10 seconds of ECG data while the patient is standing motionless but still experiencing near maximal heart rate, and then have the patient lie down. Some patients must be allowed to lie down immediately to avoid hypotension. Having the patient perform a cool-down walk after the test can delay or eliminate the appearance of ST-segment depression.[77] According to the law of Laplace, the increase in venous return and thus ventricular volume in the supine position increases myocardial oxygen demand. Data from our laboratory[78] and others suggest that having patients lie down as immediately as possible enhances ST-segment abnormalities in recovery. Therefore, the exercise testing guidelines have suggested that having the patient in the supine position in recovery is preferable to a cool-down walk. However, a cool-down walk has been suggested by some researchers in order to minimize the postexercise chances for arrhythmic events in this high-risk time when catecholamines are elevated. The supine position after exercise is less important when the test is not being performed for diagnostic purposes. When testing is not performed for diagnostic purposes, it may be preferable to have the patient walk slowly (1.0 to 1.5 mph) or continue cycling against zero or minimal resistance (0 to 25 W when testing with a cycle ergometer) for several minutes following the test.

Monitoring should continue for at least 6 to 8 minutes after exercise or until changes stabilize. An abnormal response occurring only in the recovery period is not unusual, and these responses are important to consider for optimizing the diagnostic performance of the test. All such responses are not false positives, as has been suggested. Experiments confirm mechanical dysfunction and electrophysiologic abnormalities in the ischemic ventricle following exercise. Although the supine position is preferred for diagnostic testing, a cool-down walk can be helpful for patients with an established diagnosis who are undergoing testing other than for diagnostic reasons, as well as for athletes or patients with clinically significant arrhythmias.

INDICATIONS FOR TREADMILL TEST TERMINATION

The absolute and relative indications for termination of an exercise test listed in Table 2-1 have been derived from many years of clinical experience. Absolute indications are clear-cut, whereas relative indications can sometimes be disregarded

if good clinical judgment is used. Absolute indications include a drop in systolic blood pressure despite an increase in workload, anginal chest pain becoming worse than usual, central nervous system symptoms, signs of poor perfusion (such as pallor, cyanosis, and cold skin), serious dysrhythmias, technical problems with monitoring the patient, patient's request to stop, and marked ECG changes such as 0.2-mV or greater ST-segment elevation. Relative indications for termination include other worrisome ST or QRS changes such as marked ST depression (e.g., = 2.0 mm horizontal or downsloping), increasing chest pain, fatigue, shortness of breath, wheezing, leg cramps or intermittent claudication, worrisome appearance, a hypertensive response (systolic pressure greater than 250 mmHg, diastolic pressure greater than 115 mmHg), and less serious dysrhythmias including supraventricular tachycardias. In some patients estimated to be at high risk by their clinical history, it may be appropriate to stop at a submaximal level, since the most severe ST-segment depression or dysrhythmias may occur only after exercise. If more information is required, the test can be repeated later.

EXERCISE TEST ANCILLARY TECHNIQUES

Several "add on" or ancillary imaging techniques have been shown to provide a valuable complement to exercise electrocardiography for the evaluation of patients with known or suspected CAD. Some of these methods can localize ischemia and thus help to guide interventions. These techniques are particularly helpful among patients with equivocal exercise ECGs or those likely to exhibit false-positive or false-negative responses. They are often added to confirm test results in patients with more than 1.0-mm ST depression at rest, LBBB, WPW, and paced rhythms. They are also frequently used to clarify abnormal ST-segment responses in asymptomatic individuals or those in whom the cause of chest discomfort remains uncertain. These tests can be an important complement to the standard exercise test because they can either confirm the diagnosis of CAD or obviate the need for angiography or other interventions. They can also help direct a patient to an appropriate intervention because ischemia can be localized. When an exercise ECG and an imaging technique are combined, the diagnostic and prognostic accuracy is enhanced. The major imaging procedures are myocardial perfusion and ventricular function studies using radionuclide techniques and exercise or pharmacologic echocardiography. The nonexercise stress techniques (pharmacologic stress testing using persantine or adenosine with nuclear perfusion, dobutamine or arbutamine with echocardiography) permit diagnostic assessment of patients unable to walk on the treadmill or pedal a cycle ergometer due to orthopedic or neurologic conditions. Although these newer technologies are often suggested to have better diagnostic characteristics, this is not always the case, particularly when multivariate scores are used with standard exercise testing.

Nuclear Techniques

Nuclear Ventricular Function Assessment. One of the first techniques added to exercise was radionuclear ventriculography. This involved the intravenous injection of technetium-tagged red blood cells. Using ECG gating of images obtained from a scintillation camera, images of the blood circulating within the LV chamber could be obtained. While regurgitant blood flow from valvular lesions could not be identified, ejection fraction and ventricular volumes could be estimated. The resting values could be compared to those obtained during supine exercise and criteria were established for abnormal. The most common criteria involved a drop in ejection fraction. This procedure is now rarely performed because its test characteristics appear to be inferior to newer technologies. While initially popular in the 1970s and 1980s, the blood volume techniques have come to be surpassed by perfusion techniques.

Nuclear Perfusion Imaging. The first agent used for perfusion imaging was thallium, an isotopic analog of potassium that is taken up at variable rates by metabolically active tissue. When taken up at rest, images of metabolically active muscle, such as the heart, are possible. With the nuclear camera placed over the heart after intravenous injection of this isotope, images were initially viewed using x-ray film. The normal complete donut-shaped images gathered in multiple views would be broken by "cold" spots where scar was present. Defects viewed after exercise could be due to either scar or ischemia. Follow-up imaging confirmed that the "cold" spots were due to ischemia if they filled in later. As computer imaging techniques were developed, three-dimensional imaging (single photon emission computed tomography) was possible and subtle differences could be plotted and scored. In recent years, ventriculograms based on the imaged wall as opposed to the blood in the chambers (as with radionuclear ventriculography) could be constructed. Because of the technical limitations with thallium (i.e., source and lifespan), it has largely been replaced by chemical compounds called isonitriles which could be tagged with technetium, which has many practical advantages over thallium as an imaging agent. The isonitriles are trapped in the microcirculation, permitting imaging of the heart with a scintillation camera. Rather than a single injection, as with thallium, these compounds require an injection at maximal exercise, then later in recovery. The differences in technology over the years and the differences in expertise and software at different facilities can complicate the comparisons of the results and actual application of this technology. The ventriculograms obtained with gated perfusion scans do not permit the assessment of valvular lesions or as accurate an assessment of wall motion abnormalities or ejection fraction as echocardiography.

Vasodilators, such as dipyridamole and adenosine, are commonly used to assess coronary perfusion in conjunction with a nuclear imaging agent. Dipyridamole and adenosine cause maximal coronary vasodilation in normal epicardial arteries, but not in stenotic segments. As a result, a coronary steal phenomenon occurs, with a relatively increased flow to normal arteries and a relatively decreased flow to stenotic arteries. Nuclear perfusion imaging under resting conditions is then compared with imaging obtained after coronary vasodilation. Interpretation is similar to that for exercise nuclear testing.

Echocardiography. The impact of the echocardiogram on cardiology has been considerable. This imaging technique comes second only to contrast ventriculography via cardiac catheterization for measuring ventricular volumes, wall motion, and ejection fraction. With doppler added, regurgitant flows can be estimated as well. Echocardiographers were quick to add this imaging modality to exercise, with most studies showing that supine, postexercise assessments were adequate and the more difficult imaging during exercise was not necessary. The patient must be placed supine as soon as possible after exercise and imaging begun. A problem can occur when the imaging requires removal or displacement of the important V_5 electrode, where most of the important ST changes are observed.

Dobutamine is the most common pharmacologic agent used with echocardiography. Dobutamine is a synthetic catecholamine that acts directly on β_1 and β_2 receptors. It increases the force of myocardial contractility more than it increases heart rate. It is titrated intravenously from low to higher doses while observing four views of the heart, similar to exercise echocardiography. Wall motion abnormalities are caused by the associated increased demand for myocardial oxygen and shortening of coronary artery filling time resulting from the increase in heart rate. If ischemia is induced, a wall motion abnormality appears at a specific heart rate.

Biomarkers. The latest ancillary tool to supplement the exercise ECG in an attempt to improve its diagnostic characteristics are biomarkers. The first and most logical biomarker evaluated to detect ischemia brought out by exercise was troponin. However, it has been shown that even in patients who develop ischemia during exercise testing, serum elevations in cardiac-specific troponin do not occur, demonstrating that myocardial damage does not occur.[79,80] B-type natriuretic peptide, which is released by myocardial stretching, also appears to be released by myocardial hypoxia. Armed with this knowledge, investigators have reported several studies suggesting an improvement in the diagnostic characteristics of the exercise test with B-type natriuretic peptide and its isomers.[81,82] The point of contact analysis techniques available for these assays involves a hand-held battery-powered unit that uses a replaceable cartridge. Finger stick blood samples are adequate for analyses and the results are available immediately. If validated using an appropriate study design (similar to QUEXTA), biomarker measurements could greatly improve the diagnostic characteristics of the standard office/clinic exercise test.

SUMMARY

Proper methodology is critical to patient safety and acquiring accurate results from the exercise test. Preparing the patient physically and emotionally for testing is necessary. Good skin preparation must cause some discomfort but is necessary for good conductance and to avoid artifact. Specific criteria for exclusion and termination, physician interaction with the patient,

and appropriate emergency equipment are essential. A brief physical examination is always necessary to rule out significant aortic valve disease and other contraindications for the test. Pretest standard 12-lead ECGs are needed in both the supine and standing positions. The changes caused by exercise electrode placement can be kept to a minimum by keeping the arm electrodes off the chest, placing them on the anterior deltoid instead, and by recording the baseline ECG supine. When electrode preparation and placement are properly performed, the modified exercise limb lead placement of Mason and Likar can serve well as the reference resting ECG prior to an exercise test.

Few studies have correctly evaluated the relative yield or sensitivity and specificity of different electrode placements for exercise-induced ST-segment shifts. Studies show that using other leads in addition to V_5 will increase the sensitivity; however, the specificity is decreased. ST-segment changes isolated to the inferior leads can sometimes, but not always, be false-positive responses. VCG and body surface mapping lead systems do not offer any advantage over simpler approaches for clinical purposes.

The exercise protocol should be progressive, with even increments in speed and grade whenever possible. Small, even, and frequent work increments are preferable to large, uneven, and less frequent increases, because the former yield a more accurate estimation of exercise capacity. Many investigators, rather than using the same protocol for every patient, have emphasized the value of individualizing the exercise protocol. The optimal test duration is 8 to 12 minutes, and the protocol workloads should be adjusted to permit this duration. Because ramp testing uses small increments, it permits a more accurate estimation of exercise capacity and can be individualized for every patient to yield a targeted test duration. For equipment that does not have a controller that performs such tests, the workload can be increased manually in equal increments using any treadmill.

Target heart rates based on age should not be used, because the relationship between maximal heart rate and age is poor and has a wide scatter around many different recommended regression lines. Such heart rate targets result in a submaximal test for some individuals, a maximal test for some, and an unrealistic goal for others. The Borg scales are an excellent means of quantifying an individual's effort. Exercise capacity should not be reported in total time but rather as the VO_2 or MET equivalent of the workload achieved. This practice permits the comparison of the results of many different exercise testing protocols. Hyperventilation should be avoided prior to testing. Subjects both with and without disease may or may not exhibit ST-segment changes with hyperventilation; the value of this procedure in lessening the number of false-positive responses is no longer considered useful by most researchers. The postexercise period is a critical period diagnostically, and whenever possible the patient should be placed in the supine position immediately after testing for this reason.

Key points worth emphasizing include the following:

■ The treadmill protocol should be adjusted to the patient; one protocol is not appropriate for all patients.

■ Report exercise capacity in METs, not minutes of exercise.

■ Hyperventilation prior to testing is not indicated.

■ ST measurements should be made at ST0 (J-junction), and ST depression should be considered abnormal only if horizontal or downsloping.

■ Patients should be placed supine as soon as possible after exercise. For diagnostic testing, a cool-down walk should be avoided in order for the test to have its greatest value.

■ It is critical to include the 2- to 4-minute recovery period in analysis of the ST response.

■ Measurement of systolic blood pressure during exercise is extremely important, and exertional hypotension is ominous; at this point, only manual blood pressure measurement techniques are valid.

■ Age-predicted heart rate targets are largely useless because of the wide scatter for any age; a relatively low heart rate can be maximal for a patient of a given age and submaximal for another. Thus, a test should not be considered nondiagnostic if a percentage of age-predicted maximal heart rate (i.e., 85%) is not reached.

■ The Duke treadmill score should be calculated automatically on every test.

■ Other predictive equations should be considered as part of the treadmill report.

To ensure the safety of exercise testing and reassure the noncardiologist performing the test, the following list of the most dangerous circumstances in the exercise testing lab should be considered:

■ Testing patients with aortic valvular disease should be done with great care. Consequently, a physical examination, including assessment of systolic murmurs, should be done before all exercise tests. If a significant murmur is heard, an echocardiogram should be considered.

■ ST-segment elevation without diagnostic Q waves (which is due to transmural ischemia) can be associated with dangerous arrhythmias and infarction; it occurs in about 1 out of 1000 clinical tests.

■ When a patient with an ischemic cardiomyopathy exhibits severe chest pain owing to ischemia (angina pectoris), a cool-down walk is advisable, since the ischemia can worsen in recovery.

■ A potentially dangerous situation exists when a patient develops exertional hypotension accompanied by ischemia (angina or ST depression) or when it occurs in a patient with a history of chronic heart failure, cardiomyopathy, or recent myocardial infarction.

■ When a patient with a history of sudden collapse develops frequent premature ventricular contractions, a cool-down walk is advisable (premature ventricular contractions can increase during recovery, particularly after an abrupt cessation of exercise).

Appreciation of these circumstances can help avoid any complications in the exercise lab.

REFERENCES

1. Rochmis P, Blackburn H: Exercise tests: A survey of procedures, safety, and litigation experience in approximately 170,000 tests. JAMA 1971;217:1061-1066.
2. Gibbons L, Blair SN, Kohl HW, Cooper K: The safety of maximal exercise testing. Circulation 1989;80:846-852.
3. Myers J, Voodi L, Umanu T, Froelicher VF: A survey of exercise testing: Methods, utilization, and safety in the VAHCS. J Cardiopulm Rehab 2000;20:251-258.
4. Yang JC, Wesley RC, Froelicher VF: Ventricular tachycardia during routine treadmill testing. Arch Intern Med 1991;151:349-353.
5. Irving JB, Bruce RA: Exertional hypotension and post exertional ventricular fibrillation in stress testing. Am J Cardiol 1977;39:849-851.
6. Shepard RJ: Do risks of exercise justify costly caution? Phys Sports Med 1977;5:52-58.
7. Cobb LA, Weaver WD: Exercise: A risk for sudden death in patients with coronary heart disease. J Am Coll Cardiol 1986;7:215-219.
8. Rodgers GP, Ayanian JZ, Balady GJ, Beasley JW, Brown KA, Gervino EV, Parison S, Quinnones M, Schlant RC: American College of Cardiology/American Heart Association clinical competence statement on stress testing. Circulation 2000;102:1726-1738.
9. American College of Sports Medicine: Guidelines for Exercise Testing and Prescription, 6th ed. Baltimore, Lippincott, Williams & Wilkins, 2000.

10. Astrand P, Ekblom B, Messin R, et al: Intraarterial blood pressure during exercise with different muscle groups. J Appl Physiol 1965;20:253-256.
11. Bevegard S, Freyschuss U, Strandell T: Circulatory adaptation to arm and leg exercise in supine and sitting positions. J Appl Physiol 1966;21:37-46.
12. Bobbert AC: Physiological comparison of three types of ergometry. J Appl Physiol 1960;15:1007-1014.
13. Davis JA, Vodak P, Wilmore JH, et al: Anaerobic threshold and maximal aerobic power for three modes of exercise. J Appl Physiol 1976;41:544-550.
14. Asmussen E, Nielsen M: Regulation of body temperature during work performed with arms and legs. Acta Physiol Scand 1947;14:373-382.
15. Klefbeck B, Mattsson E, Weinberg J: The effect of trunk support on performance during arm ergometry in patients with cervical cord injuries. Paraplegia 1996;34:167-172.
16. Astrand I, Guharay A, Wahren J: Circulatory responses to arm exercise with different arm positions. J Appl Physiol 1968;25:528-532.
17. Tuttle WW, Horvath SM: Comparison of effects of static and dynamic work on blood pressure and heart rate: J Appl Physiol 1957;10:294-296.
18. Wahren J, Bygdeman S: Onset of angina pectoris in relation to circulatory adaptation during arm and leg exercise. Circulation 1971;44:432-441.
19. Shaw DJ, Crawford MH, Karliner JS, et al: Arm crank ergometry: A new method for the evaluation of coronary artery disease. Am J Cardiol 1974;33:801-805.
20. DeBusk RF, Valdez R, Houston N, Haskell W: Cardiovascular responses to dynamic and static effort soon after myocardial infarction: Application to occupational work assessment. Circulation 1978;58:368-375.
21. Vander LB, Franklin BA, Wrisley D, Rubenfire M: Cardiorespiratory responses to arm and leg ergometry in women. Phys Sports Med 1984;12:101-106.
22. Fardy PS, Webb D, Hellerstein HK: Benefits of arm exercise in cardiac rehabilitation. Phys Sports Med 1977;5:30-41.
23. Asmussen E, Hemmingsen I: Determination of maximum working capacity at different ages in work with the legs or with the arms. Scand J Clin Lab Invest 1958;10:67-71.
24. Franklin BA, Vander L, Wrisley D, Rubenfire M: Aerobic requirements of arm ergometry: Implications for exercise testing and training. Phys Sports Med 1983;11:81-90.
25. Schwade J, Blomqvist CG, Shapiro WA: A comparison of the response to arm and leg work in patients with ischemic heart disease. Am Heart J 1977;94:203-208.
26. Balady GJ, Schick EC, Weiner DA, et al: Comparison of determinants of myocardial oxygen consumption during arm and leg exercise in normal persons. Am J Cardiol 1986;57:1385-1387.
27. Balady GJ, Weiner DA, McCabe CH, et al: Value of arm exercise testing in detecting coronary artery disease. Am J Cardiol 1985;55:37-39.
28. Myers J, Froelicher VF: Optimizing the exercise test for pharmacological investigations. Circulation 1990;82:1839-1846.
29. Hermansen L, Saltin B: Oxygen uptake during maximal treadmill and bicycle exercise. J Appl Physiol 1969;26:31-37.
30. Buchfuhrer MJ, Hansen JE, Robinson TE, et al: Optimizing the exercise protocol for cardiopulmonary assessment. J Appl Physiol 1983;55:1558-1564.
31. Myers J, Buchanan N, Walsh D, et al: Comparison of the ramp versus standard exercise protocols. J Am Coll Cardiol 1991;17:1334-1342.
32. Niederberger M, Bruce RA, Kusumi F, Whitkanack S: Disparities in ventilatory and circulatory responses to bicycle and treadmill exercise. Br Heart J 1974;36:377-382.
33. Wicks JR, Sutton JR, Oldridge NB, Jones NL: Comparison of the electrocardiographic changes induced by maximum exercise testing with treadmill and cycle ergometer. Circulation 1978;57:1066-1069.
34. Balke B, Ware R: An experimental study of physical fitness of Air Force personnel. US Armed Forces Med J 1959;10:675-688.
35. Astrand PO, Rodahl K: Textbook of Work Physiology. New York, McGraw-Hill, 1986, pp 331-365.
36. Bruce RA: Exercise testing of patients with coronary heart disease. Ann Clin Res 1971;3:323-330.
37. Ellestad MH, Allen W, Wan MCK, Kemp G: Maximal treadmill stress testing for cardiovascular evaluation. Circulation 1969;39:517-522.
38. Stuart RJ, Ellestad MH: National survey of exercise stress testing facilities. Chest 1980;77:94-97.
39. Sullivan M, McKirnan MD: Errors in predicting functional capacity for postmyocardial infarction patients using a modified Bruce protocol. Am Heart J 1984;107:486-491.
40. Webster MWI, Sharpe DN: Exercise testing in angina pectoris: The importance of protocol design in clinical trials. Am Heart J 1989;117:505-508.
41. Panza JA, Quyyumi AA, Diodati JG, et al: Prediction of the frequency and duration of ambulatory myocardial ischemia in patients with stable coronary artery disease by determination of the ischemic threshold from exercise testing: Importance of the exercise protocol. J Am Coll Cardiol 1991;17:657-663.
42. Redwood DR, Rosing DR, Goldstein RE, et al: Importance of the design of an exercise protocol in the evaluation of patients with angina pectoris. Circulation 1971;43:618-628.
43. Smokler PE, MacAlpin RN, Alvaro A, Kattus AA: Reproducibility of a multi-stage near maximal treadmill test for exercise tolerance in angina pectoris. Circulation 1973;48:346-351.
44. Lipkin DP, Canepa-Anson R, Stephens MR, Poole-Wilson PA: Factors determining symptoms in heart failure: Comparison of fast and slow exercise tests. Br Heart J 1986;55:439-445.
45. Guyatt GH, Sullivan MJ, Thompson PJ, et al: The sixminute walk. A new measure of exercise capacity in patients with chronic heart failure. Can Med Assoc J 1985;132:919-923.
46. Bittner V, Weiner DH, Yusuf S, et al: Prediction of mortality and morbidity with a 6-minute walk test patients with left ventricular dysfunction. SOLVD Investigators. JAMA 1994;27:661-662.
47. Curtis JP, Rathore SS, Wang Y, Krumholz KM: The association of 6-minute walk performance and outcomes in stable outpatients with heart failure. J Card Fail 2004;10:9-14.
48. Rostagno C, Olivo G, Comeglio M, et al: Prognostic value of 6-minute walk corridor test in patients with mild to moderate heart failure: comparison with other methods functional evaluation. Eur J Heart Fail 2003;5:247-252.
49. Golding LA, Myers CR, Sinning WE (eds). The Y's Way to Physical Fitness, 3rd ed. Champaign, Ill, Human Kinetics, 1989.
50. Chang JA, Frolicher VF: Clinical and exercise test markers of prognosis in patients with stable coronary artery disease. Curr Probl Cardiol 1994;19:533-538.
51. Olona M, Candell-Riera J, Permanyer-Miralda G, et al: Strategies for prognostic assessment of uncomplicated first myocardial infarction: 5-year follow up study. J Am Coll Cardiol 1995;25:815-822.
52. Borg G: Perceived exertion as an indicator of somatic stress. Scand J Rehabil Med 1970;23:92-93.
53. Borg G: Borg's Perceived Exertion Scales. Champaign, Ill, Human Kinetics, 1998.
54. Mason RE, Likar I: A new system of multiple-lead exercise electrocardiography. Am Heart J 1966;71:196-205.
55. Froelicher VF, Wolthuis R, Keiser N, et al: A comparison of two bipolar electrocardiographic leads to lead V5. Chest 1976;70:611-616.
56. Rautaharju PM, Wolf HK, Eifler WJ, Blackburn H: A simple procedure of positioning precordial ECG and VCG electrodes using an electrode locator. J Electrocardiol 1976;9:35-40.
57. Gamble P, McManus H, Jensen D, Froelicher VF: A comparison of the standard 12-lead electrocardiogram to exercise placements. Chest 1984;85:616-622.
58. Kleiner JP, Nelson WP, Boland MJ: The 12-lead electrocardiogram in exercise testing. Arch Intern Med 1978;138:1572-1573.
59. Rautaharju PM, Prineas RJ, Crow RS, et al: The effect of modified limb positions on electrocardiographic wave amplitudes. J Electrocardiol 1980;13:109-114.
60. Shapiro W, Berson AS, Pipberger HV: Differences between supine and sitting Frank-lead electrocardiograms. J Electrocardiol 1976;9:303-308.
61. Sigler LH: Electrocardiographic changes occurring with alterations of posture from recumbent to standing positions. Am Heart J 1938;15:146-152.

62. Dougherty JD: Change in the frontal QRS axis with changes in the anatomic positions of the heart. J Electrocardiol 1970;3:299-311.

63. Bruce RA, Detry JM, Early K, et al: Polarcardiographic responses to maximal exercise in healthy young adults. Am Heart J 1972;83:206-212.

64. Mimbs JW, deMello V, Roberts R: The effect of respiration on normal and abnormal Q-waves. Am Heart J 1977;94:579-584.

65. Reikkinen H, Rautaharju P: Body position, electrode level, and respiration effects on the Frank lead electrocardiogram. Circulation 1976;53:40-45.

66. Robertson D, Kostuk WJ, Ahuja SP: The localization of coronary artery stenoses by 12-lead ECG response to graded exercise test: Support for intercoronary steal. Am Heart J 1976;91:437-444.

67. Tucker SC, Kemp VE, Holland WE, et al: Multiple-lead ECG submaximal treadmill exercise tests in angiographically documented coronary heart disease. Angiology 1976;27:149-156.

68. Chaitman BR, Bourassa MG, Wagniart P, et al: Improved efficiency of treadmill exercise testing using a multiple lead ECG system and basic hemodynamic exercise response. Circulation 1978;57:71-78.

69. Miranda CP, Liu J, Kadar A, et al: Usefulness of exercise-induced ST-segment depression in the inferior leads during exercise testing as a marker for coronary artery disease. Am J Cardiol 1992;69:303-307.

70. Mirvis DM, Keller FW, Cox JW, et al: Left precordial isopotential mapping during supine exercise. Circulation 1977;56:245-252.

71. Miller WT, Spach MS, Warren RB: Total body surface potential mapping during supine exercise. Circulation 1980;62:632-645.

72. Fox KM, Selwyn AP, Shillingford JP: A method for precordial surface mapping of the exercise electrocardiogram. Br Heart J 1978;40:1339-1343.

73. Fox KM, England D, Jonathan A, et al: Precordial surface mapping of the exercise ECG. Br J Hosp Med 1982;27:291-299.

74. Yanowitz FG, Vincent GM, Lux RL, et al: Application of body surface mapping to exercise testing: ST80 isoarea maps in patients with coronary artery disease. Am J Cardiol 1982;50:1109-1113.

75. Simoons M, Block P, Ascoop C, et al: Computer processing of exercise ECGs-A cooperative study. In VanBemmel KJ, Williams JL (eds): Trends in Computer-Processed Electrocardiograms. Amsterdam, North-Holland Publishing, 1977, p. 383.

76. Mirvis DM, Ramanathan KB: Alterations in transmural blood flow and body surface ST segment abnormalities produced by ischemia in the circumflex and left anterior descending coronary arterial beds of the dog. Circulation 1987;76:697-704.

77. Gutman RA, Alexander ER, Li YB, et al: Delay of ST depression after maximal exercise by walking for two minutes. Circulation 1970;42:229-233.

78. Lachterman B, Lehmann KG, Abrahamson D, Froelicher VF: "Recovery only" ST segment depression and the predictive accuracy of the exercise test. Ann Intern Med 1990;112:11-16.

79. Akdemir I, Aksoy N, Aksoy M, et al: Does exercise-induced severe ischaemia result in elevation of plasma troponin-T level in patients with chronic coronary artery disease? Acta Cardiol 2002;57:13-18.

80. Ashmaig ME, Starkey BJ, Ziada AM, et al: Changes in serum concentrations of markers of myocardial injury following treadmill exercise testing in patients with suspected ischaemic heart disease. Med Sci Monit 2001;7:54-57.

81. Foote RS, Pearlman JD, Siegel AH, Yeo KT: Detection of exercise-induced ischemia by changes in B-type natriuretic peptides. J Am Coll Cardiol 2004;44:1980-1987.

82. Sabatine MS, Morrow DA, de Lemos JA, et al: TIMI Study Group. Acute changes in circulating natriuretic peptide levels in relation to myocardial ischemia. J Am Coll Cardiol 2004;44:1988-1995.

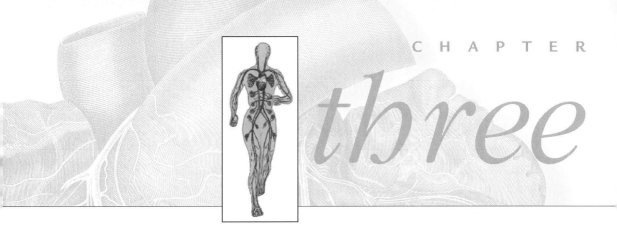

three

Ventilatory Gas Exchange

Until recent years, the use of ventilatory gas exchange techniques during exercise (commonly termed cardiopulmonary exercise testing) were generally limited to human performance laboratories or the pulmonologist's office, and applications in other clinical settings were minimal. However, technological advances have lessened the difficulty with which gas exchange analysis can be performed during exercise; thus, an increase in the application of this technology has occurred. Such measurements permit a more accurate and reproducible assessment of cardiopulmonary function than that obtained from estimations based on treadmill speed and grade.[1,2] This makes ventilatory gas exchange measurements essential when the need exists to quantify the effect of interventions with more precision.[3,4] Consequently, many clinical research protocols are now conducted using gas exchange techniques.

It is frequently argued whether the additional and more accurate information gained from exercise testing using gas exchange techniques justifies the added expense, time, and discomfort to the patient. Unfortunately, there is not a yes or no answer to this question. The answer depends upon the purpose of the test and who is conducting the test. With regard to the first consideration, if the purpose of the test is to evaluate an intervention, for example, for research purposes, the limitations of predicting exercise capacity (outlined later) mandate the use of gas exchange techniques. If a patient's symptoms are mixed and it is uncertain whether cardiovascular or pulmonary disease is limiting exercise, cardiopulmonary

techniques can help define a patient's limitations and direct therapy appropriately. In addition, a growing body of evidence suggests that gas exchange measurements are among the most important variables in risk stratification[5-7]; thus, when this is an important goal of the test, oxygen uptake (VO_2) and other gas exchange responses should be directly measured.

Alternatively, if the purpose of the test is to increase myocardial oxygen demand to an optimal level while obtaining a general estimation of metabolic equivalents (METs), gas exchange techniques would generally not be as useful. With regard to this second consideration, the absence of a good understanding of gas exchange and basic exercise physiology by clinicians continues to be a limitation to the widespread application of gas exchange technology. Cardiopulmonary exercise testing requires a degree of expertise by the technician, as proper attention to data collection and calibration are essential. At the same time, clinical application of the data requires that the physician possess a basic understanding of ventilatory gas exchange analysis. This chapter will present some basic methodology and illustrate the clinical utility of gas exchange techniques for testing patients with heart disease.

PREDICTING OXYGEN UPTAKE

As mentioned previously, the measurement of oxygen uptake requires additional cost, time, equipment, and potential discomfort to the patient, raising the question of whether these techniques are justified in clinical practice. In addition, the answer to this question may depend upon the purpose of the test and how important the added precision is to the user. With regard to measuring work with precision, it may be useful to review some of the major research studies to put this question into perspective.

Predicting oxygen uptake from treadmill or cycle ergometer workload is a common clinical practice, but such predictions can be very misleading. Although oxygen uptake and workload are directly related, with correlation coefficients ranging between 0.60 and 0.90, there is wide scatter around the regression line. Figure 3-1 illustrates the relationship between measured and predicted METs among 1110 consecutive patients referred for exercise testing in our laboratory. Note the variation in this relationship and the tendency to overpredict oxygen uptake from the work rate on the treadmill (typically 2 to 4 METs for any given work rate). This inaccuracy has been attributed to factors such as subject habituation (less variation occurs with treadmill experience), fitness (less variation occurs with increased fitness), the presence of heart disease (oxygen uptake is overpredicted for diseased individuals), handrail holding (the oxygen cost of the work is markedly reduced if the subject is allowed to hold on to the handrails), and the exercise protocol (less variation occurs when using more gradual, individualized protocols) (Table 3-1). Therefore, if quantifying work with precision is an important objective, as in research studies, a direct measurement is essential.

Studies describing the factors that affect the relationship between measured and predicted oxygen uptake are numerous. The wide scatter around the regression line between oxygen uptake and exercise time or workload is well documented yet poorly appreciated, and most pharmaceutical trials continue to report work in terms of the relatively unreliable measure, exercise time. This is of particular concern because many studies have shown that the presence of heart disease can greatly increase the error associated with predicting oxygen uptake. Sullivan and McKirnan[8] reported that among patients with coronary disease, measured oxygen uptake was 13% lower than that in normal subjects for the same treadmill work rate at higher levels of exercise. Roberts et al[9] plotted the relationship between measured and predicted oxygen uptake in a heterogeneous group of patients with heart disease and a group of normal subjects (Fig. 3-2). Measured oxygen uptake was lower at matched work rates throughout exercise among the patients. Moreover, the discrepancy between the two groups became progressively greater as the exercise progressed. Numerous other groups have reported similar findings. Dominick et al[10] reported that the American College of Sports Medicine equation overpredicted peak VO_2 by 10.0 mL/kg/min among hypertensive subjects and 8.6 mL/kg/min in subjects with fibromyalgia. Similarly, Foster et al[11] reported that the American College of Sports Medicine equations overpredicted peak VO_2 by 8.0 and 8.2 mL/kg/min for handrail supported and nonhandrail supported treadmill exercise, respectively. Berry et al[12] observed that

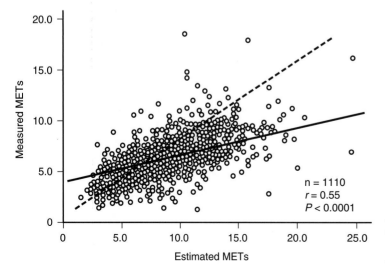

■ FIGURE 3–1

The relationship between measured and estimated oxygen uptake, expressed as peak METs, among consecutive patients referred for exercise testing for clinical reasons. The dotted line represents a line of unity, and the solid line represents the best fit of the data. *(From Myers J: Applications of cardiopulmonary exercise testing in the management of cardiovascular and pulmonary disease. Int J Sports Med 2005; 26:1-7).*

TABLE 3-1. Factors affecting the relationship between measured and predicted oxygen uptake

Factor	Effects
Habituation	Oxygen uptake and variability decrease, and reproducibility increases with treadmill experience
Fitness	Oxygen uptake and variability decrease with increased fitness
Heart disease	Oxygen uptake is overpredicted in patients with heart disease
Handrail holding	Oxygen uptake is reduced by holding handrails
Exercise protocol	Oxygen uptake is overpredicted, and variability increases with rapidly incremented, demanding protocols

peak VO_2 was overestimated by an average of 9.3 mL/kg/min among 362 patients with cardiovascular disease undergoing treadmill testing. The latter two studies also reported that the prediction of VO_2 could be significantly improved by using population-specific exercise protocols and prediction equations.

We compared the slope of the relationship between patients with heart disease and age-matched normals on a variety of treadmill and cycle ergometer protocols.[13] The slope represents a change in an independent variable (in this case, an increment in treadmill or cycle ergometer work rate) for a given change in a dependent variable (in this case, measured oxygen uptake). Thus, a slope equal to 1 would be observed if the variables changed in direct proportion to one another. However, such is never the case, even among normal subjects. Table 3-2 illustrates that patients with chronic heart failure (CHF), coronary artery disease, and those limited by angina on the treadmill have significantly reduced slopes (ranging from 0.51 to 0.53) compared to normal subjects (slope = 0.71). Many investigators have suggested that the reduced oxygen uptake values at matched work rates (sometimes called *oxygen uptake lag* or *drift*) is due to an inability of the cardiopulmonary system to adapt to the demands of the work rate. Not surprisingly, patients with CHF are particularly known to exhibit this response,

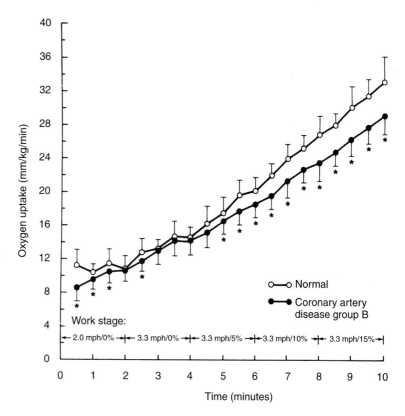

■ FIGURE 3-2

Plot of mean values of oxygen uptake for matched treadmill workloads in normal subjects and patients with coronary artery disease. At higher levels of work, oxygen uptake is significantly reduced among patients with heart disease. *(From Roberts JM, Sullivan M, Froelicher VF, et al: Predicting oxygen uptake from treadmill testing in normal subjects and coronary artery disease patients. Am Heart J 1984;108:1454-1460.)*

TABLE 3-2. Slopes in oxygen uptake versus work rate for patient subgroups performing six exercise protocols

	CAD	Angina	CHF	Normal
Slope	0.51	0.53	0.53	0.71*
SEE, mL O_2/kg/min	2.6	3.1	2.8	4.2

*$p < .001$ versus other groups. CAD, coronary artery disease; CHF, chronic heart failure; SEE, standard error of the estimate. If the change in ventilatory oxygen uptake were equal to the change in work rate; the slope would be equal to 1.0.

and the effects of beta-blockade on this response must also be considered when using workload to predict oxygen uptake.[14,15]

The choice of exercise protocol is also known to influence the relationship between measured and predicted work. Early work by Haskell et al,[16] for example, reported that estimating oxygen uptake among patients with heart disease was valid only if a gradual protocol was used. In an accelerated protocol, peak VO_2 was significantly overestimated. During the last 2 decades these findings have been replicated by many others.[8,13,17,18] Our laboratory evaluated differences between six protocols in terms of the relationship between measured and predicted oxygen uptake.[13] Three treadmill and three cycle ergometer protocols were compared. The three treadmill protocols used were: (1) a gradual (modified Balke), (2) a rapid (standard Bruce), and (3) a moderately incremented (individualized ramp) test. The three cycle ergometer protocols were: (1) a rapid (50 W/stage), (2) a gradual (25 W/stage), and (3) a moderately incremented (individualized ramp) test. Among 31 patients with heart disease and 10 normal subjects, the slope of the relationship between measured and predicted oxygen uptake was quantified throughout the exercise.

Table 3-3 presents the slopes of these relationships for each protocol. The protocols with the largest increments in work (i.e., Bruce treadmill and 50 W/stage cycle ergometer) had slopes significantly lower than those with smaller increments in work. This finding suggests that protocols that increase rapidly or have large increments in work overpredict exercise capacity. In addition, the standard error of the estimate (SEE) (oxygen uptake, mL/kg/min) was largest for the Bruce test and smallest for the individualized ramp tests, suggesting that the variability in estimating oxygen uptake from workload is greater in rapidly incremented tests than in tests that are more gradual and individualized. Similar observations have since been made by other investigators.[17]

Reproducibility. An important consideration, particularly when serially testing patients for research protocols such as pharmaceutical trials, is the reliability and reproducibility of the data. This has been one of the most important arguments in favor of the use of gas exchange techniques. The tendency to increase treadmill time with serial testing without an increase in VO_2 max is well documented. Many major multicenter drug trials in cardiology have shown significant increases in exercise time on placebo treatment that could be attributed only to repeated testing, in some cases causing a "masking" of the effects of therapy.

Changes in treadmill time with serial testing have even been observed without changes in maximal heart rate or double product.[19] Elborn et al[20] performed three consecutive treadmill tests on

TABLE 3-3. Slopes in oxygen uptake versus work rate for 41 subjects performing six exercise protocols

	Treadmills			Bicycles		
	Bruce	Balke	Ramp	25 W	50 W	Ramp
Slope	0.62	0.79	0.80	0.69	0.59	0.78
SEE	4.0	3.4	2.5	2.3	2.8	1.7

Note: Each slope ≥ 0.78 was significantly different from each slope ≤ 0.69 ($p < 0.05$ except Balke versus 25 W, $p = 0.07$). If the change in ventilatory oxygen uptake were equal to the change in work rate, the slope would be equal to 1.0. SEE, standard error of the estimate (mL O_2/kg/min); 25 W, 25 W/stage; 50 W, 50 W/stage.

separate days in patients with heart failure. They reported that the first test underestimated exercise time by approximately 20%. Pinsky et al[21] performed repeated treadmill tests among patients with heart failure until test duration on three consecutive tests varied by less than 60 seconds. This stability criterion was met within three tests on only 9 of 30 patients, whereas 13 patients required four or five tests, and eight patients required more than six tests.

Sullivan et al[1] compared the reproducibility of treadmill time and oxygen uptake among patients with angina tested on three different days within a week. Measured oxygen uptake had a higher intraclass correlation coefficient ($r = 0.88$) than treadmill time ($r = 0.70$) across the three exercise tests on different days (Table 3-4). Similarly, measured oxygen uptake was more reproducible at both the onset of angina and the ventilatory threshold than for exercise time. Russell et al[2] tested 81 patients with CHF on three different days and observed that measured peak oxygen uptake was consistent on all three tests (ranging from 1105 to 1123 mL/min, a 1.6% variation), whereas exercise time showed a progressive increase (from 419 to 470 seconds, a variation of 12.2%).

Thus, gas exchange techniques yield a more reliable, reproducible, and accurate assessment of exercise capacity and cardiopulmonary function than treadmill time or workload achieved. Therefore, this technology is important when using exercise as an efficacy parameter for studying interventions. Additional clinical applications of cardiopulmonary exercise testing are presented later.

Instrumentation

The measurement of oxygen uptake can be simply described as the product of ventilation (VE) in a given interval and the fraction of oxygen in that ventilation that has been consumed by the working muscle:

$$VO_2 \, mL/min \, (STPD) = VE \times (FiO_2 - FeO_2)$$

where FiO_2 is the fraction of inspired oxygen, and FeO_2 is the fraction of expired oxygen. FiO_2 is equal to 20.93% at sea level and 0% humidity, and ventilation is converted to *standard temperature and pressure, dry* (STPD). Thus, $FiO_2 - FeO_2$ represents the amount of oxygen consumed by the working muscle for a given sample, sometimes called "true O_2."

For the sake of explanation, the equation above is oversimplified, as it assumes that expired air is dry and that inspired and expired volumes are not different. Because these assumptions are generally not the case (unless the respiratory exchange ratio equals 1.0), several additional calculations are necessary to accurately determine oxygen uptake. First, the sample of air that is analyzed for O_2 and CO_2 content must be dried, or the humidity in the room must be measured and FiO_2 adjusted accordingly. Second, because oxygen uptake is the difference between the fraction of oxygen in the inspired and expired ventilation, both inspired and expired ventilation must be known precisely. Ventilatory volume is frequently measured only from the expired air. However, inspired volume can be determined from the expired volume and the fractions of oxygen and carbon dioxide. This is possible because nitrogen (N_2) and other inert gases do not affect the body's gas exchange processes. Thus, given that the concentrations of N_2, CO_2, and O_2 of the inspired air are known to be 0.7904, zero, and 0.2093, respectively, the fraction of inert gases (N_2) in the expired air (Fe_{N2}) becomes:

$$Fe_{N2} = 1 - FeO_2 - FeCO_2$$

Therefore, inspiratory volume (V_I) can be expressed as the difference between the fraction of

TABLE 3–4. Mean $\pm$ standard deviation of treadmill time and oxygen uptake at maximal angina-limited exercise

	Day 1	Day 2	Day 3	Intraclass correlation coefficient (ICC)	ICC, 90% confidence interval
Time (seconds)	503 ± 72	516 ± 85	526 ± 66	0.70	0.48–0.86
Oxygen uptake (L/min)	1.559 ± 0.289	1.553 ± 0.334	1.557 ± 0.294	0.88	0.76–0.95

inert gases in the expired air and the fraction of inert gases in the atmosphere:

$$V_1 = \frac{[VE \times (1 - FeO_2 - FeCO_2)]}{0.7904}$$

And the equation for oxygen uptake becomes:

$$VO_2 \text{ L/min STPD} = \frac{(1 - FeO_2 - FeCO_2)}{0.7904} \times (FiO_2 - FeO_2)$$
$$\times VE \text{ L/min STPD}$$

Collection of Expired Ventilation. The measurement of ventilation during exercise requires that the subject have either a mouthpiece in place that seals tightly and a clip sealing the nose, or a face mask that covers the nose and mouth. The masks make speaking possible, but caution must be used to ascertain that no leaking of ventilation occurs. This can sometimes be a problem at high ventilation rates. According to the preceding equation, the measurement of oxygen uptake requires that the ventilation be analyzed for total volume as well as oxygen and carbon dioxide content. This requires that the water content of the inspired air be accounted for by adjusting for standard pressure and temperature (hence the correction for STPD). As originally performed, expired gases were collected in a Tissot, which is an inverted open metal cylinder suspended in a large container filled with water. Filling the inner cylinder with expired air caused it to rise in the water, and ventilation was measured as the degree of displacement of the cylinder. Other methods of measuring air volume involved Douglas bags or weather balloons, using a turret that rotated from one bag to the next at given time intervals. These methods required a great deal of technician time and yielded limited precision, because sampling was dictated by the size of the collection bags and slowly responding analyzers. Because of the many subsequent advances in gas analysis systems, all of these methods are virtually obsolete.

Today gas analysis is commonly performed online with computer software. Various types of flowmeters are employed, including mass transducers, Fleisch pneumotachometers, hot-wire devices, small propellers or turbines, and dry-gas meters. A mixing chamber from which expired gases are sampled is usually no longer required. The Fleisch device measures a pressure drop because of the Venturi effect caused by airflow through a tube. The "hot wires" drop in temperature when cooled by air, and the propellers are spun by airflow. One of the problems with these devices is the difficulty in measuring ventilatory gas volume directly from a rapidly breathing individual.

The phasic nature of breathing can affect these devices. It has been suggested by some that many modern devices that measure flow directly from a patient are not as accurate as the older "off-line" methods. However, many technological advances have occurred in this area. These systems are now the norm commercially, and studies on their validation are available.

Most modern metabolic systems measure ventilation directly at the mouth using a light-weight, disposable flowmeter. These clever devices obviate the need for headgear, valve apparatus, and collection tubes, which can often be cumbersome. Flow is determined by a difference in pressure between the front and back of a strut or between two screens positioned in the center of the pneumotachometer. The relationship between the volume of airflow and the change in pressure is stated by Bernoulli's law (which states that flow is proportional to the square root of the pressure difference), permitting the quantification of ventilation.

Gas Exchange Data Sampling. Modern, rapidly responding gas analyzers, although facilitating precision and convenience, have led to confusion regarding data sampling because differences in sampling (i.e., breath by breath, 30 seconds, 60 seconds, or "running" breath averaging) can greatly affect precision and variability in measuring oxygen uptake. Figure 3-3 illustrates the standard deviation of various oxygen uptake samples during steady-state exercise in 10 subjects.[22] The variability in oxygen uptake is greater as the sampling interval shortens (i.e., 4.5 mL/kg/min for breath-by-breath versus 0.8 mL/kg/min for 60-second samples). Thus, a given value for oxygen uptake carries an inherent variability, and this variability depends upon the sampling interval. Shorter sampling intervals increase precision but can also increase variability.[22,23]

Data derived from small sampling intervals should be interpreted with caution, and one should resist the tendency to use breath-by-breath data simply because the technology is available. Breath-by-breath sampling can be invaluable for certain research applications, such as the measurement of oxygen kinetics, but it is inappropriate for general clinical applications. Thirty-second samples are commonly reported in the literature; for example, the majority of the studies applying peak VO_2 in a prognostic context have employed 30-second samples. Because 30-second samples can limit precision (e.g., few patients complete the test precisely at a 30-second interval), the use

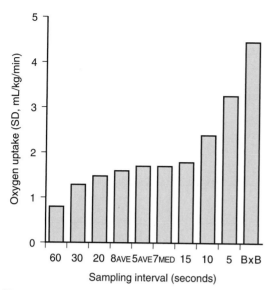

Variability in oxygen uptake expressed as a standard deviation for each sampling interval during 5 minutes of steady-state exercise. AVE, average; MED, median. *(From Myers J, Walsh D, Sullivan M, et al: Effect of sampling on variability and plateau in oxygen uptake. J Appl Physiol 1990;68: 404-410.)*

of a "rolling" or "moving" average of 30-second data, printed more frequently, is useful. Table 3-5 illustrates such an example from a patient tested in our laboratory. The 30-second moving averages were printed every 10 seconds. This method is recommended because the data are sampled frequently (increasing precision), while also reducing the variation to an acceptable level. This is an area that has not been standardized and continues to generate some controversy. Regardless of the sample chosen, investigators should report the sampling interval used, and the intervals should be consistent throughout a given trial.

Information from Ventilatory Gas Exchange Data during Exercise

Maximal oxygen uptake is the most common and most important measurement derived from gas exchange data during exercise. Unfortunately, it is frequently the only variable reported in many laboratories. Gas exchange techniques can provide a great deal of additional information regarding the capacity of the heart and lungs to deliver oxygen to the working muscle during exercise, and this information has a variety of clinical applications. In the following discussion, maximal oxygen

uptake and other gas exchange variables are outlined, with particular emphasis on their applications to testing patients with heart disease. Formulas for calculating these variables are presented in Table 3-6.

Maximal Oxygen Uptake. VO_2 max is an objective measurement of exercise capacity: it defines the upper limits of the cardiopulmonary system. It is determined by an individual's capacity to increase heart rate, augment stroke volume, and direct blood flow to the active muscles. It is often the most important variable measured, although this depends on the setting and the context of the particular patient being tested.

The term "VO_2 max" implies that an objective, maximal physiologic limit has been achieved. However, because this frequently does not occur by the criteria commonly used to define it, the term "peak VO_2" is often considered more appropriate, particularly in the clinical setting (see section on "Plateau in Oxygen Uptake" later in this chapter). VO_2 max should initially be considered in terms of what would be normal for a given individual if he or she were healthy. Determining what constitutes "normal" is no small task (this is covered in more detail under "Normal Values for Exercise Capacity" later in this chapter). However, generally the observation that VO_2 max falls within the normal range for a given gender and age makes a strong and multifactorial statement: the individual has no significant impairment in the cardiopulmonary system. Implicit in this statement, of course, is that the patient has no major limitations to cardiac output, its redistribution, or skeletal muscle metabolism or function. Changes in VO_2 max following training or detraining or reductions in VO_2 max caused by disease closely parallel changes in maximal cardiac output.[24-27] Clearly, VO_2 max is directly related to the integrated function of several systems.

Although it has been slow in coming, a better appreciation for directly measured VO_2 has evolved in clinical cardiology. For example, many pharmaceutical companies, recognizing the limitations in exercise time as a measure of cardiopulmonary work, increasingly employ gas exchange techniques in large multicenter trials.[4,28] The clinical importance of an objective and accurate measurement of exercise capacity is underscored by studies on prognosis in patients with heart disease. Exercise capacity has consistently been shown to be an important marker of prognosis. In many reviews of multivariate studies on this topic, exercise capacity appears to be chosen more

TABLE 3–5. Thirty-second "moving averages" printed every 10 seconds during last minute of maximal ramp

Time (min:sec)	Speed (mph)	Elev. (%)	METs (measured)	HR (per min)	RR (per min)	VT (mL)	VE (L/min)	VO$_2$ (per kg)	VO$_2$ (mL/min)
8:27	3.0	6.0	6.0	135	25	2607	64.5	21.1	1966
8:37	3.0	6.0	6.3	138	24	2851	67.5	21.9	2041
8:47	3.0	6.1	6.6	141	26	2878	74.1	23.1	2148
8:57	3.0	6.1	6.7	145	27	2940	78.7	23.3	2169
9:07	3.0	6.2	6.9	147	29	2816	82.9	24.1	2237
9:17	3.0	6.2	6.7	148	30	2657	79.5	23.3	2170
9:27	3.0	6.3	7.0	149	30	2816	84.6	24.5	2283

Note: This type of output provides a relatively standard sampling interval (30 seconds) while printing frequently enough to provide acceptable precision.

frequently than any other variable (including the patient's clinical history, markers of ischemia, or other exercise test variables) as a significant determinant of survival.[5,6,29,30] (See Chapter 10 for review of this topic.)

If exercise capacity is an important factor in prognosis, it follows that the more accurate and physiologic expression of exercise tolerance, peak VO$_2$, would be even more accurate in stratifying risk. There has been a burgeoning of studies (summarized in Table 10-1) applying peak VO$_2$ in the context of prognosis in the last 15 years. This issue has been of particular interest regarding patients with CHF. Peak VO$_2$ has been demonstrated repeatedly to be an independent marker for risk of death in patients with heart failure. Increased automation of gas exchange systems has made these data easier to obtain, and this objective information is replacing the former dependence on subjective measures of clinical and functional assessment. Peak VO$_2$ is now a recognized criterion for selecting patients who could potentially benefit from heart transplantation.[5-7,31-33] More powerful predictions of risk are often achieved when ventilatory gas exchange responses are combined with other clinical, hemodynamic, and exercise data.[5-7,31,32,34]

However, clearly, several specific areas require further study. In patients with heart failure, a peak VO$_2$ of 14 mL/kg/min is a widely used cutoff to separate survivors from nonsurvivors, and therefore this point is commonly used to help select patients for transplantation. Nevertheless, it is not entirely clear whether there is a specific peak VO$_2$ cutoff that optimally stratifies risk. Studies have demonstrated that each peak VO$_2$ value, ranging from 10 to 18 mL/kg/min, may represent an "optimal" cutoff point; more than likely, this value changes depending upon the severity of heart failure in the population studied.[35] In addition, because peak VO$_2$ can be subjective and somewhat difficult to define in some patients, some investigators have suggested that other ventilatory and gas exchange responses, such as VO$_2$ at the ventilatory threshold, the rate of decline in VO$_2$ during recovery from exercise (recovery kinetics), the kinetics of VO$_2$ during exercise, the VE/VCO$_2$ slope, and the oxygen uptake efficiency slope, have superior prognostic value.[5-7,31,36-46] These studies are summarized in Chapter 10 (see Table 10-3).

Minute Ventilation (VE). Minute ventilation is the volume of air moving into and out of the lungs expressed as liters per minute, *body temperature and pressure, saturated* (BTPS). VE is determined by the product of respiratory rate and the volume of air exhaled with each breath (the tidal volume). Because *true O$_2$* (the difference between inspired and expired oxygen content) differs little among individuals, even those with widely varying fitness levels, ventilation is often the major component of oxygen uptake during exercise. However, fit individuals with high maximal ventilation, and thus high maximal oxygen uptake values, must also have the ability to increase cardiac output such that the increase in ventilation matches the increase in cardiac output in the lung. The ratio of alveolar ventilation to alveolar capillary blood flow, termed the *ventilation-perfusion ratio*, is roughly 0.80 at rest. With exercise, ventilation and alveolar blood flow increase such that this ratio may approach 5.0. Abnormal ventilation is an important characteristic of patients with CHF and patients with pulmonary disease, partly because of a mismatching of the ratio of ventilation to perfusion. The ventilatory response to exercise can be

exercise test

VCO$_2$ (mL/min)	RQ	ETO$_2$ (mmHg)	ETCO$_2$ (mmHg)	VE/VCO$_2$	VE/VO$_2$	VO$_2$/HR (mL/bt)	Vd/Vt	FEO$_2$ (%)	FECO$_2$ (%)
2455	1.25	119	39	26.2	32.7	14.5	0.11	17.32	4.51
2524	1.24	118	39	26.7	33.0	14.7	0.11	17.35	4.43
2705	1.26	120	38	27.3	34.4	15.2	0.10	17.50	4.32
2814	1.30	122	36	27.9	36.2	14.9	0.10	17.67	4.23
2943	1.32	123	35	28.1	37.0	15.2	0.09	17.73	4.20
2843	1.31	123	35	27.9	36.5	14.6	0.09	17.70	4.23
2989	1.31	123	35	28.3	37.0	15.3	0.09	17.73	4.18

TABLE 3–6. Calculations for basic gas exchange data

1. Oxygen uptake (VO$_2$ L/min, STPD) = $\dfrac{(1 - \text{FeO}_2 - \text{FeCO}_2)}{0.7904} \times (\text{FiO}_2 - \text{FeO}_2) \times$ VE (STPD)

2. Minute ventilation (VE, L/min, BTPS) = respiratory rate × tidal volume.
   For calculations of VO$_2$ and VCO$_2$, VE in BTPS is converted to STPD by the following:

   $$\frac{(1 - \text{FeO}_2 - \text{FeCO}_2)}{0.7904} \times (\text{FiO}_2 - \text{FeO}_2) \times \text{VE (STPD)}$$

   or E (L/min, STPD) = VE (L/min, BTPS) × 0.826 if Pb = 760 mmHg
3. Carbon dioxide production (VCO$_2$ L/min, STPD) = VE (L/min, STPD) × FeCO$_2$

4. Respiratory exchange ratio (RER) = $\dfrac{\text{VCO}_2 \text{ (L/min, STPD)}}{\text{VO}_2 \text{ (L/min, STPD)}}$

5. Oxygen pulse (O$_2$ pulse, mL O$_2$/beat) = $\dfrac{\text{VO}_2 \text{ (mL/min, STPD)}}{\text{heart rate, beats/min}}$

6. Ventilatory equivalents for O$_2$ and CO$_2$ = $\dfrac{\text{VE (L/min, BTPS)}}{\text{VO}_2 \text{ (L/min, STPD)}}$ and $\dfrac{\text{VE (L/min, BTPS)}}{\text{VCO}_2 \text{ (L/min, STPD)}}$

7. End-tidal PCO$_2$ (PetCO$_2$, mmHg) = FetCO$_2$ × (Pb − 47)

8. Ventilatory dead space (Vd, L) = $\dfrac{\text{PaCO}_2 - \text{PeCO}_2}{\text{PaCO}_2}$ − valve dead space, (L)

   where PeCO$_2$ = FeCO$_2$ × (Pb − 47), and PaCO$_2$ is estimated using PaCO$_2$ = 5.5 + (0.90 × PetCO$_2$) − (0.0021 × Vt)
   The ventilatory dead space to tidal volume ratio (Vd/Vt) is calculated by dividing by Vt.
9. Alveolar − arterial PO$_2$ difference [P(A − a)O$_2$] = PaO$_2$ obtained from blood gas PaO$_2$ (room air) −

   $$[\text{Pb} - 47 \times 0.2093] - \frac{\text{PaCO}_2}{\text{RER}}$$

10. Breathing reserve = $\dfrac{\text{maximal VE, (L/min)}}{\text{MVV, L/min}}$

   where VE is Equation 2, and MVV is the maximal voluntary ventilation at rest.

BTPS, body temperature and pressure, saturated; gas volume at body temperature and pressure saturated with water vapor (37°C and 47 mmHg); FeCO$_2$, fraction (%) of carbon dioxide in the expired air; FeO$_2$, fraction (%) of oxygen in the expired air; FetCO$_2$, fraction (%) of end-tidal carbon dioxide; FiCO$_2$, fraction (%) of carbon dioxide in the inspired air; FiO$_2$, fraction (%) of oxygen in the inspired air; PaCO$_2$, partial pressure of carbon dioxide in arterial blood; PaO$_2$, partial pressure of alveolar oxygen; PaO$_2$, partial pressure of arterial oxygen; Pb, barometric pressure, mmHg; PeCO$_2$, mixed expired carbon dioxide pressure, mmHg; PetCO$_2$, end-tidal carbon dioxide pressure, mmHg; PetO$_2$, end-tidal oxygen pressure, mmHg; STPD, standard temperature and pressure, day; gas volume at standard temperature (0°C) and barometric pressure (760 mmHg), dry; Vt, tidal volume, mL.

important both in identifying these conditions and in gauging patients' responses to therapy.

Carbon Dioxide Production (VCO₂). Carbon dioxide produced by the body during exercise is expressed in liters per minute, STPD. VCO_2 is generated from two sources during exercise. One source, the metabolic CO_2, is produced by oxidative metabolism. Roughly 75% of the oxygen consumed by the body is converted to CO_2, which is returned to the right side of the heart by the venous blood, enters the lungs, and is exhaled as VCO_2. A second source of CO_2 is often called *nonmetabolic;* it results from the buffering of lactate at higher levels of exercise. An elevation in CO_2 in the blood can quickly result in respiratory acidosis. Fortunately, the major determinants of ventilation during exercise are these two sources of CO_2 in the blood, which are reflected in the expired air as VCO_2. Thus, VCO_2 closely matches VE during exercise, and the body maintains a relatively normal pH under most conditions. VCO_2 and VE also parallel increases in VO_2, or work rate, during exercise levels of up to roughly 50% to 70% of VO_2 max. At exercise levels beyond this, VE increases disproportionately to VO_2. This increase occurs because as exercise increases in intensity, lactate is produced at a greater rate than it is removed from the blood. The lactate must be buffered, and the buffering process yields an additional source of CO_2, which stimulates ventilation. This "ventilatory threshold" has generated a great deal of interest over the years (see discussion later in this chapter).

Respiratory Exchange Ratio (RER). The RER represents the amount of CO_2 produced divided by the amount of oxygen consumed. Normally, roughly 75% of the oxygen consumed is converted to CO_2. Thus, RER at rest generally ranges from 0.70 to 0.85. Because RER depends on the type of fuel used by the cells, it can provide an index of carbohydrate or fat metabolism. If carbohydrates were the predominant fuel, RER would equal 1.0 given the following formula:

$$C_6H_{12}O_6 \text{ (glucose)} + 6O_2 \rightarrow 6CO_2 + 6H_2O$$

$$RER = VCO_2 \div VO_2$$

$$= 6CO_2 \div 6O_2 = 1.0$$

Because relatively more oxygen is required to burn fat, the RER for fat metabolism is lower, roughly 0.70. At high levels of exercise, CO_2 production exceeds oxygen uptake; thus, an RER exceeding 1.1 to 1.2 is often used to indicate that the subject is giving a maximal effort. However, peak RER values vary greatly and generally are not a precise criterion for "maximal" exercise.

Oxygen Pulse (O₂ Pulse). Oxygen pulse is an indirect index of combined cardiopulmonary oxygen transport. It is calculated by dividing oxygen uptake (mL/min) by heart rate. In effect, O_2 pulse is equal to the product of stroke volume and a-VO₂ difference. Thus, circulatory adjustments that occur during exercise—that is, widening a-VO₂ difference, increased cardiac output, and redistribution of blood flow to the working muscle—will increase O_2 pulse. Maximal O_2 pulse is higher in fitter subjects, lower in the presence of heart disease, and more importantly, is higher at any given workload in the fitter or healthier individual. Conversely, O_2 pulse is reduced in any condition that reduces stroke volume (left ventricular dysfunction secondary to ischemia or infarction) or reduces arterial O_2 content (anemia, hypoxemia).

Ventilatory Equivalents for Oxygen and Carbon Dioxide (VE/VO₂ and VE/VCO₂). These are calculated by dividing ventilation (L/min, BTPS) by VO_2 or VCO_2 (L/min, STPD), respectively. A great deal of ventilation (25 to 40 L) is required to consume a single liter of oxygen; thus, VE/VO₂ is often in the 30s at rest. A decrease in VE/VO₂ is normally observed from rest to submaximal exercise, followed by a rapid increase at higher levels of exercise when VE increases in response to the need to buffer lactate.

VE/VO₂ reflects the ventilatory requirement for any given oxygen uptake; thus, it is an index of ventilatory efficiency. Patients with a high fraction of physiologic dead space or uneven matching of ventilation to perfusion in the lung ventilate inefficiently and therefore have high values for VE/VO₂. High VE/VO₂ values characterize the response to exercise among patients with lung disease or CHF (Fig. 3-4).

VE/VCO₂ represents the ventilatory requirement to eliminate a given amount of CO_2 produced by the metabolizing tissues. Since metabolic CO_2 is a strong stimulus for ventilation during exercise, VE and VCO_2 closely mirror one another and, after a drop in early exercise, VE/VCO₂ normally does not increase significantly throughout submaximal exercise. However, in the presence of left ventricular dysfunction, VE/VCO₂ is shifted upward compared with normal subjects, and high

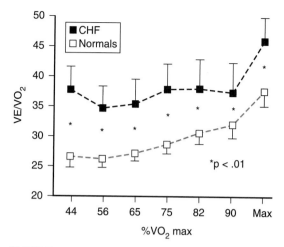

VE/VCO_2 values are one of the characteristics of the abnormal ventilatory response to exercise in this condition.

Caiozzo et al[47] compared gas exchange indices used to detect the ventilatory threshold and found that the use of the ventilatory equivalents for O_2 and CO_2 most closely reflected a lactate inflection point and thus were the best indices to detect the ventilatory threshold. Many laboratories define the ventilatory threshold as the beginning of a systematic increase in VE/VO_2 without an increase in VE/VCO_2.

Ventilatory Dead Space to Tidal Volume Ratio (Vd/Vt). Vd/Vt measured by gas exchange is an estimate of the fraction of tidal volume that represents *physiologic dead space*, the difference between minute ventilation and alveolar ventilation. Vd/Vt is an estimate of the degree to which ventilation matches perfusion in the lung and is therefore an additional measure of ventilatory efficiency. When significant ventilation-perfusion mismatching is present, Vd/Vt is high. Although Vd/Vt is commonly measured noninvasively using gas exchange techniques, the additional measurement of arterial CO_2 pressure directly from the blood is necessary to quantify Vd/Vt accurately. This is because arterial CO_2 pressure is usually not accurately estimated from end-tidal CO_2 pressure (determined from ventilation) during exercise, resulting in erroneous values for Vd/Vt.

In normal subjects, Vd/Vt falls from roughly one third to between one tenth and one fifth at peak exercise. However, in the presence of pulmonary disease or heart failure, in which there can be significant ventilation-perfusion mismatching, the Vd/Vt is elevated and often remains relatively unchanged throughout exercise. Ventilation-perfusion mismatching, and thus a high Vd/Vt, accounts in large part for the abnormally high ventilation observed in patients with pulmonary disease and heart failure. Figure 3-5 illustrates the relationship between maximal

■ **FIGURE 3-5**

The relationship between maximal estimated ventilatory dead space to tidal volume ratio (Vd/Vt max) and maximal oxygen uptake (VO_2 max) for normal subjects *(darkened squares)* and patients with chronic heart failure *(open circles)*. The correlation coefficient between the two variables was -0.73 (SEE = 6.2, $P < 0.001$).

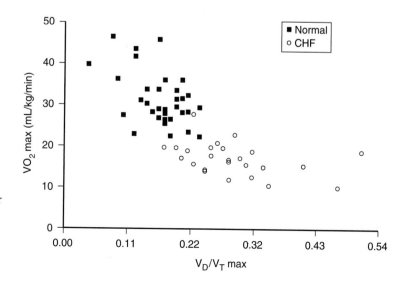

Vd/Vt and VO_2 max in a group of patients with CHF and a group of age-matched normal subjects. Not only do patients with heart failure have poorer exercise capacity, they also have markedly higher Vd/Vt values; for some patients, nearly half of the tidal volume is dead space. With such a large fraction of dead space and thus "wasted" ventilation, it is not surprising that patients with heart disease require a significantly higher ventilation for the same relative work (see Figure 3-4).

Breathing Reserve. The breathing reserve is calculated as the ratio of *maximal voluntary ventilation* (MVV) at rest to maximal exercise ventilation. Most healthy subjects achieve a maximal exercise ventilation of only 60% to 80% of the MVV at rest. One characteristic of chronic pulmonary disease is a maximal ventilation that approximates the individual's MVV. These patients reach a "ventilatory" limit during exercise, whereas normal subjects generally have a substantial ventilatory reserve (20% to 40%) at peak exercise and are limited by other factors. Therefore, the breathing reserve is commonly used to help differentiate pulmonary from cardiovascular limitations to exercise.

Ventilatory Threshold. Physiologic links between exercise capacity, lactate accumulation in the blood, and respiratory gas exchange were established by Hill and Lupton[48] more than 80 years ago. A sudden rise in the blood lactate level during exercise has long been associated with muscle anaerobiosis and has therefore been termed the *anaerobic threshold*.[49] Historically, the anaerobic threshold has been defined as the highest oxygen uptake during exercise above which a sustained lactic acidosis occurs. When this level of exercise is reached, excess H^+ ions of lactate must be buffered to maintain physiologic pH. Because bicarbonate buffering yields an additional source of CO_2, ventilation is further stimulated. This point of nonlinear increase in ventilation has been used to detect the anaerobic threshold noninvasively and is often termed the *gas exchange anaerobic threshold* or the *ventilatory threshold* (VT) (Fig. 3-6). A significant amount of disagreement continues related to the mechanism underlying this point, how it should be determined, and how it should be applied clinically.[50]

Changes in oxygen uptake at the VT have been used clinically during pharmacologic and other interventions to imply that a change in oxygen supply to the working muscle has occurred. However, the anaerobic threshold has come under scrutiny on the basis of both theoretical and pragmatic grounds.[50-55] Connett et al[55] studied dog gracilis muscle, which is a pure red fiber containing only type I and type IIA fibers, and observed lactate accumulation during fully aerobic, mild (10% VO_2 max) conditions. These investigators also observed that lactate accumulation was not altered by changes in blood flow, and that lactate accumulation occurred even though no anoxic areas were present in the muscle. This suggests that lactate production and muscle hypoxia are unrelated. Additionally, the advent of tracer technology has raised strong questions about the cause-and-effect relation between oxygen availability to the muscle and the anaerobic threshold. Many studies now suggest that lactate production occurs at all times, even in resting conditions. Further, the turnover rate of lactate (the ratio of appearance to disappearance) is linearly related to oxygen uptake during exercise.[56,57] This relationship is possible because studies have shown that lactate is "shuttled" from fibers where it is produced (presumably fast-twitch muscle) to those where it is used as an energy source (such as the heart and slow-twitch fibers). The *lactate shuttle* has engendered the concept that production, transport, and use of lactate represents an important source of energy from carbohydrates during exercise.[58]

Some arguments have also addressed whether lactate during exercise in fact increases in a pattern that is mathematically "continuous" rather than as a threshold.[59-62] The cumulative effect of these studies has led to the conclusion that the "anaerobic" threshold is not strictly related to muscle anaerobiosis, but instead reflects an imbalance between lactate appearance and disappearance. The term *ventilatory threshold* has been suggested as preferable to *anaerobic threshold*, as it does not imply the onset of anaerobiosis.

Irrespective of what causes the VT, lactate accumulates in the blood during exercise, ventilation must respond to maintain physiologic pH, a breakpoint in ventilation does appear to occur reproducibly, and this point is related to various measures of cardiopulmonary performance both in normal subjects[63-67] and in patients with heart disease.[68-75] A common argument clinically in favor of the use of the VT is that, as a submaximal parameter, it is better associated with patient's everyday activities than maximal exercise, and

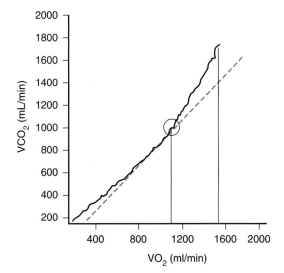

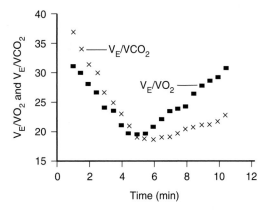

■ FIGURE 3–6

The ventilatory threshold detected using the V-slope method *(top)* and the ventilatory equivalents for oxygen and carbon dioxide *(bottom)*. The ventilatory threshold is exhibited by a nonlinear increase in VCO_2 from a computed plot using the V-slope method, and the beginning of a systematic increase in VE/VO_2 without a concomitant increase in VE/VCO_2 using the ventilatory equivalents method.

therefore using the VT avoids the increased risk and discomfort of maximal exercise. On the basis of the many studies in this area, the following suggestions might be made concerning the use of VT during exercise testing: (1) regardless of the mechanism, ventilatory changes appear strongly correlated with a lactate threshold, and (2) an alteration in the VT reflects a change in the balance between lactate production and removal, and references to muscle anaerobiosis should be avoided. Because lactate is strongly associated

with muscle fatigue, a change in this relation that can be attributed to an intervention may add important information concerning the intervention. In this context, the VT during exercise testing remains an interesting and applicable index for use during exercise studies.

An additional consideration concerns the method of choosing the VT. Our laboratory, in agreement with others, has observed that the VT can vary markedly depending upon both the observer and the method of determination. Although a number of methods of determination have been proposed, Caiozzo et al[47] reported that the use of the ventilatory equivalents for oxygen uptake (VE/VO_2) and carbon dioxide (VE/VCO_2) most closely reflected a lactate inflection point. Therefore, many laboratories have defined the VT as the beginning of a systemic increase in VE/VO_2 without a concomitant increase in VE/VCO_2. However, methods of detecting the VT that rely on minute ventilation (such as the VE/VO_2 method) may not be reliable under certain conditions (e.g., obesity, airflow obstruction, and chemoreceptor insensitivity) in which ventilation may lag behind metabolic events. Therefore, Beaver et al[76] regressed VCO_2 versus VO_2 (called the *V slope*) because CO_2 production more directly addresses lactate accumulation and is less influenced by the noise or oscillatory changes in ventilation often noted in certain patients. These investigators reported that the detection of the VT was more reliable using the V-slope method (see Fig. 3-6).

We have routinely used a method outlined by Sullivan et al[1] in which two experienced, blinded (to patient name and test purpose, i.e., whether the test represented a drug or placebo phase) observers independently chose the VT for each exercise test. When a discrepancy exists, a third observer is also blinded and chooses the VT independently. The VT is determined as the minute sample in which two of the three observers agree. The VT is not included in the analysis for that particular patient when all observers differ. We have found that two observers agree 72% of the time, and two of three observers agree 100% of the time. In a later study, this method resulted in 7% of tests being excluded.[77] This technique avoids interobserver bias and provides a means by which the VT can be determined objectively. Methods, problems, and advantages of various methods of choosing the VT or lactate inflection points have been the subjects of numerous reports.[50-55,59-62,77-82]

VE/VCO₂ Slope. The VE/VCO_2 slope has gained interest in recent years as an expression of ventilatory efficiency and a marker of prognosis in patients with cardiovascular disease. This response is usually expressed as the slope of the best-fit linear regression line relating VE and VCO_2, excluding data points beyond the VT (Fig. 3-7). While values in the 20s are typically observed among normals, values in the 30s are common in patients with mild to moderate CHF, and values greater than 40 can be observed in patients with more severe CHF. Any condition that causes heightened ventilation (e.g., early lactate accumulation in the blood, ventilation/perfusion mismatching, and deconditioning) will cause a shifting of the VE/VCO_2 relation upward and to the left, and thus an increase in the VE/VCO_2 slope. The VE/VCO_2 slope has been demonstrated to predict mortality at least as well as, and independent from, peak VO_2.[7,37-43] (See summary of studies in Table 10-3.)

Oxygen Kinetics. Although the measurement of oxygen kinetics poses some difficulties in that it often requires a specialized exercise test, is defined differently by various laboratories, and requires mathematical computations not familiar to most clinicians, this measurement is probably underutilized as an index of cardiopulmonary function clinically. Put simply, *oxygen kinetics* quantify the ability of the cardiopulmonary system to respond to the demands of a given amount of work; it is usually defined as the rate at which oxygen uptake reaches a steady-state value. Measures such as the oxygen uptake/work rate relation, the oxygen debt, the steepness of the slope of the relationship between work rate and oxygen uptake (see Table 3-2), the rate in which oxygen uptake recovers from exercise, the recently described *oxygen uptake efficiency slope*,[44-46] and various other measures of the difference between predicted and measured oxygen uptake generally describe oxygen kinetics. Although mainly limited thus far to applications in human performance laboratories among healthy subjects, this is an untapped area for quantifying interventions in patients with heart disease. Several of these indices have recently been shown to have prognostic power in patients with cardiovascular disease (see Table 10-3).

Models of oxygen kinetics have been used to study cardiovascular function before and after beta-blockade in which oxygen kinetics are slowed by propranolol and metoprolol.[83-85] Hypoxia slows oxygen kinetics and causes a greater oxygen deficit and an increase in intramuscular lactate, whereas hyperoxia appears to enhance oxygen kinetics.[86-88] Oxygen kinetics are greater below versus above

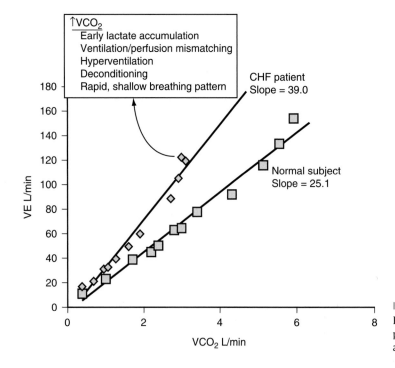

■ FIGURE 3–7

Example of the VE/VCO_2 slope in a patient with chronic heart failure (CHF) and a normal subject.

the VT,[89] and they improve after a program of physical conditioning.[90-92] A growing body of evidence suggests that these measurements are useful in classifying functional limitations in patients with heart failure.[36,93,94] De Groote et al[36] reported that oxygen kinetics during exercise and recovery are good predictors of outcome in patients with heart failure. Rickli et al[95] recently studied the mean response time, defined as the time required to reach 63% of the steady state VO_2, in patients with CHF. They observed that mean response time was the strongest univariate and multivariate predictor of mortality, and patients who exhibited an abnormal mean response time, a peak VO_2 less than 50% of the age-predicted value, and a resting systolic blood pressure less than 105 mmHg had a 1-year event rate of 59%. Other applications of oxygen kinetics for the study of pharmacologic interventions, exercise training, or other therapies in patients with heart disease are intriguing, but few such studies have been performed in the clinical setting.

Plateau in Oxygen Uptake. Maximal oxygen uptake is considered the best index of aerobic capacity and maximal cardiorespiratory function. By defining the limits of the cardiopulmonary system, it has been an invaluable measurement clinically for assessing the efficacy of drugs, exercise training, or invasive procedures. No other measure of work is as accurate, reliable, or reproducible as ventilatory maximal oxygen uptake. The collection and analysis of an expired gas sample taken during the last period of an exercise test has generally been used to determine maximal oxygen uptake. From early studies using interrupted protocols, a test was considered "maximal" only when there was no further increase in oxygen uptake despite further increases in workload. Conversely, oxygen uptake has been considered "peak" when the subject reaches a point of fatigue where no plateau in oxygen uptake was observed. Unfortunately, the many problems associated with the determination and criteria for the "plateau" in oxygen uptake make these definitions more semantic than physiologic. A brief history of this concept and its inherent problems follows.

In 1955 Taylor et al[96] established the criteria of plateauing as a failure to increase oxygen uptake more than 150 mL/min, or 2.1 mL/kg/min, with an increase in workload. Their original research was done using interrupted progressive treadmill protocols. With interrupted protocols, stages of exercise could be separated by rest periods ranging from minutes to days. Taylor et al[96] found that

75% of their subjects fulfilled these criteria. Using continuous treadmill protocols, Pollock et al[97] found that 69%, 69%, 59%, and 80% of subjects plateaued when tested using the Balke, Bruce, Ellestad, and Astrand protocols, respectively. Froelicher et al[98] found that only 33%, 17%, and 7% of healthy subjects met these criteria during testing with the Taylor, Balke, and Bruce protocols, respectively, despite the fact that there were no significant differences between the protocols in maximal heart rate, VO_2 max, or blood pressure. Taylor et al later reported that plateauing did not occur when using continuous treadmill protocols. Subsequent studies, using a variety of empirical criteria, report the occurrence of a plateau ranging from 7% to 90% of tests.

The plateau concept has been subjected to many interpretations and criteria. The newer, automated gas exchange systems, which allow breath-by-breath or any specified sampling interval, have raised new questions regarding the interpretation of a plateau. Although the definitions of plateauing vary greatly, all focus on the concept that oxygen uptake at some point will fail to continue to rise as work increases. Using ramp treadmill testing, in which work increases constantly at an individualized rate, we measured the slope of the change in work versus the change in oxygen uptake at different sampling intervals.[22,99] In this way, if oxygen uptake were no longer increasing (while work was increasing continuously) the slope of the relationship between the two variables would equal, or not differ from, zero. To increase the possibility of observing a plateau, a large sampling interval of 30 consecutive eight-breath averages was used. We observed that patients plateau on several occasions submaximally, even when some subjects do not meet these criteria at maximal exercise. This is because the slope of the relationship between oxygen uptake and work rate varies greatly, despite a constant, continuous change in external work and the use of large, averaged samples. In addition, it was found that this response was poorly reproducible, and that the occurrence of a plateau depended greatly upon which definition of a plateau was used and how the data were sampled (e.g., 30-second samples, various breath-averaging techniques, etc.). These observations would appear to preclude the determination of a plateau by common definitions.

The plateau concept is long ingrained in exercise physiology. Intuitively, it is known that the body's respiratory and metabolic systems must reach some finite limit beyond which oxygen uptake can no longer increase, and some subjects who are highly motivated may exhibit a plateau. However, the occurrence of a plateau depends as much on the criteria applied, the sampling interval, and methodology as on the subjects' health, fitness, and motivation. Studies performed in our laboratory[22,99] and others[100-103] suggest that the plateau concept has limitations for general application during standard exercise testing.

NORMAL VALUES FOR EXERCISE CAPACITY

Maximal oxygen uptake declines with increasing age, and higher values are observed among men than among women. Thus, when measuring or estimating maximal oxygen uptake, it is useful to have reference values for comparison. Numerous investigators have developed reference values for measured maximal oxygen uptake that are adjusted for age and gender, and the reader is referred to these sources for more detail.[104-115] Many clever attempts have been made to improve the prediction of what represents a "normal" exercise capacity by including height, weight, body composition, activity status, exercise mode, and clinical and demographic factors such as smoking history, heart disease, and medications. It is important to note that a "normal" value is only a number that has been inferred from some population. A predicted normal value usually refers to age

and gender, but many other factors affect one's exercise capacity. In addition to those just mentioned, these include some that are not so easily measured, such as genetics and the type and extent of disease. In the classic studies of Bruce et al,[107] gender and age were the most important factors influencing exercise capacity (compared with activity status, weight, height, or smoking). This observation has since been confirmed by our laboratory[116] and others.[117] However, the relation between age and exercise capacity is highly imprecise. Figure 3-8 illustrates the relationship between maximal oxygen uptake and age, with different levels of current physical activity considered.[118] The wide scatter around the regression lines and poor correlation coefficients underscore the common observation that a great deal of inaccuracy exists when one attempts to predict exercise capacity from age, even when considering other factors such as gender or activity level. Choosing the most appropriate reference equation is therefore critical. Table 3-7 outlines the various factors to consider when applying reference formulas.

Regression Equations. The following are commonly used generalized equations based on data published in North America and Europe in the 1950s, 1960s, and 1970s.[108-111]

Males

VO_2 max (L/min) = 4.2 − 0.032 (age) (SD ± 0.4)

VO_2 max (mL/kg/min) = 60 − 0.55 (age) (SD ± 7.5)

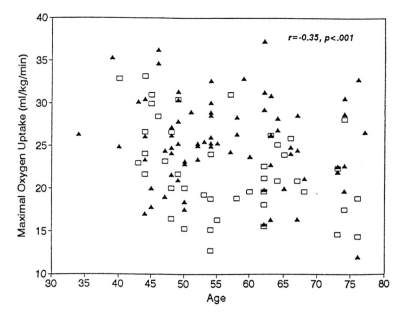

■ FIGURE 3-8

The relationship between maximal oxygen uptake and age among active ▲ and sedentary □ healthy males referred for exercise testing. *(From Myers J. Ventilatory gas exchange in heart failure: Techniques, problems and pitfalls. In Balady GJ, Pina IC (eds): Exercise and Heart Failure. Armonk, NY, Futura Publishing, 1997.)*

TABLE 3–7. **Factors to consider in reference population when applying formulas for exercise capacity**

- Population tested:
  Age
  Gender
  Anthropometric characteristics
  Health and fitness
  Heart disease
- Pulmonary disease
- Exercise mode and protocol
- Reason tested:
  Clinical referral
  Screening apparently healthy volunteers
- Exercise capacity estimated versus measured directly
- Units of measurement
- Variability of predicted values (usually 10% to 30%)

Females

VO_2 max (L/min) = 2.6 − 0.014 (age) (SD ± 0.4)

VO_2 max (mL/kg/min) = 48 − 0.37 (age) (SD ± 7.0)

Efforts have been made to improve the precision of predictive equations by considering specific populations, body size, and other demographic factors, in addition to gender. Wasserman et al[105] and Hansen et al[106] have published predicted values for maximal oxygen uptake that consider sex, age, height, weight, and whether testing was performed on a treadmill or a cycle ergometer.

Mode	Over weight	Predicted VO_2 max (mL/min)
Males		
Cycle*	No	$W \times (50.72 - 0.372 \times A)$
	Yes	$(0.79 \times H - 60.7) \times$ $(50.72 - 0.372 \times A)$
Treadmill[†]	No	$W \times (56.36 - 0.413 \times A)$
	Yes	$(0.79 \times H - 60.7) \times$ $(56.36 - 0.413 \times A)$
Females		
Cycle*	No	$(42.8 \times W) \times$ $(22.78 - 0.17 \times A)$
	Yes	$H \times (14.81 - 0.11 \times A)$
Treadmill[‡]	No	$W \times (44.37 - 0.413 \times A)$
	Yes	$(0.79 \times H - 68.2) \times$ $(44.37 - 0.413 \times A)$

A, age in years; H, height in cm; W, weight in kg.

*Overweight is $W > (0.79 \times H - 60.7)$.
[†]Overweight is $W > (0.65 \times H - 42.8)$.
[‡]Overweight is $W > (0.79 \times H - 68.2)$.

Jones et al[112] studied healthy adults on a cycle ergometer and reported the following regression equation:

VO_2 max (L/min) = 0.046 (Ht) − 0.021 (age) − 0.62 (gender) − 4.31 (r = 0.87, SEE = 0.46)

where Ht is the height in cm, and gender is coded 0 for males, 1 for females.

Although normal values were derived from studies on Scandinavian children in the 1950s,[114] Cooper and Weiler-Ravell[115] subsequently developed regression equations from studies on California schoolchildren (ages 6 to 17) that considered height rather than age:

Boys

VO_2 (mL/min) = 43.6 (Ht) − 4547

Girls

VO_2 (mL/min) = 22.5 (Ht) − 1837

where Ht is the height in cm.

Application of Nomograms. Because relatively few clinical exercise laboratories measure oxygen uptake directly, a variety of methods have been developed using estimated values from exercise times or workloads. One of the early techniques was developed by Bruce et al,[107] who suggested the use of a nomogram for estimating *functional aerobic impairment*. In this nomogram, one side depicts treadmill time using the Bruce protocol and the other side lists age. Between these two lines are percent increments of functional aerobic improvement for sedentary and active individuals. By drawing a straight line through age and the treadmill time achieved, an estimate of aerobic impairment can be read from the sloped lines. Functional aerobic improvement would be zero (100% of predicted exercise capacity) in an individual whose observed maximal oxygen uptake was the same as that predicted for age and gender; a value of 120% would indicate an exercise capacity 20% higher than predicted, and a value of 70% would indicate a capacity 30% lower than predicted. One problem with this approach is that studies have demonstrated relatively poor correlations between age and maximal oxygen uptake in healthy subjects even when activity levels were considered (see Figure 3-8). As mentioned above, this is due to the many factors that affect an individual's aerobic capacity in addition to current activity level, including past activity level, genetic endowment, mechanical efficiency, previous testing experience, and specificity of training. Thus, this nomogram is based on two relatively poor relationships, which consequently limit its ability to predict functional capacity.

Morris et al[113] developed a similar nomogram from 1388 subjects tested in a Veterans Administration hospital. These data are presented in more detail in Chapter 5, and will only be mentioned briefly here. This nomogram may be more applicable clinically than Bruce's because: (1) it is based on METs achieved from treadmill speed and grade and does not restrict one to using the Bruce protocol, and (2) it was derived from a group of males who were referred for exercise testing for clinical reasons. The regression equations derived from the group were as follows:

All Subjects
$$METs = 18.0 - 0.15 \text{ (age)}, SEE = 3.3, r = -0.46, P < 0.001$$

Active Subjects
$$METs = 18.7 - 0.15 \text{ (age)}, SEE = 3.0, r = -0.49, P < 0.001$$

Sedentary Subjects
$$METs = 16.6 - 0.16 \text{ (age)}, SEE = 3.2, r = -0.43, P < 0.001$$

When using regression equations or nomograms for reference purposes, it is important to consider several points. First, as mentioned, the relationship between exercise capacity and age is rather poor ($r = -0.30$ to -0.60). Second, nearly all equations are derived from different populations using different protocols. Thus, to some extent, they are both population- and protocol-specific. For example, the equations developed by Morris et al[113] were derived from data on a large group of Veterans Administration patients referred for testing for clinical reasons. Thus, these subjects had a greater prevalence of heart disease than those in other studies, and it is not surprising that a steeper slope was present, with a faster decline in VO_2 max with age. Finally, since treadmill time or workload tends to overpredict maximal METs, it is important to consider whether gas exchange techniques were used in developing the equations. Normal standards for *measured* VO_2 max should be used when it is measured directly, and normal standards for *estimated* exercise capacity should be used when

it is predicted from the treadmill or cycle ergometer work rate. Only a few studies have developed regression equations for measured VO_2 max. The aforementioned Veterans Administration study developed a nomogram using measured oxygen uptake among 244 active or sedentary apparently healthy males. Relative to the nomogram for estimated METs, the values are shifted downward by roughly 1.0 to 1.5 METs for any given age, reflecting the lower but more precise measures of exercise capacity:

All Subjects:
$$METs = 14.7 - 0.11 \text{ (age)}$$

Active Subjects:
$$METs = 16.4 - 0.13 \text{ (age)}$$

Sedentary Subjects:
$$METs = 11.9 - 0.07 \text{ (age)}$$

Thus, such scales are specific to both the population tested and to whether oxygen uptake was measured directly or predicted. Within these limitations, these equations and the nomograms derived from them can provide reasonable references for normal values and can facilitate communication with patients and among physicians regarding an individual's level of exercise capacity in relation to his or her peers. The figures corresponding to each of these equations, along with equations developed by other investigators, are presented in Chapter 5.

SUMMARY

The use of gas exchange techniques can greatly supplement exercise testing by adding precision and reproducibility as well as increasing the yield of information concerning cardiopulmonary function. Quantifying work from treadmill or cycle ergometer workload introduces a great deal of error and variability. In addition to some inherent variability in predicting oxygen uptake from external work, factors such as treadmill experience, the exercise protocol, and the presence of heart disease contribute further to the inaccuracy associated with predicting exercise capacity. These limitations in quantifying work in terms of exercise time or workload make gas exchange techniques essential when using exercise as an efficacy parameter in research protocols.

Maximal oxygen uptake is considered the best index of aerobic capacity and maximal cardiorespiratory function. By defining the limits of the cardiopulmonary system, maximal oxygen uptake has been an invaluable measurement clinically for assessing the efficacy of drugs, exercise training, or invasive procedures. No other measurement of work is as accurate, reliable, or reproducible.

Oxygen uptake is quantified by measuring the volume of expired ventilation and determining the difference in the oxygen content of inspired and expired air. Hemodynamically, oxygen uptake is equal to the product of cardiac output and arteriovenous oxygen difference. Historically, the maximal cardiopulmonary limits are considered to have been reached when oxygen uptake does not increase further with an increase in work (that is, when it plateaus). However, the many criteria and definitions used to describe this point and the differences that exist in data sampling limit its utility. Determining what a given patient's maximal oxygen uptake is relative to "normal" can be imprecise, because this determination is dependent not only on age and gender, but also on many clinical and demographic variables. An effort should be made to apply the most population-specific reference equation.

In addition to the measurement of oxygen uptake, the use of gas exchange techniques can provide additional information concerning cardiopulmonary function during exercise. Various methods of expressing the efficiency of ventilation, breathing patterns, physiologic dead space, and oxygen kinetics can be useful in characterizing the presence and extent of certain heart and lung diseases and in gauging their responses to therapy. A great deal of data has been published in the last 15 years documenting the prognostic utility of gas exchange techniques in patients with CHF. The additional accuracy and information provided by this technology must be balanced against potential increases in cost, time, and inconvenience to the patient. In addition, the quality of the test is dependent upon some basic skills required of the technician, who must properly calibrate the system and perform the test, and the physician, who must interpret the test. Consequently, the decision to employ gas exchange techniques should be based on the purpose of the test and the personnel available to perform the test.

REFERENCES

1. Sullivan M, Genter F, Savvides M, et al: The reproducibility of hemodynamic, electrocardiographic, and gas exchange data during treadmill exercise in patients with stable angina pectoris. Chest 1984;86:375-381.
2. Russell SD, McNeer FR, Beere PA, et al: Improvement in the efficiency of walking: An explanation for the "placebo effect" seen during repeated exercise testing of patients with heart failure. Am Heart J 1998;135:107-114.
3. Hansen JE, Sun XG, Yasunobu Y, et al: Reproducibility of cardiopulmonary exercise measurements in patients with pulmonary arterial hypertension. Chest 2004;126:816-824.
4. Myers J, Froelicher VF: Optimizing the exercise test for pharmacological studies in patients with angina pectoris. In Ardissino D, Opie LH, Savonitto S (eds): Drug Evaluation in Angina Pectoris. Norwell, Mass, Kluwer Academic Publishers, 1994, pp 41-52.
5. Myers J, Gullestad L: The role of exercise testing and gas exchange techniques in the prognostic assessment of patients with chronic heart failure. Curr Opin Cardiol 1998;13:145-155.
6. Myers J, Gullestad L, Vagelos R, et al: Hemodynamic, and cardiopulmonary exercise test determinants of survival in patients referred for evaluation of heart failure. Ann Intern Med 1998;129:286-293.
7. Corra U, Mezzani A, Bosimini E, Giannuzzi P: Cardiopulmonary exercise testing and prognosis in chronic heart failure: A prognosticating algorithm for the individual patient. Chest 2004;126:942-950.
8. Sullivan M, McKirnan MD: Errors in predicting functional capacity for postmyocardial infarction patients using a modified Bruce protocol. Am Heart J 1984;107:486-491.
9. Roberts JM, Sullivan M, Froelicher VF, et al: Predicting oxygen uptake from treadmill testing in normal subjects and coronary artery disease patients. Am Heart J 1984;108:1454-1460.
10. Dominick KL, Gullette EC, Babyak MA, et al: Predicting peak oxygen uptake among older patients with chronic illness. J Cardiopulm Rehabil 1999;19:81-89.
11. Foster C, Crowe AJ, Daines E, et al: Predicting functional capacity during treadmill testing independent of exercise protocol. Med Sci Sports Exerc 1996;28:752-756.
12. Berry MJ, Brubaker PH, O'Toole ML, et al: Estimation of VO_2 in older individuals with osteoarthritis of the knee and cardiovascular disease. Med Sci Sports Exerc 1996;28:808-814.
13. Myers J, Buchanan N, Walsh D, et al: Comparison of the ramp versus standard exercise protocols. J Am Coll Cardiol 1991;17:1334-1342.
14. Brown H, Wasserman K, Whipp BJ: Effect of beta-adrenergic blockade during exercise on ventilation and gas exchange. J Appl Physiol 1976;41:886-892.
15. Reybrouck T, Amery A, Billiet L: Hemodynamic response to graded exercise after chronic beta-adrenergic blockade. J Appl Physiol 1977;42:133-138.
16. Haskell W, Savin W, Oldridge N, DeBusk R: Factors influencing estimated oxygen uptake during exercise testing soon after myocardial infarction. Am J Cardiol 1982;50:299-304.
17. Tamesis B, Steken A, Byers S, et al: Comparison of the asymptomatic cardiac ischemia pilot and modified asymptomatic cardiac ischemia pilot versus Bruce and Cornell Exercise Protocols. Am J Cardiol 1993;72:715-720.
18. Kaminsky LA, Whaley MH: Evaluation of a new standardized ramp protocol: The BSU/Bruce Ramp protocol. J Cardiopulm Rehabil 1998;18:438-444.
19. Starling MR, Moody M, Crawford MH, et al: Repeat treadmill exercise testing: Variability of results in patients with angina pectoris. Am Heart J 1984;107:298-303.
20. Elborn JS, Stanford CF, Nichols DP: Reproducibility of cardiopulmonary parameters during exercise in patients with chronic cardiac failure: The need for a preliminary test. Eur Heart J 1990;11:75-81.
21. Pinsky DJ, Ahern N, Wilson PB, et al: How many exercise tests are needed to minimize the placebo effect of serial exercise testing in patients with chronic heart failure? Circulation 1989;80(suppl II):II-426.
22. Myers J, Walsh D, Sullivan M, Froelicher VF: Effect of sampling on variability and plateau in oxygen uptake. J Appl Physiol 1990;68:404-410.
23. Johnson JS, Carlson JJ, Vanderlaan RL, Langholz DE: Effects of sampling interval on peak oxygen consumption in patients evaluated for heart transplantation. Chest 1998;113:816-819.
24. Ehsani AA, Hagberg JM, Hickson RC: Rapid changes in left ventricular dimensions and mass in response to physical conditioning and deconditioning. Am J Cardiol 1978;42:52-56.
25. Saltin B, Blomqvist G, Mitchell JH, et al: Response to exercise after bed rest and after training. Circulation 1968; 36(suppl 7):VII1-78.
26. Blomqvist CG, Saltin B: Cardiovascular adaptations to physical training. Annu Rev Physiol 1983;45:169-189.

27. Dubach P, Myers J, Dziekan G, et al: Effect of exercise training on myocardial remodeling in patients with reduced left ventricular function after myocardial infarction. Application of magnetic resonance imaging. Circulation 1997;95:2060-2067.

28. Russell SD, Selaru P, Pyne DA, et al: Rational for use of an exercise end point and design for the ADVANCE (A Dose evaluation of a Vasopressin ANtagonist in CHF patients under going exercise) trial. Am Heart J 2003;145:179-186.

29. Chang JA, Froelicher VF: Clinical and exercise test markers of prognosis in patients with stable coronary artery disease. Curr Probl Cardiol 1994;19:533-587.

30. Morris CK, Ueshima K, Kawaguchi T, et al: The prognostic value of exercise capacity: A review of the literature. Am Heart J 1991;122: 1423-1431.

31. Myers J: Optimizing decision making in heart failure: Applications of cardiopulmonary exercise testing in risk stratification. Cardio-pulmonary Exercise Testing and Cardiovascular Health. Armonk, NY, Futura Publishing 2002, pp 103-118.

32. Mancini DM, Eisen H, Kussmaul W, et al: Value of peak exercise oxygen consumption for optimal timing of cardiac transplantation in ambulatory patients with heart failure. Circulation 1991;83:778-786.

33. Costanzo MR, Augustine S, Bourge R, et al: Selection and treatment of candidates for heart transplantation: A statement for health professionals from the Committee on Heart Failure and Cardiac Transplantation of the Council on Clinical Cardiology, American Heart Association. Circulation 1995;92:3593-3612.

34. Cohn JN, Johnson GR, Shabetai R, et al: Ejection fraction, peak exercise oxygen consumption, cardiothoracic ratio, ventricular arrhythmias, and plasma norepinephrine as determinants of prognosis in heart failure. Circulation 1993;87(suppl):VI5-16.

35. Myers J, Gullestad L, Vagelos R, et al: Cardiopulmonary exercise testing and prognosis in severe heart failure: 14 mL/kg/min revisited. Am Heart J 2000;139:78-84.

36. De Groote P, Millaire A, Decoulx E, et al: Kinetics of oxygen consumption during and after exercise in patients with dilated cardiomyopathy. J Am Coll Cardiol 1996;28:168-175.

37. Arena R, Myers J, Aslam S, et al: Peak VO_2 and VE/VCO_2 slope in patients with heart failure: A prognostic comparison. Am Heart J 2004;147:354-360.

38. Arena R, Myers J, Aslam SS, et al: Technical considerations related to the minute ventilation/carbon dioxide output slope in patients with heart failure. Chest 2003;124:720-727.

39. Bol E, de Vries WR, Mosterd WL, et al: Cardiopulmonary exercise parameters in relation to all-cause mortality in patients with chronic heart failure. Int J Cardiol 2000;72:255-263.

40. Corra U, Mezzani A, Bosimini E, et al: Ventilatory response to exercise improves risk stratification in patients with chronic heart failure and intermediate functional capacity. Am Heart J 2002;143: 418-426.

41. Francis DP, Shamim W, Davies LC, et al: Cardiopulmonary exercise testing for prognosis in chronic heart failure: Continuous and independent prognostic value from VE/VCO_2 slope and peak VO_2. Eur Heart J 2000;21:154-161.

42. Gitt A, Wasserman K, Kilkowski C, et al: Exercise anaerobic threshold and ventilatory efficiency identify heart failure patients for high risk of early death. Circulation 2002;106:3079-3084.

43. Kleber F, Vietzke G, Wernecke K, et al: Impairment of ventilatory efficiency in heart failure. Circulation 2000;101:2803-2809.

44. Baba R, Nagashima M, Goto M, et al: Oxygen uptake efficiency slope: A new index of cardiorespiratory functional reserve derived from the relation between oxygen uptake and minute ventilation during incremental exercise. J Am Coll Cardiol 1996;28:1567-1572.

45. Baba R, Tsuyuki K, Kimura Y, et al: Oxygen uptake efficiency slope as a useful measure of cardiorespiratory functional reserve in adult cardiac patient. Eur J Appl Physiol 1999;80:397-401.

46. Pardaens K, Van Cleemput J, Vanhaecke J, Fagard RH: Peak oxygen uptake better predicts outcome than submaximal respiratory data in heart transplant candidates. Circulation 2000;101:1152-1157.

47. Caiozzo VJ, Davis JA, Ellis JF, et al: A comparison of gas exchange indices used to detect the anaerobic threshold. J Appl Physiol 1982;53:1184-1189.

48. Hill AV, Lupton H: Muscular exercise, lactic acid, and the supply and utilization of oxygen. QJ Med 1923;16:135-171.

49. Wasserman K, McElroy MB: Detecting the threshold of anaerobic metabolism in cardiac patients during exercise. Am J Cardiol 1964;14:844-852.

50. Myers J, Ashley E: Dangerous curves: A perspective on exercise, lactate, and the anaerobic threshold. Chest 1997;111:787-795.

51. Noakes TD: Physiological models to understand exercise fatigue and the adaptations that predict or enhance athletic performance. Scand J Med Sci Sports 2000;10:123-145.

52. Gladden LB, Yates JW, Stremel RW, Stamford BA: Gas exchange and lactate anaerobic thresholds: Inter- and intra-evaluator agreement. J Appl Physiol 1985;58:2082-2089.

53. Yeh MP, Gardner RM, Adams TD, et al: "Anaerobic threshold": Problems of determination and validation. J Appl Physiol 1983;55: 1178-1186.

54. Shimizu M, Myers J, Buchanan N, et al: The ventilatory threshold: Method, protocol, and evaluator agreement. Am Heart J 1991;122: 509-516.

55. Connett RJ, Gayeski TEJ, Honig GR: Lactate accumulation in fully aerobic working dog gracilis muscle. Am J Physiol 1984;246: H120-H128.

56. Issekutz B, Shaw WAS, Issekutz AC: Lactate metabolism in resting and exercising dogs. J Appl Physiol 1976;40:312-319.

57. Stanley WC, Neese RA, Wisneski JA, Gertz EW: Lactate kinetics during submaximal exercise in humans: Studies with isotopic tracers. J Cardiopulm Rehabil 1988;9:331-340.

58. Brooks GA: Mammalian fuel utilization during sustained exercise. Comp Biochem Physiol B Biochem Mol Biol 1998;120: 89-107.

59. Hughson RL, Weisiger KH, Swanson GD: Blood lactate concentration increases as a continuous function during progressive exercise. J Appl Physiol 1987;62:1975-1981.

60. Myers J, Walsh D, Buchanan N, et al: Increase in blood lactate during ramp exercise: Comparison of continuous and threshold models. Med Sci Sports Exerc 1994;26:1413-1419.

61. Campbell ME, Hughson RL, Green HJ: Continuous increase in blood lactate concentration during different ramp exercise protocols. J Appl Physiol 1989;66:1104-1107.

62. Dennis SC, Noakes TD, Bosch AN: Ventilation and blood lactate increase exponentially during incremental exercise. J Sports Sci 1992;10:437-449.

63. Davis JA, Frank MH, Whipp BJ, Wasserman K: Anaerobic threshold alterations caused by endurance training in middle-aged men. J Appl Physiol 1979;46:1039-1046.

64. Ready AE, Quinney HA: Alterations in anaerobic threshold as the result of endurance training and detraining. Med Sci Sports Exerc 1982;14:292-296.

65. Tanaka K, Matsuura Y, Matsuyaka A, et al: A longitudinal assessment of anaerobic threshold and distance running performance. Med Sci Sports Exerc 1986;16:278-282.

66. Niess AM, Fehrenbach E, Strobel G, et al: Evaluation of stress responses to interval training at low and moderate altitudes. Med Sci Sports Exerc 2003;35:263-269.

67. Millet GP, Jaouen B, Borrani F, Candau R: Effects of concurrent endurance and strength training on running economy and VO(2) kinetics. Med Sci Sports Exerc 2002;34:1351-1359.

68. Sullivan MJ, Cobb FR: The anaerobic threshold in chronic heart failure. Relationship to blood lactate, ventilatory basis, reproducibility, and response to exercise training. Circulation 1990;81:1147-1158.

69. Matsumura N, Nishijima H, Kojima S, et al: Determination of anaerobic threshold for assessment of functional state in patients with chronic heart failure. Circulation 1983;68:360-367.

70. Weber KT, Kinasewitz GT, Janicki JS, Fishman AP: Oxygen utilization and ventilation during exercise in patients with chronic cardiac failure. Circulation 1982;65:1213-1223.

71. Myers J, Atwood JE, Sullivan M, et al: Perceived exertion and gas exchange after calcium and β-blockade in atrial fibrillation. J Appl Physiol 1987;63:97-104.

72. Sullivan M, Atwood AE, Myers J, et al: Increased exercise capacity after digoxin administration in patients with heart failure. J Am Coll Cardiol 1989;13:1138-1143.

73. Brubaker PH, Marburger CT, Morgan TM, et al: Exercise responses of elderly patients with diastolic versus systolic heart failure. Med Sci Sports Exerc 2003;35:1477-1485.

74. Guazzi M, Tumminello G, Matturri M, Guazzi MD: Insulin ameliorates exercise ventilatory efficiency and oxygen uptake in patients with heart failure-type 2 diabetes comorbidity. J Am Coll Cardiol 2003;42:1044-1055.

75. Auricchio A, Stellbrink C, Butter C, et al: Clinical efficacy of cardiac resynchronization therapy using left ventricular pacing in heart

failure patients stratified by severity ventricular conduction delay. J Am Coll Cardiol 2003;42:2109-2116.

76. Beaver WL, Wasserman K, Whipp BJ: A new method for detecting anaerobic threshold by gas exchange. J Appl Physiol 1986;60: 2020-2027.

77. Shimizu M, Myers J, Buchanan N, et al: The ventilatory threshold: Method, protocol, and evaluator agreement. Am Heart J 1991;122: 509-516.

78. Dickstein K, Barvik S, Aarsland T, et al: A comparison of methodologies in detection of the anaerobic threshold. Circulation 1990; 81(suppl II):38-46.

79. Hughes EF, Turner SC, Brooks GA: Effects of glycogen depletion and pedaling speed on "anaerobic threshold." J Appl Physiol 1982; 52:1598-1607.

80. Whipp BJ, Ward SA, Wasserman K: Respiratory markers of the anaerobic threshold. Adv Cardiol 1986;35:47-64.

81. Gaesser GA, Poole DC: Lactate and ventilatory threshold: Disparity in time course of adaptations to training. J Appl Physiol 1986; 61:999-1004.

82. Beaver WL, Wasserman K, Whipp BJ: Improved detection of lactate threshold during exercise using a log-log transformation. J Appl Physiol 1985;59:1936-1940.

83. Hughson RL: Alterations in the oxygen deficit-oxygen debt relationships with beta-adrenergic receptor blockade in man. J Physiol (Lond) 1984;349:375-387.

84. Petersen ES, Whipp BJ, David JA, et al: Effects of β-adrenergic blockade on ventilation and gas exchange during exercise in humans. J Appl Physiol 1983;54:1306-1313.

85. Twentyman OP, Disley A, Gribbin HR, et al: Effect of β-adrenergic blockade on respiratory and metabolic responses to exercise. J Appl Physiol 1981;51:788-792.

86. Linnarsson D: Dynamics of pulmonary gas exchange and heart rate changes at start and end of exercise. Acta Physiol Scand 1974;415:1-68.

87. Linnarsson D, Karlsson J, Fagraeus L, Saltin B: Muscle metabolites and oxygen deficit with exercise in hypoxia. J Appl Physiol 1974;36:399-402.

88. Peltonen JE, Tikkanen HO, Ritola JJ, et al: Oxygen uptake response during maximal cycling in hyperoxia, normoxia and hypoxia. Aviat Space Environ Med 2001;72:904-911.

89. Sietsema KE, Daly JA, Wasserman K: Early dynamics of O_2 uptake and heart rate as affected exercise work rate. J Appl Physiol 1989;67:2535-2541.

90. Hickson RC, Bomze HA, Holloszy JO: Faster adjustment of O_2 uptake to the energy requirement of exercise in the trained state. J Appl Physiol 1978;44:877-881.

91. Caputo F, Denadai BS: Effects of aerobic endurance training status and specificity on oxygen uptake kinetics during maximal exercise. Eur J Appl Physiol 2004;93:87-95.

92. Millet GP, Libiez S, Borrani F, et al: Effects of increased intensity of intermittent training in runners with differing VO_2 kinetics. Eur J Appl Physiol 2003;90:50-57.

93. Sietsema K: Analysis of gas exchange dynamics in patients with cardiovascular disease. In Wasserman K (ed.): Exercise Gas Exchange in Heart Disease. Armonk, NY, Futura Publishing, 1996, pp 71-81.

94. Toyofuku M, Takaki H, Sugimachi M, et al: Reduced oxygen uptake increase to work rate increment (Delta VO2/Delta WR) is predictable by VO2 response to constant work rate exercise in patients with chronic heart failure. Eur J Appl Physiol 2003;90:76-82.

95. Rickli H, Kiowski W, Brehm M, et al: Combining low-intensity and maximal exercise test results improves prognostic prediction in chronic heart failure. J Am Coll Cardiol 2003;42:116-122.

96. Taylor HL, Buskirk E, Heuschel A: Maximal oxygen intake as an objective measurement of cardiorespiratory performance. J Appl Physiol 1955;8:73-80.

97. Pollock ML, Bohannon RL, Cooper KH, et al: A comparative analysis of four protocols for maximal treadmill stress testing. Am Heart J 1976;92:39-46.

98. Froelicher VF, Brammell H, Davis G, et al: A comparison of the reproducibility and physiologic response to three maximal treadmill exercise protocols. Chest 1974;65:512-517.

99. Myers J, Walsh D, Buchanan N, Froelicher VF: Can maximal cardiopulmonary capacity be recognized by a plateau in oxygen uptake? Chest 1989;96:1312-1316.

100. Katch VL, Sady SS, Freedson P: Biological variability in maximum aerobic power. Med Sci Sports Exerc 1982;14:21-25.

101. Noakes TD: Implications of exercise testing for prediction of athletic performance: A contemporary perspective. Med Sci Sports Exerc 1988;20:319-330.

102. Duncan GE, Howley ET, Johnson BN: Applicability of VO2max criteria: Discontinuous versus continuous protocols. Med Sci Sports Exerc 1997;29:273-278.

103. Noakes TD: Maximal oxygen uptake: "Classical" versus "contemporary" viewpoints: A rebuttal. Med Sci Sports Exerc 1998; 30:1381-1398.

104. Jones NL: Clinical Exercise Testing. Philadelphia, WB Saunders, 1997, pp 243-247.

105. Wasserman K, Hansen JE, Sue DY, Whipp BJ: Principles of Exercise Testing and Interpretation. Baltimore, Lippincott, Williams & Wilkins 1999, pp 143-162.

106. Hansen JE, Sue DY, Wasserman K: Predicted values for clinical exercise testing. Am Rev Respir Dis 1984;129(suppl): 549-555.

107. Bruce RA, Kusumi F, Hosmer D: Maximal oxygen uptake and nomographic assessment of functional aerobic impairment in cardiovascular disease. Am Heart J 1973;85:546-562.

108. Shephard RJ: Endurance Fitness. Toronto, University of Toronto Press, 1969.

109. Astrand P: Human physical fitness, with special reference to sex and age. Physiol Rev 1956;36(suppl 2):307-335.

110. Astrand I: Aerobic work capacity in men and women with special reference to age. Acta Physiol Scand 1960;49(suppl 196):1-92.

111. Lange-Anderson K, Shephard RJ, Denolin H, et al: Fundamentals of exercise testing. Geneva, World Health Organization, 1971.

112. Jones NL, Markrides L, Hitchcock C, et al: Normal standards for an incremental progressive cycle ergometer test. Am Rev Respir Dis 1985;131:700-708.

113. Morris CK, Myers J, Kawaguchi T, et al: Nomogram based on metabolic equivalents and age for assessing aerobic exercise capacity in men. J Am Coll Cardiol 1993;22:175-182.

114. Astrand P-O. Experimental Studies of Physical Working Capacity in Relation to Sex and Age. Copenhagen, Muskgaard, 1952.

115. Cooper CM, Weiler-Ravell D: Gas exchange response to exercise in children. Am Rev Respir Dis 1984;129(suppl):547-548.

116. Myers J, Do D, Herbert W, et al: A nomogram to predict exercise capacity from a specific activity questionnaire and clinical data. Am J Cardiol 1994;73:591-596.

117. Kline GM, Porcari JP, Hintermeister R, et al: Estimation of VO2max from a one-mile track walk, gender, age, and body weight. Med Sci Sports Exerc 1987;19:253-259.

118. Myers J: Ventilatory gas exchange in heart failure: Techniques, problems, and pitfalls. In Balady GJ, Pina IL (eds): Exercise and Heart Failure. Armonk, NY, Futura Publishing, 1997, pp 221-242.

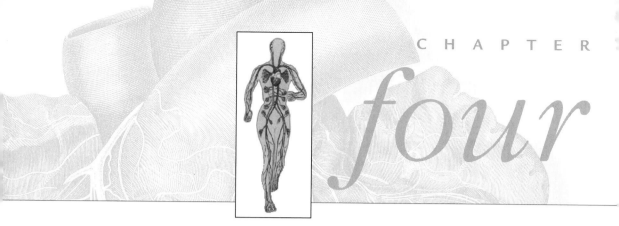

four

Special Methods: Computerized Exercise ECG Analysis

INTRODUCTION

While debate surrounds the role of Edmund Waller[1] in the invention of the electrocardiogram, ECG (he can claim precedence to the term in 1897[2]), Willem Einthoven[3] was certainly the first to document ST changes in the ECG with exercise. Einthoven made his observations in 1908, almost 90 years after Charles Babbage, the man scholars credit with the origination of computing, abandoned construction of his Difference Engine due to lack of funds.[4] In fact, progress towards mechanical calculation was slow until the turn of the century, when Lord Kelvin[5] built one of the earliest analog computers at the University of Glasgow, Scotland. Meanwhile, 6 years before Einthoven won a Nobel Prize for the "discovery of the mechanism of the electrocardiogram" (1924), Bousfield[6] associated ST-segment changes with myocardial ischemia. Four years later, Feil and Siegel[7] reported exercise induced ECG changes, but it was not until 1932 that Goldhammer and Scherf[8] proposed exercise ECG testing as a diagnostic tool for angina. In the intervening period, physicists had been gradually replacing mechanical calculators with electronic versions although it took a further 10 years before the first all-electronic digital computer was constructed by Alan Turing, considered by many to be the founder of modern digital computing.

The evolution of the microprocessor was critical to the success of the exercise ECG. Particularly important was the ability of computer processing to capture the large volume of raw data provided and present it in a format suitable for analysis either by clinician or computer. In addition, our best predictors of coronary artery disease (CAD) are multivariate equations derived only through computer processing of data stored in digital form. Finally, the ready availability of personal computers has allowed the development of "expert" systems, which can pool demographic and exercise test data, calculate risk scores, and prompt the noncardiologist with advice on appropriate management.

PRINCIPLES AND HISTORICAL ORIGINS

It is an observation pertinent to many biological tests that their ultimate aim is the reduction of an almost infinite data output into a small number of variables with significance for clinical decision-making. The first step in this process for the ECG is analog-to-digital conversion. The concept of analog-to-digital conversion has, in recent times, entered public commerce with the replacement of the audiocassette by the compact disc. The "natural" form of an electrical signal is analog, that is, a continuous signal varying in amplitude with time. However, computers deal with discrete not continuous data and to facilitate storage and analysis, conversion is required. Converting the analog signal into digital form requires periodic sampling at fixed time intervals with conversion of the amplitude at any given point in time into a binary number. The closeness of the converted signal to the original is governed by three factors. The *resolution* of the measurement is governed primarily by the number of bits per byte (see Glossary in this chapter). This can be thought of as the number of "gradations" on the "ruler". The *sampling frequency* is simply the number of measurements per second, expressed in Hertz. Finally, the *size of the input voltage window* must be large enough to accommodate the largest possible range of signal amplitudes. It is apparent that within the confines of the minimum acceptable analog voltage window, the greater the number of bits and higher the sampling frequency, the more true to the analog signal the digital representation will be.

The development of analog-to-digital converters was critical to the progression of clinical electrocardiography. In fact, a digital computer was first used for ECG analysis in 1957 by Pipberger et al.[10] This was one of the first practical applications for computers in medicine. Hardware for analog-to-digital conversion was limited and thus a special purpose system for the ECG had to be developed. These authors outlined some advantages of the digital system, including more precise and accurate measurements, less distortion, rapid mathematical manipulation, and no degradation with repetitive playback or long-distance transmission. With these advantages, applications were soon developed and in 1959, a system for separating normal and abnormal ECGs came into use.[10] By 1961, the first program capable of ECG wave recognition was available.[11] These systems analyzed data from three orthogonal ECG leads (Frank XYZ), and it was not until later that the first system capable of analyzing 12-lead ECG data was produced.[12] Since 1962, a large number of programs have been written making use of increasingly sophisticated analysis techniques and exponential increases in computing power.

As the ability to convert analog signals to digital was critical to the progression of clinical electrocardiography, the exercise ECG benefited from this technology. Three critical problems were solved by computer processing: data volume, electrical noise, and movement artifact. The major advantages of computerization of exercise testing are summarized in Table 4-1.

PROBLEMS SOLVED BY COMPUTERIZATION

Data Reduction

Since the total period of an exercise test can exceed 30 minutes, and many physicians want to analyze all 12 leads during and after testing, the resulting quantity of ECG data and measurements can quickly be substantial. One approach to data reduction is to use the three-lead vectorcardiogram (based on the Frank XYZ lead system), which makes use of signals from only three leads to construct a three-dimensional electrical image of the heart. This has been shown to be equivalent to the 12-lead system[13] and although each can be calculated from the other, clinicians favor the l2-lead version. From the point of view of the cardiologist, data volume can be reduced by the process of waveform averaging (discussed later), which allows "snapshot" average summary reports and measurement plots. Computerization can further reduce the raw data by a variety of compression techniques similar to the Hoffman encoding. One simple method of compression involves concentrating on bit *changes* in amplitude only. For example, the series 4,4,4,4,4,5,5, 5,5,8 can be stored as $4^{\times5}$, $5^{\times4}$, 8.

Noise Reduction

Noise is defined as any electrical signal that distorts or is foreign to the waveform of interest. It can be caused by any combination of line-frequency interference, skeletal muscle activation, respiration, or skin contact as summarized in Table 4-2.

TABLE 4–1. Advantages of digital versus analog data processing

More precise and more accurate measurements
Less distortion in recording
Direct accessibility to digital computer analysis and storage techniques
Rapid mathematical manipulation (for averaging and filtering)
Avoidance of the drift inherent in analog components
Digital algorithm control permitting changing analysis schema with software rather than hardware changes
No degradation with repetitive playback or long distance transmission
Data output advantages include higher plotting resolution and facile repetitive manipulation

TABLE 4-2.	**Causes of noise**

Line-frequency (60 [power line AC frequency in the US]
  or 50 Hz [Europe]))
Muscle
Respiration
Skin contact
Electrical continuity artifact

High-frequency Noise

Activation of skeletal muscle groups and movement of skin or electrodes produces noise which is usually of high frequency and overlaps with that of the ECG. The latter is associated with changes in contact resistance. The effects of both of these high-frequency noise sources can be reduced by signal averaging.

Low-frequency Noise

Contact noise appears as low-frequency noise or sometimes as step discontinuity baseline drift. It can be caused either by poor skin preparation resulting in high skin impedance, or through disruption of the electrode gel. It is reduced by meticulous skin preparation and rejection of beats that show significant baseline drift. Using the median rather than the mean for signal averaging can also reduce this.

Line-frequency Noise

Line-frequency noise is generated by interference of the 50- or 60-Hz electrical energy that powers most ECG machines and every electrical device (including fluorescent lights) in the environment of the ECG. Shielding the device and patient cables with grounded metal materials can reduce this, but persistent noise may need to be removed by a 50- or 60-Hz notch filter. Applied in series with the ECG amplifier, a notch filter removes only the line frequency, that is, it attenuates all frequencies in a narrow band around 50 or 60 Hz. An example of 60-Hz noise and its removal by a notch filter is given in Figure 4-1.

Baseline Wander

Respiration causes an undulation of the waveform amplitude and the baseline varies with the respiratory cycle. Baseline wander can be reduced by low-frequency filtering. Since the clinically relevant portion of the ECG power spectrum has most of its energy at frequencies above those of the

baseline drift, this simple technique can work fairly well and is still popular. However, low-frequency filtering results in distortion of the ST segment and can cause artifactual ST-segment depression and slope changes. Other baseline removal approaches have been used, including linear interpolation between isoelectric regions, high-order polynomial estimates, and cubic-spline techniques, which can each smooth the baseline to various degrees (Fig. 4-2). In the case of the cubic-spline, the fundamental limit is the lack of sufficient baseline estimation points to unambiguously specify the form of baseline wander.

Methods of Noise Reduction

Filters

Several different electronic filters have been developed by the industry to accomplish the task of noise reduction in the ECG. One example is the source consistency filter which reduces ECG noise without reducing bandwidth by enforcing a measured spatial consistency between recording electrodes. The linear phase, high-pass filter has a cut-off frequency lower than heart rate for baseline wander and a time-varying filter employing a combination of linear and nonlinear techniques for muscle artifact. The most powerful method of reducing noise, known as "signal averaging", has the disadvantage of removing beat-to-beat differences.

Signal Averaging

Signal averaging can be applied to any discrete, regularly repeating pattern embedded within a more complex one in order to eliminate extraneous information. There are several components to this process requiring the use of a number of processes starting with locating the QRS complex and then applying mathematical processes.

Several methods are available for the detection of the QRS complex. It is possible simply to use a threshold amplitude or rate-of-voltage-change of a low-pass and high-pass, filtered signal (this is normally the case with single-lead detection). However, a common technique, when data from more leads are available, is first to apply a transformation function, in order to generate a derived waveform more suitable for analysis and measurement. One of the most common transformation functions is the Absolute Spatial Vector Velocity

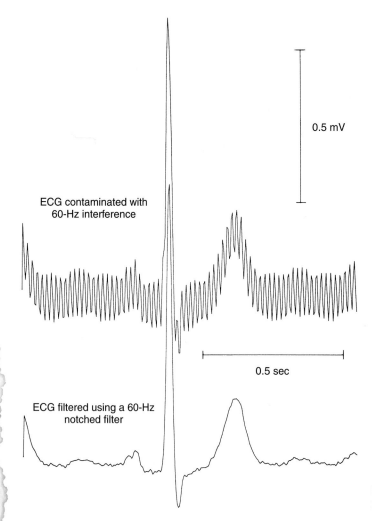

0.5 mV

ECG contaminated with
60-Hz interference

0.5 sec

ECG filtered using a 60-Hz
notched filter

▒ FIGURE 4–1
Example of the effect of a 60-Hz notched filter.

(ASVV), normally calculated from three orthogonal leads (Fig. 4-3). Using three perpendicular and statistically independent leads maximizes the yield of electrical information, improving the validity of the subsequent transformation. The ASVV is calculated from the formula[14]:

$$ASVV = \left[(\Delta X / \Delta t)^2 + (\Delta Y / \Delta t)^2 + (\Delta Z / \Delta t)^2 \right]^{\frac{1}{2}}$$

where ΔX, ΔY, and ΔZ are the changes in amplitude of leads X, Y, and Z during the time interval Δt. This produces the detection function $d(i)$ which can be expressed in the following form:

$$d(i) = \sum_k \left| X_k(i + 1) - X_k(i - 1) \right|$$

The derived waveform accentuates the directional properties of the electrical signal; it does not disturb the ECG data itself. This effect is an improvement in the detection of onsets and offsets of the major ECG waveform components, which can then be related back to the unfiltered ECG signals from individual, simultaneously recorded leads.

Some workers discovered empirically that a greater immunity to noise is preserved by separately filtering the slope calculations from each of the orthogonal leads prior to the nonlinear operation of taking the absolute value of this sum. This can be demonstrated by contrasting the results of the computationally faster method of first summing the absolute slopes and then filtering only the sums (i.e., the ASVV curve itself). In order to reduce the computational requirements of this multiple-lead-filtering operation, the filter can be redesigned into a prefilter/equalizer form. The prefilter is a simple moving average (recursive running sum), which does much of the stopband attenuation (see Glossary in this chapter) at an insignificant cost in processing time.

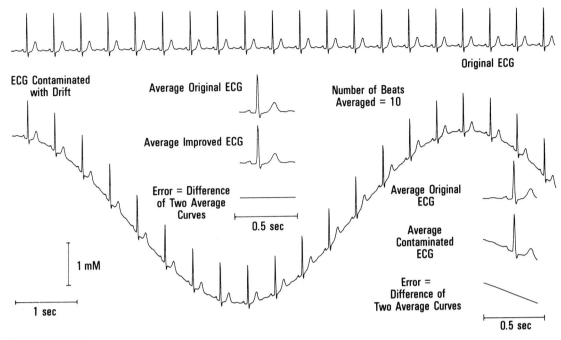

■ FIGURE 4–2

Example of the effect of a cubic spline filter on baseline wander.

The equalizer is a standard filter designed to improve the passband and stopband performance where needed. This optimization results in the same filter performance while using only 60% of the coefficients required for the more conventional approach.

The primary function of the ASVV waveform is to allow identification of components of the ECG; however, before the algorithms which achieve this are implemented, an intermediary process is required to exclude premature ventricular contractions, aberrances, and regions of excessive noise. Methods of accomplishing this vary from recognition of R-R interval duration and classification by multivariate cluster analysis to calculation of area differences, template comparison, and cross-correlation of complexes.

The source consistency filter is a patented filter that reduces ECG noise without reducing bandwidth by enforcing a measured spatial consistency between recording electrodes. No torso geometry or electrode placement assumptions are required.[15] Other filter approaches widely adapted by industry are the linear phase high-pass filter having a cut-off frequency lower than heart rate for baseline wander and a time-varying filter employing a combination of linear and nonlinear filtering techniques for removing muscle artifact.[16]

The American Heart Association and others have recommended that 16-bit resolution and 500 samples per second are minimal digitizing specifications for computer processing of an ECG. Higher sampling rates are needed for resolution of high-frequency components such as late potentials.

Averaging removes changes that occur from beat to beat such as T-wave alternans. Cambridge Heart, a Boston Company involved in innovative ECG technologies, has received a patent for an exercise system that uses special electrodes and software to detect this phenomenon.

Instead of simple mean beat averages, a technique of averaging was introduced for the early on-line systems that did not require as much computer power as averaging sequential windows of raw data. Called incremental averaging by the developer (David Mortara, PhD), it is a method well suited to a continuous input with slow changes. In this method of averaging, each digital sample of a new, time-aligned QRS complex is compared with its corresponding member in the current average. Alignment is accomplished using frequency components of the QRS complex. Wherever the average is low (or high), it is incremented (or decremented) by a small, fixed amount (3.5 μV) independent of the size

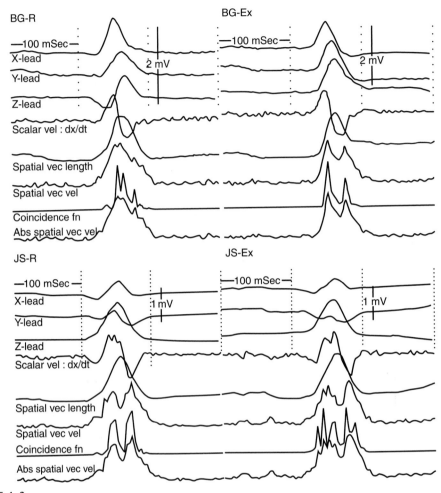

■ **FIGURE 4–3**
ASVV mathematical construct.

of the difference. ST-level and slope measurements can be displayed and recorded. These measurements are made from the average cycle, using the onset and offset of QRS determined during initialization. ST-slope measurements were made to correlate with visual impressions by dynamically adjusting the ST-slope interval with heart rate. The ST interval for slope measurement was one eighth of the average RR interval. The incremental average was a major breakthrough, almost simulating how the human reader learns from previous complexes what to look for even with noise present. In addition, it was implemented when practical computer chips available to manufacturers did not have the power to on-line average the waveforms as was previously done off-line. Though there is some concern that the average may not follow changes quickly enough, this does not seem to be a problem in the clinical setting.

While beat averaging can effectively reduce most of the sources of noise, two types of artifact that can actually be caused by the signal averaging process are due to:

- Introduction of beats that are morphologically different than others in the average and
- Misalignment of beats during averaging (exemplified in Fig. 4–4).

As the number of beats included in the average increases, the level of noise reduction is greater. ECG waveforms change in morphology over time; however, consequently, the time over which averaging takes place and the number of beats included in the average has to be compromised.

Waveform Recognition

Recognition algorithms identify waveform complexes and intervals in different ways, but three mechanisms are in common use. One involves identifying the peak of the R wave or the nadir of the S wave. Another identifies the onset or offset of a complex by using time derivatives from a single lead such as V_5. A third method demarcates the beginning and end of the QRS complex using a variety of mathematical constructs, such as change in spatial velocity. Whichever method is used, accurate labeling is vital to all time-dependent (horizontal axis) measurements. The vertical axis is calibrated with reference to an isoelectric baseline located within the PR segment, which can be identified by using a fixed interval before the Q or R wave, or by algorithms that search for a flat region.

Waveform Alignment

A process critical to signal averaging is the time-alignment of serial beats. This can only be achieved accurately with reference to a recognizable feature or point in each complex. This point is known as the fiducial point. An obvious candidate for such a point is the peak of the R wave; however, it was found that because of rapid amplitude changes at each peak, different peak regions could be sampled during digitizing, resulting in misalignment of complexes. A better option turns out to be the point of most rapid change in ECG amplitude (dx/dt), which usually occurs in the downslope of the R wave or in upslope of QS. This point can be consistently found and, particularly for one-lead analysis, works reliably and efficiently. The process of alignment is further refined by cross-correlation of 200 msec regions of the ASVV curve containing the candidate QRS complexes. Correlations are computed for alignments at every point from −20 to +20 msec of each initial point considered. The point at which the maximum correlation is achieved is considered to be the final alignment fiducial for the complexes being correlated (a minimum correlation coefficient of + 0.90 is set for a beat to be included). This method is more accurate than threshold-selected alignment and lends increased immunity to noise. A short burst of noise in a critical spot (e.g., near the temporary alignment point selected earlier) may cause the alignment point to be missed, since thresholds use properties of the signal which are local to only a few points. Cross-correlation, on the other hand, uses

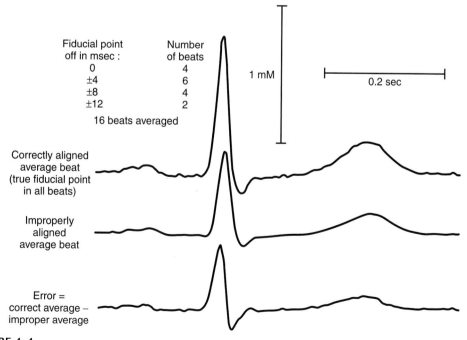

■ FIGURE 4–4

Example of the effect of misalignment of QRS complexes on the resultant averaged waveform.

properties of the signal which are distributed over the entire range being correlated, making it more robust.

EVALUATION OF COMPUTER ALGORITHMS

An Italian group evaluated the accuracy of a microcomputer-based exercise test system comparing the ST computer output with the measurements obtained by two experienced cardiologists.[17] Six hundred ECG strips were randomly selected from the exercise test recordings of 60 patients. The ST shift (at J + 80 msec) was blindly assessed by two observers (with the aid of a calibrated lens) and compared with computer measurements. Correlation coefficients, linear regression equations, percent of discrepant measurements, and 95% confidence limits of the mean error were calculated for all leads. The computer did not analyze five samples from a total of 600 (0.8%) ECG strip recordings because of excessive noise or signal loss, while 51 (9%) were considered unreadable by both observers and 67 (11%) were rejected by at least one observer. Correlation between the measurements taken by computer and observer(s) measurements was statistically significant, no systematic measurement bias was found, and the mean difference was lower than human eye resolution. They concluded that their computer algorithms provided results as good as those provided by trained cardiologists in measuring ST changes occurring during exercise test. However, this study did not evaluate whether computer improvement of the signal-to-noise ratio (SNR) would allow accurate measurements even on cardiologists' uninterpretable ECG. Only a dedicated exercise test database, in which different patterns of noise are superimposed on noise-free recordings previously annotated for ST level, could assess this potential advantage of computer-assisted analysis.

COMPUTER-DERIVED CRITERIA FOR ISCHEMIA

A number of investigators have proposed various computer-derived criteria for detecting ischemia during exercise testing. Some of these are shown in Figure 4-5 and Table 4-3.

In 1965, Blomqvist[18] reported a computerized quantitative study of the Frank vector leads. He divided the PR, QRS, and ST-T segments into eight subsegments of equal duration (i.e., time-normalized). He found that the maximal information for differentiation of patients with angina pectoris from normal subjects was obtained by measuring the ST amplitude at the time-normalized midpoint (ST4) of the ST-T segment.

In 1969, Hornsten and Bruce[19] reported using a computer of average transients to analyze exercise ECG data gathered from bipolar lead CB5 (similar in configuration and amplitude to V_5). They reported that in apparently healthy middle-aged men, ST-segment depression with exercise was found to be more prevalent and of greater magnitude than anticipated. They concluded that a single bipolar precordial lead appeared to be as reliable as the three-dimensional Frank lead system.

McHenry et al[20] (at USAFSAM) reported results with a computerized exercise ECG system developed at USAFSAM and later applied at the University of Indiana. ST-segment amplitude was measured over the 10-msec interval of the ST segment, starting at 60 msec after the peak of the R wave. The slope of the ST segment was measured from 70 to 110 msec beyond the R-wave peak. The PQ, or isoelectric, interval was found by scanning before the R wave for the 10-msec interval with the least slope (rate of change). If the ST-segment depression was 1.0 mm or greater and if the sum of ST-segment depression in millimeters and ST slope in millivolts per second equaled or was less than 1.0 during or immediately after exercise, the response was defined as abnormal. By comparing two groups of subjects, one with angina pectoris and the other consisting of age-matched clinically normal people, this measurement, called the ST index, was developed. This evaluation broke the rule of "no limited challenge" and so it was not surprising that when the integral was applied in clinical practice, it did not outperform standard criteria.

Some investigators have expressed the magnitude of the ST-segment deviation from the baseline in terms of the ST area or integral. Sheffield et al[21] measured the area from the end of the QRS to either the beginning of the T wave or to where the ST segment first crossed the isoelectric baseline. In this study, normal subjects demonstrated a modest increase in ST integral with increasing heart rate, with the mean integral at maximal heart rate being −4.3 μV (for a reference comparison, 25 mm/sec paper speed and gain of 1 cm equals 1 mV; a 1 mm block thus equals 4 μVsec. Patients with angina pectoris had a mean integral

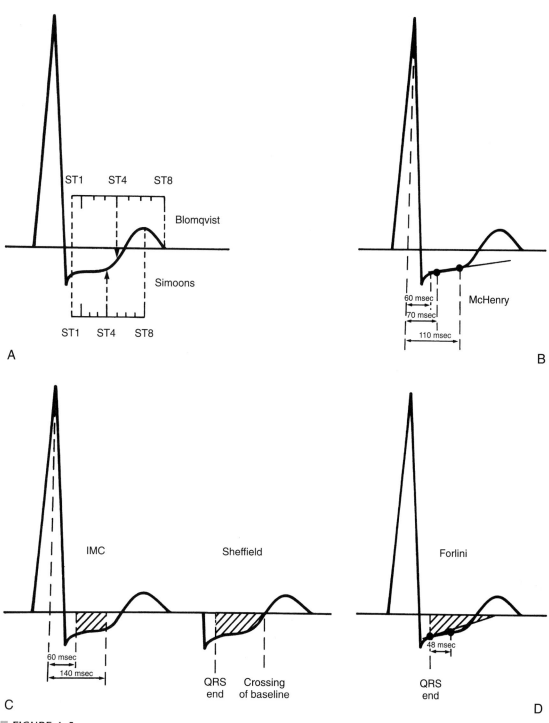

■ **FIGURE 4–5**
Illustration of some of the computer-derived criteria for myocardial ischemia.

TABLE 4–3. Some computer-derived criteria for diagnosing coronary artery disease (CAD)

Criterion	Description
ST depression	ST depression is the deviation of the ST segment from the PQ (isoelectric) interval. Measurements are usually made at 0 (ST_0-junction point) or 60 msec (ST_{60}) after QRS. Standard visual criteria consider 0.1 mV of ST_0 depression with horizontal or downsloping as abnormal.
ST slope	ST slope is the change in ST depression during the ST-T time interval (units are in millivolts per second). Slope measurements are generally made using ST amplitudes at two time points.
ST integral	ST integral is the calculated area bounded by the isoelectric baseline and the ST segment (units are in microvolt-seconds). Sheffield et al originally described measuring the ST integral from the end of the QRS complex to the beginning of the T wave or where the ST segment crosses the isoelectric line.
ST index	ST index, as implemented by McHenry, is the sum of abnormal ST-segment depression in millimeters and of ST slope in millivolts per second. Ascoop used a linear combination of ST slope and ST depression.
ST/HR index	ST/HR index, as defined by Kligfield et al, is the division of the change in the ST-segment depression from baseline value to maximum exercise by the change in heart rate over the same time period (units are in microvolts per beat per minute).
ST/HR slope	ST/HR slope, as proposed by Elamin et al, consisted of plotting ST-segment depression against heart rate and finding the steepest slope of the resulting curve.
Treadmill exercise score (TES)	Hollenberg et al developed TES as an empirical multivariable score combining ECG and hemodynamic measurements. TES is derived by summing the areas of the time curves of the ST-segment amplitude and slope changes in the two leads (aV_F and V_5) corrected by R-wave height, divided by exercise duration (in minutes) and percent maximal predicted heart rate.
Discriminant function analysis	Discriminant function analysis is a multivariate approach that collectively considers clinical, hemodynamic, and exercise variables. The first portion of the analysis is a stepwise regression that ranks variables according to diagnostic value. The most diagnostic variables are then selected in an equation that functions as a score (discriminant) or a probability (logistic) for the presence of CAD.
ST depression with baseline adjustment	ST depression with baseline adjustment is the correction of the recorded ST-depression measurement for the amount of baseline ST depression.
ST depression with R wave adjustment	ST depression with R-wave adjustment is the division of the ST depression by the R-wave amplitude or the multiplication of the ST shift by R-wave amplitude divided into the population average R-wave amplitude to normalize.

of −15.3 µVsec and this occurred at significantly lower heart rates. They computed the time-voltage integral of the ST segment beginning at QRS end and continued until they crossed the isoelectric line or reached 80 msec after QRS end. This integral expresses the area of ST-segment deviation from the baseline. An ST integral greater than −10 µVsec was found to be an abnormal exercise ECG response, and the normal range was from 0 to −7.5 µVsec. By arbitrarily taking −7.5 µVsec as the cut-off range for normal subjects, Sheffield obtained a sensitivity of 81% and a specificity of 95% on 41 normal and 31 angina patients. This measurement has the advantage of "combining" slope and depression in one measurement. Using a cutpoint of −16 µVsec, the MRFIT

group found a sensitivity of 34% and specificity of 96%.[22]

Simoons et al[23] reported using a PDP-8E computer on-line to process the Frank orthogonal leads. The interactive computer system also controlled the exercise test that allowed the physician and technician to interact with the patient. A range of amplitudes for exercise heart rates was established by considering the response of the normal group to adjust for the normal ST-segment depression increase in proportion to heart rate. He obtained a sensitivity of 81% and a specificity of 93% using this new criterion. In comparison, previous computer criteria were not superior to this ST-amplitude measurement adjusted for heart rate.

Sketch et al[24] studied 107 patients referred for evaluation of chest pain, who had coronary angiography using a commercial system. Patients who had a previous myocardial infarction (MI) and who were on digitalis were excluded. Lead V_5 was continuously sampled at 500 samples per second, and 16 complexes were averaged sequentially. They measured the ST integral over an interval from 60 to 140 msec after the peak of the R wave and chose −6 μVsec as the cut-off point for normal subjects. This area measurement began at 60 msec after the peak of the R wave and extended for 80 msec. Postexercise areas were more specific, whereas areas measured during exercise were more sensitive.

In an attempt to test the diagnostic value of an isolated ST integral, Forlini et al[25] exercise-tested 133 subjects. In this study, there were 62 normal subjects, 29 patients with coronary disease and an abnormal visual exercise test (CAD-ST+) and 42 patients with CAD but with normal visual exercise tests (CAD-ST−). Using the isolated ST-integral measurement, Forlini et al found an overall sensitivity of 85% and a specificity of 90%. In group CAD-ST−, 79% of the patients were diagnosed as abnormal despite having normal or nondiagnostic exercise tests as determined by visual criteria.

In 1977, Ascoop et al[26] reported on the diagnostic performance of automatic analysis of the exercise ECG studied in 147 patients with coronary angiography. The computer-determined results were compared with visual analyses of the same recordings. Two bipolar thoracic leads were computer-processed at maximal exercise. A single, averaged beat was obtained and the onset and offset of the QRS complex were determined using a template method. The ST depressions at 10 and 50 msec after the QRS end, ST slope, and ST integral were measured. A group of patients with a mean age of 48 were divided into learning and testing set. Of the 87 patients in the learning set, 57 had abnormal coronary angiograms and 30 essentially had no coronary lesions. In the test population of 60 patients, 39 had significant coronary disease, while 21 had no angiographic disease. These researchers concluded that the bipolar leads were superior to vector leads and that the computer criteria performed better than visual analysis.

In 1979, Turner et al[27] reported their findings in 125 consecutive patients who had treadmill tests and coronary angiography. The Quinton model 740 computer analyzed V_5 and calculated ST index. Of the 125 patients studied, 38 had normal coronary arteries and the rest had significant disease. Unfortunately, their results were confounded by consideration of angina in the determination of abnormal results and a vague classification of "inadequate test."

A Dutch group evaluated a new exercise test score based on changes in Q, R, and S waves.[28] The study population did not include consecutive patients but consisted of 155 persons with 53 normals (group I) and 102 patients with documented CAD (group II). Another 20 patients (group III) with proven CAD and a positive exercise test by ST-segment criteria were studied for the influence of beta-blockade on the QRS score. For the QRS score, Q-, R-, and S-wave amplitudes, which could be recovered immediately, were subtracted from pretest values: delta Q, delta R, and delta S, respectively. The score was calculated by the formula: (delta R − delta Q − delta S) AVF + (delta R − delta Q − delta S) V_5. Using a cut-off point more than 5 as normal, the QRS score resulted in a sensitivity of 88%, a specificity of 85%, and a predictive accuracy of 87%. For ST-segment depression these values were 55%, 83%, and 65%, respectively. Applying Bayes' theorem, the combination of an abnormal QRS score and ST-segment depression resulted in the highest post-test risk for CAD and a normal QRS score without ST-segment depression in the lowest post-test risk. The QRS score and the maximal ST-segment depression changed significantly with beta-blockade.

Hollenberg et al[29] developed a treadmill score which graded the ST-segment response to exercise by combining the total of all changes in ST amplitude and slope measured during the entire exercise test and throughout recovery. This treadmill score was empirically derived by summing the areas of the time curves that describe the ST-segment amplitude and slope changes in two leads (AV_F and V_5). This summed area is then divided by the duration of exercise (in minutes) and the percent maximal predicted heart rate achieved during the exercise test. These area measurements were obtained using a Marquette CASE-I computerized exercise system. In their first study, 70 patients who had coronary angiography and 46 healthy volunteers were studied (a population with limited challenge). Using the treadmill exercise score (TES) shown below, sensitivity and specificity were 85% and 98%, respectively.

TES = J-point amplitude and ST-slope curve areas score/Duration of exercise × percent predicted max HR achieved

This score includes the following measures of severity: depth of J-point depression, slope, occurrence of depression in relation to heart rate, decreased heart rate response to exercise, and functional capacity. Subsequent refinements by this group included validation of adjusting the amplitude of ST depression by R-wave amplitude using a thallium ischemia score.[30] They then applied the modified TES to asymptomatic army officers with the usual results expected in a low-risk population.[31] Unfortunately other investigators could not reproduce or validate their results with their score.[32] The problem with the TES is that it is based on empirical choice of variables rather than using biostatistical techniques to choose variables that are significantly and independently associated with CAD.

ST/HR Slope

Though accomplished originally manually, this measurement is included with computer measurements because its measurement is more practical when performed by computer. In 1980, Elamin et al[33] reported results with a new exercise test criterion proposed to detect the presence and severity of CAD. In 206 patients with anginal pain and using recordings from the standard 12 plus a bipolar lead, the maximal rate of progression of ST-segment depression relative to increases in heart rate (maximal ST/HR ratio) was measured. Displacement of the ST segment was measured at 80 msec after the QRS end. Curves were constructed, relating values of the ST segment to heart rate during rest and exercise in each of the 13 leads. Rate of development of ST-segment depression with respect to increments in heart rate observed in any one lead was represented as the slope of a computed regression line. The ranges of maximal ST/HR slopes in the 38 patients with no disease, 49 with single-vessel, 75 with double-vessel, and 44 with triple-vessel disease were different from each other and there was no overlap; that is, perfect results. This procedure required 3 hours of analysis time per test by a skilled person and ramped exercise that resulted in a linear heart rate increase of 10 bpm per stage.

Thwaites et al[34] performed a study to determine whether the maximal ST/HR slope using a bicycle ergometer is better than the standard 12-lead analysis using a Bruce treadmill protocol. The maximal ST/HR slope was calculated in 81 patients and compared with the results of a standard 12-lead exercise test. In 21 patients (26%), the ST/HR slope could not be calculated. In 60 patients with ST/HR slope values, the extent of the CAD was predicted in 24 patients (40%). The sensitivity and specificity of the ST/HR slope compared to standard ST analyses was 91% versus 81% and 27% versus 64%, respectively.

Kligfield et al[35] from Cornell compared the exercise ECG with radionuclide ventriculography and coronary angiography in 35 patients with stable angina to assess the value of the ST/HR slope. An ST/HR slope of 6.0 or more identified three-vessel coronary disease with a sensitivity and specificity of 90%. The exercise ST/HR slope was directly, but weakly, related to the exercise ejection fraction. Poorer results were obtained when they enlarged their series, and they have demonstrated marked variability in the maximal slope measurement, particularly as affected by the rate of heart rate changes and the frequency with which the ST measurements are made. Quyyumi et al[36] assessed this criterion in 78 patients presenting with chest pain and found the maximum ST/HR slope had a sensitivity of 90%, but a specificity of only 40%, and was not useful in predicting the extent of coronary disease.

Sato et al[37] have reported applying the Leeds methods with the Bruce protocol and computerized ECG analysis. They selected 142 patients out of 1026 who had undergone coronary angiography and exercise testing and 402 low-risk normals without symptoms (limited challenge). For any disease, they used standard criteria of 1 mm if horizontal or downsloping and 1.5 mm at 80 msec post-J-junction if upsloping. For the ST/HR slope, AV_F and V_5 changes appeared to be combined, resulting in slope values twice as high as reported by other investigators. ST/HR slope could not be calculated for technical reasons in nearly 20% of their patients. They chose slope values of 7.5 and 16 μV/bpm as partition criteria for any and left main/three-vessel disease, respectively. Okin and Kligfield[38-40] from Cornell have reported increased discriminant power for the diagnosis of CAD.

ST/Heart Rate Index

Kligfield et al[41] from Cornell subsequently obtained similar results to that obtained with the ST/HR slope by simply dividing the change in the ST segment from baseline to maximum exercise by the change in heart rate over the same time period. This measurement has been called the ST/HR index and in Figure 4-6 it is compared

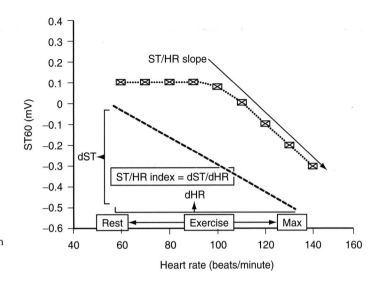

FIGURE 4-6

Comparison of the ST/HR slope and the ST/HR index. Note that ····⊠···· starts with early repolarization at rest while –––– starts at the isoelectric line.

to the ST/HR slope. The Cornell group excluded tests with upsloping ST segments from standard visual analysis; such results occurred in 17% of their patients. As is advisable from a biostatistical point of view and done in clinical practice, such tests should be considered borderline or normal. By excluding them, the Cornell group found the standard criteria of 1 mm to have a significantly poorer performance than the ST/HR index or slope. When we applied this measurement in our laboratory we could not repeat their results: the diagnostic characteristics of the ST measurements were not improved by dividing by heart rate.[42]

Meta-Analysis of ST/HR Studies

Differences in test performance between studies can be explained by population selection, particularly "limited challenge" and by methodological differences. Only half of the published studies have supported heart rate adjustment and most of these positive studies came from Leeds and Cornell.[43] Morise and Duvall[44] found no difference in test performance when comparing standard criteria and the heart rate index in an appropriate clinical population.

Concern must be directed to the populations that have been used to study this measurement from Cornell. Separating the most sick from the most well is not a fair evaluation; in fact, this is a biostatistical error called limited challenge. In addition, they included patients with prior MIs, normal subjects who did not present a diagnostic

problem, angina patients without catheterization, and some patients with confirmed angiographic disease. This mixture of patients explains why their receiver operating characteristic (ROC) curves have such large areas. It is inappropriate to use specificity from a group of normal subjects and sensitivity from an abnormal group to define test performance. They could argue that limited challenge is not a problem if you are just comparing criteria, but it is a problem if it causes other differences that affect one of the measurements and not the other. This happens when comparing ST/HR index to ST measurements. There is a difference in mean maximal heart rate between their three groups; that is, 165 bpm for the normal subjects versus 134 bpm for the angina patients versus 115 bpm for the catheterization-confirmed coronary disease patients. ROC curves based on heart rate alone have comparable areas to ST measurements. Inclusion of normal subjects exaggerates the performance of heart rate correction schemes because of the differences in maximum heart rate between normal subjects and diseased patients.[45,46]

ST Amplitude at ST60 or ST0?

The Cornell group[47] suggested that one of the reason for differing results[41] was the ST measurement point used. Whereas they used the ST amplitude at ST60 without considering slope, others made ST measurements at ST0, and then only when the ST segment was horizontal or downsloping. These results were obtained using visual measurements and a personal computer[48], similar to what Okin et al reported using a Quinton workstation. We performed a similar analysis to test this hypothesis by analyzing 202 patients with cardiac catheterization and exercise tests referred initially for evaluation of possible CAD but without a history or ECG evidence of a prior MI. They were tested using a modified Balke-Ware or ramp protocol resulting in nearly linear increases in heart rate. All were males, with a mean age of 60 years, 71 (35%) had no significant coronary disease and 60 (30%) had three-vessel or left main disease. We considered the actual ST/HR slope, summed depression in all leads, and chose the lead with the greatest depression for division by change in heart rate. The measurement point did not affect the ST-measurement characteristics when made without slope considerations. Measurements of exercise-induced ST-segment depression at either the J-junction or 60 msec after the J-junction, regardless of slope, were reliable markers for coronary disease. There was no significant difference between measurements made at the J-junction or 60 msec later, when only horizontal or downsloping ST-segment depression was considered as an abnormal response. Slope considerations significantly improve diagnostic accuracy when measurements are made at the J-junction, but not for measurements made 60 msec after J-junction.

ST60 or ST0 with or without Slope Being Considered

A uniform criterion for an abnormal exercise-induced ST-segment response that maximizes its diagnostic accuracy is essential, not only for obvious clinical reasons, but also to allow internal consistency in direct comparisons of the exercise response in different populations. Unfortunately, a single method of interpretation has never been uniformly accepted in clinical practice.[49] There have been proponents of patterns of ST-segment depression that include upsloping as an abnormal response,[50] and others believe that the consideration of horizontal or downsloping ST-segment depression significantly impacts the accuracy of exercise testing beneficially. Savvides et al[51] demonstrated little difference in the classification of patients between measurements made at the J-point and 70 msec later. A meta-analysis performed by Gianrossi et al[52] revealed that the consideration of slope had a significant impact on the accuracy of exercise testing, but a study by Stuart and Ellestad[50] suggests that upsloping ST-segment depression should still be considered

an abnormal response. Kurita et al[53] evaluated 230 patients referred for angiography and found that 60% (46/77) of patients with equal or greater than 1.5-mm junctional and upsloping ST-segment depression had significant coronary disease. Stuart and Ellestad[50] found that of 70 patients with upsloping ST-segment depression 40 (57%) had multivessel coronary disease.

The issue of whether the consideration of slope, in other words excluding upsloping as an abnormal response, significantly improves diagnostic accuracy is another question. Rijneke et al[54] studied 623 patients with bicycle exercise testing and coronary angiography. The criterion for an abnormal response was ST-segment depression of 0.1 mV or greater at ST60. There was no significant difference between measurements that included upsloping ST-segment depression as an abnormal response and measurements that only considered horizontal or downsloping ST-segment depression as abnormal. When quantitating the depth of horizontal or downsloping exercise-induced ST-segment depression, there was no significant difference between measurements made at the J-junction or 60 msec after the J-junction as markers for CAD. Slope considerations were a significant improvement in the identification of CAD when measurements were made at the J-junction, but not when made 60 msec after the J-junction. When using the computer-generated analysis of ST-segment depression measured at ST0 and slope, the cutpoint of 0.7 mm or greater of ST-segment depression had the best combination of sensitivity and specificity, not 1.0 mm or greater of ST-segment depression, which was the best cutpoint for visual interpretation of the exercise ECG. The computer can measure the ST segments more accurately than the human eye and when evaluating ST segments visually there is a "rounding-off" of values, for example, 0.7 mm of ST-segment depression is often rounded up to 1.0 mm visually. For ST60 and slope the cutpoint of 0.6 mm, for ST0 without slope considered the cutpoint of 1.4 mm, and for ST60 without slope considered the cutpoint of 0.9 mm of exercise-induced ST-segment depression yielded the highest predictive accuracy.

Which Leads Should be Analyzed by a Computer?

A Finnish group compared the diagnostic characteristics of the individual exercise ECG leads, three different lead sets comprising standard leads and the effect of the partition value in the detection of CAD.[55] ST-segment depression was considered at peak exercise in 101 patients with CAD and 100 patients with a low likelihood of the disease (limited challenge). The lead system used was the Mason-Likar modification of the standard 12-lead system and exercise performed on a bicycle. The comparisons were performed by means of ROC area under the curve and sensitivities at 95% specificity. Leads I, aV_R, V_4, V_5, and V_6 had the greatest diagnostic capacity while leads aV_L, aV_F, III, V_1, and V_2 were quite poor.

This same group compared the diagnostic performances of ST/HR hysteresis, ST/HR index, ST-segment depression 3 minutes after recovery from exercise, and ST-segment depression at peak exercise in a study population of 128 patients with angiographic CAD and 189 patients with a low likelihood of the disease.[56] ST/HR hysteresis, which integrates the ST/HR depression of the exercise and recovery phases, appeared to be relatively insensitive to the lead selection and exhibited relatively high area under the curves (invalidated by limited challenge, i.e., taking the most well and most sick, and not the intermediate group who present to the physician for diagnosis).

DIRECT COMPARISON OF COMPUTER CRITERIA

An extensive library and Medline search was conducted to find all exercise ECG research papers that compared multiple computerized criteria for diagnosing the presence of CAD. Most of the studies described previously considered only one criterion or compared only one criterion to visual analysis, and thus they were excluded. The search resulted in eight studies: Ascoop et al (1977),[26] Simoons and Hugenholtz (1977),[57,58] Detry et al (1985),[59] Deckers et al (1989),[60] Detrano et al (1987),[61,62] Pruvost et al (1987),[63] Froelicher et al[65] and Atwood et al.[66] The following computerized ECG criteria were investigated in these studies: ST depression, ST slope, ST integral, ST index, ST/HR index, ST/HR slope, Hollenberg's TES, and discriminant function analysis. Patient selection, exercise test type, and test methodologies were noted along with the results and conclusions of each study (Table 4-4).

Ascoop (the Netherlands)

In 1977, Ascoop et al[26] recorded ECG tracings from two bipolar thoracic leads (CM5, CC5) and compared the visual ECG readings to computerized measurements. One hundred forty seven males suspected of ischemic heart disease underwent a cycle ergometer exercise test. ST depressions (at 0, 10, and 50 msec after QRS), ST slopes over multiple intervals, and the ST integral were measured at maximal exercise. Ascoop et al divided their patient population into training and test groups. The computerized criteria yielded higher sensitivities than visual analysis. Visual analysis had sensitivities of 25% and 28% in the training and test groups, respectively, while computerized criteria generated sensitivities from 42% to 70% at comparable specificity. Furthermore, results using the CC5 lead were consistently better than those from the CM5 lead. Among the computerized criteria, the ST integral yielded the lowest sensitivity and specificity with 42% to 49% and 93% to 95%, respectively. The best separation was actually achieved using the criterion consisting of a linear combination of the ST_{10-50} slope (slope in the 10–50-msec interval) and ST_{10} depression in the CC5 lead. The sensitivities were 70% and 64% in the learning and testing group, respectively. Independent ST slope criteria resulted in sensitivities of 65% and 54%, while using ST depression alone yielded 56% and 67% sensitivities at similar specificities.

Simoons (Rotterdam)[64]

In 1977, Simoons[57] reported using a PDP-8E on-line computer to process the Frank orthogonal leads during a cycle ergometer exercise test. In their study, they analyzed the exercise ECGs of 95 male patients with CAD and 129 healthy normal males. Standard visual ECG readings were compared to the following computerized ECG measurements recorded at maximal heart rate: ST depression and slopes at fixed intervals after the end of QRS, negative ST area, ST index, polar coordinates, and Chebyshev waveform vectors. Using ECGs from a training group (86 normal subjects, 52 patients) and a test group (43 normal subjects, 43 patients), they observed that ST-depression measurements at fixed intervals after QRS were more diagnostic than the time-normalized ST amplitudes, the negative ST area, or the Chebyshev waveform vectors. ST slopes and the transformation to polar coordinates did not improve diagnostic performance. Simoons obtained their best results with HR-adjusted ST_{60} measurements in lead X (similar to V_5). They documented sensitivities of 81% and 70% in the training and test groups, respectively, with 93% specificity. Standard visual criteria had significantly lower results; 50% and 51% sensitivities at

TABLE 4–4. Summary of all available exercise ECG studies that compare multiple computerized criteria for diagnosing CAD

Investigator	Total no. of subjects	No. of healthy normals	No. patients (% with disease)	Criterion	Sensitivity (%)	Specificity (%)
Ascoop et al (1977)[26]	Training group: 87	0	87 (66%)	Combination of ST slope and depression	70	90
				ST slope	65	90
				ST_{50}	56	90
				ST integral	42	93
				Visual	25	100
	Test group: 60	0	60 (65%)	Combination of ST slope and depression	64	95
				ST_{50}	67	95
				ST slope	54	95
				ST integral	49	95
				Visual	28	100
Simoons (1977)[57,58]	Training group: 138	86	52 (100%)	ST_{60} adjusted for HR	81	93
				Discriminant function analysis	88	84
				ST integral	52	94
				Visual	50	94
	Test group: 86	43	43 (100%)	ST_{60} adjusted for HR	70	93
				Discriminant function analysis	79	79
				ST integral	51	95
				Visual	51	95
Detry et al (1985)[59]	387	103	284 (81%)	Discriminant function analysis	82	92
				ST_{60}	64	82
				ST slope	93	66
Detrano et al (1987)[61]	271	0	271 (45%)	Visual—ST_{80}	67	72
				Max ST/HR index in V_5 and aV_F	65	70
				Hollenberg's treadmill score	59	71
Pruvost et al (1987)[63]	558	0	558 (56%)	Discriminant function analysis	68	83
				ST depression	59	71

Study				Method	Sensitivity	Specificity
Deckers et al (1989)[60]	345	123	222 (53%)	Discriminant function of Detry	84	90
				ST_{80}/HR index	78	90
				HR adjusted	74	90
				ST amplitudes and slope		
				Hollenberg's treadmill score	67	90
QUEXTA (1998)[65]	814	0	411 (51%)	Visual	45	85
				ST/HR index and slope	49	85
				Hollenberg's treadmill score	35	85
Atwood et al (1998)[66]	1384	0	825 (60%)	ST integral	37	85
				Visual	52	80
				ST/HR index and slope	51	80
				Hollenberg's treadmill score	42	80

Note: Any of the studies above that included healthy or low-risk normals broke the "limited challenge" rule for evaluating a diagnostic test.

94% and 95% specificities in the training group and test group, respectively. Simoons also investigated linear discriminant function analysis, which exhibited only modest improvements.

Detry (Belgium)

Detry et al[59] used multivariate analysis for diagnosing CAD in a population of 284 symptomatic and 103 "healthy" men (unfortunately, this breaks the rule of "no limited challenge"). Computer-averaged ECG signals from the Frank leads were recorded at maximal exercise. Their multivariate analysis chose five variables in the discriminant function equation: heart rate, ST_{60} segment level, onset of angina during the test, workload, and the ST slope in lead X. ST_{60} alone had a sensitivity of 64% at an 82% specificity. ST slope was highly sensitive (93%) at a specificity of 66%. However, the multivariate approach outperformed both ST criteria with 82% sensitivity at a specificity of 92%. They asserted that by interpreting the exercise test response in a compartmental and probabilistic model, the diagnostic value of the exercise test was enhanced.

Detrano (Cleveland Clinic)

Detrano et al[61] compared visual analysis to both the Hollenberg TES and ST index. Treadmill tests and coronary angiography were performed on 271 patients (185 male, 86 female) suspected of having coronary heart disease. Patients were excluded if they had any of the following conditions: valvular disease or cardiomyopathy, unstable angina, serious arrhythmia, left bundle branch block, extreme obesity, and disorder affecting mobility. The following ECG-derived computer variables were calculated: ST depression in lead V_5 relative to rest, maximal ST index in V_5 and aV_F, and the area formula or TES developed by Hollenberg. Detrano et al observed that neither the TES nor ST index outperformed the visual analysis. Visual analysis yielded a sensitivity of 67% at a specificity of 72%, while maximal ST index and TES measurements yield sensitivities of 65% and 59%, respectively, at a similar specificity.

Pruvost (France)

In 1987, Pruvost et al[63] performed stepwise discriminant function analysis on 12 exercise variables on patients who underwent coronary angiography and a treadmill test. The multivariate analysis was compared to independent univariate analysis of ST-depression measurements. Twelve clinical and exercise parameters were ranked according to discriminant power. The top five variables (exercise duration, history of angina, angina during exercise, age, and maximal heart rate), using stepwise multivariate regression, had the most diagnostic value. Inclusion of the remaining seven variables in the discriminant function provided little enhancement. Pruvost found that multivariate analysis, with 68% sensitivity at a specificity of 83%, was more accurate than the visual ST-segment measurements (sensitivity 59%, specificity 76%). ST depression was not selected as an independent predictor of CAD in their multivariate analysis.

Deckers (Rotterdam)

Deckers et al[60] studied 345 men in 1989 for the diagnosis of CAD. None had a prior MI or were taking digoxin, but half were receiving beta-blockers. Two hundred twenty-two of the subjects had undergone catheterization for chest pain, while the other 123 were apparently healthy men (unfortunately representing a limited challenge population). Patients with at least one 50% occlusion were considered as having CAD; they used bicycle ergometry and recorded orthogonal Frank-lead ECG. The following variables were evaluated: ST-segment measurements adjusted for instantaneous heart rate, TES, the Detry Score, and the ST/HR index. The Detry discriminant function model and the ST/HR index functioned the best (i.e., sensitivity 70% to 80% at a specificity 90%) and were least influenced by beta-blocker therapy. The ST-segment measurements adjusted for instantaneous heart rate yielded results of 74% sensitivity at 90% specificity. They found the diagnostic value of the TES score to be low, but it was improved when the ST amplitude and slope time-areas were considered without adjustment for heart rate or time. Visual readings were not considered. These favorable results with HR-adjusted variables could be due to their failure to avoid limited challenge.

Quantitative Exercise Testing and Angiography (QUEXTA)

QUEXTA was performed to compare the diagnostic utility of scores, measurements, and equations with that of visual ST-segment measurements in patients with reduced workup bias.[65] Included were 814 consecutive male patients who presented with angina pectoris and agreed to undergo both exercise testing and coronary angiography. Digital ECG recorders and angiographic calipers were used for testing at each site, and test results were sent to core laboratories. Workup bias was reduced, as shown by comparison with a pilot study group. This reduction was responsible for a dramatically different sensitivity and specificity for the traditional criterion of 1-mm horizontal or downsloping ST depression than from meta-analysis of 150 studies that did not try to do so (i.e., 45% sensitivity/85% specificity). Computerized measurements and visual analysis had similar diagnostic power. Equations incorporating nonECG variables and either visual or computerized ST-segment measurement had similar discrimination and were superior to single ST-segment measurements. These equations correctly classified five more patients of every 100 tested (area under the curve of 0.80 for equations and 0.68 for visual analysis). Computerized ST-segment measurements were similar to visual ST-segment measurements made by cardiologists.

The VA-Hungarian Computer Measurement Comparison Study

We performed a study to compare computer-measured with visual exercise ECG measurements.[66] A retrospective analysis was accomplished on consecutive patients referred to two university-affiliated Veteran's Affairs Medical Centers and the Hungarian Heart Institute for evaluation of chest pain. Both patients underwent both exercise testing with digital recording of their exercise ECGs and coronary angiography. Patients with previous cardiac surgery, valvular heart disease, left bundle branch block, or Wolff-Parkinson-White syndrome on their resting ECG were excluded from the study. Prior cardiac surgery was the predominant reason for exclusion of patients who underwent exercise testing during this time period. There were 1384 consecutive male patients without a prior MI and with complete data who had undergone exercise tests between 1987 and 1997. Measurements included clinical, exercise test data and visual interpretation of the ECG recordings collected using a computer program, over 100 computed measurements

from the digitized ECG recordings, and compilation of angiographic data from clinical reports.

Computer Analysis

Microprocessor-based exercise ECG devices were used at three sites to simultaneously record all 12 ECG leads through exercise and recovery at 500 samples per second (Mortara Electronics, Milwaukee, Wis) on optical discs. Optical disc recordings were processed off-line using standard personal computers. Averaging of the raw data from three leads (II, V_2 and V_5) and determination of QRS onset and offset points were performed using software developed by Sunnyside Biomedical (Los Altos, Calif). The computer-chosen isoelectric line and QRS onset and offset points were confirmed visually for their accuracy. The following measurements and calculations were evaluated: (1) ST_0 (J-junction) and ST_{60} (60 msec after the J-junction) 2 minutes prior to maximal exercise, at maximal exercise, and at 1, 3.5, and 5 minutes of recovery; (2) ST slope, based on a least squares fit between ST_0 and ST_{60}, at the same times as the amplitude measurements; (3) ST integral; (4) ST index; (5) the sum of and the maximum ST depression in II, V_2, and V_5 at maximal exercise and 3.5 minutes of recovery; (6) ST_0 and ST_{60}/HR index and slope; (7) Hollenberg's TES (which includes time-amplitude plots for the three leads in exercise and recovery [six separate areas]); and (8) ST_{60} in V_5 during exercise at heart rates of 100 and 110 bpm. Several empirical composite adjustments were made in an attempt to simulate visual analysis by adjusting for baseline depression and using slope criteria changing with heart rate. R-wave amplitude was available at all of the time periods and results obtained adjusting the ST measurements by this amplitude are reported.

Population Characteristics

The mean age of this male population was 59 (±10) years. Age, presenting chest pain, hypercholesterolemia, diabetes, and abnormal resting ECG were significantly different between those with and without CAD. Table 4-5 lists all of the important clinical variables in the VA-Hungarian study.

Postexercise Test Hemodynamic, nonECG and visual ECG Results

Table 4-6 compares the exercise test data between those with and without any obstructive

TABLE 4-5. Clinical characteristics of population in VA-Hungarian study

Variables	No CAD N = 559	Any CAD N = 825 (60%)	p values
Age	55 ± 11	62 ± 9	<0.0001
Symptom status			
Typical angina	115 (21)	357 (43)	<0.0001
Atypical angina	351 (63)	360 (44)	<0.0001
Nonanginal chest pain	48 (9)	62 (8)	NS
No chest pain	45 (8)	46 (6)	NS
Chest pain score (1–4 [none])	2.0 ± 0.8	1.8 ± 0.8	<0.0001
Diabetes	61 (11)	142 (17)	0.001
Abnormal resting ECG	122 (22)	244 (30)	0.001
Resting ST depression (ST <0)	71 (13)	157 (19)	0.002
Hypercholesterolemia	162 (29)	343 (42)	<0.0001
Currently or ever smoked	374 (67)	543 (66)	NS
Body mass index (kg/m^2)	28 ± 5	28 ± 5	NS
Peripheral vascular disease	47 (8)	73 (9)	NS
Congestive heart failure	25 (5)	23 (3)	NS
Chronic obstructive pulmonary disease	34 (6)	55 (7)	NS
Family history of coronary artery disease	246 (44)	349 (42)	NS
Hypertension	271 (49)	454 (55)	0.02
Stroke	12 (2)	29 (3.5)	NS
Digoxin	21 (4)	24 (3)	NS
Beta-blocker	132 (24)	246 (30)	0.01

Note: Data are presented as mean ± standard deviation or number (percent) of subjects.
NS, nonsignificant.

angiographic coronary disease. The Duke treadmill angina score and all of the hemodynamic measurements were significantly different except for maximal systolic blood pressure.

ST Criteria Performance and Validation

The diagnostic performance of the ST variables that exhibited an average ROC area within the 95% confidence intervals associated with visual analysis when tested within five randomly selected one half population samples are tabulated in Table 4-7 and illustrated in Figure 4-7. The most

stable computerized ST measurements with the highest discriminating power are listed in Table 4-7. They included visual ST analysis, the sum of the depression at ST_{60} in II, V_5 and V_2, the maximum ST_{60} depression in these three leads, the time area in recovery of the slope and ST60 for V_5 (part of the Hollenberg score), HR index (ST_{60} or ST_0 V_5), and ST_{60} in V_5 at 3.5 minutes of recovery. Measurements made at 3.5 minutes of recovery and use of V_5 predominated compared to other leads or at other time points. Thus, only these seven measurements out of the 100 that were calculated by the exercise ECG analysis

TABLE 4-6. Exercise test results in VA-Hungarian study

Variables	No CAD N = 559	Any CAD N = 825 (60%)	p value
Maximal heart rate (bpm)	137 ± 24	125 ± 22	<0.0001
Delta heart rate (bpm)	56 ± 24	48 ± 20	<0.0001
Maximal SBP (mmHg)	170 ± 27	168 ± 30	NS
Delta SBP (mmHg)	46 ± 26	38 ± 31	<0.0001
Maximal double product (×1000)	23.5 ± 6.5	21.3 ± 6.1	<0.0001
Delta double product (×1000)	13.8 ± 6.2	11.4 ± 5.5	<0.0001
METs	8.5 ± 3.4	6.9 ± 3.8	<0.0001
Exercise angina score (0–2)	0.37 ± 0.60	0.69 ± 0.77	<0.0001
Abnormal ST depression	115 (21%)	426 (52%)	<0.0001

Note: Data are presented as mean ± standard deviation or number (percent) of subjects.

TABLE 4–7. The diagnostic characteristics of the computerized ST measurements with results comparable to visual analysis with sensitivity at a cut point associated with a specificity matching 1-mm visual analysis (80%) in the VA-Hungarian study

ST measurement	ROC (± one SE)	Sensitivity (± one SE)	Average ROC (± 1 SD)	Average sensitivity (± 1 SD)	Cutpoint
V5 slope 3.5-min rec	0.68 ± 0.02	45 ± 2	0.68 ± 0.02	44 ± 2	0.064 mV/ms
V5 ST60 3.5-min rec	0.68 ± 0.01	49 ± 2	0.67 ± 0.02	49 ± 4	−0.055 mV
Sum ST60 3.5-min rec	0.68 ± 0.02	48 ± 2	0.67 ± 0.01	47 ± 4	−0.084 mV
Most ST60 3.5-min rec	0.67 ± 0.02	49 ± 2	0.67 ± 0.01	48 ± 2	−0.053 mV
V5 ST60 5-min rec	0.67 ± 0.02	43 ± 2	0.67 ± 0.02	44 ± 4	−0.054 mV
V5 slope 5-min rec	0.67 ± 0.02	42 ± 2	0.67 ± 0.02	41 ± 2	−0.016 mV/msec
ST/Heart Rate Index	0.69 ± 0.01	51 ± 2	0.66 ± 0.02	47 ± 4	−0.0022 mV/bpm
Visual ST analysis	0.67 ± 0.01	52 ± 2	0.67 ± 0.03	51 ± 3	1 mm

Rec, recovery; ROC, range of characteristics curve areas.

program had ROC curve areas greater than 0.65. While several of the ST time areas that are part of the Hollenberg score had ROC curve areas comparable to visual analysis, the score itself had an ROC area of 0.65 (sensitivity of 42% at a specificity of 80%). The independent areas are not listed since their complexity exceeds that of the other measurements. In addition, the sensitivity of the measurements at specificity of 80%, matching visual analysis, is also listed. Note that the ST slope cutpoint is slightly upward rather than being zero for horizontal.

Other Leads

Review of the 12-lead visual ECG interpretations confirmed that changes isolated to the inferior and anterior leads, as well as changes isolated to V_4 or V_6, were rare and there were no significant ST changes that were not reflected in V_5. As in a prior study based on visual analysis,[67] in our patients without Q waves, changes isolated to leads other than V_5 were rare and did not improve or add to the diagnostic ability of the exercise ECG. Using the computerized measurements, the sum of ST depression or the maximum depression in the three leads representing the three main areas of the myocardium (leads II, V_2, and V_5) failed to improve the diagnostic accuracy of the test compared to visual or computer analysis of a single lead.

Recovery Measurements

While the visual analysis considered abnormal ST depression in exercise and/or recovery (sensitivity 52%, specificity 79%; ROC 0.67), a separate analysis of the data set revealed that 110 of the 541 abnormal ST responders achieved the 1-mm ST criteria only in exercise and 60 were abnormal in recovery only. If the ST response was considered abnormal and if the criteria were achieved in exercise, regardless of the status in recovery, the sensitivity was 46% and the specificity was 81% (ROC 0.65). If the ST response was considered abnormal when the 1-mm criteria were achieved in recovery, regardless of the result during exercise, the sensitivity was about 43% and the specificity was 87% (ROC 0.67). If 0.5 mm was the criterion for abnormal (similar to the cutpoint of 0.054 mV for ST_{60}), the sensitivity was 57% and the specificity 73%. In addition, the ROC values for measurements in recovery were greater than comparable measurements during maximal exercise (see Table 4-7). The importance of recovery measurements was consistent with previous experience from visual analysis.[68] That is, recovery changes are not generally false positives as previously thought and they have excellent diagnostic value. In addition, the ROC values for other ST measurements in recovery tended to be greater than comparable measurements during maximal exercise. Therefore, the recovery time is probably important because the conflicting impact of increasing heart rate during exercise "pulling" up the ST segment (resulting in a trend towards a positive slope) is no longer present. It is important to have the patient lie down immediately after exercise and not perform a cool-down walk for this measurement to function as it did in this study. Because it is a simple measurement, less contaminated by noise, ST_{60} in V_5 at 3.5 minutes of recovery has much to recommend it. Furthermore, it was also identified as diagnostic for severe disease in an earlier study.[69]

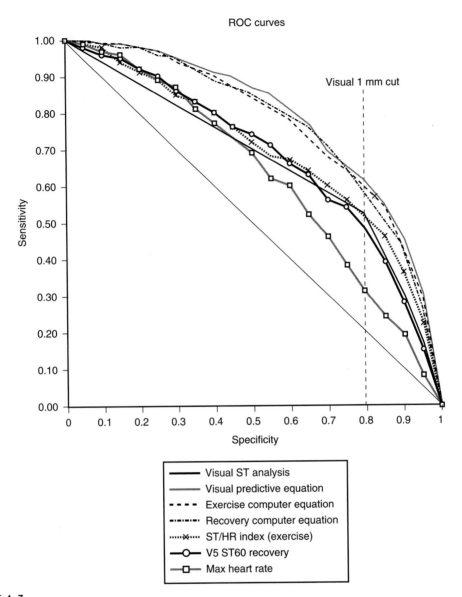

ROC curves

Visual 1 mm cut

Legend:
- Visual ST analysis
- Visual predictive equation
- Exercise computer equation
- Recovery computer equation
- ST/HR index (exercise)
- V5 ST60 recovery
- Max heart rate

■ **FIGURE 4–7**
The diagnostic performance of the ST variables that exhibited an average ROC area within the 95% confidence intervals associated with visual analysis when tested within five randomly selected one-half population samples.

R-Wave Adjustment

Dividing the computer measurements by the computer-measured R-wave amplitude at the time of the measurement failed to significantly improve the ROC areas (the highest [0.68] was obtained by adjusting ST_{60} in lead V_5 at 3.5 minutes of recovery). Prior studies have suggested that adjusting ST-depression measurements by R-wave amplitudes may yield greater diagnostic results than ST-depression measurements alone.[70]

We did not observe any differences in the ROC areas using the computer measurements in V_5 at maximal exercise or during recovery, on dividing by R-wave amplitude.

Effect of Medication Status and the Resting ECG

Beta-blocker administration did not affect the diagnostic characteristics of the standard visual criteria in agreement with previous findings.[71] LVH and visually classified resting ST depression had a similar association with a lowered specificity, also in agreement with previous findings.[72] The exclusion of all patients with resting ECG abnormalities and those patients taking digoxin significantly lowered sensitivity and raised specificity.

Summary of the VA-Hungarian Computer Study

The computer measurements had similar diagnostic power compared to visual interpretation. Computerized measurements from lead V_5 at 60 msec after the QRS end (ST60) during 3.5 minutes of recovery or adjusted by heart rate at maximal exercise was equivalent or superior to all other measurements. Measurements from leads II and V_2 or at multiple other times during recovery or exercise did not add to or improve diagnostic performance. Beta-blockers had no effect on test characteristics, whereas resting ST depression decreased specificity. Computerized exercise ST measurements are comparable to visual ST measurements; neither heart rate adjustment nor the Hollenberg score were superior to simpler measurements; prediction equations, including clinical and exercise test results, exhibited the greatest diagnostic power. Since computer analysis was equivalent to visual ST interpretation by the physician, it can supplement and facilitate exercise ECG interpretation similar to the widely utilized computer programs for the resting ECG.[73]

THE SUNNYSIDE BIOMEDICAL EXERCISE ECG PROGRAM

The advancement of digital integrated circuit technology has made it possible to use increasingly sophisticated methods to process exercise ECGs in real time. This section describes a combination of techniques developed by Olson, Froning and Froelicher for beat classification and temporal alignment, baseline removal, and representative beat extraction that can be incorporated into a microprocessor system. Our signal-processing techniques used for processing of exercise ECG were refined over a period of several years in a number of off-line minicomputer test-bed systems. These techniques have been applied in a real-time microprocessor-based exercise system (commercially available in the QUEST [Quinton/Burdick Corporation]) and now run under the Windows operating system (Microsoft, Redmond, Wash). Four areas of signal processing for the exercise ECG are described: (1) Absolute Spatial Vector Velocity generation, (2) baseline removal, (3) beat classification and temporal alignment, and (4) representative beat extraction.

Absolute Spatial Vector Velocity

Determination of onset and offset of waves should be based on the earliest onset and latest offset seen in any lead. This necessitates the use of a mathematical construct or combination waveform derived from three orthogonal (i.e., statistically independent) leads where electrical activity in all orientations will be represented. The approach we use is a filtered ASVV curve as the basis for all similarity measures and temporal alignments.

Submitting a low- and high-pass filtered signal derived from one or more ECG leads to a threshold detection algorithm is a standard technique for R-wave detection. The low-pass filter tends to minimize effects of power-line interference and high-frequency muscle noise while the high-pass filter reduces low-frequency baseline drift and wander.

It was discovered empirically that a greater immunity to noise is preserved by separately filtering the slope calculations from each of the orthogonal leads prior to the nonlinear operation of taking the absolute value of this sum. This is apparent when this approach is contrasted to the results of performing the computationally faster method of first summing the absolute slopes and then filtering only the sums (i.e., the ASVV curve itself). In order to reduce the computational requirements of this multiple-lead filtering operation, the filter was redesigned into a prefilter/equalizer form. The prefilter is a simple moving average (recursive running sum) that does much of the stopband attenuation at an insignificant cost in processing time. The equalizer is a standard filter designed to act in concert with the prefilter to improve the passband and stopband performance where needed. This optimization resulted in the same filter performance characteristics while using only 60% of the coefficients required for the more conventional approach.

These filtering operations do not disturb the ECG data itself; they are used to generate a derived waveform (the ASVV) which is convenient for internal processing. The ASVV curve is subsequently used to detect R waves, align beats for fiducial marking, and determine onsets and offsets of the major ECG waveform components. Later measurements on the unfiltered ECG signals from individual, simultaneously recorded leads are made in relation to these detected fiducial points and markers along the ASVV curve.

Baseline Removal

The baseline for the ECG often wanders or drifts in an unpredictable and undesirable manner during exercise. This wander can take several forms such as sharp discontinuities, ramps, or cyclical swings. Such baseline wander can be induced by electrode impedance changes resulting from perspiration, motion, respiration, or other sources.

A commonly used technique for removing unwanted baseline fluctuations is to pass the ECG signal through a high-pass filter. The low end of the passband of this type of filter is designed to remove much of the baseline wander. Since the clinically relevant portion of the ECG power spectrum often has most of its energy at frequencies above those of the baseline drift, this simple technique can work fairly well and is still popular. However, if this type of filter design attenuates frequencies that are clinically relevant, then the diagnostic accuracy of many measurements can be affected.

Another method of dealing with baseline wander takes advantage of an a priori knowledge of the underlying morphology of the ECG signal. The degree of baseline wander present in an individual QRS complex is estimated by measuring the relative levels of the TP segments both before and after the QRS complex. If the amplitude difference between these levels exceeds some threshold, the beat is discarded from further processing. This technique has the advantage of not introducing any distortion into the waveform, and works best for detecting and avoiding QRS complexes that have sharp discontinuities or ramps in their baseline.

Removing an estimate of the baseline wander from the signal is not the same as removing the true baseline wander. All baseline compensation methods have theoretical and practical limits, and all are capable of introducing a certain amount of distortion. In the case of the cubic-spline, the fundamental limit is the lack of sufficient baseline estimation points to unambiguously specify the form of the baseline wander. In other words, it is likely that the set of PR-segment values and their locations does not contain enough points to satisfy the Nyquist sampling criterion, given the power spectra of the baseline wander.

Beat Classification and Alignment

The improvement in SNR is achieved by coherent processing of the ECG signal by QRS fiducial alignment and averaging point by point. Thus, a representative ECG complex is extracted from many beats that have been temporally aligned. It is imperative that only similar beats be used in this extraction process. Distorted complexes, arrhythmic or aberrant complexes and noise must be excluded. Cross-correlation of segments of the ASVV is used both to determine which template a QRS complex will be assigned to and also to adjust the final temporal alignment point for each classified QRS complex.

A threshold detection algorithm applied earlier to the ASVV curve generates several candidate R waves. Computing the cross-correlation of 200-msec regions of the ASVV curves containing the candidate QRS complexes then forms templates. The cross-correlation are computed for alignments at every point from −20 to +20 msec of each initial point considered. The point at which the maximum correlation is achieved is then considered to be the final alignment fiducial for the complexes being correlated. In addition, a minimum correlation coefficient of +0.90 is needed to classify a beat into a template. Choosing the alignment corresponding to the maximum correlation is more accurate than using the threshold-selected alignment and gives increased immunity to the template selection process from noise. A short burst of noise in a critical spot (e.g., near the temporary alignment point selected earlier) may cause the alignment point to be missed, since thresholds use properties of the signal which are local to only a few points. Cross-correlation, on the other hand, uses properties of the signal which are distributed over the entire range being correlated, and thus is more immune to the effects of short bursts of noise which may be present.

Representative Beat Extraction

The software should produce, from the set of aligned and similar beats, one ECG complex which is representative of the set. This composite

ECG complex should emphasize those characteristics which are representative of the set and minimize those characteristics which appear only in a few ECG complexes in the set. Thus, such a composite, representative ECG complex would have an increased SNR, largely because most of the noise in the signal should not be aligned consistently between all of the ECG complexes and is effectively "averaged" out.

An arithmetic mean is the linear process that produces the greatest increase in SNR when the noise satisfies several constraints, including that it be Gaussian distributed. However, in the case of exercise ECG data, the noise is not distributed in a Gaussian manner particularly due to the presence of skeletal muscle artifact. In addition, the noise often contains significant transient components that are due to sharp discontinuities in the baseline or the "hump" effect of cyclical baseline swing. Taking a point-by-point mean from a set of QRS complexes with this type of noise would pass $1/N$ of the noise level to the representative complex (where N is the number of QRS complexes in the original set).

A process which gives less of an increase in the SNR for Gaussian-type noise, but which is relatively immune to the effects of sharp discontinuities or "humps", is the median. In addition, the attenuation of muscle noise by using the median seems adequate for consistent measurements. However, the median is a computationally expensive operation, requiring a sorting procedure on each of the representative beat epochs on a point-by-point basis. An algorithm that uses an estimate based on the previous median point index can speed-up the sorting for the next point. In most cases, this implementation of the median operation is five times faster than a standard median computation implementation, thus allowing use of this attractive extraction method.

A hybrid method, sometimes referred to as a trimmed mean, combines some advantages of both the methods described above. It computes an arithmetic mean based only on the "center" points surrounding the median point, throwing out several extreme points on both the high and low side. However, we use the median because it better attenuates muscle artifact.

Summary of the Sunnyside Biomedical Program

This program has been under continual development and refinement for over 2 decades. It started with NASA technology and then incorporated features of Simoons program, which he wrote himself and generously shared with the medical community. As part of incorporation into medical devices, the FDA has approved it several times. Initially DOS based, it now runs under the Windows operating system with requirements met by most desktop personal computers. We have used it in our lab for all of our studies and feel it is the most reliable ECG signal-processing program available.

EXPERT SYSTEMS

We have discussed in this chapter the role that computerization has played in the measurement, presentation, storage, and analysis of the exercise ECG. In this section, we describe a computer approach that takes a broader view and can help the healthcare provider apply insights from epidemiological trials and specialists to clinical management.

While many of the commercial devices provide printed summaries at the completion of the exercise test, these reports are limited and require extensive additional comments and editing. To expand on report generation and to provide an interpretive program similar to the programs for interpreting the resting ECG, we have developed an expert system called EXTRA. It operates as an aid to physician interpretation of the exercise test, and as a teaching tool for students. There are five modules: data entry, database, report generator, summary statistics, and test performance analysis. Data entry has evolved over the years from the use of a specialized scan sheet, directly on screen via mouse or touch-screen using Windows-based programs, to now being available for screen entry on the web (www.sunnysidebiomedical.com). Although the entry is simple and intuitive, help is offered with definitions of words and error-checking. After this, the information is logged into the database, which also contains examples of abnormalities to demonstrate how the expert system interprets unusual cases. The report generator organizes the patient data in a clear, legible report that is ready to be placed in the medical record. The expert system incorporated in EXTRA automatically applies many of the published rules for interpreting the exercise test, and reports this information. A sample report is provided as Figure 4-8. Clearly, this report obviates the need for dictation or hurried handwritten

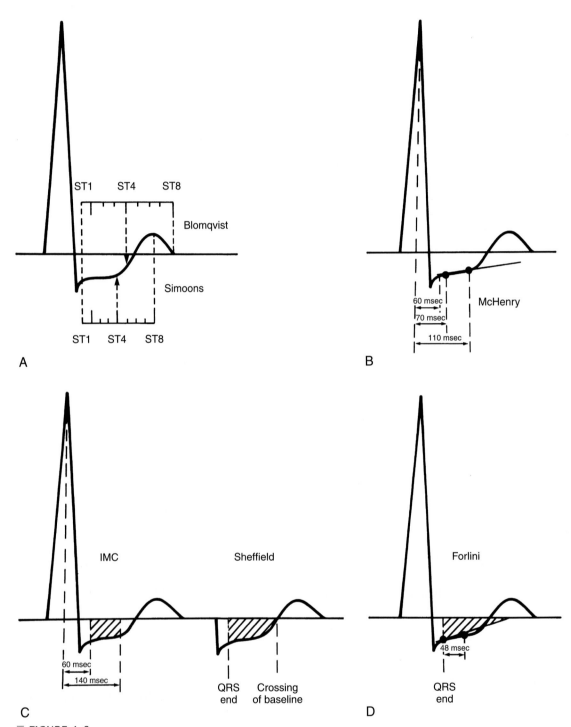

■ FIGURE 4–8
A sample report using the expert system incorporated in EXTRA which automatically applies many of the published rules for interpreting the exercise test, and reports this information. This report obviates the need for dictation, replaces illegible handwritten reports, and is immediately generated by the software.

notes, and is ready immediately. The summary module provides a standard statistical analysis of any specified or all treadmill tests entered. It can also list and print a report of all patients with complications associated with testing. If angiographic data is entered, then ROC areas can be calculated.

Powerful multivariate analysis of both exercise test and epidemiological data has led to tools which can improve the predictive accuracy of the exercise test and predict overall risk with much greater accuracy than a single test alone. The drawback of this approach is that the multivariate equations derived are often unwieldy, and the complex task of calculation proves just too much for most clinicians to fit it into their standard patient workup. The automation of this calculation represents the ideal deployment of computer-processing power. Furthermore, with the current emphasis on general practitioners to lower the cost of healthcare, the combination of expert systems and prediction equations helps the non-specialist to correctly direct patients to appropriate levels of care.

COMMERCIAL EXERCISE TESTING SYSTEMS

Computers are being widely utilized as part of commercial exercise testing systems for processing exercise ECGs gathered during clinical testing. We just list some of the major manufacturers below.

Burdick

Burdick Instruments made the biggest technological jump in exercise testing technology in 1994 with the release of the QUEST. Touching the color screen can help perform all control functions. The capacitance touch-screen keeps attention to the ECG output and cleverly changes colors through the phases of testing. This machine is so intuitive and powerful that all functions can be performed without ever referring to a manual. Burdick was recently purchased by Quinton which has moved its manufacturing unit to the Burdick plant in Michigan, where the Quest is still being manufactured.

General Electric (Marquette Electronics)

Started in a Milwaukee garage by Michael Cudahy and Norman Cousins in 1967, this innovative

company went public in 1992 and was then bought by GE in 1998. They continue a tradition of mechanical and technical excellence that has made them popular around the world. Watch out though for their output called "linked medians." This presentation links averages to look like raw data so that the unsuspecting reader would consider the raw data to be of good quality, while it really could be too noisy to process.

Mortara Instruments

Dr. Mortara left Marquette in 1982 to found his own medical electronics company, also in Milwaukee, but with subsidiaries in Italy and Rotterdam. He has established himself as a major innovator in ECG technology, often driving the entire industry with his vision of better and less expensive equipment.

Quinton Instrument

Founded by Wayne Quinton, an award-winning medical inventor with numerous patents to his credit, Quinton broke into the exercise field early with the development of the first treadmill used by Bob Bruce at the University of Washington.

Schiller

Founded and still directed by the ingenuous Alfred Schiller, this amazing Swiss company has 30 years tradition of providing healthcare professionals with innovative and reliable equipment. They build their own printed circuit boards in their Baar factory using robotics and have QA techniques not matched in the medical industry. They have become the number one supplier of ECG machines in Europe.

Though cardiologists agree that computerized analysis simplifies the evaluation of exercise ECG, there has been less agreement as to whether or not accuracy is enhanced.[73] A recent comparison of computerized resting ECG analysis programs led to the conclusion that physician over-reading is necessary.[74]

SUMMARY

While computer processing of the exercise ECG can be helpful it can also result in false-positive

ST depression. In order to avoid this problem, the physician should always be provided ECG recordings of the raw unprocessed ECG data for comparison to any averages the exercise test monitor generates. It is preferable that averages always be contiguously preceded by the raw ECG data. The degree of filtering and preprocessing should always be presented along with the ECG recordings and this should be contrasted to the American Heart Association recommendations (0 to 100 Hz using notched power line frequency filters). It is preferable that the American Heart Association standards be the default setting. All averages should be carefully labeled and explained, particularly those that simulate raw data. Simulation of raw data with averaged data should be avoided ("linked medians"). Obvious breaks should be inserted in between averaged ECG complexes. Averages should be checkmarked so that the PR isoelectric line is indicated as well as the ST-measurement points. Often the ST-amplitude measurements are incorrect because the isoelectric line is set in the P wave. None of the computerized scores or measurements has been sufficiently validated to recommend their widespread adoption.

Though computers can record very clean representative ECG complexes and neatly print a wide variety of measurements, the algorithms they use are not perfect and can result in serious differences from the raw signal. The physician who uses commercially available computer-aided systems to analyze the results of exercise tests should be aware of the problems and always review the raw analog recordings to see if they are consistent with the processed output. Even if computerization of the original raw analog ECG data could be accomplished without distortion, the problem of interpretation still remains. Numerous algorithms have been recommended for obtaining the optimal diagnostic value from the exercise ECG. These require validation before wide-spread adaptation.

Unfortunately, in spite of sales in the thousands, none of the commercial units have had validation of their signal-processing or measurement algorithms. Nor have their diagnostic capacities been adequately compared to standard visual techniques or with angiography or outcomes. However, most manufacturers use digital databases to improve their software and should soon be presenting the performance of their machines on validated patient data.

The ECG has come a long way since Einthoven and Waller first presented their findings around the turn of the century. Obviously the histories of the computer and the exercise ECG have been intertwined, the latter dependent on the former to provide solutions to critical problems of data volume and storage, to play its part in improving discrimination, and to make available the knowledge of the specialist and the results of sophisticated prediction equations in expert systems. The exercise test continues to be in a dominant position in the workup of cardiac patients because of its speed, low cost, multiple applications, and vast quality and quantity of data generated.

GLOSSARY/ABBREVIATIONS

Impedance: A measure of opposition to electrical flow represented as R for resistance as one of the three components of Ohm's Law (I = E/R). It is in fact a complex ratio of sinusoidal voltage to current in an electric circuit or component.

Bits and bytes: A byte can be thought of as the computer "word". The size of the word relates to the maximum size of number that the computer can deal with. Bits are subsections of bytes, and the number of "gradations" or measurement units can be calculated from $2^n -1$ where n is the number of bits. Thus 8-bit digitization would divide the input into $2^8 - 1$, or 255 V in the range −127 to +127. Current desk top computers operate with 32 bit bytes, but this will shortly increase to 64.

Authorities such as the American Heart Association recommend a minimum of 500-Hz sampling and 16-bit resolution. Music compact discs are generally digitized at 16 bit and 44 kHz.

Passband: The frequency range within which a filter allows signals to pass with minimum attenuation

Stopband: The frequency range in which a filter highly attenuates signals

SNR: Signal to noise ratio

REFERENCES

1. Waller A: Introductory address on the electromotive properties of the human heart. BMJ 1888;2:751-754.
2. Rautaharju PM: A hundred years of progress in electrocardiography. 1: Early contributions from Waller to Wilson. Can J Cardiol 1987; 3:362-374.
3. Einthoven W: Weiteres uber das elektrokardiogramm. Arch fd ges Physiol 1908;122:517.
4. Hyman A: Charles Babbage – pioneer of the computer. Princeton, NJ, Princeton University Press, 1982.
5. Kelvin WT-L: Evening Lecture To The British Association at the Southampton Meeting Friday, August 25, 1882. Scientific papers: physics, chemistry, astronomy, geology, with introductions, notes and illustrations. New York, P. F. Collier, 1910.

6. Bousfield G: Angina pectoris: Changes in the electrocardiogram during paroxysm. Lancet 1918;2:457.
7. Feil H, Siegel M: Electrocardiographic changes during attacks of angina pectoris. Am J Med Sci 1928;175:256.
8. Goldhammer S, Scherf D: Elektrokardiographische untersuchungen bei kranken mit angina perctoris ("ambulatorischer Typus"). Ztschr f klin Med 1932;122:134.
9. Taback L, Marden E, Mason H, et al: Digital recording of electrocardiographic data for analysis by digital computer. Med Electronics 1959;6:167-171.
10. Pipberger H, Arms R, Stallmann F: Automatic screening of normal and abnormal electrocardiograms by means of a digital electronic computer. Proc Soc Exp Biol Med 1961;106:130-132.
11. Stallmann F, Pipberger H: Automatic recognition of electrocardiographic waves by digital computer. Circ Res 1961;9:1138-1143.
12. Caceres C, Steinberg C, Abraham S, et al: Computer extraction of electrocardiographic parameters. Circulation 1962;25:356-362.
13. Willems J, Lesaffre E, Pardaens J: Comparison of the classification ability of the electrocardiogram and vectorcardiogram. Am J Cardiol 1987;59:119-124.
14. Willems J: Computer analysis of the electrocardiogram. In Macfarlane P, Lawrie TV (eds): Comprehensive Electrocardiology – Theory and Practice in Health and Disease. New York, Pergamon Press, 1989, pp 1139-1176.
15. Mortara D: A new ECG filter for dynamic ECG signals. J Electrocardiol 1992;25(suppl):200-206.
16. Pinto V: Filters for reduction of baseline wander and muscle artifact in the ECG. J Electrocardiol 1992;25(suppl):40-48.
17. Petrucci E, Ghiringhelli S, Balian V, et al: Clinical evaluation of algorithms for ST measurement during exercise test. Clin Cardiol 1996;19:248-252.
18. Blomqvist G: The Frank lead exercise electrocardiogram. Acta Med Scand 1965;178:1-98.
19. Hornsten TR, Bruce RA: Computed ST forces of Frank and bipolar exercise electrocardiograms. Am Heart J 1969;78:346-350.
20. McHenry PL, Stowe DE, Lancaster MC: Computer quantitation of the ST segment response during maximal treadmill exercise. Circulation 1968;38:691-702.
21. Sheffield LT, Holt TH, Lester FM, et al: On-line analysis of the exercise ECG. Circulation 1969;40:935-944.
22. Rautaharju PM, Prineas RJ, Eifler WJ, et al: Prognostic value of exercise electrocardiogram in men at high risk of future coronary heart disease: Multiple risk factor intervention trial experience. J Am Coll Cardiol 1986;8:1000-1010.
23. Simoons ML, Boom HD, Smallenberg E: On-line processing of orthogonal exercise electrocardiograms. Comput Biomed Res 1975;8:105-117.
24. Sketch MH, Mohiuddin MS, Nair CK, et al: Automated and nomographic analysis of exercise tests. JAMA 1980;243:1053-1057.
25. Forlini FJ, Cohn K, Langston ME: ST segment isolation and quantification as a means of improving diagnostic accuracy in treadmill stress testing. Am Heart J 1975;90:431-438.
26. Ascoop CA, Distelbrink CA, DeLang PA: Clinical value of quantitative analysis of ST slope during exercise. Br Heart J 1977;39:212-217.
27. Turner AS, Nathan MC, Watson OF, et al: The correlation of the computer quantitated treadmill exercise electrocardiogram with cinearteriographic assessment of coronary artery disease. NZ Med J 1979;89:115-118.
28. van Campen CM, Visser FC, Visser CA: The QRS score: A promising new exercise score for detecting coronary artery disease based on exercise-induced changes of Q-, R- and S-waves: A relationship with myocardial ischemia. Eur Heart J 1996;17:699-708.
29. Hollenberg M, Budge WR, Wisneski JA, Gertz EW: Treadmill score quantifies electrocardiographic response to exercise and improves test accuracy and reproducibility. Circulation 1980;61:276-285.
30. Hollenberg M, Wisneski JA, Gertz EW, Ellis RJ: Computer-derived treadmill exercise score quantifies the degree of revascularization and improved exercise performance after coronary artery bypass surgery. Am Heart J 1983;106:1096-1104.
31. Hollenberg M, Zoltick JM, Go M, et al: Comparison of a quantitative treadmill exercise score with standard electrocardiographic criteria in screening asymptomatic young men for coronary artery disease. N Engl J Med 1985;313:600-606.

32. Vergari J, Hakki H, Heo J, Iskandrian AS: Merits and limitations of quantitative treadmill exercise score. Am Heart J 1987;114:819-826.
33. Elamin MS, Mary DASG, Smith DR, Linden RJ: Prediction of severity of coronary artery disease using slope of submaximal ST segment/heart rate relationship. Cardiovasc Res 1980;14:681-691.
34. Thwaites BC, Quyyumi AA, Raphael MJ, et al: Comparison of the ST/heart rate slope with the modified Bruce exercise test in the detection of coronary artery disease. Am J Cardiol 1986;57:554-556.
35. Kligfield P, Okin PM, Ameisen O, Borer JS: Evaluation of coronary artery disease by an improved method of exercise electrocardiography: The ST segment/heart rate slope. Am Heart J 1986;112:589-598.
36. Quyyumi AA, Raphael MJ, Wright C, et al: Inability of the ST segment/heart rate slope to predict accurately the severity of coronary artery disease. Br Heart J 1984;51:395-398.
37. Sato I, Keta K, Aihara N, et al: Improved accuracy of the exercise electrocardiogram in detection of coronary artery and three vessel coronary disease. Chest 1989;94:737-744.
38. Okin PM, Ameisen O, Kligfield P: Recovery-phase patterns of ST segment depression in the heart rate domain: Identification of coronary artery disease by the rate-recovery loop. Circulation 1989;3:533-541.
39. Okin PM, Kligfield P: Heart rate adjustment of ST segment depression and performance of the exercise electrocardiogram: A critical evaluation. J Am Coll Cardiol 1995;25:1726-1735.
40. Okin PM, Chen J, Kligfield P: Effect of baseline ST segment elevation on test performance of standard and heart rate-adjusted ST segment depression criteria. Am Heart J 1990;119:1280-1286.
41. Kligfield P, Ameisen O, Okin PM: Heart rate adjustment of ST segment depression for improved detection of coronary artery disease. Circulation 1989;79:245-255.
42. Lachterman B, Lehmann KG, Detrano R, et al: Comparison of ST segment/heart rate index to standard ST criteria for analysis of exercise electrocardiogram. Circulation 1990;83:44-50.
43. Bobbio M, Detrano R: A lesson from the controversy about heart rate adjustment of ST segment depression. Circulation 1991;84:1410-1413.
44. Morise AP, Duvall RD: Accuracy of ST/heart rate index in the diagnosis of coronary artery disease. Am J Cardiol 1992;69:603-606.
45. Rodriguez M, Froning J, Froelicher V: ST0 or ST60. Am Heart J 1993;126:752-754.
46. Morris CK, Myers J, Froelicher VF, et al: Nomogram based on metabolic equivalents and age for assessing aerobic exercise capacity in men. J Am Coll Cardiol 1993;22:175-182.
47. Okin PM, Bergman G, Kligfield P: Effect of ST segment measurement point on performance of standard and heart rate-adjusted ST segment criteria for the identification of coronary artery disease. Circulation 1991;84:57-66.
48. Froning JN, Froelicher VF: Detection and measurement of the P-wave and T-wave during exercise testing using combined heuristic and statistical methods. J Electrocardiol 1987;20(suppl):145-156.
49. Miranda CP, Lehmann KG, Froelicher VF: Indications, criteria for interpretation, and utilization of exercise testing in patients with coronary artery disease: Results of a survey. J Cardiopulm Rehabil 1989;9:479-484.
50. Stuart RJ Jr, Ellestad MH: Upsloping S-T segments in exercise stress testing. Six year follow-up study of 438 patients and correlation with 248 angiograms. Am J Cardiol 1976;37:19-22.
51. Savvides M, Ahnve S, Bhargava V, Froelicher VF: Computer analysis of exercise-induced changes in electrocardiographic variables: comparison of methods and criteria. Chest 1983;84:699-706.
52. Gianrossi R, Detrano R, Mulvihill D, et al: Exercise-induced ST depression in the diagnosis of coronary artery disease: A meta-analysis. Circulation 1989;80:87-98.
53. Kurita A, Chaitman BR, Bourassa MG: Significance of exercise-induced junctional S-T depression in evaluation of coronary artery disease. Am J Cardiol 1977;40:492-497.
54. Rijneke RD, Ascoop CA, Talmon JL: Clinical significance of upsloping ST segments in exercise electrocardiography. Circulation 1980;61:671-678.
55. Viik J, Lehtinen R, Turjanmaa V, et al: Correct utilization of exercise electrocardiographic leads in differentiation of men with coronary artery disease from patients with a low likelihood of coronary

artery disease using peak exercise ST-segment depression. Am J Cardiol 1998;81:964-969.

56. Viik J, Lehtinen R, Turjanmaa V, et al: The effect of lead selection on traditional and heart rate-adjusted ST segment analysis in the detection of coronary artery disease during exercise testing. Am Heart J 1997;134:488-494.

57. Simoons M: Optimal measurements for the detection of coronary artery disease by exercise electrocardiography. Comput Biomed Res 1977;10:483-499.

58. Simoons M, Hugenholtz PG: Estimation of the probability of exercise-induced ischemia by quantitative ECG analysis. Circulation 1977;56:552-559.

59. Detry JMR, Robert A, Luwaert RJ, et al: Diagnostic value of computerized exercise testing in men without previous myocardial infarction. Eur Heart J 1985;6:227-238.

60. Deckers JW, Rensing BJ, Tijssen JGP, et al: A comparison of methods of analyzing exercise tests for diagnosis of coronary artery disease. Br Heart J 1989;62:438-444.

61. Detrano R, Salcedo E, Leatherman J, Day K: Computer-assisted versus unassisted analysis of the exercise electrocardiogram in patients without myocardial infarction. J Am Coll Cardiol 1987;10:794-799.

62. Detrano R, Salcedo E, Passalacqua M, Friis R: Exercise electrocardiographic variables: A critical appraisal. J Am Coll Cardiol 1986;8:836-847.

63. Pruvost P, LaBlanche JM, Beuscart R, et al: Enhanced efficacy of computerized exercise test by multivariate analysis for the diagnosis of coronary artery disease. A study of 558 men without previous myocardial infarction. Eur Heart J 1987;8:1287-1294.

64. Simoons ML, Hugenholtz PG, Ascoop CA, et al: Quantitation of exercise electrocardiography. Circulation 1981;63:471-475.

65. Froelicher VF, Lehmann KG, Thomas R, et al: The electrocardiographic exercise test in a population with reduced workup bias: Diagnostic performance, computerized interpretation, and multivariable prediction. Veterans Affairs Cooperative Study in Health Services #016 (QUEXTA) Study Group. Quantitative Exercise Testing and Angiography. Ann Intern Med 1998;128 (12 Pt 1):965-974.

66. Atwood J, Do D, Froelicher V: Can computerization of the exercise test replace the cardiologist? Am Heart J 1998;136: 543-552.

67. Miranda CP, Liu J, Kadar A, et al: Usefulness of exercise-induced ST-segment depression in the inferior leads during exercise testing as a marker for coronary artery disease. Am J Cardiol 1992;69: 303-308.

68. Lachterman B, Lehmann KG, Abrahamson D, Froelicher VF: "Recovery only" ST-segment depression and the predictive accuracy of the exercise test. Ann Intern Med 1990;112:11-16.

69. Ribisl PM, Liu J, Mousa I, et al: A comparison of computer ST criteria for diagnosis of severe CAD. Am J Cardiol 1993;71: 546-551.

70. Berman JA, Wynne J, Mellis G, Cohn PF: Improving diagnostic accuracy of the exercise test by combining R wave changes with duration of ST segment depression in a simplified index. Am Heart J 1983;105:60-66.

71. Herbert WG, Lehmann KG, Dubach P, et al: Effect of beta blockade on exercise ECG: ST level versus delta ST/HR index. Am Heart J 1991;122:993-1000.

72. Miranda CP, Lehmann KG, Froelicher VF: Correlation between resting ST-depression, exercise testing coronary angiography, and long-term prognosis. Am Heart J 1991;122:1617-1628.

73. Milliken JA, Abdollah H, Burggraf GW: False-positive treadmill exercise tests due to computer signal averaging. Am J Cardiol 1990; 65:946-948.

74. Willems JL, Abreu-Lima C, Arnaud P, et al: The diagnostic performance of computer programs for the interpretation of ECGs. N Engl J Med 1991;325:1767-1773.

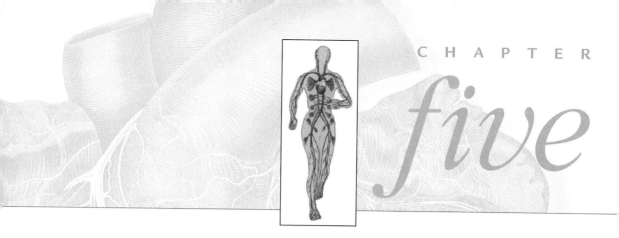

five

Interpretation of Hemodynamic Responses to Exercise Testing

In this chapter, hemodynamic responses to exercise are reviewed, with some notable examples from the literature used to underscore particularly important points. The purview of *hemodynamics* not only includes normal and abnormal heart rate and blood pressure responses to exercise, but also cardiac output and its determinants, and how cardiac output is influenced by cardiovascular disease. Because exercise capacity is such an important measurement clinically and is influenced so strongly by exercise hemodynamics, this chapter also includes factors affecting exercise capacity, as well as the important issue of how normal standards for exercise capacity are expressed.

When interpreting the exercise test, it is important to consider each of its responses separately. Each type of response has a different impact on making a diagnostic or prognostic decision and must be considered along with an individual patient's clinical information. A test should not be called abnormal (or positive) or normal (or negative), but rather the interpretation should specify which responses were abnormal or normal. Neither should the results be called subjectively or objectively positive or negative, but the particular responses should be recorded. Both the objective responses to exercise testing (exercise capacity, heart rate, blood pressure, electrocardiographic changes, and dysrhythmias) and subjective responses (patient appearance, the results of the physical examination, and symptoms, particularly angina) require interpretation and each will be discussed in this chapter. The final report should be directed to the physician who ordered the test and

who will receive the report. It should contain clear information that helps in patient management rather than vague "med-speak." Interpretation of the test is highly dependent upon the application for which the test is used and on the population tested, so this chapter should be considered a preface for information available in later chapters.

EXERCISE CAPACITY VERSUS FUNCTIONAL CLASSIFICATION

The functional status of patients with heart disease is frequently classified by symptoms during daily activities (New York Heart Association, Canadian, or Weber classifications are common examples). However, as pointed out in Chapter 3, *there is no validated substitute for directly measured maximal oxygen uptake*. Table 5-1 illustrates correlation coefficients between various functional measures, including symptom questionnaires, and maximal oxygen uptake in 66 patients with chronic heart failure tested in our laboratory. Note that although these functional measures are widely used as estimates of exercise capacity, their association with VO_2 max is only modest, with correlation coefficients ranging in the order of 0.25 to 0.50.

VO_2 max is the greatest amount of oxygen that a person can extract from the inspired air while performing dynamic exercise involving a large portion of the total body muscle mass. Since maximal ventilatory oxygen uptake is equal to the product

TABLE 5–1. Correlation coefficients between various functional measures in 66 patients with heart failure

	Age	Rest HR	EF	FVC	FEV_1	Estimated METs	VSAQ METs	VO_2 peak	VO_2@VT	PE@VT	DASI	NYHA	6MWT	KC Phys Lim	KCQL	KC Sym Tot
Age	1															
Rest HR	0.30	1														
EF	0.13	0.23	1													
FVC	-0.03	0.30	0.21	1												
FEV_1	-0.10	0.30	0.21	0.90**	1											
Estimated METs	-0.30	-0.02	0.30	0.40*	0.34*	1										
VSAQ METs	-0.11	0.15	0.25	0.32	0.35	0.80**	1									
VO_2 Peak	-0.42*	0.10	0.45*	0.54**	0.63**	0.70**	0.50**	1								
VO_2@VT	-0.30	0.10	0.51**	0.60**	0.61**	0.50**	0.40*	0.91**	1							
PE@VT	0.40	0.52*	0.24	0.30	0.25	-0.35	-0.25	-0.20	-0.10	1						
DASI	-0.10	0.20	0.15	0.35*	0.31	0.50**	0.40*	0.31	0.42*	0.10	1					
NYHA	0.10	0.01	-0.10	0.03	-0.04	-0.30	-0.30	-0.20	-0.30	0.31	-0.70**	1				
6MWT	-0.30*	0.10	0.30*	0.45**	0.34*	0.60**	0.50**	0.50**	0.44*	0.24	0.42**	-0.5**	1			
KC Phys Limitation	0.10	0.10	0.15	0.32	0.41*	0.50**	0.44**	0.35	34	-0.30	0.70***	-0.50**	0.50**	1		
KCQL	0.20	0.30	0.25*	-0.15	-0.04	0.32	0.30	0.23	0.10	-0.03	0.50***	-0.40**	0.22*	0.64**	1	
KC SymTot	0.04	0.40*	0.23	-0.04	0.10	0.40*	0.34*	0.32	0.30	0.05	0.60***	-0.50**	0.40**	0.70**	0.72**	1
KC ClinSum	0.10	0.24	0.22	0.20	0.30	0.50**	0.43*	0.40*	0.33	-0.12	0.71**	-0.60**	0.50**	0.90***	0.80***	0.92**

$*p < 0.05; **p < 0.01$

DASI, duke activity status index; EF, ejection fraction; Estimated Mets, Mets calculated from peak treadmill speed and grade; FEV_1, forced expiratory volume in 1 second; FVC, forced vital capacity; HR, heart rate; KC ClinSum, Kansas City clinical summary score; KC PhyLim, Kansas City physical limitation score; KCQL, Kansas City quality of life score; KC SymTot, Kansas City total symptom score; 6MWT, 6 minute walk test; NYHA, New York Heart Association Functional Class; VSAQ Mets, Mets determined from Veterans Specific Activity Questionnaire; VT, Ventilatory threshold.

of cardiac output and arteriovenous oxygen (a-VO$_2$) difference, it is a measure of the functional limits of the cardiovascular system. In general, maximal a-VO$_2$ difference is physiologically limited to roughly 15 to 17 mL/dL. Thus, in many individuals maximal a-VO$_2$ difference widens up to fixed limit, making maximal oxygen uptake an indirect estimate of maximal cardiac output. VO$_2$ max is dependent upon many factors, including natural physical endowment, activity status, age, and gender, but it is the best index of exercise capacity and maximal cardiovascular function. As a rough reference, the maximal oxygen uptake of the normal sedentary adult typically falls within the range of 25 to 45 mL O$_2$/kg/min, but a "normal" reference should always be considered relative to age and gender, as discussed in Chapter 3. Aerobic training can generally increase maximal oxygen uptake up to 25%, but this also varies widely. The degree of increase depends upon the initial level of fitness and age as well as the intensity, frequency, and duration of training. Individuals performing aerobic training, such as distance running, can have maximal oxygen uptake values as high as 60 to 80 mL O$_2$/kg/min. For convenience, oxygen uptake is often expressed in multiples of basal resting requirements (metabolic equivalents; METs). The MET is a unit of basal oxygen uptake equal to approximately 3.5 mL of O$_2$/kg/min. This value is the oxygen requirement to maintain life in the resting state.

Figure 5-1 illustrates the relationship between maximal oxygen uptake, exercise habits, and age.[1] Although the three activity levels have different regression lines that fit the data as one would expect, there is a great deal of scatter around the lines, and the correlation coefficients are relatively poor. This shows the inaccuracy associated with predicting maximal oxygen uptake from age and habitual physical activity. It is preferable to estimate an individual's maximal oxygen uptake from the workload reached while performing an exercise test. Maximal oxygen uptake is, of course, most precisely determined by direct measurement using ventilatory gas exchange techniques (Chapter 3).

Patterson et al[2] were among the first to use measured VO$_2$ to functionally classify patients with coronary disease and relate these responses to angiographic data. They studied 43 patients with cardiac disease and compared their functional classification by maximal oxygen uptake and clinical assessment. When a discrepancy occurred, the hemodynamic data from cardiac catheterization usually indicated that maximal oxygen uptake more accurately reflected the degree of impairment. Patients began to experience limiting symptoms when maximal oxygen uptake was less than 22 mL O$_2$/kg/min (6 METs) and considered themselves severely limited when maximal oxygen uptake was 16 mL O$_2$/kg/min (4 METs) or less. Many studies have shown that when a patient's exercise capacity

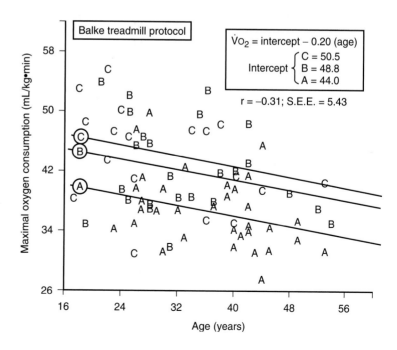

■ FIGURE 5–1

Relationship between maximal oxygen uptake, current exercise status, and age. A, sedentary subjects; B, moderate exercise; C, heavy exercise.

is estimated to be less than 4 or 5 METs, prognosis is poor compared to those with normal exercise capacity. The direct measurement of maximal oxygen uptake is now widely used to estimate prognosis in patients with chronic heart failure (this issue is addressed in detail in Chapter 10).

Questionnaire Assessment. Functional classifications have been found to be relatively limited and poorly reproducible. One problem is that "usual activities" can decrease so that an individual can become greatly limited without having a change in functional class. An alternative approach is to use specific activity scales such as that of Goldman et al,[3] shown in Table 5-2, and the Duke Activity Status Index, shown in Table 5-3, or to question a patient regarding usual activities that have a known MET cost. Hlatky et al[4] developed the Duke Activity Status Index, a brief, self-administered questionnaire to estimate functional capacity and assess aspects of quality of life. Fifty subjects undergoing exercise testing with measurement of peak oxygen uptake were studied. All subjects were questioned about their ability to perform a variety of common activities by an interviewer blinded to exercise test findings. A 12-item scale was then developed that correlated well with peak oxygen uptake. We use a similar approach to estimate a patient's exercise capacity prior to undergoing exercise testing in order to individualize the test and target a test duration.[5] The Veterans Specific Activity Questionnaire (VSAQ) is shown in Table 5-4.

EXERCISE CAPACITY AND CARDIAC FUNCTION

Exercise capacity determined by exercise testing has been proposed as a means to estimate ventricular function. A direct relationship between the two would appear to be supported by the fact that: (1) cardiac output is the major determinant of peak VO_2 in most individuals and (2) both resting ejection fraction (EF) and exercise capacity have prognostic value in patients with cardiovascular disease. However, a poor relationship between resting ventricular function and exercise performance has been reported by many investigators, both among patients with coronary artery disease (CAD) and those with reduced ventricular function. Exercise-induced ischemia could limit exercise even in the presence of normal resting ventricular function; thus, patients with angina would have to be excluded when assessing this relationship. In addition, silent ischemia must be considered when evaluating the interaction between ventricular function and exercise tolerance. During the 1980s, there was considerable interest in attempting to explain exercise capacity based on hemodynamic responses.

TABLE 5–2. Specific activity scale (SAS) of Goldman	

Class I (≥7 METs)	A patient can perform any of the following activities:
	    Carrying 24 pounds up eight steps
	    Carrying an 80-pound object
	    Shoveling snow
	    Skiing
	    Playing basketball, touch football, squash, or handball
	    Jogging/walking 5 mph

Class II (≥5 METs)	A patient does not meet class I criteria but can perform any of the following activities to completion without stopping:
	    Carrying anything up eight steps
	    Having sexual intercourse
	    Gardening, raking, weeding
	    Walking 4 mph

Class III (≥2 METs)	A patient does not meet class I or class II criteria but can perform any of the following activities to completion without stopping:
	    Walking down eight steps
	    Taking a shower
	    Changing bedsheets
	    Mopping floors, cleaning windows
	    Walking 2.5 mph
	    Pushing a power lawnmower
	    Bowling
	    Dressing without stopping

Class IV (≤2 METs)	None of the above

TABLE 5-3. Duke activity status index (DASI)	
Activity	**Weight**
Can you?	
1. Take care of yourself, that is, eating, dressing, bathing, and using the toilet?	2.75
2. Walk indoors, such as around your house?	1.75
3. Walk a block or two on level ground?	2.75
4. Climb a flight of stairs or walk up a hill?	5.50
5. Run a short distance?	8.00
6. Do light work around the house like dusting or washing dishes?	2.7
7. Do moderate work around the house like vacuuming, sweeping floors, or carrying in groceries?	3.50
8. Do heavy work around the house like scrubbing floors or lifting and moving heavy furniture?	8.00
9. Do yard work like raking leaves, weeding, or pushing a power mower?	4.5
10. Have sexual relations?	5.25
11. Participate in moderate recreational activities like golf, bowling, dancing, doubles tennis, or throwing a basketball or football?	6.00
12. Participate in strenuous sports like swimming, singles tennis, football, basketball, or skiing?	7.50

DASI, sum of weights for "yes" replies; VO_2, $0.43 \times DASI + 9.6$.

A few of the more notable studies are discussed in the following.

At the University of California, San Diego, the relationship between resting ventricular function and exercise performance in patients with a wide range of resting EF values who were able to exercise to volitional fatigue was investigated.[6] Radionuclide measurements of left ventricular perfusion and EF were compared with treadmill responses in 88 patients who had coronary heart disease but were free of angina pectoris. The exercise tests included supine bike radionuclide ventriculography, thallium scintigraphy, and treadmill testing with expired gas analysis. The number of abnormal Q-wave locations as well as the EF, end-diastolic volume, cardiac output, exercise-induced ST-segment depression, and thallium scar and ischemia scores were considered. Resting and exercise EF were highly correlated with thallium scar score but not with maximal oxygen uptake. Fifty-five percent of the variability in predicting treadmill time was explained by the combination of change in heart rate (39%), thallium ischemia score (12%), and resting cardiac output (4%). The change in heart rate induced by the treadmill test explained only 27% of the variability in measured

TABLE 5-4. Veterans specific activity questionnaire
Before beginning your treadmill test today, we need to estimate what your usual limits are during daily activities. Following is a list of activities that increase in difficulty as you read down the page. Think carefully, then underline the first activity that, if you performed it for a period of time, would typically cause fatigue, shortness of breath, chest discomfort, or otherwise cause you to want to stop. If you do not normally perform a particular activity, try to imagine what it would be like if you did.

1 MET:	Eating; getting dressed; working at a desk
2 METs:	Taking a shower; shopping; cooking; walking down eight steps
3 METs:	Walking slowly on a flat surface for one or two blocks; doing moderate amounts of work around the house like vacuuming, sweeping the floors, or carrying in groceries
4 METs:	Doing light yard work (e.g., raking leaves, weeding, sweeping, or pushing a power mower); painting; light carpentry
5 METs:	Walking briskly; social dancing; washing the car
6 METs:	Playing nine holes of golf, carrying your own clubs; heavy carpentry; mowing lawn with a push mower
7 METs:	Carrying 60 pounds; performing heavy outdoor work, i.e., digging, spading soil, etc.; walking uphill
8 METs:	Carrying groceries upstairs; moving heavy furniture; jogging slowly on flat surface; climbing stairs quickly
9 METs:	Bicycling at a moderate pace; sawing wood; jumping rope (slowly)
10 METs:	Briskly swimming; bicycling up a hill; jogging 6 mph
11 METs:	Carrying a heavy load (e.g., a child or firewood) up two flights of stairs; cross-country skiing; bicycling briskly and continuously
12 METs:	Running briskly and continuously (level ground, 8 mph)
13 METs:	Performing any competitive activity, including those that involve intermittent sprinting; running competitively; rowing competitively; bicycle racing

maximal oxygen uptake. Myocardial damage predicted resting EF, but the ability to increase heart rate with treadmill exercise was the most important determinant of exercise capacity. Exercise capacity was only minimally affected by asymptomatic ischemia and was relatively independent of ventricular function.

A plot of resting EF versus measured maximal oxygen uptake is shown in Figure 5-2. This poor relationship ($r = 0.25$) confirms many other studies among patients with chronic heart failure and coronary heart disease. The relationship was not improved by excluding patients with a peak exercise respiratory exchange ratio less than 1.1 or with a maximal perceived exertion less than 17. However, maximal exercise EF, maximal end-diastolic volume, and thallium ischemia were significantly correlated with exercise capacity. Resting EF correlated negatively with the sum of Q-wave areas on the resting ECG ($r = -0.40$), and thallium scar score explained most of the variability in resting EF (44%), with ST depression adding only 6%. The change in EF with exercise poorly correlated with the amount of ST-segment depression and thallium ischemia score. When routine treadmill parameters were considered alone, change in rate-pressure product was selected first but could explain only 6% of the variability in resting EF.

Among cardiac parameters used to predict treadmill time or VO_2 max, it was found that thallium ischemia, resting cardiac output, and maximal end-diastolic volume, sequentially, explained 19% of the variability. When the patients were separated into those with normal and those with abnormal resting EF (0.50 being the discriminant value), the predictive variables changed, but there was no appreciable improvement in explaining the variability in exercise capacity. When treadmill parameters were added, the change in heart rate during treadmill exercise was entered first, explaining 39% of the variability, followed by the thallium ischemia score (12%), and resting cardiac output (4%) to account for 55% of the variability in exercise capacity. Again, separating patients by normal and abnormal resting EF did not improve the prediction. When treadmill parameters alone were considered, the change in heart rate with exercise alone explained 38% of the variance in exercise capacity.

Ehsani et al[7] published a similar study. Extensive measurements of systolic ventricular function were considered, but none of these were found to be good predictors of maximal oxygen uptake. Resting EF did not correlate with maximal oxygen uptake, and there was a weak correlation between peak exercise EF and maximal oxygen uptake. However, in contrast to our study, these researchers observed that the change in EF from rest to maximal exercise ($r = 0.77$) and maximal heart rate ($r = 0.61$) correlated significantly with maximal oxygen uptake. It is not clear why different findings were made with regard to the change in EF. Both studies indicated that chronotropic incompetence was a significant factor in determining maximal oxygen uptake, but considerable variance in maximal oxygen uptake remained unexplained.

In a seminal study among patients with heart failure, Weber et al[8] classified 62 patients with chronic stable congestive heart failure into functional classes based on peak VO_2. Pulmonary capillary wedge pressure and direct Fick measurements of cardiac output were made at rest and during upright exercise. The most limited patients increased cardiac output by heart rate alone and had lower maximal heart rates, lower oxygen pulse values, and a lesser change in oxygen pulse from rest to maximal exercise. Patients were symptom-limited by exercise cardiac output rather than high filling pressures. A normal exercise capacity was achieved by increasing both heart rate and stroke volume and tolerating a very high filling pressure during upright exercise. These findings were supported by those of Litchfield et al[9] in a study of six patients with severe ventricular dysfunction. Other compensatory mechanisms included an increase in end-diastolic volume and elevated circulating catecholamines. Higginbotham et al[10] also examined determinants of upright exercise performance

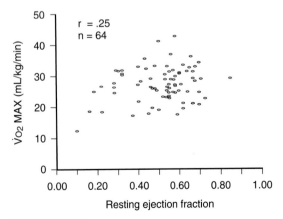

■ FIGURE 5-2

A plot of resting ejection fraction versus measured maximal oxygen uptake, illustrating the poor relationship even in patients not limited by angina.

in 12 patients with severe left ventricular dysfunction using radionuclide angiography and invasive measurements. Multivariate analysis identified changes in heart rate, cardiac output, and a-VO_2 difference with exercise to be important predictors of VO_2 max. Resting EF did not correlate with VO_2 max, nor did changes in EF, stroke counts, or end-diastolic counts during exercise. Wilson et al[11] observed that despite widely varying wedge pressure and cardiac output responses to exercise, patients with chronic heart failure had similar levels of fatigue and dyspnea responses at comparable workloads, as well as similar quality-of-life measurements. This finding suggests that the level of exercise intolerance in patients with heart failure has little relation to objective measures of circulatory, ventilatory, or metabolic dysfunction during exercise.

Together these observations demonstrate that: (1) exercise capacity is largely explained by the extent to which cardiac output increases (this appears to be true among both normal subjects and patients with cardiovascular disease, even those with widely ranging measures of ventricular function) and (2) the relation between exercise capacity, symptoms, and ventricular function is poor, and with the exception of maximal cardiac output, hemodynamic data contribute minimally to the explanation of variance in exercise capacity.

The discrepancy between ventricular function and exercise capacity is now well known. Studies have employed radionuclide, angiographic, and echocardiographic measures of ventricular size and function to document this finding in patients with heart disease. Correlations between exercise capacity and various indices of ventricular function have generally ranged from −0.10 to 0.25.[12] Increasing heart rate and cardiac index appear to be the most important determinants of exercise capacity, but they often leave more than 50% of the variance in exercise capacity unexplained. Radionuclide techniques add little to the explanation of variance in exercise capacity. The change in EF from rest to maximal supine exercise has no predictive power, probably because of the complex nature of this response. The established clinical impression today is that good ventricular function does not guarantee normal exercise capacity, and vice versa. Thus, even in patients free of angina, exercise limitations or expectations should not be determined by ventricular function but rather by the patient's symptomatic response to exercise. If knowledge concerning a patient's ventricular function is necessary for treating the patient,

it must be measured directly, not predicted from the exercise response.

Adaptations in anaerobic metabolism may contribute to the poor ability of cardiac and treadmill parameters to predict measured and estimated VO_2 max. However, differences in a-VO_2 difference may more simply explain these findings. The fact that patients with severely limited ventricular function can improve their exercise capacity after training without altering resting ventricular function[13-15] further underscores the poor relationship between resting ventricular function and exercise capacity. The hypothesis that exercise training could be used to increase exercise capacity and improve the poor prognosis associated with cardiac dysfunction has recently been suggested by a meta-analysis of randomized trials (the ExTraMATCH Trial).[16] This analysis demonstrated a 35% reduction in mortality and a 28% reduction in hospital admissions among patients with CHF randomized to exercise training versus controls, despite the fact that it is well established that training has little, if any, effect on ventricular function.

MYOCARDIAL DAMAGE AND EXERCISE CAPACITY

The relationships between myocardial damage, ventricular function, and exercise capacity are poorly understood. Pfeiffer et al[17] reported that ventricular performance was directly related to the amount of myocardium remaining after myocardial infarctions (MIs) were induced in rats. Yet, rats with smaller infarctions (4% to 30% of the left ventricle) had no discernible impairment in either baseline hemodynamics or peak indices of pumping and pressure-generating ability when compared with sham-operated controls. This result suggests that considerable damage to the left ventricle can occur before pump performance or oxygen transport is affected.

Carter and Amundsen[18] reported an inverse correlation ($r = -0.68$) between infarct size estimated from serum creatinine phosphokinase and exercise capacity at approximately 3 months post-MI. This relationship improved ($r = -0.84$) after exercise training, implying that infarct size affects the response to training. In contrast, Grande and Pedersen[19] reported an insignificant correlation between the enzyme estimate of infarct size and exercise duration ($r = -0.15$) performed within 2 months after an infarction. They observed significant correlations between infarct size and maximal heart rate ($r = 0.39$), maximal systolic blood pressure (SBP) ($r = -0.32$), the increases in both SBP ($r = -0.46$), and heart rate ($r = 0.39$) from rest to 100 W. In our study, the thallium scar score, an estimate of myocardial damage, did not significantly correlate with VO_2 max or change in heart rate. However, there was a significant negative correlation between peak VO_2 and maximal SBP, rate-pressure product, and change in rate-pressure product from rest to maximal exercise.

DePace et al[20] studied resting left ventricular function, thallium-201 scintigraphy, and a QRS-scoring scheme in patients who had suffered MIs. For patients remote from their MI, significant correlations between resting EF and QRS score ($r = -0.51$) and between resting EF and thallium score ($r = 0.61$) were similar to the values for Q wave areas ($r = -0.40$) and thallium scar score ($r = -0.72$) that we obtained. Thallium score correlated poorly with QRS score in the DePace study, but Q-wave sum was significantly correlated to thallium scar in our study ($r = 0.48$). The thallium scar score was highly correlated to resting EF. Both parameters had very poor correlations with exercise capacity. Thus, although cardiac output and VO_2 max are strongly related, data reported from both animal and human studies suggest that resting cardiac function has only a minor impact on VO_2 max.

USE OF NOMOGRAMS TO EXPRESS EXERCISE CAPACITY

As experience with exercise testing has progressed, many protocols have been developed to assess various patient populations. As discussed in Chapter 2, rapidly paced protocols may be suited to screening younger or more active individuals (i.e., Bruce, Ellestad), whereas more moderate ones are appropriate for older or deconditioned patients (i.e., Ramp, Naughton, Balke-Ware, United States Air Force School of Aerospace Medicine [USAF-SAM]). The main disadvantage to having so many techniques has been determining equivalent workloads between them (e.g., what does 5 minutes on a modified Bruce protocol mean relative to a Balke-Ware protocol or in terms of real-life activities such as hiking or grocery shopping?). An estimation of maximal ventilatory oxygen uptake from treadmill or ergometer workload during dynamic exercise (expressed as METs) has been the common language with which investigators and

clinicians communicate when assessing these widely different exercise protocols and everyday physical activities of their patients.

It has been well established that peak VO_2 can be reasonably estimated from the workload achieved on a given protocol, although there are notable limitations in doing so (see discussions in Chapters 2 and 3). As mentioned earlier, the term *metabolic equivalent* (MET) has been commonly used to describe the quantity of oxygen consumed by the body from inspired air under basal conditions. The MET is equal on average to 3.5 mL O_2/kg/min.[21] A multiple of the basal metabolic rate, or MET, is a useful clinical expression of a patient's exercise capacity. Directly measured VO_2 may be translated into METs by dividing by 3.5, thus providing a unit-less and convenient method for expressing a patient's exercise capacity. Despite the practicality and acceptance by exercise physiologists of the MET concept, exercise capacity is more commonly expressed as exercise time. This practice can lead to confusion, since there are so many different protocols, and a given exercise time can represent a good exercise capacity on one protocol but a poor exercise capacity on another.

Because VO_2 is dependent upon age, gender, activity status, and disease states, tables that take these factors into account must be referred to in order to accurately categorize a certain MET value as either normal or abnormal. Morris et al,[22] from our group, developed a nomogram in order to make it more convenient for physicians to translate a MET level into a percentage of normal exercise capacity for males based on age and activity status, similar to that published earlier by Bruce et al,[23] except that we utilized METs instead of time. We retrospectively reviewed the exercise test results of 3583 male patients referred to our laboratory for the evaluation of possible or probable CAD. Excluded were those who had a submaximal test, a prior MI as indicated by history or Q wave, a history of congestive heart failure, beta-blocker or digitalis use, prior coronary artery bypass surgery (CABS) or coronary angioplasty, valvular heart disease, chronic obstructive pulmonary disease, or claudication (i.e., only normal subjects with maximal efforts were included). This left us with a male "referral" population of 1388 with a mean age of 57 (range 21 to 89). For those who could be so classified, a further subgrouping was done into sedentary and physically active groups. An additional grouping was made of those under age 54, with similar subgroupings.

A separate nomogram was developed from data on 244 normal males who volunteered for maximal exercise testing with ventilatory gas exchange analysis. These subjects differed from the former in that they were a healthy, younger (mean age 45 ± 14 years, range 18 to 72) free-living population. Exercise testing was performed for research purposes in these subjects and not for clinical reasons. They were also classified into sedentary and active groups.

All referred patients underwent exercise testing using the USAFSAM treadmill protocol.[24] The MET values were calculated using commonly used equations based on speed and grade.[25] Standard criteria for terminating the test were followed,[26] but no heart rate or time limits were imposed, and a maximal effort was encouraged. Among volunteers who performed exercise testing with ventilatory gas exchange, an individualized ramp treadmill protocol was employed.[27] Only subjects who were limited by fatigue, leg fatigue, or shortness of breath were included. Simple univariate linear regression was performed, with age as the independent variable and METs achieved as the dependent variable. This was done separately for the entire group as well as for the "sedentary" and "active" groups. All equations are numbered in sequence in the following for convenience.

Percentage exercise capacity was obtained from the following equation:

$$\text{exercise capacity} = \frac{\text{observed MET level}}{\text{predicted METs}} \times 100 \quad 1.$$

Exercise capacity represents the actual percentage capacity for a given age based on METs performed, with 100% being the average for a given age. Values for percent exercise capacity were calculated for various ages using this equation. A nomogram was fashioned by plotting specific ages and observed MET levels for differing values of exercise capacity. A "best fit" line was then drawn through the various intercepts to complete the nomogram (Figs. 5-3 and 5-4).

Among patients tested for clinical reasons ("referrals"), regression analyses of METs against age for the entire group and for each of the two subgroups yielded the following equations:

All "Referrals":

predicted METs = 18.0 − 0.15 (age), $n = 1388$,
   SEE = 3.3, $r = -0.46$, $p < 0.001$ 2.

Active:

predicted METs = 18.7 − 0.15 (age), $n = 346$,
   SEE = 3.0, $r = -0.49$, $p < 0.001$ 3.

Sedentary:

predicted METs = 16.6 − 0.16 (age), $n = 253$,
   SEE = 3.2, $r = -0.43$, $p < 0.001$ 4.

The nomogram for Equation 2 is illustrated in Figure 5-3, the nomogram for Equations 3 and 4 is illustrated in Figure 5-4, and a plot of the relationship reflecting Equation 2 is presented in Figure 5-5.

For the entire group of 1388 referrals, the mean maximum Borg score and mean maximal heart rate were 18 and 144, respectively, which are consistent with a maximal effort. Maximal heart rate regressed with age (shown in Fig. 5-6) led to the following equation:

maximal heart rate = 196 − 0.9 (age),
   SEE = 21.2, $r = -0.43$, $p < 0.001$ 5.

The relationships were then reanalyzed, excluding referrals 54 years of age or older in order to match a prior study population. Examination of this new grouping (mean age 43, $n = 442$) yielded regression equations not appreciably different from those shown for all ages.

Healthy Volunteers Tested with Ventilatory Gas Exchange Analysis. Regression analysis of measured METs against age for the normal subjects

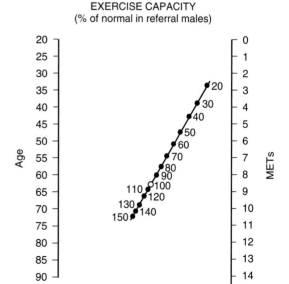

■ FIGURE 5–3

Nomogram of percent normal exercise capacity for age in total population of referral males.

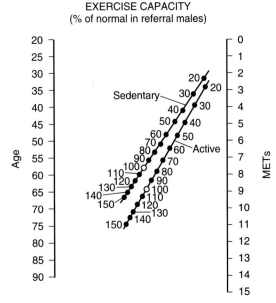

EXERCISE CAPACITY
(% of normal in referral males)

■ **FIGURE 5–4**

Nomogram of percent normal exercise capacity in sedentary and active referral males.

and for active and sedentary subgroups yielded the following equations:

All "Normals":

$$predicted\ METs = 14.7 - 0.11\ (age),\ n = 244,$$
$$SEE = 2.5,\ r = -0.53,\ p < 0.001 \qquad 6.$$

Active:

$$predicted\ METs = 16.4 - 0.13\ (age),\ n = 122,$$
$$SEE = 2.5,\ r = -0.58,\ p < 0.001 \qquad 7.$$

Sedentary:

$$predicted\ METs = 11.9 - 0.07\ (age),\ n = 74,$$
$$SEE = 1.8,\ r = -0.47,\ p < 0.001 \qquad 8.$$

The nomogram for Equation 6 is illustrated in Figure 5-7, and the nomogram for Equations 7 and 8 is illustrated in Figure 5-8. For these subjects, the values observed for maximal heart rate and maximal perceived exertion were 167 ± 19 and 19.0 ± 1.2, respectively, consistent with a maximal effort.

Maximal heart rate regressed with age yielded the following equation:

$$Maximal\ heart\ rate = 200 - 0.72\ (age),$$
$$SEE = 15.3,\ r = -0.55,\ p < 0.001 \qquad 9.$$

Comparison with Other Populations. The regression equation from the Morris et al[22] study differs from that developed by Froelicher et al[28] in 1975 using United States Air Force (USAF) military personnel. The latter group regressed measured VO_2 against age, and the following equations for 710 asymptomatic men of all activity levels were obtained (age range 20 to 53 years):

$$predicted\ METs = 13.1 - 0.08\ (age),\ n = 710,$$
$$SEE = 1.7,\ r = -0.32 \qquad 10.$$

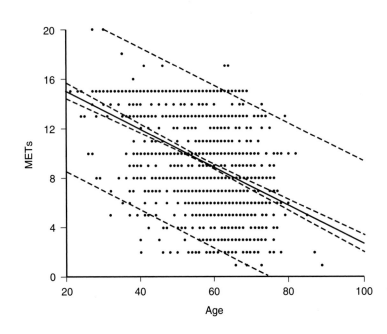

■ **FIGURE 5–5**

Graph illustrating regression equation of METs versus age for all referral patients. *Inner lines* represent 95% confidence limits; *outer lines* represent 95% prediction limits ($r = -0.49; p < 0.001$).

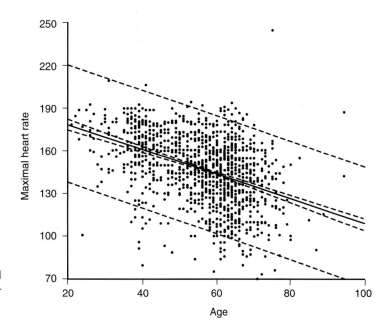

■ FIGURE 5-6

Graph illustrating regression equation of maximal heart rate versus age for referral patients. *Inner lines* represent 95% confidence limits; *outer lines* represent 95% prediction limits ($r = -0.43$; $p < 0.001$).

This is contrasted by the Morris et al[22] population of patients who were less than 54 years old, in which the equation was as follows:

$$\text{predicted METs} = 18.8 - 0.17 \text{ (age)}, n = 442,$$
$$\text{SEE} = 3.3, r = -0.33, p < 0.001 \qquad 11.$$

The slope and intercept are apparently different, which reflects the different populations (discussed later). In an early and widely cited paper, Bruce et al[23] derived a nomogram for functional capacity from 138 healthy men (mean age 49) and calculated the observed exercise capacity from the following equation:

$$\text{observed MET level} = 1.11 + 0.016$$
$$\text{(duration in seconds, Bruce test)} \qquad 12.$$

They then obtained the predicted exercise capacity for age by regressing treadmill duration on age in order to obtain this equation:

$$\text{predicted METs} = 13.7 - 0.08 \text{ (age)},$$
$$\text{SEE} = 1.37 \qquad 13.$$

From the values for observed MET levels and predicted METs, they calculated the relative impairment. Their group consisted of healthy volunteers, like those in the USAF study and healthy volunteers from Long Beach, and all three populations were roughly the same age (Equations 6, 10, and 13). Thus, these equations yield approximately

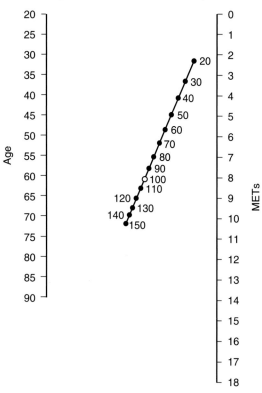

MEASURED MAXIMAL OXYGEN UPTAKE
(% of normal in volunteer males)

■ FIGURE 5-7

Nomogram of percent normal exercise capacity among normal subjects tested using ventilatory oxygen uptake.

MEASURED MAXIMAL OXYGEN UPTAKE
(% of normal in volunteer males)

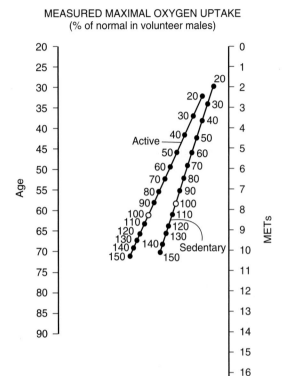

■ **FIGURE 5–8**

Nomogram of percent normal exercise capacity among active and sedentary normal subjects tested using ventilatory oxygen uptake.

the same results for any given age. These contrast the population of patients who were referred to our hospital-based laboratory for evaluation of possible CAD (Equation 2).

Dehn and Bruce[29] conducted a review of the literature related to VO_2 max and its variation with age and activity, and derived the following regression equation from a compilation of 17 previous studies encompassing 700 observations in healthy males of all ages:

$$\text{predicted METs} = 16.2 - 0.11 \, (\text{age}) \quad 14.$$

All of these equations are listed in Table 5-5 for comparison.

Several factors account for the differences between the regression equations obtained from the referred group in the Veterans Administration (VA) and those obtained by Froelicher et al[28] and Bruce et al.[23] The steeper slope in the VA population

is consistent with a faster decline in VO_2 max with age than that found in the previous studies. Regression equations can vary as a result of population differences, including age, activity status, state of health, definition of normal or healthy individuals, and gender. The latter is not an issue in this context, as all studies involved males. There are significant differences in the mean ages and age ranges of the studies cited, with the VA population being the oldest. For this reason, we included a separate analysis of patients under 54 years of age, but a steeper slope was still obtained. The decline in maximal heart rate with age is also steeper in our referrals, paralleling that for the slope in VO_2. Thus, maximal heart rate decreased with age at a greater rate than in prior studies,[30] which could be attributed to a submaximal effort or complicating illnesses in older patients, or it may simply be due to the wide scatter that has been observed for this measurement in past studies.

The classifications of the study populations were done by a "cardiac screening exam" in Bruce's study,[23] by exclusion criteria in our study, and, most stringently, by having to fulfill criteria to achieve "flying status" in the USAF study. Cardiac patients have lower VO_2 max values than normal subjects; therefore, failure to adequately exclude such patients could cause variations in the results. Activity status was not classified in the study by Bruce; it was classified by a similar method in the VA and USAF studies. Varying levels of conditioning could also be a factor in the divergence of the regression equations.

One must also consider differences in methodology when examining divergent results. Only the healthy volunteers at the VA and USAF study used measured VO_2 values. Additionally, the treadmill protocols were quite different, and it has been demonstrated that some protocols are more accurate than others when estimating METs. For instance, more gradual protocols may favor the elderly, and thus alter the regression line. Nevertheless, the mean MET levels for age in our study agree quite well with those of prior investigations (Table 5-6).

It would be difficult to sort out which study has produced the most "universal" regression equations, as all have weaknesses in either population selection or methodology. Ours applies to a typical population referred to a hospital or clinic for evaluation of possible heart disease, excluding those with obvious medical problems that might compromise their exercise capacity. The earlier studies by Bruce et al and Froelicher et al consisted primarily of apparently healthy "normals"

TABLE 5–5. Equations for predicting maximal METs from age

Investigator	Equation	No. patients	Mean age (range)	Assessment of activity	Definition of normal	Oxygen uptake	Protocol
Morris et al[22]	METs = 18.0 − 0.15 (age)	1388	57 (21–89)	Simple questionnaire	No history of CABS, CHF, BB, digoxin, COPD, claudication, angina, prior MI, arrhythmias, or >1 Q wave on ECG	Estimated	USAFSAM
Morris et al[22]	METs = 18.7 − 0.15 (age)	346 (Active)	N/A	Simple questionnaire	As above	Estimated	USAFSAM
Morris et al[22]	METs = 16.6 − 0.16 (age)	479 (Sedentary)	N/A	Simple questionnaire	As above	Estimated	USAFSAM
Morris et al[22]	METs = 14.7 − 0.11 (age)	244	45 (20–72)	Simple questionnaire	Apparently healthy	Measured	Ramp
Froelicher et al[28]	Pred METs = 13.1 − 0.08 (age)	710	N/A (20–53)	None	Normal exam, normal resting and exercise ECG, no HTN	Measured	3.3 mph 1% grade increment per minute
Bruce et al[23] Wolthuis et al[24]	METs = 13.7 − 0.08 (age) METs = 13 − 0.05 (age)	2092 704	44.4 (N/A) 37 (25–54)	None Questionnaire interview	Cardiac screening exam Normal history and physical exam, CXR, resting and exercise ECG and Holter. No arrhythmias, HTN, or medications	Estimated Measured 3.3 mph 1%	Bruce Balke (long) 1% grade increment per minute
Dehn and Bruce[29]	METs = 16.2 − 0.11 (age)	700	52.2 (40–72)	—	—	Mixed	Mixed

BB, beta-blocker; CABS, coronary artery bypass surgery; CHF, chronic heart failure; COPD, chronic obstructive pulmonary disease; HTN, hypertension; MI, myocardial infarction; USAFSAM, United States Air Force School of Aerospace Medicine.

TABLE 5-6. MET levels for age decades from previous studies

	Froelicher[28]	Hossack[36]	Pollock[108]	Morris (referrals)[22]
20–29	11 ± 2	13 ± 1	12 ± 2	—
30–39	10 ± 2	12 ± 2	12 ± 2	—
40–49	10 ± 2	11 ± 2	11 ± 2	11 ± 4
50–59	—	10 ± 2	10 ± 2	9 ± 4
60–69	—	8 ± 2	8 ± 2	8 ± 3
70–79	—	5 ± 1	8 ± 2	7 ± 3
80–89	—	—	—	5 ± 3

and volunteers, so their findings may not be applicable to patients seen by practicing physicians. The regression lines from our referred group may differ from those done on "free-living populations" because of varying levels of disease prevalence and activity. This difference in subject population seems a more likely explanation for the differences than protocol selection, as the regression lines were almost identical when obtained by Froelicher et al using the Balke and Bruce protocol.

The aforementioned factors likely combine to explain the upward shift in the slope of the nomogram scale among volunteers whose oxygen uptake was determined directly from ventilatory gas exchange analysis. It is well established that estimating MET levels from treadmill work results in an overestimation of exercise capacity.[25,27,31,32] The approximate 1.0 to 1.5 higher predicted MET values for any given age among referred patients, whose exercise capacity was estimated from treadmill workload, is not surprising given that differences of this magnitude between measured and estimated maximal oxygen uptake have been reported previously.[27,32] Moreover, the fact that the larger group was referred for testing for clinical reasons naturally makes it a group more inclined to have disease, even though "obvious" disease was excluded. Not only did the presence of cardiovascular disease exacerbate the overprediction of oxygen uptake, but the slope of the maximal heart rate versus age relationship was also steeper in this group of patients. The resultant lower maximal heart rate contributed to the lower measured oxygen uptake at a given work rate for any given age. These data underscore two important points: (1) the scales are population-specific and (2) although measured oxygen uptake is the more precise measure of work, the scales are also specific to whether oxygen uptake was measured or predicted.

An advantage to using nomograms is that they are relatively simple to use: a line drawn between values for age and observed MET levels gives the percent normal exercise capacity. For instance, if a patient were to complete 6 minutes of a Bruce protocol (stage 2), he would have achieved an exercise capacity of 7 METs. If he were 55 years old, this would be calculated as an age-related exercise capacity of 122%, using the nomogram. Similarly, if the same patient completed 8 minutes of a Balke protocol, he would also have achieved 7 METs and would have an age-related exercise capacity of 122%.

Values below 100% indicate exercise impairment relative to one's age group, whereas values above 100% indicate better than normal performance. In addition, equations to obtain particular MET levels may be based on *time* in a protocol, that is, METs = 1.11 + 0.016 (duration in seconds) for the Bruce protocol. Equations to estimate METs based on *speed and grade* from the ACSM[25] are widely used: METs = (mph × 26.8) × [0.1 + (grade × 0.018) + 3.5] / 3.5. The equation for METs based on *cycle ergometer* workload is: METs = [10.8 × W × body weight in kg] + 7]/3.5. The total-population nomograms are appropriate if activity status is unknown. The referral patient nomograms (see Figs. 5-3 and 5-4) may be used for patients referred for testing for clinical reasons, and the normal subject nomograms would be more appropriate for individuals tested for screening or pre-exercise program evaluations with VO_2 measured directly (see Figs. 5-7 and 5-8).

The term *METs* is a more meaningful and useful expression of exercise capacity than the various expressions of protocol times and stages often used. Use of the term facilitates comparisons of data using different protocols and tailoring of protocols for particular patients. MET levels can be used for exercise prescription and for estimating levels of disability by using tables listing the MET demands of common activities (Table 5-7). Many clinicians find exercise capacity relative to peers in an age group to be a useful means of assessing a patient's cardiovascular status. Despite the limitations

TABLE 5-7. MET demands for common daily activities

Activity	METs
Mild	
Baking	2.0
Billiards	2.4
Bookbinding	2.2
Canoeing (leisurely)	2.5
Conducting an orchestra	2.2
Dancing, ballroom (slow)	2.9
Golfing (with cart)	2.5
Horseback riding (walking)	2.3
Playing a musical instrument	2.0
Volleyball (noncompetitive)	2.9
Walking (2 mph)	2.5
Writing	1.7
Moderate	
Calisthenics (no weights)	4.0
Croquet	3.0
Cycling (leisurely)	3.5
Gardening (no lifting)	4.4
Golfing (without cart)	4.9
Mowing lawn (power mower)	3.0
Playing drums	3.8
Sailing	3.0
Swimming (slowly)	4.5
Walking (3 mph)	3.3
Walking (4 mph)	4.5
Vigorous	
Badminton	5.5
Chopping wood	4.9
Climbing hills	7.0
Cycling (moderate)	5.7
Dancing	6.0
Field hockey	7.7
Ice skating	5.5
Jogging (10-minute mile)	10.0
Karate or judo	6.5
Roller skating	6.5
Rope skipping	12.0
Skiing (water or downhill)	6.8
Squash	12.0
Surfing	6.0
Swimming (fast)	7.0
Tennis (doubles)	6.0

Note: These activities can often be done at variable intensities if one assumes that the intensity is not excessive and that the courses are flat (no hills), unless otherwise specified.

From Fletcher GF, Balady GJ, Amsterdam EA, et al: Exercise standards for testing and training: A statement for healthcare professionals from the American Heart Association. Circulation 2001;104:1694-1740.

associated with estimating METs from treadmill or bicycle workloads,[25-27,31,32] exercise capacity estimated from work rate has been repeatedly shown to be an independent predictor of mortality.[33,34]

Estimating a patient's functional status relative to age and gender is an important exercise test result that should be included in the test report. A more detailed discussion of "normal" estimates of exercise capacity and their limitations is presented in Chapter 3. *METs* is a term that can improve communication between physicians, and expressing exercise capacity as a percentage of what is understood to be normal can do the same for dialogue between physicians and their patients regarding functional status, prognosis, and disability.

MAXIMAL CARDIAC OUTPUT

Maximal cardiac output has long been considered the major factor limiting maximal oxygen uptake; numerous studies have demonstrated a linear relation between cardiac output and oxygen uptake during exercise. The rate of increase in cardiac output is commonly judged to be roughly 6 L per 1 L increase in oxygen uptake. However, there is a wide biologic scatter between maximal cardiac output and VO_2 max in healthy persons, even when age, gender, and activity status are considered. Because both maximal cardiac output and maximal oxygen uptake decline with age, the effects of age and disease are usually difficult to separate.

McDonough et al[35] measured maximal cardiac output in a group of patients and found a decline in maximal cardiac output to be the major hemodynamic consequence of symptomatic CAD and one that resulted in exercise impairment. Reductions in left ventricular performance at high levels of exercise, manifested by decreasing stroke volume and increasing pulmonary artery pressure, appeared to be the mechanism limiting cardiac output. Hossack et al[36] studied 100 patients with coronary disease (89 men, 11 women) to characterize their aerobic and hemodynamic profiles at rest and during upright treadmill exercise. The mean maximal cardiac output, measured using the direct Fick equation, was 57 ± 14% of average normal values. The reduction in maximal heart rate (63 ± 13% of normal) was a greater factor influencing the reduction in cardiac output than stroke volume (88 ± 16% of normal). Peak VO_2 was 48 ± 15% of normal, and the greater reduction in peak VO_2 compared with cardiac output was due to lower peripheral extraction in the patients with CAD. Variables that correlated with maximal cardiac output in a univariate analysis included angina severity ($r = -0.45$), peak VO_2 ($r = 0.67$), maximal heart rate ($r = -0.31$), degree of left ventricular dysfunction ($r = -0.45$), maximal SBP ($r = -0.31$), and number of vessels with 50% or greater diameter reduction ($r = -0.30$). Resting EF did not correlate with maximal cardiac output using a multivariate analysis, but four variables correlated significantly ($r = 0.77$) with maximal cardiac output in the following order: VO_2 max, number of vessels with 50% or greater stenosis, magnitude of ST depression, and gender. These data were used to estimate limits of maximal cardiac output and stroke volume in normal subjects, and these normal standards were then used to evaluate the results in the patients. Patients with an EF of less than 50% had significantly impaired age-adjusted cardiac output and stroke volume.

Many similar studies were performed during the 1980s and 1990s, and while they varied greatly in terms of populations and methods used to measure cardiac output (echocardiographic, nuclear, impedence cardiography, or direct Fick), collectively they confirm that cardiac output is the major hemodynamic factor influencing exercise capacity. Therefore, a disruption in any of the factors that define cardiac output (e.g., maximal heart rate achieved, stroke volume, filling pressure, ventricular compliance, contractility, or afterload) will limit exercise tolerance.

MAXIMAL HEART RATE

Methods of Recording. From many hemodynamic studies performed over the years, maximal heart rate has emerged as clearly the most important determinant of cardiac output during exercise, particularly at high levels. One issue of concern in the past was the method of maximal heart rate measurement. Although measuring a patient's maximal heart rate should be a simple matter, the different ways of recording it and differences in the type of exercise used can pose problems. The best way to measure maximal heart rate is to use a standard ECG recorder and calculate instantaneous heart rate from the RR intervals. Methods using the arterial pulse or capillary blush techniques are much more affected by artifact than ECG techniques. Some investigators have used averaging over the last minute of exercise or in immediate recovery; both of these averaging methods are inaccurate. Heart rate drops quickly in recovery and can climb steeply even in the last seconds of exercise. Premature beats can affect averaging and must be eliminated in order to obtain the actual heart rate. Cardiotachometers are available but may fail to trigger or may trigger inappropriately on T waves, artifact, or aberrant

beats, thus yielding inaccurate results. Not all cardiotachometers have the accuracy of the ECG paper technique.

Atwood et al[37] compared nine different sampling intervals (1, 2, 3, 6, 10, 15, 20, 30, and 60 seconds) using calipers at rest and during exercise to determine the "ideal" method of measurement in subjects with normal sinus rhythm and patients with atrial fibrillation. This task is particularly difficult in patients with atrial fibrillation because of the irregularity of the ventricular response. The heart rate obtained from each interval was compared with true heart rate (determined by a 4-minute sample at rest and by the last 30 seconds of each minute during exercise). Among patients with atrial fibrillation, large differences were observed between the heart rate obtained and true heart rate, both at rest and during exercise, using small sampling intervals. The mean of these differences ranged between 16 ± 11 beats per minute (range 14 to 22) using 1-second sampling intervals and 2.2 ± 2.0 beats per minute (range 1.6 to 4.4) using 20-second sampling intervals during progressive exercise. Variability of the heart rate obtained from random heart rate samples was also high when short sampling intervals were used among patients with atrial fibrillation. These observations were contrasted by subjects in normal sinus rhythm, among whom neither variability nor measurement error was influenced remarkably by changing the sampling interval or increasing heart rate. It was concluded that the number of RR intervals from a 6-second rhythm strip at the end of each minute multiplied by 10 represented a reasonable balance between convenience and precision for measuring heart rate during exercise, both in patients with atrial fibrillation and those in normal sinus rhythm.

Factors Limiting Maximal Heart Rate. Several factors may affect maximal heart rate during dynamic exercise (Table 5-8). Maximal heart rate declines with advancing years and is affected only minimally by gender. Height, weight, and even lean body weight apparently are not independent factors

---

TABLE 5–8. Factors affecting maximal heart rate in response to dynamic exercise

Age	Bed rest
Gender	Altitude
Level of fitness	Type of exercise
Cardiovascular disease	True maximal exertion

affecting maximal heart rate. Sheffield et al[38] tested 100 asymptomatic females 19 to 69 years old on a treadmill and concluded that the regression of maximal heart rate based on age in women was different than in men, being about 5 beats per minute lower for any given age. However, for practical purposes, gender is not generally considered an important factor that affects maximal heart rate during exercise testing. Some investigators have reported significant decreases in maximal heart rates among well-trained athletes. It has been speculated that blood volume changes and cardiac hypertrophy can explain this lower heart rate. However, this finding has not been consistent; in one study, a group of elite marathon runners underwent maximal exercise testing and were found to have maximal heart rates similar to age-matched sedentary controls. Although this point remains unsettled, it is possible that training in early life may result in cardiac hypertrophy or dilation. Perhaps cardiac dimensions contribute to the determination of the maximal heart rate in individuals with a healthy sinus node.

Age, Fitness, and Cardiovascular Disease. Many studies have assessed maximal heart rate during treadmill testing in a variety of subjects, with and without cardiovascular disease. Regressions with age have varied depending on the population studied and other factors. Table 5-9 and Figure 5-9 summarize these studies of maximal heart rate; note the wide variation among the regression equations based on age.

A consistent finding in these studies has been a relatively poor relationship between maximal heart rate and age. Correlation coefficients in the order of −0.40 are typical, with standard deviations in the range of 10 to 15 beats per minute. In general, this relationship has not been "tightened" by considering activity status, weight, cardiac size, maximal respiratory exchange ratio, or perceived exertion. An exercise program most likely has divergent effects on this relationship at the age extremes. Younger individuals may be able to achieve larger changes in cardiac dimensions than older subjects, and those larger changes may affect maximal heart rate. Among older individuals, there may be a significant learning effect, whereby the individual is less afraid to exert themselves maximally, and therefore a higher maximal heart rate is achieved on later testing when they are less apprehensive. Given the inconsistencies associated with age-related maximal heart rate, indiscriminant use of age-predicted maximal heart rate in making exercise

prescriptions or in setting goals for treadmill performance should be avoided.

The physiologic limits on maximal heart rate in normal men are determined by rapidity of sinus node recovery, cardiac dimensions, left ventricular filling, and contractile state. Systole has a relatively fixed time interval; when heart rate increases, relatively less time during the cardiac cycle is spent in diastole. It seems logical that a limit would be approached at which an increase in heart rate would not effectively increase cardiac output as a result of decreased diastolic filling; not only would the heart receive less blood to pump, thereby imposing mechanical limitations, but the degree of coronary artery perfusion would decrease, imposing metabolic constraints. Although this theoretic limitation is reasonable, there is little experimental work to support it. In the following, some of the major population studies assessing the relationships among age, heart rate, and other hemodynamic factors are discussed.

Bruce et al[39] attempted to separate the effects of age from the effects of cardiovascular disease on maximal heart rate by analyzing data on over 2000 healthy middle-aged men and subgroups of over 2000 ambulatory male patients with hypertension, coronary heart disease, or both. All underwent maximal treadmill tests, and the data from each subgroup were regressed with age and compared. Any substantial difference in slope would imply that disease, independent from age, influenced maximal heart rates. These investigators found an age-related decline in all groups, with correlation coefficients ranging from −0.3 to −0.5. Applying the derived equations for a 50-year-old man would yield an estimated maximal heart rate of 177 beats per minute for healthy men, 168 for hypertensives, and 151 for those with CAD.

Cooper et al[40] examined the maximal heart rate response to treadmill testing in over 2500 men ranging in age from 10 to 80 years with a mean of 43. Patients with abnormal resting ECGs and those unable to give a maximal effort were excluded from the study. Levels of cardiovascular fitness were determined by age-adjusted treadmill times using the Balke-Ware protocol; subjects were grouped as below average, above average, or average based on their results. Although this population as a whole showed a regression line and a slope similar to those of other studies, the data based on cardiovascular fitness showed significantly different slopes. These data suggested that those with lower fitness achieved lower maximal

TABLE 5–9. Summary of studies assessing maximal heart rate

Investigator	No. subjects	Population studied	Mean age ± SD (range)	Mean hr max (SD)	Regression line	Correlation coefficient	Standard error of the estimate (beats/min)
Astrand*	100	Asymptomatic men	50 (20–69)	166 ± 22	y = 211 − 0.922 (age)	NA	NA
Bruce	2091	Asymptomatic men	44 ± 8	181 ± 12	y = 210 − 0.662 (age)	−0.44	14
Cooper	2535	Asymptomatic men	43 (11–79)	181 ± 16	y = 217 − 0.845 (age)	NA	NA
Ellestad†	2583	Asymptomatic men	42 ± 7 (10–60)	173 ± 11	y = 197 − 0.556 (age)	NA	NA
Froelicher	1317	Asymptomatic men	38 ± 8 (28–54)	183	y = 207 − 0.64 (age)	−0.43	10
Lester	148	Asymptomatic men	43 (15–75)	187	y = 205 − 0.411 (age)	−0.58	NA
Robinson	92	Asymptomatic men	30 (6–76)	189	y = 212 − 0.775 (age)	NA	NA
Sheffield	95	Men with CHD	39 (19–69)	176 ± 14	y = 216 − 0.88 (age)	−0.58	11‡
Bruce	1295	Men with CHD	52 ± 8	148 ± 23	y = 204 − 1.07 (age)	−0.36	25‡
Hammond	156	Men with CHD	53 ± 9	157 ± 20	y = 209 − 1.0 (age)	−0.30	19
Morris	244	Asymptomatic men	45 (20–72)	167 ± 19	y = 200 − 0.72 (age)	−0.55	15
Graettinger	114	Asymptomatic men	46 ± 13 (19–73)	168 ± 18	y = 199 − 0.63 (age)	−0.47	NA
Morris	1388	Men referred for evaluation for CHD, normals only	57 (21–89)	144 ± 20	y = 196 − 0.9 (age)	−0.43	21

*Astrand used bicycle ergometry; all other studies were performed on a treadmill.
†Data compiled from graphs in reference cited.
‡Calculated from available data.
CHD, coronary heart disease; HR max, maximal heart rate; NA, not able to calculate from available data.

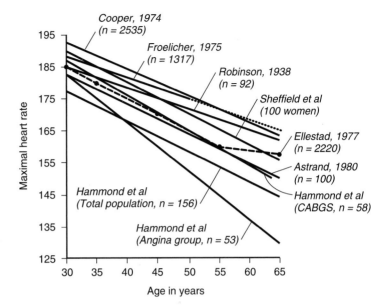

FIGURE 5-9

Regression lines from studies in the literature assessing maximal heart rate versus age during dynamic exercise, including population size. See Table 5-9 for additional details.

heart rates and that these differences were more divergent at older ages. Those who had better cardiovascular fitness tended to show less rapid declines in their maximal heart rates with age.

In an effort to clarify the relationship between maximal heart rate and age, Londeree and Moeschberger[41] performed a comprehensive review of the literature, compiling information on more than 23,000 subjects aged 5 to 81 years. Stepwise multiple regression analysis revealed that age alone accounted for 75% of the variability in maximal heart rate; other factors added only an additional 5% and included mode of exercise, level of fitness, and continent of origin, but not gender. The 95% confidence intervals, even when accounting for these factors, ranged 45 beats per minute. Heart rates at maximal exercise were lower during bicycle ergometry than on the treadmill and even lower with swimming. In addition, trained individuals had significantly lower maximal heart rates than untrained subjects.

At USAFSAM, the cardiovascular responses to maximal treadmill testing were compared using three different popular treadmill protocols to evaluate reproducibility among tests.[42] The Bruce, Balke, and Taylor protocols were used in the evaluation of healthy men; each subject performed one test per week for 9 weeks, repeating each protocol three times in randomized order. The maximal heart rates achieved were reproducible within each protocol, and no significant differences in heart rate were achieved among the three protocols. In addition, larger numbers of normal subjects were studied, as shown in Figure 5-10, which also shows the

wide scatter. In general, these findings agree with subsequent data from our laboratory in Long Beach. In the latter study, Graettinger et al[43] assessed clinical, echocardiographic, and functional determinants of maximal heart rate. Despite controlling for age, activity status, gender, and hypertension, it was reported that measures of cardiac size and function added little to the prediction of maximal heart rate. Most of the variance in maximal heart rate was accounted for simply by age. Given the large degree of individual variability in cardiac size and function, as well as the variance in the relationship between maximal heart rate and age, maximal heart rate may always be a difficult variable to explain.

Bed Rest. Another factor that affects maximal heart rate, and one that is important clinically, is bed rest. Among the many adverse physiologic effects of bed rest are substantial increases in heart rate at rest, submaximal work levels (35 to 40 beats per minute) and maximal exercise.[44] In a classic paper, Convertino et al[45] examined the cardiovascular responses to maximal exercise in normal men following 10 days of bed rest. A significant increase in maximal heart rate was found following bed rest as compared to before bed rest. It was suggested that lack of gravitational forces on baroreceptor mechanisms might have played a role in this accentuated heart rate response. Measurements of peak VO$_2$ in both the supine and upright positions revealed lower values with upright exercise. Oxygen uptake during maximal supine exercise was not impaired compared with pre-bed rest measurements. Since maximal heart

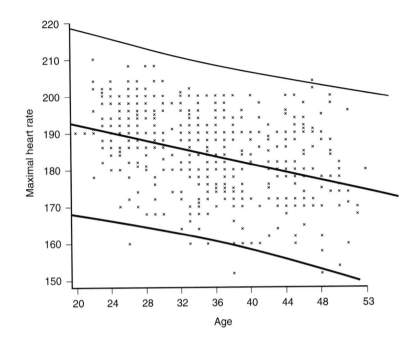

USAFSAM (United States Air Force School of Aerospace Medicine) study of healthy pilots illustrating the relationship between maximal heart rate and age, along with the normal scatter.

rates increased significantly, but VO_2 max decreased, changes in heart volume were likely involved and likely reflect changes in plasma volume during prolonged bed rest.

Altitude. Altitude affects the heart rate response to exercise. During acute exposure to altitude, heart rate increases at matched submaximal levels. Maximal heart rate decreases after prolonged exposure to altitude. Cunningham et al[46] have shown that catecholamine levels are elevated in plasma and urine at high altitudes. At sea level, atropine administration does not impair maximal heart rate, implying that parasympathetic withdrawal is complete at maximal exercise. However, Hartley et al[47] examined maximal heart rate before and after the administration of atropine in normal, untrained men who had lived at sea level all of their lives. The subjects were studied with bicycle ergometry at sea level and at a 15,000-foot altitude. Maximal heart rate decreased a mean of 24 beats per minute, and maximal oxygen uptake decreased by 26% at the higher altitude. Atropine administration did not affect maximal heart rate at sea level but significantly increased maximal heart rate at high altitude (165 to 176 beats per minute). Mean maximal heart rate did not increase with the administration of supplemental oxygen, so the impaired heart rate response was not due to hypoxia alone. At high altitude, there is a reduction in sympathetic nervous system activity, likely due to a reduction in beta-receptor sensitivity, which underlies the reduction in maximal heart rate.

Motivation. A final factor affecting maximal exercise heart rate is motivation to exert oneself maximally. Motivation is, of course, a difficult factor to quantify. Older patients may be restrained by poor muscle tone, pulmonary disease, claudication, orthopedic problems, and other noncardiac causes of limitation. The usual decline in maximal heart rate with age is not as steep in people who are free from myocardial disease and stay active, but it still occurs.

CHRONOTROPIC INCOMPETENCE OR HEART RATE IMPAIRMENT

Chronotropic incompetence (CI) and *heart rate impairment* are terms that have been used to describe inadequate heart rate responses to exercise. In a seminal study on this issue, Ellestad and Wan[48] analyzed the results from 2700 patients tested in their treadmill laboratory. They defined a group of patients who achieved below the 95% confidence limits for maximal heart rate regressed with age as having CI. Patients with no ST-segment depression who had CI had a four times greater incidence of CAD than did those without CI in the

4 years after the test. In a similar followup study of 1500 patients who underwent angiography and treadmill testing, McNeer et al[49] found that those with a maximal exercise heart rate less than 120 beats per minute had a 60% survival rate at 4 years versus 90% for those who exceeded a maximal heart rate of 160 beats per minute. Bruce et al[50] followed 2000 clinically healthy men after screening them with treadmill testing and found that the inability to achieve a maximal heart rate 90% of that predicted for age had a fourfold risk for CAD after 5 years.

In recent years, a number of studies performed at the Cleveland Clinic have confirmed the strong prognostic value of inadequate heart rate responses to exercise. Lauer et al[51] studied 146 men and 85 women who were not taking beta-blocking agents and exhibited CI defined as (1) failure to achieve 85% of age-predicted maximal heart rate or (2) a low *chronotropic index*, a measure that expresses heart rate achieved accounting for age, functional capacity, and resting heart rate. The patients were followed for a mean of 41 months. Both indices were strong predictors of cardiac events (death, MI, unstable angina, or revascularization); the relative risks for failure to achieve 85% predicted heart rate and a low chronotropic index were 2.47 and 2.44, respectively. An inadequate heart rate response to exercise predicted cardiac events even after exercise-induced ischemia was adjusted for by echocardiography. Similar findings were made in the Framingham cohort[52] during a 7-year followup among 1575 males. An inadequate heart rate response to exercise was associated with nearly twice the risk for total mortality and cardiac events, even after adjustments were made for age and other CAD risk factors. Researchers from the Cleveland Clinic have also observed that a low chronotropic index was as strong a predictor of mortality as an abnormal nuclear perfusion scan,[53] and was a better predictor of mortality than angiographic results in a multivariate analysis.[54]

Few studies in this area considered the prevalence of exercise test-induced angina or evaluated other factors in their patients with CI. From previous studies of normal subjects and in evaluating patients with CAD, we have noted no distinguishing features in those with heart rate impairment. Hammond et al[55] initiated a study in our laboratory to better characterize patients with CI. These subjects represented a cross-section of patients with CAD, including those who had had an MI, CABS, or angina pectoris. Because the definition of CI required that patients have an impaired

heart rate on two separate tests, the sample group was more rigidly defined than in other studies. Patients who met the criteria for CI had both a significantly lower prevalence of CABS and a greater prevalence of exercise-induced angina than did the other patients. It appeared that the limited maximal heart rates were due to angina-limited effort; in addition, it appeared that patients who had undergone CABS had less heart rate impairment. Because of these differences, the 156 men were divided into subgroups based on whether or not they had angina or had undergone CABS. The mean heart rate of patients with CI was significantly lower than that of the other patients at a submaximal workload (5% grade), except for those in the angina group (see Fig. 5-9). There was a lower mean maximal oxygen uptake in all of the patients with CI except for the surgical bypass group. This difference retained significance in the group without angina; therefore, symptom limitation is not the only explanation. These findings demonstrate that patients with CI are functionally impaired.

Is exercise-induced angina or myocardial dysfunction the cause of CI? Much of what had been called CI in early studies is related to early termination of exercise because of angina pectoris. Nevertheless, a significant number of patients are not limited by angina, yet have heart rate impairment. These patients also have significantly lower aerobic capacity than do age-matched patients with a normal heart rate response. In the study by Hammond et al,[55] two groups of patients with CI were characterized: those limited by angina and those limited by other factors. From radionuclide testing, it appeared that the patients with CI *and* angina had good mechanical myocardial reserve with less scarring, higher EFs, and lower end-diastolic volumes. In contrast, the patients with CI but without angina had more scarring, lower EFs, and higher end-diastolic volumes. This difference in the state of the myocardium was not apparent from clinical features, such as history of congestive heart failure, MI, or pathologic Q waves, but was apparent only from the results of radionuclide testing.

Because the heart rate response to exercise reflects the balance between central nervous system withdrawal of vagal tone and an increase in sympathetic tone, an abnormal heart rate response to exercise is also likely related to abnormal autonomic balance.[56] There has a been a great deal of interest in recent years in the role of the autonomic nervous system as a predictor of risk,[57-60] and clearly autonomic imbalance is one reason CI has repeatedly been shown to be a predictor of mortality. Nevertheless, from a clinical perspective, one would also expect abnormal radionuclide studies and poor prognostic features to be concentrated in patients with CI. We were surprised to find that most patients with CI stopped the test because of angina; in those without angina, the extent of myocardial damage was correlated with the impaired heart rate response. Many previous studies overlooked the occurrence of angina and evidence of prior MI in their examination of patients with heart rate impairment. Patients with CI most likely represent a mixed group with a variety of explanations for the impaired heart rate response, including impaired autonomic function, angina, myocardial dysfunction, and simply normal variation.

HEART RATE RECOVERY

A faster recovery of heart rate after exercise has long been associated with higher levels of fitness. Studies in this area date back to the 1930s and the work of Cotton and Dill[61] in the Harvard fatigue laboratory. Recent studies have suggested that the rate in which heart rate recovers from exercise is mediated by autonomic factors, particularly the rate at which vagal tone is reactivated.[62] As mentioned in the above discussion on CI, many studies have been published over the last decade indicating a strong association between autonomic balance and mortality, with a deficiency in vagal tone being a primary marker of increased risk.[57-60] Because heart rate recovery is thought to be primarily a vagal phenomenon, investigators have recently used measures of heart rate recovery to study its potential as an easily measured marker of risk.

Several provocative studies were published between 1999 and 2004 addressing the diagnostic/prognostic utility of heart rate in recovery. Cole et al[63] studied 2428 patients referred for thallium scintigraphy over a 6-year period. They found that, using a decrease equaling 12 beats per minute or less at 1 minute into recovery as the definition of an abnormal response, a relative risk of 4.0 for mortality was observed. Even when adjusted for other potential confounders (such as age, fitness, gender, and other cardiac risk factors), abnormal heart rate recovery was associated with a doubling of the risk of mortality. These investigators then addressed this issue among 5000 subjects in the Lipid Research Clinics Prevalence study.[64] Abnormal heart rate recovery

was defined in this study by a decrease equaling 42 beats per minute or less at 2 minutes postexercise. Patients with an abnormal response had 2.5 times the mortality rate of those with a normal response. In a third study, Nishime et al,[65] studied 9454 patients who underwent exercise testing and followed them for a median of 5.2 years. Using the original 12 beats per minute or less at 1 minute of recovery as the cutoff for abnormal, they observed a fourfold greater mortality among abnormal responders. Comparing the heart rate recovery response to the Duke prognostic score, heart rate recovery produced survival curves similar to the Duke score, and among patients with abnormal scores on both tests, survival was even further compromised.

Our group attempted to validate heart rate recovery as a prognostic marker, addressed whether it had any diagnostic value, and tried to clarify some of the methodological issues surrounding its use (e.g., what is the optimal recovery rate and what time point postexercise should it be measured?).[66] Among 2193 patients who underwent both treadmill testing and coronary angiography over a 13-year period, we found that a decrease in heart rate equaling 22 beats per minute or less at 2 minutes in recovery best identified high-risk patients (hazard ratio of 2.6). It was also observed that beta-blockers had no significant impact on the prognostic value of heart rate recovery. By multivariate analysis, the combination of a low exercise capacity (<5 METs) and an abnormal heart rate recovery response yielded a particularly poor prognosis, with these patients having a fivefold risk of mortality. Kaplan-Meier survival curves from this study illustrating the combination of heart rate responses in recovery and exercise capacity are illustrated in Figure 5-11. Interestingly, heart rate recovery did not add any *diagnostic* value.

Given these and other recent results documenting the prognostic power of heart rate recovery, it would seem prudent to include heart rate recovery routinely as part of the test summary. However, additional studies are needed to clarify a number of practical issues, such as population specificity, optimal criteria, and whether or not heart rate recovery is best defined using a cooldown walk versus the supine position.

MEASURES OF MAXIMAL EFFORT

Various objective measurements have been used in efforts to confirm that a maximal effort was performed. These measurements are important

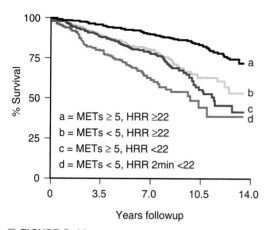

FIGURE 5–11

Kaplan-Meier survival curves among patients exhibiting normal and abnormal heart rate recovery responses. (*From Shetler K, Marcus R, Froelicher VF, et al: Heart rate recovery: Validation and methodologic issues. J Am Coll Cardiol 2001;38:1980-1987).*

TABLE 5–10. Indicators of maximal effort used in exercise studies
Patient appearance and breathing rate
Borg scale
Age-predicted heart rate and exercise capacity
Systolic blood pressure
Expired gas measurements: respiratory exchange ratio, plateau, and exceeding the ventilatory threshold
Venous lactate concentration

because they can provide information as to whether patients have exerted themselves maximally, something that has a number of relevant diagnostic and prognostic clinical implications. Historically, a decrease or failure to increase oxygen uptake by 150 mL per minute with an increase in workload has defined a *plateau* and has been thought to accurately reflect a maximal physiologic effort when interrupted protocols are used. Although this definition remained popular over several decades, the conditions under which this criterion was developed were quite different from the way clinical exercise testing was performed. Gradually, this marker of maximal physiologic effort fell into disfavor among many physiologists.[67-69] It is infrequently seen in continuous treadmill protocols among patients with heart disease, and when it occurs, it may actually be due to: (1) the patient holding on to the handrails, (2) incomplete expired air collection, (3) the criteria used for plateau, (4) differences in the gas exchange sampling interval used, or (5) differences in the equipment used. This issue is discussed in more detail in Chapter 3. Indicators of maximal effort that have been used are listed in Table 5-10; it should be noted that all of them have limitations.

The Borg scale has been developed to subjectively grade levels of exertion. This method is best applied to match levels of perceived exertion during comparison studies. The linear scale ranges from 6 (very, very light) to 20 (very, very hard); the nonlinear scale ranges from 0 to 10, and both

correlate with the percentage of maximal heart rate during exercise. *Respiratory exchange ratio*, defined as the ratio of carbon dioxide production to oxygen utilization, increases in proportion to exercise effort. Values greater than 1.10 are reached by most individuals at the point of maximal dynamic exercise. However, this ratio varies greatly, and its determination requires gas exchange analysis during exercise. Blood lactate levels have also been used (i.e., >7 or 8 mmol), but this requires mixed venous samples, and they also vary greatly between individuals. All objective criteria that have been proposed in the past are problematic because of intersubject variability and definition. Clinically, the indications outlined by the American Heart Association and American College of Sports Medicine for stopping an exercise test along with clinical judgment (see Table 2-2) should take precedence over any other reason for stopping.

TYPE OF DYNAMIC EXERCISE

Although steps, escalators, ladders, and other devices have been used over the years, the three predominant types of exercise testing used clinically are the treadmill and supine or upright bicycle ergometry. Position and type of exercise influence the physiologic response to exercise. We and other groups have found maximal heart rate to be fairly consistent in a wide range of patients with various treadmill and upright cycle ergometer protocols. (See Chapter 2 for discussion of comparison of exercise modes.) Supine bicycle ergometry is commonly used for radionuclide studies and for cardiac catheterization studies. Because of changes in venous return and filling pressures, the supine position results in a lower resting heart rate and higher end-diastolic volumes. When supine, there is little change in stroke volume or end-diastolic volume during exercise from values obtained at rest. As a result of the unusual position and positional disadvantage, there usually is an element of isometric exercise and a lower mechanical efficiency in the supine position. In general, patients are less able to give maximal efforts in the supine position, and maximal heart rate is usually significantly lower, whereas SBP is often higher. In patients with significant CAD, angina may develop at a lower double product in the supine compared to the upright position, which may also contribute to a lower maximal heart rate.

BLOOD PRESSURE RESPONSE

SBP should rise with increasing treadmill or cycle ergometer workloads. Diastolic blood pressure usually remains about the same, but the fifth Korotkoff sound can sometimes be heard all the way to zero in healthy young subjects. Although a rising diastolic blood pressure can be associated with CAD, more likely it is a marker for labile hypertension, which leads to CAD. The highest SBP should be achieved at maximal workload. When exercise is stopped, some individuals will experience an abrupt drop in SBP owing to peripheral pooling. For this reason, patients should not be left standing on the treadmill when the test is terminated. The SBP usually normalizes shortly after the patient is placed in the supine position during recovery, but it may remain below normal for several hours after the test. As mentioned earlier, the product of heart rate and SBP (double product), determined by cuff and auscultation, correlates highly with measured myocardial oxygen uptake during exercise. Usually, an individual patient's angina symptoms will be precipitated at approximately the same double product. Double product has also been used as an estimate of the maximal workload that the left ventricle can perform.

It should be emphasized that the automated devices for measuring SBP, although popular, are not as reliable as manual methods. While the available devices generally correlate with manual methods, they have not been adequately validated, particularly for the detection of exertional hypotension. In one study assessing the performance of many of the automated devices, it was reported that only half had acceptable accuracy and reliability.[70] Thus, the major guidelines on exercise testing continue to recommend manual methods for measuring blood pressure during exercise.

In a seminal study assessing clinical correlates and the prognostic applications of blood pressure responses to exercise, Irving et al[71] examined six groups of subjects: 5459 men and 749 women classified into three categories each: 2532 men and 244 women who were asymptomatic and healthy, 592 men and 158 women who were hypertensive, and 1586 men and 347 women who had clinical manifestations of CAD. None had undergone cardiac surgery; all had their followup status ascertained by periodic mail questionnaires. Reported deaths were reviewed and classified by three cardiologists; 140 deaths were attributed to CAD, 118 of them occurring in the men classified as having such disease.

Retesting of 156 persons from 1 to 32 months later showed that blood pressure values agreed within 10% in two thirds; the overall mean difference was only 8.6 mmHg, and the correlation at maximal exercise was superior to that of the resting observations obtained just before exercise. Hypertensive patients had a significantly greater body weight than normotensive persons. Among men, the lowest maximal systolic pressure was observed in the group with CAD; among women, the lowest maximal systolic pressure was found in the healthy group.

Patients with CAD were slightly older, and only the women showed a significant correlation between maximal systolic pressure and age. Only 5% of the variation in maximal systolic pressure in the patients with CAD was due to a shortened duration of exercise. Maximal systolic pressures correlated fairly well ($r = 0.46$ to 0.68 for the various groups) with resting systolic pressure, and this relation was independent of the diagnosis of cardiovascular disease in both men and women. Relations between blood pressure, the number of stenotic coronary arteries, and EF at rest were examined in 182 men with CAD and 22 without such disease. Lower maximal systolic pressures were often associated with two- or three-vessel disease or reduced EF, or both. The prognostic value of maximal systolic pressure for subsequent death resulting from CAD was examined in the men. The annual rate of sudden cardiac death increased from 6.6 per 1000 men with maximal systolic pressure of 200 mmHg or more to 25.3 and 97.9 per 1000, respectively, for those with 140 to 199 mmHg and less than 140 mmHg maximal systolic pressure. Cardiomegaly, Q waves on the resting ECG, and persistent postexertional ST depression were more common in men with the lowest systolic pressure at maximal exercise.

Over the last 3 decades, many other studies have reported that a comparatively low SBP response to exercise is associated with a poor prognosis.

This is particularly true among patients with chronic heart failure.[72] It would appear that the capacity to achieve an adequate SBP requires a relatively normal functioning left ventricle such that cardiac output increases in proportion to the increase in work rate, and that it can be sustained even when exertion is near-maximal.

Exertional Hypotension. *Exercise-induced hypotension* (EIH) has been demonstrated in most studies to be associated with either a poor prognosis or a high risk of angiographically documented CAD. Although studies on EIH have varied widely in terms of population, definition of EIH, and endpoints for followup, this abnormal SBP response has consistently been found to indicate an increased risk for cardiac events. In addition, EIH has been associated with cardiac complications during exercise testing and appears to be corrected by CABS.[73-76]

The normal blood pressure response to dynamic upright exercise is characterized by a progressive increase in SBP, no change or a decrease in diastolic blood pressure, and a widening of the pulse pressure.[77] Even when tested to exhaustion, normal individuals do not exhibit a reduction in SBP.[78] Exercise-induced decreases in SBP can occur in patients with CAD, valvular heart disease,[79] chronic heart failure, and arrhythmias. Occasionally, patients without clinically significant heart disease will exhibit EIH during exercise owing to antihypertensive therapy including beta-blockers, prolonged strenuous exercise, vasovagal responses, and on rare occasions it has been reported to occur in normal females. Pathophysiologically, EIH could be due to left ventricular dysfunction, exercise-induced ischemia causing left ventricular dysfunction, or papillary muscle dysfunction and mitral regurgitation. Rich et al[80] described a patient in whom EIH was found to be due to right ventricular ischemia.

Numerous studies have addressed the diagnostic and prognostic implications of EIH. Their important findings regarding definition, prevalence, high-risk subgroups, intervention, and mortality are summarized in Table 5-11.[71, 73-75, 81-91] One difficulty encountered in interpreting these studies is that although EIH is usually related to CAD and a poor prognosis, various criteria have been used to define it. This variation probably explains why the significance of EIH ranges from life-threatening in some studies to benign in others.

To further investigate the causes, definition, and predictive power of EIH, Dubach et al[81] analyzed patients referred for exercise testing at the Long Beach VA Medical Center. This prospective study included all patients referred for clinical reasons to the treadmill laboratory and who were the followed-up for a 2-year period for cardiac events. The population consisted of 2036 patients, 131 (6.4%) of whom exhibited a drop below the standing rest value.

To clarify the uncertainty regarding the definition of EIH, the following criteria were applied: (1) a drop of 20 mmHg or more in SBP after an initial rise but no fall below the value at rest and (2) a drop in SBP below the standing rest value. A drop of 20 mmHg was felt to be sufficient to avoid the technical limitations associated with ascertaining a true drop in blood pressure during treadmill testing. It was demonstrated that the definition of "a drop below rest" was clearly a better criterion than "a drop of 20 mmHg" for predicting increased risk for deaths and MIs. Therefore, the odds (risk) ratio of EIH for death was calculated using only the criterion of an SBP drop below rest.

While the average prevalence of EIH in previous studies was 8% (553/6693), the prevalence at LBVAMC was 5%. The predictive value for left main or three-vessel disease ranged from 20% to 100% in previous studies, with an average of 48% for the prevalence and 68% for the predictive value (see Table 5-11). In our study, the prevalence of severe CAD in those with EIH was 45% and the predictive value was 61%. The wide scatter of prevalences of EIH and of left main and three-vessel disease, and consequently in the predictive value of EIH, is the result of the variability in patient selection and methodologies used in the studies. In the reported studies, varying percentages of patients underwent cardiac catheterization, and it was not always possible to distinguish between left main and triple-vessel disease or to determine whether the right coronary artery was also involved when left main disease was present. Patients with valvular heart disease, cardiomyopathy, and women were not consistently included or excluded. In spite of these limitations, a consistent finding among the studies is that slightly more than half of the patients with known or suspected CAD and EIH had left main or three-vessel disease.

Fifteen percent of our patients with EIH had neither a history of MI nor an ischemic response during treadmill testing. There was no bradycardia, as is usually associated with a vasovagal reaction, nor could we find a relationship between beta-blocker therapy and EIH. Therefore, our results suggested that factors other than those

TABLE 5–11. Summary of major studies on significance of exercise-induced hypotension (EIH)

Investigator	No. subjects	Incidence of EIH* (%)	Definition of EIH	Predictive value of EIH for lm/3vd (%)	Findings
Thomson and Kelemen (1975)[75]	17	—	Fall in SBP below resting levels accompanied by chest pain and ST-segment depression	100	Multivessel CAD was found in all patients with EIH. All six patients who had CABS normalized exercise BP response
Irving et al (1977)[71]	6	—	Decrease or limited increase (<10 mmHg) in SBP	—	EIH was associated with ventricular fibrillation post exercise in all six cases
Levites et al (1978)[88]	1105	2.7	Decrease in SBP below resting level	20	Extent of CAD was not different between those with and without EIH
Morris et al (1978)[74]	1020	2.5	Decrease in SBP ≥10 mmHg	78	EIH was highly specific for multivessel CAD
Sanmarco et al (1980)[84]	378	24	Failure of SBP to rise ≥10 mmHg or a decrease ≥20 mmHg during exercise	70	Sensitivity, specificity, and predictive value of EIH were 38.6%, 87.4%, and 70% for 3VD or LM disease, respectively; values were similar to ST-segment depression
Weiner et al (1982)[82]	436	10.8	Decrease in SBP during exercise below pre-exercise standing level	55	EIH was not associated with exercise-induced complications, but most subjects had severe ischemic responses. EIH was reversed with CABS and has 8% 3-year mortality
Hammermeister et al (1983)[83]	557	6.3	Decrease in exercise SBP below resting SBP	50	EIH was associated with CAD and LV dysfunction
Hakki et al (1986)[85]	127	13.4	Decrease in SBP of ≥10 mmHg	—	Prior MI, abnormal EF, multivessel CAD, and Tl[201] perfusion were defects more common with EIH
Mazzotta et al (1987)[86]	224	20.0	Failure of BP to increase or overt decrease of BP during exercise testing	—	EIH was related to severity of LV dysfunction only when symptoms and hemodynamic decompensation existed
Gibbons et al (1987)[87]	820	3.0	Decrease in SBP at peak exercise ≥10 mmHg from SBP at rest	—	Of 27 patients with EIH, 22 had 3VD or LM CAD: most had decreased EF and wall motion abnormalities with exercise
Dubach et al (1988)[81]	2036	6.4	Decrease in SBP during exercise below standing pre-exercise value	61	EIH was associated with 3.2 times the risk for cardiac events during 2-year followup. EIH was defined as drop in SBP of only 20 mmHg, not associated with increased risk
Morrow et al (1993)[89]	2546	3.1	Fall in SBP below standing rest	—	Degree of decrease or failure to raise SBP graded by 1 to 4 used as part of multivariate score to predict mortality
Frenneaux et al (1992)[90]	129 (HCM)	33	Decrease in SBP ≥20 mmHg	—	EIH due to lower systemic vascular resistance at peak exercise
Iskandrian et al (1992)[91]	25 (CAD)	—	Decrease in SBP ≥20 mmHg	—	Extent of CAD and thallium ischemia similar between those with and without EIH

*Percent incidence of EIH among cohort of exercise test referrals.

CABS, coronary artery bypass surgery; CAD, coronary artery disease; DCM, dilated cardiomyopathy; EF, ejection fraction; EIH, exercise-induced hypotension; HCM, hypertrophic cardiomyopathy; LM, left main; LV, left ventricular; MI, myocardial infarction; SBP, systolic blood pressure; 3VD, three-vessel disease.

just mentioned can cause EIH, such as abnormal peripheral vasodilation during exercise or exercise-induced mitral regurgitation.

All of the patients with EIH who died had either a history of MI or an ischemic response during the exercise test. Since no deaths occurred in patients with EIH who had neither a prior MI nor ischemia, there could be two hypothetical mechanisms for EIH: (1) a primary cardiac cause owing to left ventricular dysfunction or ischemia that is associated with an increased risk of death or (2) an unknown, noncardiac cause probably resulting from an abnormal but benign peripheral vascular response. Patients with EIH clearly have an increased risk of death. In all the study sub-groups, the risk of death was at least two times greater in patients with EIH than in those without EIH, with the exception of patients recovering from a recent MI. The patients recovering from a recent MI had the highest death rate, suggesting that the degree of left ventricular dysfunction must predominate over other predictors, including EIH.

Weiner et al,[82] Thompson and Kelemen,[75] and Morris et al[74] found a lower mortality in patients with EIH who received an intervention—CABS or percutaneous transluminal coronary angioplasty—than in those who were medically treated. Our results confirmed this, but were even more striking: we found 12 deaths in 95 medically treated patients and no deaths in 22 patients who had an intervention. This suggests that percutaneous transluminal coronary angioplasty or CABS in patients with EIH can reduce mortality. However, it should be noted that the patients were not randomized to surgery in any of those studies. Li et al,[76] Thompson and Kelemen,[75] and Morris et al[74] reported a reversing of EIH with CABS. Eighteen of our patients had EIH that was reversed by revascularization.

In the Seattle Heart Watch,[83] EIH was defined as a drop in SBP below rest. The study was performed in 1241 patients who had treadmill testing and angiography. As defined, EIH had a limited sensitivity for severe forms of CAD and a risk ratio of 2 or less. However, the predictive value was high when EIH did occur—50% for triple-vessel or left main disease. Of course, predictive value is directly related to the prevalence of left main disease in the population. It is interesting to note that EIH was equally accurate for diagnosing triple-vessel disease, left main disease, or left ventricular dysfunction, but the differences in predictive value for these findings were due to the different prevalences of these abnormalities.

These results were confirmed by Weiner et al,[82] who found that a fall in SBP occurred in 23% of patients with left main disease versus 17% of those with triple-vessel disease and 6% of those with milder forms of disease. As an indicator of either left main or three-vessel disease, a fall in SBP had a predictive value of 66% and a sensitivity of 19%. Irving and Bruce[73] described six men clinically diagnosed with CAD and having postexertional ventricular fibrillation after maximal exercise testing. The common feature of their treadmill test was exertional hypotension, that is, a decrease or a limited increase (10 mmHg) in SBP. All six men were successfully cardioverted. The researchers concluded that close monitoring of changes in systolic pressure during and shortly after exercise testing is as important as the evaluation of ST changes. This study underscores the importance of closely monitoring blood pressure during an exercise test for safety reasons.

The limitations of the studies on EIH include the following: invasive measurements have not been made during exercise to clarify the causes of EIH; the reproducibility of EIH has not been adequately explored; inadequate numbers of patients have had data on ventricular function; and the pre-exercise SBP was the reference value rather than a true "resting" systolic pressure. In addition, left ventricular function was often only indirectly assessed by a history of MI, and thallium scintigraphy was not available to confirm silent ischemia. Finally, patients with EIH were not randomized to interventions, so conclusions regarding the impact of revascularization on survival need to be confirmed by a randomized trial. It is important to note that EIH has mainly been described during treadmill testing, and limited data are available with bicycle ergometer testing. Nevertheless, studies are reasonably consistent in regard to the prevalence, prognosis, and predictive value of EIH.

The following conclusions can be made regarding EIH:

1. The definition of EIH is of crucial importance in the evaluation of the exercise test response. A drop in SBP below pre-exercise values is the most ominous criterion; a drop of 20 mmHg or more without a fall below pre-exercise values has a significantly lower predictive value. However, the exercise test should be stopped when a drop of 10 to 20 mmHg is detected, as suggested in the American Heart Association/American College of Cardiology and American College of Sports Medicine guidelines.

2. EIH can be due to either left ventricular dysfunction (as reflected by MI status) or ischemia. In the roughly 10% of patients in which EIH occurs without association with either of these two factors, EIH appears to be benign. Although speculative, other potential mechanisms of EIH that deserve further investigation include exercise-induced mitral regurgitation and a (noncardiac) peripheral vasodilatory mechanism.
3. Although the risk of mortality is increased in patients with EIH, two subgroups in our cohort did not show this increased risk. EIH was not associated with increased risk in those tested within 3 weeks after an MI nor in those without a prior myocardial infarction or ischemia during the exercise test.

While it is important to note that the definitions for EIH have varied widely, it is an exercise test response that clearly indicates a significantly increased risk for cardiac events. EIH is usually related to myocardial ischemia, and the increased risk associated with this response has frequently been associated with three-vessel or left main CAD. Although EIH appears to be reversed by revascularization procedures, confirmation of a beneficial effect on survival requires a randomized trial.

Excessive Rise in Systolic Blood Pressure During Exercise. An excessive rise in SBP during an exercise test, frequently termed *exercise-induced hypertension*, has received much less attention than the aforementioned blood pressure decreases during exercise. Hypertensive responses, often defined as an increase in SBP to levels exceeding 220 to 250 mmHg, have generally been associated with lower mortality rates relative to normal blood pressure responses.[71,89,92] Those exhibiting hypertensive responses to exercise have been shown to have a lower prevalence of angiographic CAD.[92] Exaggerated SBP responses to exercise have been reported to be more common in elderly subjects and those with hypertension, even when blood pressure is well-controlled at rest, and has been suggested to be a predictor of future resting hypertension and the development of left ventricular hypertrophy.[93-96] Ha et al[97] recently reported that an SBP response to an exercise test of more than 220 mmHg in men or 190 mmHg in women (or a diastolic blood pressure increase >10 mmHg or exceeding 90 mmHg) was associated with a greater likelihood of echocardiographic wall motion abnormalities during exercise, even in the absence of angiographic CAD. Some of the major studies in this area are outlined in Table 5-12.

The clinical significance of exercise-induced hypertension has not been fully clarified. This response may be associated with resting hypertension, may be a normal variant, or may have another underlying cause such as a neurogenic abnormality in peripheral vascular regulation.

TABLE 5-12. Summary of major studies on significance of excessive blood pressure (EBP) responses to exercise

Investigator	No. subjects	Incidence of EBP (%)*	Definition of ebp	Findings
Irving (1977)	—	—	—	—
Lauer (1995)[92]	9608	33	>210 mmHg in men, >190 mmHg in women	EBP associated with lower prevalence of severe CAD and lower mortality rate (RR = 0.20)
Chatterjee (1994)	100	26	Any increase in DBP with exercise	80% of abnormal responders had CAD vs. 45% of normal responders
Wilson (1990)	35	35	≥230 mmHg SBP, ≥100 mmHg DBP	EBP subjects had similar cardiac output responses to exercise, but higher peripheral resistance
Allison (1999)	150	—	≥214 mmHg systolic	Subjects with EBP were 3.6 times more likely to have a CV event, and 2.4 times more like to have future diagnosis of hypertension
Ha (2002)[97]	132	24	>220 mmHg SBP in men; >190 SBP in women, or DBP >10 or above 90 mmHg	82% of those with EBP had positive exercise tests. EBP associated with wall motion abnormalities by echo even in absence of CAD

*Usually a selected group or included only those referred for angiography. Actual overall incidence of EBP is much lower.
DBP, diastolic blood pressure; EBP, excessive blood pressure response to exercise; SBP, systolic blood pressure.

It appears to be associated with more favorable outcomes. The long-standing recommendation in the American Heart Association/American College of Cardiology and American College of Sports Medicine guidelines to stop an exercise test when SBP reaches 250 mmHg or more represents an intuitive and reasonable limit rather than one based on clinical studies.

Exercise-Recovery Ratio for Systolic Blood Pressure. A body of data has been published in recent years suggesting that the ratio of SBP in recovery to peak exercise SBP is a marker of CAD. However, this ratio is not widely used, perhaps because the mechanism for this response and its association with disease has not been fully defined. Another problem has been differences in the criteria used and the time point in recovery used to derive the ratio. Several studies have used a ratio of SBP at 3 minutes into recovery to peak exercise of 0.90 as a cutpoint for abnormal, and have demonstrated a diagnostic accuracy for CAD similar to that for ST depression.[98-100] Others have found significantly higher ratios for normal subjects than for patients with CAD or heart failure[101-105] or have shown an abnormal ratio to be a marker for more severe heart failure.[102,106] Kato et al[100] found an abnormal response to be a strong predictor of cardiac death in post-MI patients. Laukkanen et al[105] reported that an abnormal recovery response was associated with a 69% higher incidence of MI during a mean 13-year followup. Amon et al[107] divided the SBP at 1, 2, and 3 minutes after exercise by the peak exercise SBP. These three ratios declined steadily during recovery among normal subjects, from 0.85 to 0.79 at 2 minutes and to 0.73 at 3 minutes. The ratios in patients with CAD remained elevated at 0.97 to 0.93. Abnormal ratios were more frequent in patients with CAD than in those with either ST-segment depression or angina.

NORMAL HEART RATE AND BLOOD PRESSURE VALUES

The early emphasis placed on the exercise ECG tended to de-emphasize other exercise responses. As outlined above, considering heart rate and blood pressure responses during exercise and recovery may improve the diagnostic and prognostic value of exercise testing and may be useful for identifying the presence or the severity of CAD. The value of any measurement in providing diagnostic information from exercise testing depends on (1) the accuracy and completeness with which a measurement has been made in healthy individuals (reference values) and (2) the effectiveness with which certain limits of the measurement (discriminant values) separate healthy individuals from those with disease. The reference values presented in Figure 5-12 were developed to determine discriminant values for separating patient groups. Many exercise test responses do not have a Gaussian distribution and require that nonparametric statistical tests be used. Therefore, discriminant values should be determined as percentiles rather than as standard deviations or confidence limits.

USING HEMODYNAMIC MEASUREMENTS TO ESTIMATE MYOCARDIAL OXYGEN CONSUMPTION

Although heart rate and stroke volume are important determinants of both maximal oxygen uptake and myocardial oxygen consumption, myocardial oxygen consumption has other independent determinants. It has been demonstrated that the relative metabolic loads of the entire body and those of the heart are determined separately and may not change in parallel with a given intervention. The heart receives only 4% of cardiac output at rest, but it utilizes 10% of systemic oxygen uptake. In the myocardium, the wide arteriovenous oxygen difference of 10 to 20 vol% at rest reflects the fact that oxygen in the blood passing through the coronary artery circulation is nearly maximally extracted. This value can be compared to the 4 to 6 vol% difference across the systemic circulation. When the myocardium requires a greater oxygen supply, coronary blood flow must be increased by coronary artery dilatation. During exercise, coronary blood flow can increase through normal coronary arteries up to five times the normal resting flow.

The increased demand for myocardial oxygen required by dynamic exercise is the key to the use of exercise testing as a diagnostic tool for CAD. Myocardial oxygen consumption cannot be directly measured in a practical manner, but its relative demand can be estimated from its determinants, such as heart rate, wall tension (left ventricular pressure and diastolic volume), contractility, and cardiac work. Although all of these factors increase during exercise, increased heart rate is particularly important in patients who have obstructive CAD. An increase in heart rate

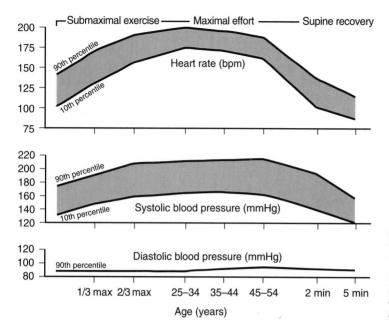

THE RESPONSE OF HEALTHY MEN TO TREADMILL EXERCISE

FIGURE 5-12
The hemodynamic responses of over 700 healthy men to maximal treadmill exercise. *Bands* represent 80% of the population; 10% had values *above the band*, and 10% had values *below the band*.

results in a shortening of the diastolic filling period, the time during which coronary blood flow is the greatest. In normal coronary arteries, dilation occurs. However, in obstructed vessels, dilation is limited and flow can be decreased by the shortening of the diastolic filling period. This causes inadequate blood flow and therefore insufficient oxygen supply.

SUMMARY

Hemodynamic information, including heart rate, blood pressure, and exercise capacity, are important features of the exercise test. Because it can objectively quantify exercise capacity, exercise testing is now commonly used for disability evaluation rather than reliance on functional classifications. No questionnaire or submaximal test can provide as reliable a result as a symptom-limited exercise test. Age-predicted maximal heart rate targets are relatively useless for clinical purposes, and they should not be used for exercise testing endpoints. It is surprising how much steeper the age-related decline in maximal heart rate is in clinically referred populations as compared with age-matched normal subjects or volunteers. Nomograms greatly facilitate the description of exercise capacity relative to age and enable comparisons among patients. However, numerous different regression equations

have been used to express exercise capacity relative to gender and age.

When expressing exercise capacity as a relative percentage of what is deemed normal, careful consideration should be given to population specificity. Exercise capacity is influenced by many factors other than age and gender, including health, activity level, body composition, and the exercise mode and protocol used. Additional studies are needed to develop normal standards for exercise capacity in women. Although exertional hypotension has been defined in many different ways, it has been shown to predict severe angiographic CAD and is associated with a poor prognosis. A failure of SBP to adequately increase is particularly worrisome in patients who have sustained a myocardial infarction. The exercise test should always be stopped when a sustained reduction in systolic pressure occurs. Recent studies have documented the prognostic power of CI during exercise and the rate in which heart rate recovers following an exercise test. Although many laboratories now routinely include these responses as part of the exercise test report, several methodological issues need to be standardized. The diagnostic and prognostic value of the recovery/peak exercise SBP ratio requires further study. Until automated devices are adequately validated, we strongly recommend that blood pressure be taken manually with a cuff and stethoscope.

REFERENCES

1. Froelicher VF, Thompson AJ, Noquero I, et al: Prediction of maximal oxygen consumption. Comparison of the Bruce and Balke treadmill protocols. Chest 1975;68:331-336.
2. Patterson J, Naughton J, Pietras R, et al: Treadmill exercise in assessment of the functional capacity of patients with cardiac disease. Am J Cardiol 1972;30:757-762.
3. Goldman L, Hashimoto B, Cook EF, Loscalzo A: Comparative reproducibility and validity of systems for assessing cardiovascular functional class: Advantages of a new specific activity scale. Circulation 1981;64:1227-1234.
4. Hlatky M, Boineau R, Higgenbotham M, et al: A brief, self-administered questionnaire to determine functional capacity (The Duke Activity Status Index). Am J Cardiol 1989;64:651-654.
5. Myers J, Do D, Herbert W, et al: A nomogram to predict exercise capacity from a specific activity questionnaire and clinical data. Am J Cardiol 1994;73:591-596.
6. McKirnan D, Sullivan M, Jensen D, Froelicher VF: Treadmill performance and cardiac function in selected patients with coronary heart disease. J Am Coll Cardiol 1984;3:253-261.
7. Ehsani AA, Biello D, Seals DR, et al: The effects of left ventricular systolic function on maximal aerobic exercise capacity in asymptomatic patients with coronary artery disease. Circulation 1984;70:552-560.
8. Weber KT, Kinasewitz GT, Janicki J, Fishman AP: Oxygen utilization and ventilation during exercise in patients with chronic cardiac failure. Circulation 1982;65:1213-1222.
9. Litchfield RL, Kerber RE, Benge JW, et al: Normal exercise capacity in patients with severe left ventricular dysfunction: Compensatory mechanisms. Circulation 1982;66:129-134.
10. Higginbotham MB, Morris KG, Conn EH, et al: Determinants of variable exercise performance among patients with severe left ventricular dysfunction. Am J Cardiol 1983;51:52-60.
11. Wilson J, Rayos G, Yeoh TK, et al: Dissociation between exertional symptoms and circulatory function in patients with heart failure. Circulation 1995;92:47-53.
12. Myers J, Froelicher VF: Hemodynamic determinants of exercise capacity in chronic heart failure. Ann Intern Med 1991;115:377-386.
13. Sullivan MJ, Green HJ, Cobb FR: Exercise training in patients with severe left ventricular dysfunction: Hemodynamic and metabolic effects. Circulation 1988;78:506-515.
14. Dubach P, Myers J, Dziekan G, et al: Effect of high-intensity exercise training on central hemodynamic responses to exercise in men with reduced left ventricular function. J Am Coll Cardiol 1997;29:1591-1598.
15. Piepoli MF, Flather M, Coats AJS: Overview of studies of exercise training in chronic heart failure: The need for a prospective randomized multicentre European trial. Eur Heart J 1998;19:830-841.
16. Piepoli MF, Davos C, Francis DP, Coats AJ: ExTraMATCH Collaborative. Exercise training meta-analysis of trials in patients with chronic heart failure. BMJ 2004;328:189-196.
17. Pfeiffer MA, Pfeffer JM, Fishbein MC, et al: Myocardial infarction size and ventricular function in rats. Circ Res 1979;44:503-512.
18. Carter CL, Amundsen LR: Infarct size and exercise capacity after myocardial infarction. J Appl Physiol 1977;42:782-785.
19. Grande P, Pedersen A: Myocardial infarct size and cardiac performance during exercise soon after myocardial infarction. Br Heart J 1982;47:44-50.
20. DePace NL, Iskandrian AS, Hakki A, et al: Use of QRS scoring and thallium-201 scintigraphy to assess left ventricular function after myocardial infarction. Am J Cardiol 1982;50:1262-1268.
21. Jette M, Sidney K, Blumchen G: Metabolic equivalents (METs) in exercise testing, exercise prescription, and evaluation of functional capacity. Clin Cardiol 1990;13:555-565.
22. Morris C, Myers J, Kawaguchi T, et al: Nomogram based on metabolic equivalents and age for assessing aerobic capacity in men. J Am Coll Cardiol 1993;22:175-182.
23. Bruce RA, Kusumi F, Hosmer D: Maximal oxygen intake and nomographic assessment of functional aerobic impairment in cardiovascular disease. Am Heart J 1973;85:546-562.
24. Wolthuis RA, Froelicher VF, Fischer J, et al: New practical treadmill protocol for clinical use. Am J Cardiol 1977;39:697-700.
25. American College of Sports Medicine: Guidelines for Exercise Testing and Prescription, 6th ed. Baltimore, Lippincott, Williams & Wilkins, 2000.
26. Gibbons RJ, Balady GJ, Beasley JW et al: ACC/AHA guidelines for exercise testing. A report of the American College of Cardiology/American Heart Association Task Force on Practice Guidelines (Committee on Exercise Testing). J Am Coll Cardiol 1997;30:260-315.
27. Myers J, Buchanan N, Walsh D, et al: Comparison of the ramp versus standard exercise protocols. J Am Coll Cardiol 1991;17:1334-1342.
28. Froelicher VF, Allen M, Lancaster MC: Maximal treadmill testing of normal USAF aircrewmen. Aerosp Med 1974;45:310-315.
29. Dehn MM, Bruce RA: Longitudinal variations in maximal oxygen intake with age and activity. J Appl Physiol 1972;33:805-807.
30. Hammond HK, Froelicher VF: Normal and abnormal heart rate responses to exercise. Prog Cardiovasc Dis 1985;27:271-296.
31. Sullivan M, McKirnan D: Errors in predicting functional capacity for post-myocardial infarction patients using a modified Bruce protocol. Am Heart J 1984;107:486-491.
32. Roberts JM, Sullivan M, Froelicher VF, et al: Predicting oxygen uptake from treadmill testing in normal subjects and coronary artery disease patients. Am Heart J 1984;108:1454-1460.
33. Morris CK, Ueshima K, Kawaguchi T, et al: The prognostic value of exercise capacity: A review of the literature. Am Heart J 1991;122:1423-1430.
34. Mark DB, Lauer MS: Exercise capacity. The prognostic variable that doesn't get enough respect. Circulation 2003;108:1534-1536.
35. McDonough JR, Danielson RA, Willis RE, Vine KL: Maximal cardiac output during exercise in patients with coronary artery disease. Am J Cardiol 1974;33:23-29.
36. Hossack KF, Bruce RA, Kusumi F, Kannagi T: Prediction of maximal cardiac output in preoperative patients with coronary artery disease. Am J Cardiol 1983;52:721-726.
37. Atwood JE, Myers J, Sandhu S, et al: Optimal sampling interval to estimate heart rate at rest and during exercise in atrial fibrillation. Am J Cardiol 1989;63:45-48.
38. Sheffield LT, Malouf JA, Sawyer JA, et al: Maximal heart rate and treadmill performance of healthy women in relation to age. Circulation 1978;57:79-84.
39. Bruce RA, Gey GO Jr., Cooper MN, et al: Seattle Heart Watch: Initial clinical, circulatory and electrocardiographic response to maximal exercise. Am J Cardiol 1974;33:459-469.
40. Cooper KH, Purdy JG, White SR, et al: Age-fitness adjusted maximal heart rates. Med Sport 1977;10:78-88.
41. Londeree BR, Moeschberger ML: Influence of age and other factors on maximal heart rate. J Cardiopulm Rehabil 1984;4:44-49.
42. Froelicher VF, Brammel H, Davis G, et al: A comparison of three maximal treadmill exercise protocols. J Appl Physiol 1974;36:720-725.
43. Graettinger W, Smith D, Neutel J, et al: Influence of left ventricular chamber size on maximal heart rate. Chest 1995;107:341-345.
44. Myers J: Physiologic adaptations to exercise and immobility. In SL Woods, E Sivarajan-Froelicher, CJ Holpenny, S Underhill-Motyer (eds): Cardiac nursing, 3rd ed. Philadelphia, JP Lippincott, 1995, pp. 147-162.
45. Convertino V, Hung J, Goldwater D, et al: Cardiovascular responses to exercise in middle-aged man after 10 days of bed rest. Circulation 1982;65:134-140.
46. Cunningham WL, Becker ES, Kreuzer F: Catecholamines in plasma and urine at high altitudes. J Appl Physiol 1965;20:607-610.
47. Hartley LH, Vogel JA, Cruz JC: Reduction of maximal exercise heart rate at altitude and its reversal with atropine. J Appl Physiol 1974;36:362-365.
48. Ellestad MH, Wan MKC: Predictive implications of stress testing—Follow-up of 2700 subjects after maximal treadmill stress testing. Circulation 1975;51:363-369.
49. McNeer JF, Margolis JR, Lee KL, et al: The role of the exercise test in the evaluation of patients for ischemic heart disease. Circulation 1978;57:64-70.
50. Bruce RA, Fisher FD, Cooper MN, et al: Separation of effects of cardiovascular disease and age on ventricular function with maximal exercise. Am J Cardiol 1974;34:757-763.
51. Lauer M, Mehta R, Pashkow F, et al: Association of chronotropic incompetence with echocardiographic ischemia and prognosis. J Am Coll Cardiol 1998;32:1280-1286.

52. Lauer M, Okin P, Martin G, et al: Impaired heart rate response to graded exercise: Prognostic implications of chronotropic incompetence in the Framingham Heart Study. Circulation 1996;93:1520-1526.

53. Lauer MS, Francis GS, Okin PM, et al: Impaired chronotropic response to exercise stress testing as a predictor of mortality. JAMA 1999;28:565-566.

54. Dresing TJ, Blackstone EH, Pashkow FJ, et al: Usefulness of impaired chronotropic response to exercise as a predictor of mortality, independent of the severity of coronary artery disease. Am J Cardiol 2000;86:602-609.

55. Hammond HK, Kelly TL, Froelicher VF: Radionuclide imaging correlates of heart rate impairment during maximal exercise testing. J Am Coll Cardiol 1983;2:826-833.

56. Colucci WS, Ribeiro JP, Rocco MB, et al: Impaired chronotropic response to exercise in patients with congestive heart failure. Role of postsynaptic beta-adrenergic desensitization. Circulation 1989;80:314-323.

57. Lauer MS: Heart rate response in stress testing: Clinical implications. ACC Curr J Rev 2001;10:16-19.

58. Schwartz PJ: The autonomic nervous system and sudden death. Eur Heart J 1998;19:F72-80.

59. La Rovere MT, Bigger JT, Marcus FI, et al: Baroreflex sensitivity and heart rate variability in prediction of total cardiac mortality after myocardial infarction. Lancet 1998;351:478-484.

60. Tsuji H, Venditti FJ Jr., Manders ES, et al: Reduced heart rate variability and mortality risk in an elderly cohort. The Framingham Heart Study. Circulation 1994;90:878-883.

61. Cotton FS, Dill DB: On the relation between the heart rate during exercise and that of immediate post exercise period. Am J Physiol 1935;111:544-556.

62. Imai K, Sato H, Hori M, et al: Vagally medicated heart rate recovery after exercise is accelerated in athletes but blunted in patients with chronic heart failure. J Am Coll Cardiol 1994;24:1529-1535.

63. Cole CR, Blackstone EH, Pashkow FJ, et al: Heart-rate recovery immediately after exercise as a predictor or mortality. N Engl J Med 1999;341:1351-1357.

64. Cole RC, Foody JM, Blackstone EH, Lauer MS: Heart rate recovery after submaximal exercise testing as a predictor of mortality in a cardiovascularly healthy cohort. Ann Intern Med 2000;132:552-555.

65. Nishime EO, Cole CR, Blackstone EH, et al: Heart rate recovery and treadmill exercise score as predictors of mortality in patients referred for exercise ECG. JAMA 2000;284:1392-1398.

66. Shetler K, Marcus R, Froelicher VF, et al: Heart rate recovery: Validation and methodologic issues. J Am Coll Cardiol 2001;38:1980-1987.

67. Myers J, Walsh D, Sullivan M, Froelicher VF: Effect of sampling on variability and plateau in oxygen uptake. J Appl Physiol 1990;68:404-410.

68. Noakes TD: Maximal oxygen uptake: "Classical" versus "contemporary" viewpoints: A rebuttal. Med Sci Sports Exerc 1998;30:1381-1398.

69. Day JR, Rossiter HB, Coats EM, et al: The maximally attainable VO2 during exercise in humans: The peak vs. maximum issue. J Appl Physiol 2003;95:1901-1907.

70. Bailey RH, Bauer JH: A review of common errors in the indirect measurement of blood pressure. Sphygmanometry. Arch Intern Med 1993;153:2741-2748.

71. Irving JB, Bruce RA, DeRouen TA: Variations in and significance of systolic pressure during maximal exercise (treadmill) testing. Am J Cardiol 1977;39:841-848.

72. Myers J, Gullestad L, Vagelos R, et al: Clinical, hemodynamic, and cardiopulmonary exercise test determinants of survival in patients referred for evaluation of heart failure. Ann Intern Med 1998;129:286-293.

73. Irving JB, Bruce RA: Exertional hypotension and postexertional ventricular fibrillation in stress testing. Am J Cardiol 1977;39:849-851.

74. Morris SN, Phillips JF, Jordan JW, McHenry PL: Incidence of significance of decreases in systolic blood pressure during graded treadmill exercise testing. Am J Cardiol 1978;41:221-226.

75. Thomson PD, Kelemen MH: Hypotension accompanying the onset of exertional angina. Circulation 1975;52:28-32.

76. Li W, Riggins R, Anderson R: Reversal of exertional hypotension after coronary bypass grafting. Am J Cardiol 1979;44:607-611.

77. Wolthuis RA, Froelicher VF, Fischer J, Triebwasser JH: The response of healthy men to treadmill exercise. Circulation 1977;55:153-157.

78. Saltin B, Sternberg J: Circulatory response to prolonged severe exercise. J Appl Physiol 1964;19:833-838.

79. Atwood JE, Kawanashi S, Myers J, Froelicher VF: Exercise testing in patients with aortic stenosis. Chest 1988;93:1083-1087.

80. Rich MW, Keller A, Chouhan L, Fischer K: Exercise-induced hypotension as a manifestation of right ventricular ischemia. Am Heart J 1988;115:184-186.

81. Dubach P, Froelicher VF, Klein J, et al: Exercise-induced hypotension in a male population—Criteria, causes, and prognosis. Circulation 1988;78:1380-1387.

82. Weiner DA, McCabe CH, Cutler SS, Ryan TJ: Decrease in systolic blood pressure during exercise testing: Reproducibility, response to coronary bypass surgery and prognostic significance. Am J Cardiol 1982;49:1627-1631.

83. Hammermeister KE, DeRouen TA, Dodge HT, Zia M: Prognostic and predictive value of exertional hypotension in suspected coronary heart disease. Am J Cardiol 1983;51:1261-1265.

84. Sanmarco M, Pontius S, Selvester R: Abnormal blood pressure response and marked ischemic ST-segment depression as predictors of severe coronary artery disease. Circulation 1980;61:572-578.

85. Hakki AH, Munley B, Hadjimiltiades S, et al: Determinants of abnormal blood pressure response to exercise in coronary artery disease. Am J Cardiol 1986;57:71-75.

86. Mazzotta G, Scopinara G, Falcidieno M, et al: Significance of abnormal blood pressure response during exercise-induced myocardial dysfunction after recent acute myocardial infarction. Am J Cardiol 1987;59:1256-1260.

87. Gibbons R, Hu D, Clements I, et al: Anatomic and functional significance of a hypotensive response during supine exercise radionuclide ventriculography. Am J Cardiol 1987;60:1-4.

88. Levites R, Baker T, Anderson G: The significance of hypotension developing during treadmill exercise testing. Am Heart J 1978;95:747-753.

89. Morrow K, Morris CK, Froelicher VF, et al: Prediction of cardiovascular death in men undergoing noninvasive evaluation for coronary artery disease. Ann Intern Med 1993;118:689-695.

90. Frenneaux MP, Counihan PJ, Caforio A, et al: Abnormal blood pressure response during exercise in hypertrophic cardiomyopathy. Circulation 1990;82:1995-2002.

91. Iskandrian AS, Kegel JG, Lemlek J, et al: Mechanism of exercise-induced hypotension in coronary artery disease. Am J Cardiol 1992;69:1517-1520.

92. Lauer MS, Pashkow FJ, Harvey SA, et al: Angiographic and prognostic implications of an exaggerated exercise systolic blood pressure response and rest systolic blood pressure in adults undergoing evaluation for suspected coronary artery disease. J Am Coll Cardiol 1995;26:1630-1636.

93. Dlin RA, Hanne N, Silverberg DS, Bar-Or O: Follow-up of normotensive men with exaggerated blood pressure response to exercise. Am Heart J 1983;106:316-320.

94. Benbassat J, Froom P: Blood pressure response to exercise as a predictor of hypertension. Arch Intern Med 1986;146:2053-2055.

95. Jackson AS, Squires WG, Grimes G, Beard EF: Prediction of future resting hypertension from exercise blood pressure. J Cardiac Rehabil 1983;3:263-268.

96. Gottdiener JS, Brown J, Zoltick J, Fletcher RD: Left ventricular hypertrophy in men with normal blood pressure: Relation to exaggerated blood pressure response to exercise. Ann Intern Med 1990;112:161-166.

97. Ha JW, Juracan EM, Mahoney DW, et al: Hypertensive response to exercise: A potential cause for new wall motion abnormality in the absence of coronary artery disease. J Am Coll Cardiol 2002;39:323-327.

98. Taylor AJ, Beller GA: Postexercise systolic blood pressure response: Clinical application to the assessment of ischemic heart disease. Am Fam Physician 1998;58:1126-1130.

99. Tsuda M, Hatano K, Hayashi H, et al: Diagnostic value of postexercise systolic blood pressure response for detecting coronary artery disease in patients with or without hypertension. Am Heart J 1993;125:718-725.

100. Kato K, Saito F, Hatano K, Tsuzuki J, et al: Prognostic value of abnormal postexercise systolic blood pressure response: Prehospital discharge test after myocardial infarction in Japan. Am Heart J 1990;119:264-271.
101. Acanfora D, De Caprio L, Cuomo S, et al: Diagnostic value of the ratio of recovery systolic blood pressure to peak exercise systolic blood pressure for the detection of coronary artery disease. Circulation 1988;77:1306-1310.
102. Nezuo S, Inoue S, Kawahara Y, et al: Clinical significance of abnormal postexercise systolic blood pressure response in patients with hypertrophic cardiomyopathy. Am J Cardiol 1996; 27:65-71.
103. Miyahara T, Yokota M, Iwase M, et al: Mechanism of abnormal postexercise systolic blood pressure response and its diagnostic value in patients with coronary artery disease. Am Heart J 1990; 120:40-49.
104. Abe K, Tsuda M, Hayashi H, et al: Diagnostic usefulness of postexercise systolic blood pressure response for detection of coronary artery disease in patients with electrocardiographic left ventricular hypertrophy. Am J Cardiol 1995;76:892-895.
105. Laukkanen JA, Kurl S, Salonen R, et al: Systolic blood pressure during recovery from exercise and the risk of acute myocardial infarction in middle-aged men. Hypertension 2004;44:820-825.
106. Kitaoka H, Takata J, Furuno T, et al: Delayed recovery of postexercise blood pressure in patients with chronic heart failure. Am J Cardiol 1997;79:1701-1704.
107. Amon KW, Richards KL, Crawford MH: Usefulness of the postexercise response of systolic blood pressure in the diagnosis of coronary artery disease. Circulation 1984;70:951-956.
108. Pollock ML, Bohannon RL, Cooper KH, et al: A comparative analysis of four protocols for maximal treadmill stress testing. Am Heart J 1976;92:39-46.
109. Irving JB, Bruce RA: Exertional hypotension and postexertional ventricular fibrillation in stress testing. Am J Cardiol 1977; 39:849-851.

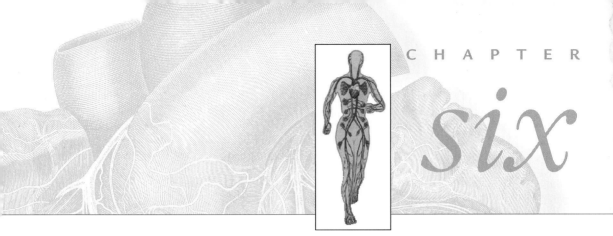

C H A P T E R

six

Interpretation of ECG and Subjective Responses (Chest Pain)

INTRODUCTION

This chapter will present information regarding the electrocardiographic (ECG) response to exercise. There is some duplication with the diagnostic chapter, but this chapter provides the basis for the later chapters by featuring the normal ECG responses to exercise and specific waveform behaviors. ECG responses to exercise with potential, but without established diagnostic value, such as alternans and frequency components, are also discussed. The three ST responses to exercise associated with ischemia: elevation, normalization, and depression will be presented in both chapters.

STUDIES OF THE COMPLETE ELECTROCARDIOGRAPHIC RESPONSE TO EXERCISE

The key historical studies describing the ECG response to progressive, dynamic exercise are outlined by the year of their presentation:

1908 – Einthoven[1] reported the first attempt to evaluate the response of the ECG to exercise. He made a number of accurate observations in a postexercise ECG, including an increase in the amplitude of the P and T waves and depression of the J junction.[1]

1953 – Simonson[2] reported the ECG response to treadmill testing of a wide age range of normal subjects.

1965 – Blomqvist[3] reported his classic description of the response of the Frank vectorcardiographic leads to bicycle exercise using computer techniques.

1973 – Rautaharju et al[4] analyzed P-, ST- and T-vector functions in the Frank leads in response to exercise. They reported that all P-wave vector measurements increased during exercise and were compatible with right atrial overload, whereas T-wave vectors decreased slightly. The ST-segment vector shifted clockwise to the right and upward.

1975 – Simoons and Hugenholtz[5] reported Frank lead vectorcardiographic changes during exercise in normal subjects. The direction and magnitudes of time-normalized P, QRS and ST vectors and other QRS parameters were analyzed during and after exercise in 56 apparently healthy men, aged 23 to 62 years of age. The PR interval and the P-wave amplitude increased during exercise. Direction of the P vectors did not change, differing with the previous reports that had noted changes consistent with right atrial overload. No significant change in QRS magnitude was observed, and the magnitude in spatial orientation and the maximum QRS vectors remained constant. QRS onset to T-wave peak shortened. The terminal QRS vectors and the initial ST vectors gradually shortened and shifted to the right and upward. The T-wave amplitude lessened during exercise. In the first minute of recovery, the P and T magnitudes markedly increased and then all measurements gradually returned to the resting level. There was an increase in S-wave duration in leads X and Y, and right-axis shift in the QRS complex was heart rate dependent. The ST-segment shifted upward to the right and posteriorly, and T-wave magnitude increased markedly in the first minute of recovery. The QRS complex shortened in some young individuals during exercise.

1979 – USAFMC Normal Aircrewmen Study was based on digital data from 40 low-risk normal subjects, processed and analyzed across treadmill times on the basis of waveform component and lead.[6] Emphasis will be given to this study because of our intimate knowledge of its findings.

USAFMC Normal Aircrewmen Study

Figure 6-1 illustrates the waveforms produced using median values of the measurements of all 40 subjects for leads V_5, Y, and Z. These figures demonstrate the specific waveform alterations that occur in response to maximal treadmill exercise. Supine, exercise to HR 120, maximal exercise, 1-minute recovery, and 5-minute recovery were chosen as representative times. There is depression of the J junction and peaking of the T waves at maximal exercise and at 1-minute recovery. Along with the J-junction (QRS end or ST_0) depression, marked ST upsloping is seen. J-junction depression did not occur in Z lead (which is equivalent to and of the same polarity as V_2). As the R wave decreases in amplitude, the S wave increases in depth. The QS duration shortens minimally, but the RT duration decreases in a larger amount.

Q-, R-, and S-Wave Amplitudes

In leads CM_5, V_5, CC_5, and Y, the Q-wave shows very small changes from the resting values; however, it does become slightly more negative at maximal exercise. Q-wave changes were not noted in the Z lead. Changes in median R-wave amplitude are not detected until near maximal and maximal effort is approached. At maximal exercise and on into 1-minute recovery, a sharp decrease in R-wave amplitude is observed in CM_5, V_5, and CC_5. These changes are not seen in the Z lead. The lowest median R-wave value in Y occurred at maximal exercise, with R-wave amplitude increasing by 1-minute recovery. In leads CM_5, V_5, and CC_5 the lowest R-wave amplitude was seen at 1-minute recovery. This different temporal response in R-waves in the lateral versus

inferior leads is unexplained. There is little change in S-wave amplitude in Z. However, in the other leads, the S-wave became greater in depth or more negative, showing a greater deflection at maximal exercise, and then gradually returning to resting values in recovery. A decrease in the QS interval occurred and it was shortest at maximal exercise. By 3 minutes of recovery, the QS interval returned to normal. A steady decrease in the duration of the RT interval decreased during exercise. The shortest interval was seen at maximal exercise and 1-minute recovery.

ST-Slope, J-Junction Depression and T-Wave Amplitude

The first amplitude measurement of the ST segment is made at the beginning of the ST segment, known as ST_0 or the J junction, and it is also the end of the QRS complex. This measurement has the widest range of responses to changes of heart rate of any ECG waveform and distinguishing this normal response from its response to ischemia is key to the diagnostic application of the exercise ECG. The amplitude of the J junction in lead Z was very little changed through exercise, but elevated slightly in recovery. It appears that the lead system affects the anterior-posterior presentation of the ST vector more than anticipated. The J junction was depressed in all other leads to a maximum depression at maximal exercise, and then it gradually returned toward pre-exercise values slowly in recovery. There was very little difference between the three left precordial leads. A dramatic increase in ST-segment slope was observed in all leads and was greatest at 1-minute recovery.

These changes returned toward pretest values during later recovery. The greatest or steepest slopes were seen in lead CM_5, which did not show the greatest ST-segment depression. A gradual decrease in T-wave amplitude was observed in all leads during early exercise. At maximal exercise the T wave began to increase, and at 1-minute recovery the amplitude was equivalent to resting values, except in leads Y and Z, where they were greater than at rest.

BLOOD COMPOSITION SHIFTS AND THE ECG

During exercise, there are elevations in plasma osmolality, potassium, sodium, calcium, phosphate, lactate, and proteins. There is a constant

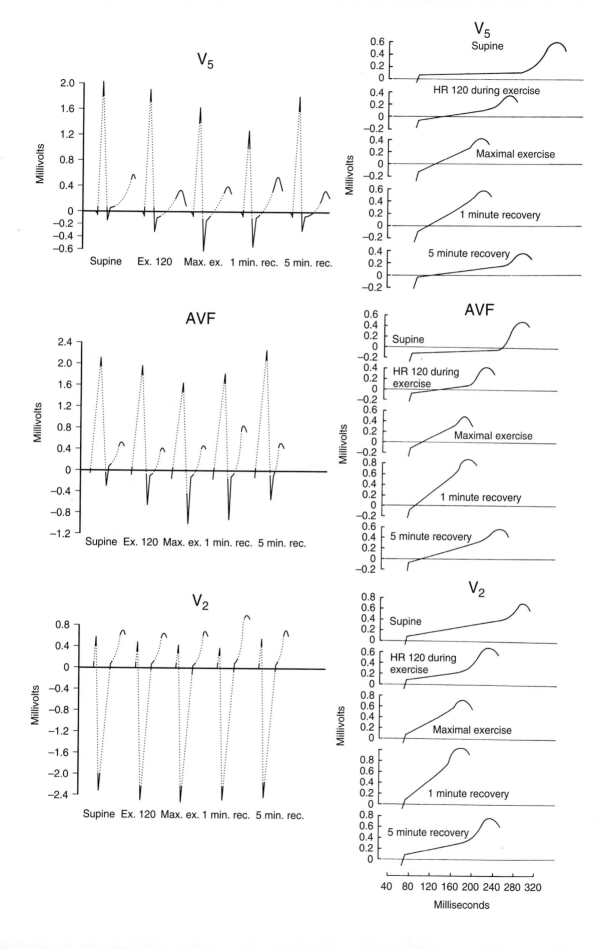

The waveforms produced using median values of the measurements of all 40 subjects for leads V_5, Y, and Z. These figures demonstrate the specific waveform alterations that occur in response to maximal treadmill exercise. Supine, exercise to HR 120, maximal exercise, 1-minute recovery, and 5-minute recovery were chosen as representative times for presentation of these median-based simulated waveforms.

and gradual increase in these measurements for both males and females, regardless of environmental conditions. Sodium and potassium rapidly return to normal after exercise. During respiratory acidosis, there is a loss of potassium from the musculoskeletal system that is increased by muscular activity. Potassium enters the myocardium during acidosis and exits after exercise. The mechanism for this variance between myocardial and skeletal muscle is not known. Serum potassium increases immediately postexercise and this increase may be related to postexercise T-wave changes. The increase in potassium during exercise contrasts with the decrease in T waves during exercise.

Coester et al[7] drew arterial samples for blood gases and electrolytes at rest, during the last minute of maximal bicycle exercise, and at recovery. The amplitude of the T- and P-waves increased in bipolar lead CH_5 reached a maximum in the first 2 minutes after exercise. All electrolytes measured were increased at the end of exercise, with potassium raised by 60% and phosphorus by 53%. Potassium dropped the most rapidly below resting values, along with plasma bicarbonate. ECG alterations were not closely related in time with any single factor such as potassium, but they appeared to reflect an interaction of the changes in mineral balance. The normal right-axis and posterior-axis deviation of the QRS complex and decreasing R-wave amplitude could be due to right ventricular overload, respiratory-induced descent of the diaphragm, changes in thoracic impedance, or changes in ventricular blood volume. The decreased T-wave amplitude may be related to decreased end-systolic volume, changes in sympathetic tone, electrolyte concentration changes, or shifts in the T-wave vector. Other factors may also contribute to the changes in the exercise ECG, such as positional changes in the electrodes, changes in action potentials, electrolyte or hematocrit changes, changes in intracardiac blood volume, and augmentation of the atrial repolarization wave. The effect of age must be considered because there is extensive normal variation related to age. For example, greater ST-segment depression and greater right-axis deviation occur in older persons.

Wilkerson et al[8] studied five healthy males during exercise for 20 minutes on a motor-driven treadmill at five submaximal intensities. Peripheral venous blood samples were drawn from an indwelling catheter prior to and during each exercise bout. Blood samples were assayed for whole-blood hemoglobin, total plasma protein concentrations, and hematocrit, with plasma water concentration calculated from these values. The plasma concentration of the electrolytes sodium (Na^+), potassium (K^+), total calcium (Catot), ionized calcium (Ca^{2+}), chloride (Cl^-), and inorganic phosphorus (Pi) were also determined. With plasma and blood volumes, the total plasma contents of each of the measured constituents and the concentration of each electrolyte per liter of water were calculated. Statistically significant linear increases in plasma concentrations of Na^+, K^+, and Cl^- relative to exercise intensity were observed, with linear decreases in plasma contents of Na^+ and Cl^- and linear increases in K^+ content. Plasma Pi concentration decreased with a Pi increased content, with plasma Catot concentration elevated at the highest two work loads. Plasma Catot content increased linearly with exercise intensity and duration. Plasma water concentration and content decreased with exercise intensity, resulting in no change in electrolyte concentration per liter of water except at the highest two exercise intensities. Changes in plasma volume and plasma water must be considered when postulating a role for electrolytes in the physiological responses of humans to exercise.

To investigate the effect of acute graded increases in plasma volume on fluid and regulatory hormone levels, Grant et al[9] studied eight untrained men who performed prolonged cycle exercise with and without plasma volume expansion. The exercise plasma levels of aldosterone, arginine vasopressin, and atrial natriuretic peptide were all altered by acute plasma volume increases. A pronounced blunting of the aldosterone response during exercise was observed, the magnitude of which was directly related to the amount of hypervolemia. In contrast, the lower arginine vasopressive and the higher atrial natrimetic peptide observed during exercise appeared to be due to the effect of plasma volume expansion on resting concentrations. Because osmolality did not vary among conditions, the results indicate that plasma volume represents an important primary stimulus in the response of aldosterone to exercise. The lower exercise blood concentrations of both epinephrine and norepinephrine observed with plasma volume expansion would suggest that a lower sympathetic drive might be implicated at least in the lower aldosterone responses.

Nordsborg et al[10] studied changes in gene expression during recovery from high-intensity, intermittent, one-legged exercise before and after 5.5 weeks of training. Genes related to metabolism, as well as Na[+], K[+], and pH homeostasis, were selected for analyses. After the same work was performed before and after the training period, several muscle biopsies were obtained from vastus lateralis muscle. In the untrained state, the Na[+],K[+]-ATPase alpha1-subunit mRNA level was approximately threefold higher at 0, 1, and 3 hours after exercise, relative to the pre-exercise resting level. After 3 to 5 hours of recovery in the untrained state, pyruvate dehydrogenase kinase 4 and hexokinase II mRNA levels were elevated 13-fold and sixfold, respectively. However, after the training period, only pyruvate dehydrogenase kinase 4 mRNA levels were elevated during the recovery period. No changes in resting mRNA levels were observed as a result of training. It appears from this study that cellular adaptations to high-intensity exercise training may, in part, be induced by transcriptional regulation. After training, the transcriptional response to an exercise bout at a given workload is diminished.

Potassium release from contracting skeletal muscle cells facilitates ongoing muscle contraction but may also lead to muscular fatigue. McKenna[11] reviewed the effects of altered physical activity on K[+] regulation during exercise. Endurance and sprint training specifically enhance prolonged and high-intensity exercise performance, respectively. Both forms of training reduce the exercise-induced rise in plasma (K[+]) at the same absolute exercise work rate and duration and increase the total concentration of Na[+],K[+] pumps in trained human muscle by approximately 15%. However, the increased pump density has not been proven to account directly for either the reduced hyperkalemia or the improved exercise performance after training. The most likely factor accounting for the improved K[+] regulation after training is an increased activation of Na[+],K[+] pumps during exercise, but this is not due to increased circulating catecholamine concentrations after training.

A chronic reduction in physical activity reduced the muscle Na[+],K[+] pump concentration in animal models, with an augmented exercise-induced rise in plasma [K[+]]. They found that while physical training enhances, inactivity impairs K[+] regulation during exercise.

RESPONSE OF SPECIFIC PORTIONS OF THE ECG TO EXERCISE

Studies on Q-wave Changes

Ellestad's group[12] analyzed the response of Q waves in lead CM5 in 50 patients with coronary artery disease (CAD) and in 50 normal subjects before and immediately after exercise. The septal Q wave in lead CM_5 was smaller in patients with coronary disease than it was in normal subjects at rest and immediately after exercise. Disappearance of the Q wave in lead CM5 along with ST-segment depression after exercise was 100% specific for CAD. They felt that low Q-wave voltage and its failure to increase after exercise indicated abnormal septal activation and reflected loss of contraction due to ischemia. Loss of the septal Q could also be due to septal fibrosis secondary to coronary disease.

Studies on R-Wave Changes

Exercise-induced R-wave amplitude changes were studied by Kentala and Luurela[13] in healthy individuals and in patients with known coronary disease. Physically active normal subjects and patients with coronary disease who responded well to an exercise program demonstrated an increased R-wave amplitude in lead V5 relative to pre-exercise supine rest measurements both on assumption of an upright posture and in response to exercise. The R-wave amplitude then decreased in the supine position postexercise. Such changes were not found in patients who did not benefit from physical conditioning. Bonoris et al[14] compared exercise-induced R-wave amplitude changes and ST-segment depression in 266 patients, many of who were specifically chosen as false-positive or false-negative responders. Using R-wave criteria, the sensitivity was improved. Uhl and Hopkirk[15] examined R-wave amplitude changes in 44 asymptomatic men with left bundle branch block (LBBB). Among the seven men with angiographically significant CAD, all demonstrated an increase in the amplitude of the R wave from rest to maximal exercise. In only 10 of the 37 men with normal angiograms did exercise induce an increase in R-wave amplitude, resulting in a sensitivity of 100% and a specificity of 73%.

Yiannikas et al[16] used the sum of the change in R-wave amplitudes in V_4, V_5, and V_6 to investigate the response of 50 men with ST-T wave changes on their resting ECGs. Four of six subjects who increased R-wave amplitude during exercise had angiographically significant CAD, and the other two had cardiomyopathy. Greenberg et al[17] were able to improve the sensitivity of the exercise test from 50% to 76% by including R-wave criteria in 50 patients without compromising specificity or predictive value. Baron et al[18], using the mean of the R-wave changes inferiorly and laterally, reported that of 62 patients with CAD, 61 (98%) increased the amplitude of the R wave with exercise. Nearly as many studies have been unable to demonstrate that changes in the R-wave amplitude during exercise are useful clinically. Particularly defining was the study from the Thorax Center in Rotterdam: they could not improve sensitivity using R-wave amplitude changes as compared to ST-segment changes.[19] This was despite the use of several lead systems, clinical subsets of patients, and different criteria for abnormal.

R-Wave Amplitude Changes and Left Ventricular Function

We found poor correlations between ejection fraction (EF) and R-wave amplitude at rest and during exercise in 60 patients ($r = 0.50$ and 0.51, respectively).[20] Further, there was no significant relationship between changes in R-wave amplitude and changes in left ventricular ejection fraction (LVEF) during exercise in these patients or in 18 normals. Luwaert et al[21] studied 252 patients, evaluated for chest pain, and demonstrated a significant, although low, correlation between the sum of the orthogonal R waves and resting EF ($r = 0.22$). Eenige van et al studied the value of R-wave amplitude changes during exercise in determining EF, end-diastolic pressures, and left ventricular wall motion. No useful diagnostic information was obtained using R-wave changes in this study.

Mechanism of R-Wave Amplitude Changes

The direct relationship between left ventricular volume and R-wave amplitude was defined as the unsubstantiated "Brody effect."[22] Research cited above demonstrated a poor correlation between

changes in R-wave amplitude and left ventricular volume and others have reported an inverse association between end-diastolic volume and R-wave voltage. Levken et al[23] reported that the endocardial QRS amplitude decreased during volume increases in dogs. Deanfield et al[24] reported that R-wave amplitude was essentially unaffected by either increases or decreases in left ventricular volume.

The association of cardiac enlargement secondary to congestive heart failure with a decrease in R-wave amplitude also contradicts the Brody hypothesis. Furthermore, if R-wave amplitude changes were strictly the result of changes in volume, one would expect R-wave amplitude to increase when changing from standing to supine, since diastolic volume would increase. Since the R wave has been shown to correlate with systolic volume and EF, an association with contractility has been suggested. Axis shifts have been implicated as the cause of changes in R-wave amplitude. However, the shift of the QRS and ST-segment vector toward the right and posteriorly is a normal response to exercise. David et al[25] performed an experiment that was strongly against the concept that R-wave amplitude changes are due mainly to changes in ventricular volume. After inducing ischemia in dogs, R-wave amplitude continued to increase despite clamping of the vena cava, which reduced ventricular volume.

If the R-wave/volume relationship does not explain the increase in R-wave amplitude which accompanies myocardial infarction (MI), exercise, or coronary spasm, then it could be due to ischemia-induced changes in the electrical properties of the myocardium. The biphasic R-wave changes directly correlated with changes in intramyocardial conduction times, whereas intracardiac dimensional changes and R-wave changes were unrelated.

University of California, San Diego, R-Wave Study

We used digitized exercise ECGs to relate R-wave changes with ischemic ST-segment shifts.[26] The ECG changes were analyzed spatially in three dimensions, enabling optimal representation of global myocardial electrical forces. Patients were separated into groups achieving maximal heart rates higher and lower than the mean maximal heart rate achieved of 161 beats per minute (bpm). Data on asymptomatic normals has demonstrated that the R-wave amplitude typically increases from rest to submaximal exercise, perhaps to a heart rate of 140 bpm and then decreases to the maximal exercise endpoint (Figure 6-2). Therefore, if a patient were limited by exercise intolerance, whether due to objective or subjective symptoms or signs, the R-wave amplitude would increase from rest to such an endpoint. Such patients may be demonstrating a normal R-wave response but can be classified "abnormal," since the severity of disease results in a lower exercise capacity and heart rate. Thus, exercise-induced changes in R-wave amplitude have no independent predictive power but are associated with CAD because patients with coronary disease are often submaximally tested,

where R-wave amplitude normally increases from baseline. If they had been exercised further, the normal decrease in R wave at maximal exercise would be observed.

Percent R-Wave Changes

Figure 6-2 illustrates the percent change of R-wave amplitude for each individual compared with R wave at supine rest in V_5 and lead Y (similar to leads II or aV_F). At lower exercise heart rates, the great variability of R-wave response was apparent, and many normal individuals had significant increases in R-wave amplitude. Though most showed a decline at maximum exercise, some normal subjects had an increase, whereas others showed very little decrease. At 1-minute recovery there was a greater tendency toward a decline in lead V_5, but not in Y. Further into recovery, R-wave amplitude remained decreased in lead V_5, but increased in Y.

Studies on S-Wave Changes

During exercise there is an increase in the S wave in the lateral precordial leads. It was hypothesized that this increase in the S wave reflects the normal increase in cardiac contractility during exercise and that its absence is indicative of ventricular dysfunction. However, it is more likely that the increase in S wave is caused by exercise-induced axis shifts and conduction alterations.

Studies on U-Wave Changes

In 1980, Gerson et al[27] reported 248 patients who underwent exercise testing with leads CC_5 and V_L monitored, 36 of who had exercise-induced U-wave inversion. Of 71 patients with significant left anterior descending (LAD) or left main disease and no prior MI, 35% had U-wave inversion compared to only 4% of 57 patients without LAD or left main disease and only 1% of 82 patients who had no CAD. U-wave inversion was diagnosed if a discrete negative deflection within the TP segment relative to the PR segment occurred during or after exercise. Inverted U waves were not diagnosed if the exercise heart rate increased to a level such that the QT interval could not be accurately measured.

While other case reports have occasionally noted U-wave changes with exercise, other unconfirmed observations include the following. Kodama et al[28]

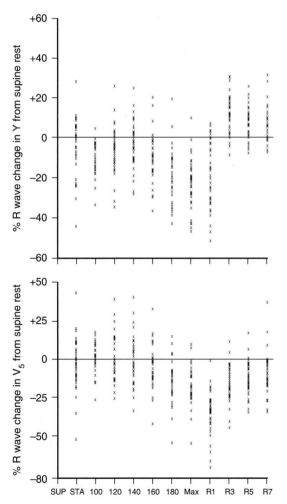

FIGURE 6–2

R-wave changes relative to heart rate during progressive treadmill exercise in a group of low-risk normals. This figure illustrates the percent change of R-wave amplitude for each individual compared with his R wave at supine rest in V_5 and Y.

performed treadmill tests on 60 patients with angina pectoris whose culprit lesion was located only in the LAD. They concluded that the exercise-induced U-wave inversion in patients with one-vessel disease of the LAD indicates the severe degree of myocardial ischemia induced in the territory perfused by the LAD. However, it did not have independent significance since it closely corre-lates with the presence of S-T segment shift. Hayat et al[29] reported exercise-induced positive U-waves to be an infrequent, but specific, marker of significant single coronary (circumflex or right) artery stenosis that disappeared after percutaneous coronary intervention. In a study of 20 patients recovering from an anterior wall MI, Miwa et al[30] concluded that exercise-induced negative U waves in precordial leads were specific markers for the presence of a viable myocardium. In another study, these same authors concluded that exer-cise-induced U-wave alterations were a marker for well-developed collateral circulation in patients with stable, but severe, effort angina.[31]

Junctional ST-Segment Depression

Mirvis et al[32] reported their observations regard-ing junctional ST depression during exercise using left precordial isopotential mapping. During exercise, junctional depression was maxi-mal along the left lower sternal border. In the early portion of the ST segment, they found a minimum isopotential along the lower left sternal border that was continuous with terminal QRS forces in both intensity and location. The late por-tion of the ST-segment had a minimum isopoten-tial located in the same areas as those observed at rest (i.e., the upper left sternal border). Thus, junctional depression is the result of competition between normal repolarization and delayed termi-nal depolarization forces. Junctional depression was most marked along the left lower sternal border. In addition, the slope of the ST segment varied from site to site and was directly correlated to magnitude and direction of the J-point devia-tion. This classic study demonstrates that junc-tional depression is the result of the presence of negative potentials over the left lower sternal border during early repolarization. These nega-tive potentials responsible for physiologic junc-tional depression could be caused by delayed activation of basal areas of the left and right ven-tricles, which leads to accentuated depolariza-tion-repolarization overlap.

ABNORMAL ST-SEGMENT CHANGES

Epicardial electrode mapping usually records ST-segment elevation over areas of severe ischemia and ST-segment depression over areas of lesser ischemia. ST-segment depression is the reciprocal of the injury effect occurring in the endocardium, as viewed from an electrode overly-ing normal epicardium. ST-segment elevation seen from the same electrode reflects transmural injury or, less frequently, epicardial injury. On the ECG recorded from the skin, exercise-induced myocardial ischemia can result in one of three ST-segment manifestations: elevation, normaliza-tion, or depression. These will be discussed in depth in the following sections.

ST-Segment Elevation

Variant angina with its associated ST-segment elevation was first described by Prinzmetal et al[33] in 1959 and explained as being secondary to coro-nary artery spasm. They reported 32 patients with rest angina and ST elevation with reciprocal ST-segment depression. The chest pain termi-nated, spontaneously but arrhythmias often occurred which could lead to ventricular fibrilla-tion (VF) and death. While many of these patients had normal coronary arteries on cardiac catheter-ization, subsequent studies showed that approxi-mately half of them had significant fixed lesions.[34-36] Patients with variant angina can also have typical ST depression during exercise testing.[37] Four patients with Prinzmetal angina were reported who only developed ST-segment depression in recovery after a treadmill test.[38]

Variant Angina

Variant angina, also referred to as Prinzmetal's angina, is a distinct syndrome of ischemic chest pain classically occurring at rest, associated with transient ST-segment elevation on the ECG, and relieved promptly by nitroglycerin. Although its complex pathophysiology is poorly understood, it is believed to occur as a result of coronary artery spasm and has traditionally been associated with a benign prognosis. The concept of coronary artery spasm as the trigger of Prinzmetal's syn-drome was furthered during the 1970s, when a number of investigators identified patients with variant angina and found that there was no relation between the degree of coronary stenosis or myocardial oxygen demand and the patients' chest pain.[39,40] Instead, a diminished myocardial blood supply, presumably resulting from coronary artery spasm, was more closely related to the onset of symptoms.

With the advent of coronary angiography and a provocative test[41] to diagnose variant angina in the 1970s, investigators had the opportunity to study the pathophysiology, treatment and prognosis of this syndrome. Table 6-1 outlines the definition of variant angina and Table 6-2 lists the historical highlights.

The traditional belief that variant angina has a benign prognosis may only apply to patients without CAD who receive appropriate treatment; the Bory study[42] shows that even this group has a greater morbidity than initially appreciated. Because of the complex pathophysiology and the variable degree of CAD in patients who present with variant angina, the prognosis changes depending on the subgroup analyzed. Prognosis probably could be better defined if the three clinical groups outlined in Table 6-3 could be identified and studied separately.

Prevalence of Exercise-Induced ST Elevation

The most common ECG abnormality seen in the exercise laboratory is ST-segment depression, while ST elevation is relatively rare (Table 6-4, studies of exercise-induced ST elevation). Its prevalence depends upon the population tested but occurs more frequently in patients who have had a Q-wave MI.

Fortuin and Friesinger[43] reported the angiographic and clinical findings and 2-year follow-up of 12 patients with 0.1 mV or more ST-segment elevation during or after exercise. These patients were selected from 400 patients who had coronary angiography and exercise testing. Seven of them had previous MIs, and 9 of the 10 with angina developed it during the exercise test. One patient with atypical chest pain had normal coronary arteries and improved during the follow-up.

TABLE 6-2. Brief history of variant angina in medical literature
Heberden: "Disorders of the Breast" 1772, first mention of nonexertional angina Printzmetal[33]: "A Variant Form of Angina Pectoris," *American Journal of Medicine*, 1959: 32 cases—first case a 42-year-old physician; from 1928 to 1958, 250 articles were published on atypical angina; Printzmetal cites 11 articles discussing a total of 12 cases of probable variant angina Schroeder[41]: *Journal of the American College of Cardiology*, 1983—43 patients treated successfully with a calcium antagonist Bory[42]: *European Heart Journal*, 1996—follow-up of more than 100 patients with variant angina and normal coronary angiograms

Seven of eight with exercise-induced ST-segment elevation in lead V_3 had LAD coronary disease. All four with inferior elevation had right coronary disease. None had ST-segment elevation at rest, but many had Q waves or T-wave inversion or both. Within 2 years, four of the patients died, one had a documented MI, and two became unstable.

Hegge et al[44] found 11% of the patients they studied with maximal treadmill testing and coronary angiography to have exercise-induced ST-segment elevation in the postexercise 12-lead ECG. This relatively high prevalence of ST-segment elevation is probably explained by inclusion of V_1 and V_2, where ST elevation can be normal. The ST-segment elevation was present in precordial leads only in 12 patients, in the inferior leads only in five patients, and in both in one patient. Seventeen patients had severe CAD in the arteries supplying the appropriate area and the remaining patient had a normal coronary angiogram.

Chahine et al[45] reported the prevalence of exercise-induced ST-segment elevation in 840 consecutive patients to be 3.5%. CM_5 and CM_6 were the only leads monitored, so lateral wall ST-segment elevation was all that could be detected. Only about 20% of those who had CAD showed ST-segment elevation. Sixty-four percent

TABLE 6-1. Definition of variant angina
Burning or squeezing type of retrosternal chest pain occurring at rest, usually in the early morning Transient ST-segment elevation on ECG with the pain Relief of the pain with sublingual nitroglycerin within 5 minutes Focal coronary artery spasm without evidence of subsequent myocardial infarction

TABLE 6-3. Variant angina subgroups of patients with different prognoses
Patients with pure endothelial dysfunction (young women, Japanese) Patients with endothelial dysfunction resulting from early atherosclerosis Patients with fixed atherosclerotic lesions whose coronary artery spasm (increased coronary arterial tone) occurs in proximity to subtotal atherosclerotic lesions

TABLE 6–4. Studies of exercise-induced ST-segment elevation during standard clinical testing

Study	Size of population tested	Type of population	Percent population with prior MI	No. of leads measured for elevation	Criteria for elevation	Prevalence of abnormal elevation (%)	Percent prior MI in patients with elevation
Bruce (1988)	3050	Angina (CASS)	47	11	1 mm	4.7	83
Bruce (1988)	1136	CHD (SHW)	47	CB_5	>0	0.5	57
Sriwattankomen (1980)	1620	All referred	—	11	1 mm	3.8	47
Longhurst (1979)	6040	All referred	—	12 + XYZ	0.5 mm	1.6	0
Chahine (1976)	840	VAMC	—	V_5, V_6	1 mm	3.5	80
Stiles (1980)	650	541 patients with ST-segment depression versus 109 with ST-segment elevation	10	11	1 mm	4	61
Waters (1980)	720	Mixed	1	$12/CM_5$	—	6.5	76

All referred, all patients referred to exercise lab; CASS, Coronary Artery Surgery Study; CHD, coronary heart disease; MI, myocardial infarction; SHW, Seattle Heart Watch; VAMC, Veterans Affairs Medical Center.
Modified from Nostratian FJ, Froelicher VF: Exercise-induced ST elevation. Am J Cardiol 1989;63:986-987.

of the patients with left ventricle dyskinesia displayed ST-segment elevation. Manvi and Ellestad[46] presented results in 29 patients with CAD who had abnormal left ventriculograms. ST-segment elevation occurred in 48%, 33% developed ST-segment depression, and the remaining 19% had no changes. ST-segment elevation occurred in 1.3% of 2000 exercise tests.

Simoons et al[47] investigated the spatial orientation of exercise-induced ST-segment changes in relation to the presence of dyskinetic areas, as demonstrated by left ventriculography. In patients with an anterior infarct, the ST vectors were widely scattered, but were most often directed to the left, anterior, and superior. Patients with an inferior MI had ST-segment vectors directed rightward and anteriorly, and also inferiorly if inferior dyskinesia was present. Anteriorly orientated ST-segment changes were associated with anterior or apical scars in patients with anterior infarcts. Thus, ST-segment vector shifts associated with dyskinesia resulted in ST-segment elevation over the dyskinetic area. In patients with dyskinetic areas, the direction of the ST-segment changes varied so widely that only the magnitude of the changes could be used as a criterion for exercise-induced ischemia.

Sriwattanakomen et al[48] reviewed 1620 exercise tests and found 3.8% to have ST-segment elevation, when all leads except aVR were evaluated. They then correlated exercise-induced ST-elevation with the coronary arteriography and left ventriculograms of 38 patients, 37 of which had significant coronary disease. In 27 patients with Q waves, 25 had significant disease and ventricular aneurysms, whereas among 11 patients with no Q waves and significant disease, only two had ventricular aneurysms. One patient had a ventricular aneurysm but no coronary disease. The sites of ST elevation correctly localized the area of ventricular aneurysm in 30 of 33 instances and determined the diseased vessels in 38 of 40 instances. They concluded that ST elevation during exercise in the absence of Q waves indicates significant proximal disease without ventricular aneurysm, whereas with Q waves, ST elevation is indicative of ventricular aneurysm in addition to significant proximal disease. Ischemia and abnormal wall motion may independently or together underlie the mechanism for ST-segment elevation during exercise.

Longhurst and Kraus[49] reviewed 6,040 consecutive exercise tests and found 106 patients (1.8%) without previous MIs who had exercise-induced ST-segment elevation. Their criterion was 0.5-mm elevation in a 15-electrode array. Forty-six of

these patients with ST-segment elevation had ventriculography and coronary angiography. Coronary disease was detected in 40 of 46, with nearly equal numbers having one-, two-, and three-vessel disease. Ventriculograms were normal in 36 of 40 patients. Of 21 patients with anterior ST-segment elevation, 86% had LAD obstruction. There was no anatomic correlation in those with lateral or inferior-posterior exercise-induced elevation.

Dunn et al[50] performed exercise thallium scans on 35 patients with exercise-induced ST-segment elevation and coronary artery obstruction. Ten patients developed exercise ST-segment elevation in leads that showed no Q waves on the resting ECG. The site of elevation corresponded to a reversible perfusion defect and a severely obstructed coronary artery. Associated ST-segment depression in other leads occurred in seven patients, but only one had a second perfusion defect at the site of depression. Three of the 10 patients had a wall motion abnormality at the same site. Twenty-five patients developed exercise ST-segment elevation in leads with Q waves. The site of the elevation corresponded to a severe stenosis and a thallium perfusion defect that persisted on the 4-hour redistribution scan. Associated ST-segment depression in other leads occurred in 11 patients and eight had a second perfusion defect at the site of the depression. In all 25 patients, there was a wall motion abnormality at the site of the Q wave. Without a previous infarct, they found ST-segment elevation to indicate the site of severe transient ischemia; associated ST-segment depression was usually reciprocal. In patients with Q waves, exercise-induced ST-segment elevation may be due to ischemia around the infarct, abnormal wall motion, or both. Associated ST-segment depression may be due to a second area of ischemia rather than being reciprocal.

Braat et al[51] assessed the value of lead V_{4R} during exercise testing for predicting proximal stenosis of the right coronary artery. In 107 patients, a Bruce exercise test with the simultaneous recording of leads I, II, V_{4R}, V_1, V_4 and V_6 was followed by coronary angiography. ST-segment changes were recorded in the conventional leads and in lead V_{4R}. Seventy-nine of the 107 patients were studied because of inadequate control of angina pectoris. In the 46 patients who had a previous MI, the infarct location was inferior in 28 and anterior in 18. Seven of the 14 patients without MI and significant proximal stenosis in the right coronary artery showed an ST-segment deviation of 1 mm or greater in lead V_{4R} during exercise. This was also observed in 11 of 18 patients with an old inferior wall infarction and proximal occlusion of the right coronary artery. None of the 53 patients without significant proximal stenosis in the right coronary artery showed exercise-related ST-segment changes in lead V_{4R}. Exercise-related ST-segment deviation in lead V_{4R} (elevation in 17 and depression in 4 patients) had a sensitivity of 56%, a specificity of 96%, and a predictive accuracy of 84% in recognizing proximal stenosis in the right coronary artery.

Mark et al[52] studied 452 consecutive patients with one-vessel disease that underwent treadmill testing to determine if patterns of ST depression or elevation during exercise testing provide reliable information about the location of an underlying coronary lesion. Exercise ST changes were classified as elevation or depression and by lead groups involved. The ST depression occurred most commonly in leads V_5 or V_6 regardless of which coronary artery was involved. In contrast, anterior ST elevation indicated LAD coronary disease in 93% of cases, and inferior ST elevation indicated a lesion in or proximal to the posterior descending artery in 86% of cases. Furthermore, anterior ST elevation in leads without diagnostic Q waves usually indicated a high-grade, often proximal, LAD stenosis, whereas anterior ST elevation in leads with Q waves usually indicated a totally occluded LAD coronary artery. Thus, they found ST elevation during exercise testing, although uncommon, to be a reliable guide to the underlying coronary lesion, whereas ST depression was not.

Waters et al[53] reported that 47 patients out of 720 who underwent treadmill testing developed ST elevation. Chahine et al[45] found 29 patients with ST-segment elevation among 840 patients who had an exercise test. Bruce et al[54] reported a prevalence of 0.5% in the Seattle Heart Watch Study in 1974 but later[55] reported a prevalence of 5% in 1136 patients observed in Seattle community practice. Part of this increase would be due to the quantitative measurements made using signal averaging. De Feyter et al[56] in his study of 680 patients reported a prevalence of 1% but a multilead system was not used. Bruce also analyzed the Coronary Artery Surgery Study registry data[57] and compared it to the results of the Seattle Heart Watch Study. He found that although the two groups were relatively matched, patients in the Coronary Artery Surgery Study had more left ventricular dysfunction and less ST elevation than in the Seattle study. However, the Coronary Artery Surgery Study used visual analysis of 12-lead ECGs and the Seattle study used computer analysis of lead CB5. However, in both groups, the 6-year mortality for patients with ST elevation was significantly higher than patients with ST depression (29% versus 14%).

Methods of ST-Elevation Measurement

ST-segment depression is measured from the isoelectric baseline, or when ST segment depression is present at rest, the amount of additional depression is measured. However, ST-segment elevation is always considered from the baseline ST level. Whether the elevation occurs over or adjacent to Q waves or in non-Q wave areas is important. Unfortunately, many of the studies do not provide the methods of measurement or the condition of the underlying ECG. Table 6-5 lists some of the factors that should be considered when assessing studies of ST elevation. Figure 6-3 illustrates the points of measurement.

Multiple causes for ST elevation during treadmill testing have been suggested. These include left ventricular aneurysm, variant angina, severe ischemic heart disease, and left ventricular wall motion abnormalities. Left ventricular aneurysm after MI is the most frequent cause of ST-segment elevation on the resting ECG and occurs over Q waves or in ECG leads adjacent to Q waves. Early repolarization is a normal variant pattern of ST elevation that occurs in normal individuals who rarely exhibit diagnostic Q waves.

Is ST Elevation Due to Ischemia or Wall Motion Abnormality?

There is controversy regarding whether ischemia or wall motion abnormalities are the major cause of ST-segment elevation. Fortuin et al[43] studied 12 patients and concluded that severe CAD found on angiography was the cause of ST-segment elevation. The location of elevation also correlated

TABLE 6–5. Some factors in assessing studies of exercise-induced ST-segment elevation

Population tested (prevalence of patients with myocardial infarction, variant angina, or spasm)
Baseline (resting) ECG
ECG leads monitored
Leads in which elevation occurs relative to Q waves
Criteria for elevation
Methods of ST-shift detection (visual or computerized)

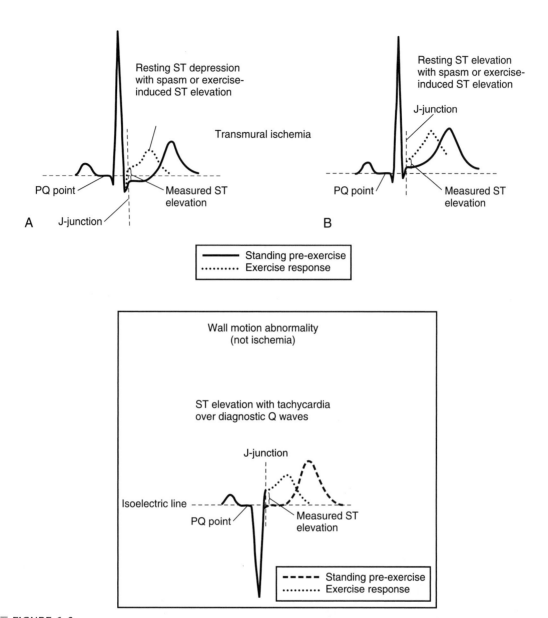

■ FIGURE 6–3

An illustration of the points of measurement of ST elevation in the presence and absence of Q waves and ST abnormalities at rest. *B* represents the early repolarization often seen in normal resting ECGs.

with the coronary obstruction. They noted that temporary ligation of an artery in dogs produced reversible ST elevation and these changes do not occur unless the blood flow is decreased to at least 70%. Hegge et al[58] studied 158 patients, 18 of whom had ST elevation on treadmill testing. Seventeen of these patients were found to have significant CAD correlating anatomically with the area where ST-segment elevation occurred. Lahiri et al[59] reported five patients who presented

with ST-segment elevation during exercise and chest pain at rest. These patients also had positive thallium tests with reversible defects. Three of these patients subsequently had MI and two died. However, Caplin and Banim[60] and Hill et al[61] have shown that such ECG changes can occur in patients with normal coronary arteries who develop spasm and have an excellent prognosis. Fox et al[62] reported the results of coronary artery bypass surgery on 24 patients post-MI, who had exercise-induced ST elevation. Fifteen of these patients had loss of both symptoms and exercise-induced ST-segment elevation. Since this ST elevation was abolished by coronary bypass surgery, they felt the underlying mechanism was myocardial ischemia.

Waters et al[53] found that 36 of 47 patients who presented with ST elevation on exercise testing had Q waves in inferior or anterior leads on their resting ECG. Ninety-four percent of their patients had evidence of wall motion abnormality on cardiac catheterization. In the remaining 11 patients, 10 had Prinzmetal's angina and no Q wave or wall motion abnormalities. They concluded that ST-segment elevation was caused directly by a segmental wall motion abnormality in patients with a previous MI, but by spasm in patients with variant angina. Gerwitz et al[63] studied 28 patients with a previous anterior MI with thallium exercise testing. Fifteen of the patients had evidence of ST elevation while 13 did not. They found that patients with ST elevation had larger anterior lateral or septal thallium defects and lower EFs. They concluded that myocardial ischemia was not required for exercise-induced ST-segment elevation to occur and that exercise-induced ST elevation primarily reflects the extent of previous anterior wall damage and to a lesser extent an increase in heart rate.

Chahine et al[45] arrived at similar conclusions after studying 29 patients who had ST elevation during exercise testing. Twenty-five of their patients had ECG evidence of anterior MI. Eighteen of the 21 patients who had an angiogram showed left ventricular aneurysm and 19 had critical LAD lesions. They reviewed all patients with anterior MI or critical LAD disease and found that only 22% and 18%, respectively, showed exercise-induced ST-segment elevation, while 64% of the cases with left ventricular aneurysm displayed this phenomenon. They concluded that exercise-induced ST elevation is usually due to left ventricular aneurysms.

Stiles et al[64] and Longhurst and Kraus[49] reviewed a large number of patients with ST elevation during exercise. Their conclusion was that most of these patients had previous Q-wave infarcts and regional wall motion abnormalities. If there was no previous MI, then ST elevation was related to the severity of CAD. Dunn et al[50] correlated thallium and angiography results and concluded that in patients without previous MI, the site of ST elevation correlates with severe CAD. ST-segment depression in these patients represents either reciprocal changes or two areas of ischemia independent of each other. However, in patients with Q-wave infarcts, ST elevation was due to wall motion abnormality, peri-infarction ischemia, or both. They also found that ST elevation in V1 and AVL in patients without evidence of MI correlates well with significant lesions in the LAD artery and ischemia in the anterior wall. Shimokawa et al[65] arrived at similar conclusions. They found that in patients with ST elevation, the degree of perfusion defect might be larger on the nuclear scan than in patients with ST depression.

Retrospective studies by Arora et al[66] and Sriwattanakomen et al[48] found that the patients with ST-segment elevation on exercise testing and no previous Q waves on the resting ECG, usually stop due to angina, have reversible thallium defects, and single-vessel disease on cardiac catheterization. On the other hand, patients with abnormal Q waves had multivessel disease, fixed thallium defects, and stopped due to fatigue and shortness of breath.

In conclusion, in patients with ST elevation during exercise when no abnormal Q wave is seen on the baseline ECG, there is a very high likelihood of a significant proximal narrowing in the coronary artery supplying the area where it occurs. It is also likely to be associated with serious arrhythmias. When elevation occurs in an ECG with abnormal Q waves, it is usually due to a wall motion abnormality and the elevation can conceal ST depression due to ischemia. Figure 6-4 is an example of ST elevation in a normal baseline ECG and Figure 6-5 illustrates the typical ST elevation over Q waves that occurs after an MI. This patient is unusual in that the elevation occurs in multiple areas.

ST-Segment Normalization or Absence of Change

Another manifestation of ischemia can be no change or normalization of the ST segment due to cancellation effects. Electrocardiographic abnormalities at rest, including T-wave inversion and ST-segment depression, have been reported to return to normal during attacks of angina and during exercise in some patients with ischemic heart disease. This cancellation effect is a rare occurrence, but it should be kept in mind. The ST-segment and T-wave represent the portion of ventricular repolarization that is not cancelled. Since ventricular geometry can be roughly approximated by a hollow ellipsoid open at one

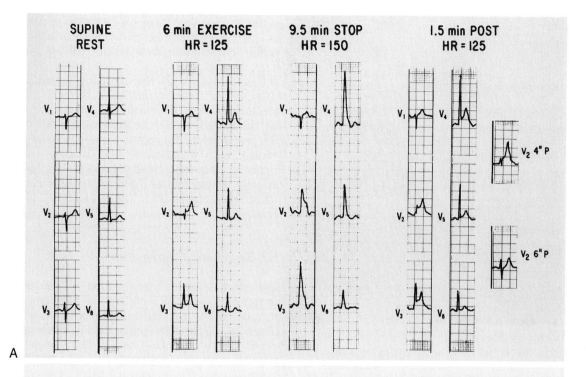

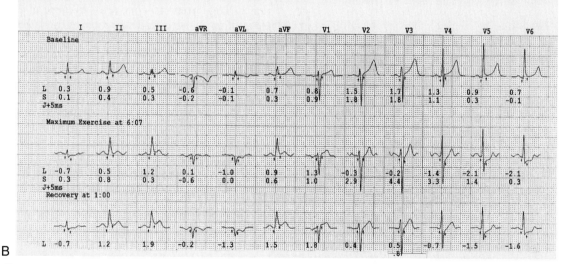

■ FIGURE 6–4

Example of ST elevation in two patients with a normal resting ECG. *A,* The anterior ST elevation is due to transmural anterior ischemia associated with a tight proximal left anterior descending coronary artery lesion that responded to PTCA. *B,* The inferior ST elevation with reciprocal lateral depression is due to a total right coronary artery occlusion.

end, the widespread cancellation of the relatively slowly dispersing electrical forces during repolarization is understandable. Patients with severe CAD would be most likely to have cancellation occur; yet, they have the highest prevalence of abnormal tests. Nobel et al[67] reported normalization of both inverted T waves and depressed ST segments in 11 patients during exercise-induced angina. When exercise testing fails to produce ST-segment depression or elevation in a patient with known CAD, this could be due to two or more severely ischemic myocardial segments causing canceling

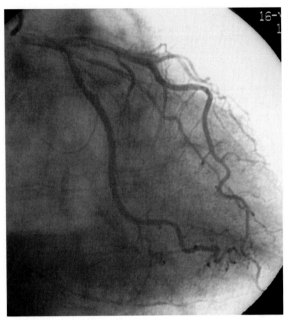

C

■ **FIGURE 6–4** *continued*
C, The left coronary angiogram showing a normal left coronary system with collateral filling of the distal right coronary artery found in the referred to in patient *B.*

ST-segment vectors. Sweet and Sheffield[68] reported a patient with minor ST-segment depression and T-wave inversion in lead V5 who normalized, or "improved" his ECG during treadmill testing only to have an acute infarction 10 minutes after the test. This normalization of ST-segment depression should thus be considered ischemic ST-segment elevation.

Lavie et al[69] from the Mayo Clinic studied 84 consecutive patients with resting T-wave inversion. Radionuclide angiography revealed significant new wall motion abnormalities in 13 (28%) of the 47 patients with persistent T-wave inversion and in 23 (62%) of the 37 patients with T-wave pseudonormalization during exercise. The response of the EF to exercise was better in patients with persistent T-wave inversion than in those with pseudonormalization. Mechanical evidence of ischemia was seen in 14 of the 23 patients with T-wave pseudonormalization (60%) but without ST-segment depression. In patients with resting T-wave inversion, pseudonormalization was slightly more sensitive but less specific than a positive exercise test for predicting significant new wall motion abnormalities or decreases in the EF with exercise. Thus, although pseudonormalization is not extremely useful alone, the presence or absence

of this finding can increase the diagnostic accuracy of exercise electrocardiography in patients with resting T-wave inversion and suspected ischemic heart disease.

The prevalence of the canceling of surface ST-segment changes by multiple ischemic ST vectors is not known. The inability of patients to give an adequate effort are more likely explanations for the majority of false-negative exercise tests in patients with multivessel CAD. In those with single-vessel disease, the decreased sensitivity of exercise testing is most likely due to insufficient myocardial ischemia to cause surface ECG changes.

ST-Segment Depression

The most common manifestation of exercise-induced myocardial ischemia is ST-segment depression. The standard criterion for this type of abnormal response is horizontal or downward sloping ST-segment depression of 0.1 mV or more for 60 to 80 msec. It appears to be due to generalized subendocardial ischemia. A "steal" phenomenon is likely from ischemic areas because of the effect of extensive collateralization in the subendocardium. ST depression does not localize the area of ischemia, as does ST elevation or help to indicate which coronary artery is occluded. The normal ST-segment vector response to tachycardia and to exercise is a shift rightward and upward. The degree of this shift appears to have a fair amount of biologic variation. Most normal individuals will have early repolarization at rest, which will shift to the isoelectric PR-segment line in the inferior, lateral, and anterior leads with exercise. This shift can be further influenced by ischemia and myocardial scars. When the later portions of the ST-segment are affected, flattening or downward depression can be recorded. Both local effects and the direction of the spatial changes during repolarization cause the ST segment to have a different appearance at the many surface sites that can be monitored. The more leads with these apparent ischemic shifts, the more severe the disease.

The probability and severity of CAD are directly related to the amount of J-junction depression and are inversely related to the slope of the ST segment. Downsloping ST-segment depression is more serious than horizontal depression, and both are more serious than upsloping depression. However, patients with upsloping ST-segment

a baseline ECG with early repolarization. Abnormal elevation is measured from the upward shift from the baseline level (normally the ST segment sinks with increasing heart rate). Abnormal depression is measured only from when it crosses the isoelectric line. The drop from baseline elevation is not counted as abnormal. Figure 6-7 illustrates how ST shifts are measured when the baseline ECG shows depression. The additional depression is measured from the baseline level of the ST segment and not from the isoelectric line. Elevation is measured from the baseline depression and can actually result in "normalization" of the ST segment.

Exercise-Induced ST-Segment Depression Not Due to Coronary Artery Disease

Table 6-9 lists some of the conditions that can possibly result in false-positive responses. In a population with a high prevalence of heart disease other than CAD, an abnormal ST response would be as diagnostic for that disease as it would be for CAD in populations with a high prevalence of CAD. Digitalis and other drugs can cause exercise-induced repolarization abnormalities in normal individuals. Patients who have had abnormal responses and who have anemia, electrolyte abnormalities, or are on medications should be retested when these conditions are altered. Meals and even glucose ingestion can alter the ST segment and T wave in the resting ECG and can potentially cause a false-positive response. To avoid this problem, all ECG studies should be

performed after at least a 4-hour fast. This requirement is also important because of the hemodynamic stress put on the cardiovascular system by eating—after eating, exercise capacity is decreased and angina occurs at lower hemodynamic stress levels.

Women

Gender has an effect on the exercise ECG that is not explained by hormones alone. Estrogen given to men does not increase the rate of false-positive responses.[86] It has been suggested that the lower specificity of exercise-induced ST-segment depression in women is due to hemodynamic or hemoglobin concentration differences. The diagnostic characteristics of exercise-induced ST depression in woman will be discussed later. It appears that exercise-induced ST depression is more common in adolescent girls than boys.[87]

Digoxin

Sundqvist et al[88] reported the effect of digoxin on the ECG at rest and during and after exercise in 11 healthy subjects. Exercise was performed on a heart rate-controlled bicycle ergometer with stepwise increased loads up to a heart rate of 170 bpm. The subjects were studied after digoxin at two dose levels and after withdrawal of digoxin. Administration of digoxin induced significant ST-T depression at rest and during exercise even at the small dose. The ST-T changes were numerically small and dose dependent. There was usually junctional depression and no downsloping but six individuals had as much as a millimeter of ST depression. The most pronounced ST depression occurred at a heart rate of 110 to 130 bpm. At higher heart rates the ST depression was less pronounced but still statistically significant. During the first minutes after exercise no significant digitalis-induced ST-T depression was seen. This type of reaction is not usually seen in myocardial ischemia. Fourteen days after withdrawal of the drug there were no significant digitalis-induced ST-T changes. In a subsequent study in 20 normals, they concluded that the digoxin-induced ST depression during exercise mimics exercise-induced changes in patients with CAD, but could be discerned by the analysis of ST/HR loops.[89]

This is in agreement with observations by Tonkon et al[90] who studied 15 normal subjects, before and after the administration of digoxin, with exercise testing. Fourteen subjects developed 0.1 to 0.5 mV of ST-segment depression with

TABLE 6–9.   Some conditions that can result in false-positive responses

Valvular heart disease	Left ventricular hypertrophy
Congenital heart disease	Wolff-Parkinson-White syndrome
Vasoregulatory abnormality	Pre-excitation variants
Cardiomyopathies	Mitral valve prolapse syndrome
Pericardial disorders	Hyperventilation repolarization abnormality
Drug administration	
Electrolyte abnormalities	Hypertension
Bundle branch block	Excessive double product
Nonfasting state	Improper lead systems
Anemia	Incorrect criteria
Sudden excessive exercise	Improper interpretation
Inadequate recording equipment	Interventricular conduction defect with T-wave inversion

exercise, but the ST segments normalized at maximal exercise and remained normal throughout recovery. Sketch et al[91] studied 98 healthy males, aged 22 to 70 years, who were administered digoxin at 0.25 mg per day for 14 days and then underwent daily exercise testing until it was interpreted as normal. Twenty-four subjects had an abnormal ST response to exercise, and in 20 of them the ST-segment depression resolved less than 4 minutes into recovery.

Digoxin has been shown to produce abnormal ST depression in response to exercise in 25% to 40% of apparently healthy individuals.[92] The prevalence of abnormal responses is directly related to age and perhaps digoxin uncovers subclinical coronary disease.

Left Bundle Branch Block

Whinnery et al[93] reported 31 asymptomatic men who serially developed LBBB and who were studied with both maximal treadmill testing and coronary angiography. They demonstrated that there could be a marked degree of exercise-induced ST-segment depression in addition to that found at rest in healthy men with LBBB. No difference was found between the ST-segment response to exercise in those with or those without significant CAD. Thus, the ST-segment response to exercise testing cannot be used to make diagnostic decisions in patients with LBBB. Ellestad's group[94] recently reported exercise testing in 41 patients with LBBB. Seven were nonischemic and 34 had coronary artery obstruction. ST depression equaling 0.5 mm or more from baseline, when measured at the J point in leads II and AVF, and an increase of R-wave amplitude in lead II significantly identified ischemia.

Exercise-Induced Left Bundle Branch Block

Vasey et al[95] reviewed the records of 2584 consecutive patients who underwent both treadmill testing and coronary angiography to determine the relation between exercise-induced acceleration-dependent LBBB and the presence of CAD. Rate-dependent LBBB during exercise was identified in 28 patients (1.1%) who were categorized according to their presenting symptoms: classic angina pectoris, atypical chest pain, symptomatic arrhythmias, and asymptomatic. Asymptomatic individuals were being screened for silent CAD. CAD was present in 7 of 10 patients who presented with classic angina pectoris, but 12 of 13 patients presenting with atypical chest pain had normal coronary arteries. All 10 patients in whom LBBB

developed at a heart rate of 125 bpm or higher were free of CAD, whereas 9 of 18 patients in whom LBBB developed at a heart rate of less than 125 bpm had CAD. Normal coronary arteries were present in three patients who presented with angina and in whom both chest pain and LBBB developed during exercise. They concluded that: (1) patients who presented with atypical chest pain and have rate-dependent LBBB are significantly less likely to have CAD than patients who presented with classic angina, (2) the onset of LBBB at a heart rate of 125 bpm or higher is highly associated with the presence of normal coronary arteries, regardless of patient presentation, and (3) patients with angina in whom both chest pain and LBBB develop during exercise may have normal coronary arteries.

From their exercise testing experience at Mayo Clinic, Grady et al[96] estimated a 0.5% prevalence of the development of transient LBBB during exercise. They performed a matched control cohort study to determine whether exercise-induced LBBB is an independent predictor of mortality and cardiac morbidity. Seventy cases of exercise-induced LBBB were identified and matched with 70 controls based on age, test date, sex, prior history of CAD, hypertension, diabetes, smoking, and beta-blocker use. A total of 37 events occurred in 25 patients during a mean follow-up period of 3.7 years. There were seven deaths, of which five occurred among patients with exercise-induced LBBB. Exercise-induced LBBB independently was associated with a three times higher risk of death and major cardiac events.

Right Bundle Branch Block

Whinnery et al[97] also reported the response to maximal treadmill testing in 40 asymptomatic men with acquired right bundle branch block. There was no exercise-induced ST-segment depression in the inferior and lateral leads. Exercise-induced ST-segment depression in the anterior precordial leads is frequently noted in patients with right bundle branch block. This is most apparent in the right precordial leads with an rSR' or a notched R wave; these leads often show a downsloping ST segment at rest, and such a finding is thus not indicative of myocardial ischemia. Figure 6-8 shows ST depression in lateral leads in patients with angina and Figure 6-9 shows the absence of ST depression in lateral leads in a patient without coronary heart disease (CHD), but with both showing anterior ST depression.

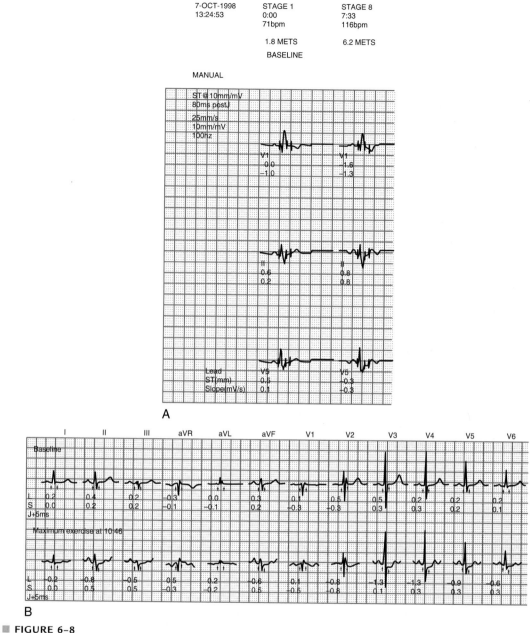

■ FIGURE 6–8

Examples of abnormal exercise-induced ST depression in two patients, one with right bundle branch block with coronary artery disease and the other with ischemia. *a*, Patient with abnormal ST depression in the lateral leads. *b*, Patient with ST depression in V_2 that represents ischemia because the T waves are not inverted in V_2, like they normally are in V_2. Both are true positives.

Wolfe-Parkinson-White Syndrome (WPW)

WPW is a conduction disturbance in which atrial impulses are transmitted to the ventricle by an accessory pathway in addition to normal atrioventricular conduction. The result of depolarization reaching the ventricles by two wave fronts is the delta wave (ventricular activation due to the accessory pathway), a short PR interval and a widened QRS complex.[98] During exercise, increases in sympathetic tone, decreases in vagal tone, and subsequent changes in the automaticity of conductive tissues may result in ECG changes.

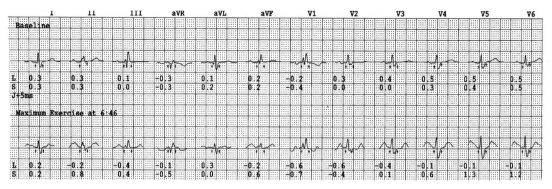

■ FIGURE 6–9

Example of exercise-induced ST depression in the anterior leads, but not in the lateral leads, in a patient with right bundle branch block without evidence for ischemia or coronary artery disease (i.e., a negative ST response).

ST-segment depression typical for ischemia occurs in approximately 50% of patients.[99,100]

Jezior et al[101] from Walter Reed have identified 176 patients with pre-excitation reported in eight studies who were exercise tested with ischemic appearing changes occurring in 86 (49%) (Table 6-10).[102–107] Although the majority of these patients did not undergo angiography, most were felt to be clinically at low risk for significant CAD. The ischemic-appearing ST segments during exercise are hypothesized to be the result of increasing sympathetic tone leading to modification of the different electrophysiologic properties of the ventricle and accessory pathway but they could be due to the memory effect of abnormal depolarization.

The complete block of the accessory pathway can be brought out by exercise resulting in disappearance of the delta wave. However, the ischemic-appearing ST segments may persist despite delta-wave disappearance. In a population felt to have false-positive exercise tests, Poyatos et al[100] demonstrated normalization of ST segments in 20 of 28 patients whose delta wave disappeared, with eight continuing to display ST-segment depression. A proposed mechanism for this phenomenon is the concept of "cardiac memory" with persistence of abnormal repolarization, as can be seen with the cessation of pacing or resolution of a bundle branch block.[108]

While nuclear perfusion imaging is usually relied on to confirm a false-positive ST response, several studies have demonstrated a high frequency of perfusion abnormalities in patients with WPW. In a review of false-positive thallium studies, Paquet et al[103] identified 47 patients in the literature with WPW who underwent exercise myocardial perfusion imaging. Only 24 patients (51%) were reported as having a normal study with the majority of abnormal studies being false positives. They concluded that exercise myocardial perfusion imaging may be of limited benefit in such patients. The mechanism of perfusion abnormalities in WPW has been compared to that seen in LBBB. Ventricular asynchrony leading to regional differences in perfusion has been proposed as the cause.

Disappearance of the delta wave has been used to stratify those patients at risk for developing rapid tachyarrhythmias and sudden death. Jezior[109–111] identified 238 patients in seven studies in whom the behavior of the delta wave was described (Table 6-11). Complete disappearance is described in 98 patients (41%). Of these patients, 43 (18%)

TABLE 6–10. Case studies of patients with Wolff-Parkinson-White syndrome who underwent exercise testing

Study	Number of patients studied	ST depression	Nuclear testing performed	Abnormal nuclear perfusion
Gazes et al	23	20	-	-
Poyatos et al	58	31	18	9
Strasberg et al	54	19	-	-
Paquet et al	1	1	1	1
Archer et al	8	7	8	2
Tawarahara et al	20	-	20	2
Pattoneri et al	11	7	-	-
Greenland et al	1	1	-	-
Total	176	86 (49%)	47	14 (30%)

TABLE 6-11. Seven studies where the behavior of the delta wave was described during exercise testing

Study	Baseline delta wave	Gradual loss of delta wave	Sudden loss of delta wave	Loss of delta wave (gradual+sudden)	Partial loss of delta wave
Gaita et al	65	10	8	18	-
Poyatos et al	48	7	16	23	-
Strasberg et al	36	14	4	18	16
Pattoneri et al	9	-	-	2	-
Sharma et al	56	9	13	22	-
Daubert et al	10	4	2	6	3
Lévy et al	14	-	-	9	-
Total	238	44 (18%)	43 (18%)	98 (41%)	19 (8%)

exhibited sudden complete disappearance and 44 (18%) gradual disappearance. Nineteen patients (8%) demonstrated incomplete disappearance.

Current consensus opinion is that gradual disappearance of the delta wave represents facilitated and preferential conduction through the AV node over the accessory pathway as sympathetic tone increases.[6] However, sudden disappearance of the delta wave from one beat to the next suggests a complete block of conduction in the accessory pathway, therefore identifying pathways with a long anterograde effective refractory period.

Attempts have been made to stratify patients at risk of sudden death by using this classification system. Patients with short accessory pathway refractory periods are able to sustain the fastest heart rates during atrial fibrillation, which can lead to VF in the susceptible patient.[112] Patients with a shortest RR interval between consecutive pre-excited beats, equaling 250 msec or less during atrial fibrillation induced in electrophysiology study (EPS), have the shortest accessory pathway refractory periods, and are felt to be at highest risk for sudden death. Sharma et al[109] studied 56 patients with both EPS and exercise testing. Thirty-four patients without disappearance of the delta wave had a mean shortest RR interval of 236 ± 64 msec. In nine patients with a gradual loss of delta wave, mean shortest RR interval was 242 ± 37 msec. Sudden loss of the delta wave occurred in 13 patients and was associated with a mean shortest RR interval of 410 ± 148 msec. The authors suggested that sudden loss of the delta wave during exercise, therefore, identified patients at low risk for the development of VF. Gaita et al[113] studied 65 patients without heart disease with EP testing, eight of whom had sudden complete disappearance of the delta wave. Seven of these eight patients had a shortest RR interval of more than 250 msec and were felt to be

at low risk for sudden death. They concluded that the exercise test has a high negative predictive value in the setting of sudden, complete disappearance of the delta wave. In contrast, gradual or incomplete loss of the delta wave during exercise did not reliably predict high-risk patients. Pappone et al[114] have proposed the routine use of EP testing to risk-stratify young asymptomatic patients for sudden death. If such a screening strategy were employed, exercise testing prior to EPS would potentially eliminate the need for invasive risk stratification in approximately 20% of asymptomatic patients with sudden, complete disappearance of the delta wave.

Atrial Repolarization

Riff and Carleton[115] demonstrated in patients with atrioventricular dissociation that the duration of atrial repolarization (the atrial T wave) can play a role in the normal rate-related depression of the J junction in inferior leads (AVF, II) and can increase S-wave amplitude. The effect of atrial repolarization on the ST segments in lateral leads is less important, but it affects a bipolar lead such as CM_5, which contains anterior and inferior forces.

Sapin et al[116] postulated that exaggerated atrial repolarization waves during exercise could produce ST-segment depression mimicking myocardial ischemia. The P waves, PR segments and ST segments were studied in leads II, III, aV_F and V_4 to V_6 in 69 patients whose exercise ECG suggested ischemia (100 μV horizontal or 150 μV upsloping ST depression 80 msec after the J point). All had a normal ECG at rest. The exercise test in 25 patients (52% male, mean age 53 years) were false positives based on normal coronary angiograms or normal nuclear studies. Forty-four patients with a similar age and gender distribution, anginal chest pain, and at least one significant coronary lesion served as a true-positive control group. The false-positive group was characterized by (1) markedly downsloping PR segments at peak exercise, (2) longer exercise time and more rapid peak exercise heart rate than those of the true-positive group, and (3) absence of exercise-induced chest pain. The false-positive group also displayed significantly greater absolute P-wave amplitudes at peak exercise and greater augmentation of P-wave amplitude by exercise in all six ECG leads than were observed in the true-positive group. Multivariable analysis revealed that exercise duration and downsloping PR segments in the inferior ECG leads were independent predictors of a false-positive test.

Greek investigators analyzed exercise-induced ST-segment depression in subjects with a 120-msec or shorter PR segment and normal coronary arteries.[117] A population of 86 individuals who demonstrated ST-segment depression of 1.5 mm or more on treadmill testing and had a subsequent normal coronary angiography was classified into two groups: those ($n = 71$) with a normal PR interval and those ($n = 15$) with a 120-msec or shorter PR interval. All subjects had abnormal ST depression of 1.5 mm or more and normal coronary angiograms. In subjects with short PR segments and normal coronaries, a trend of greater exercise induced-ST-segment depression during treadmill testing was observed in V_5.

Hyperventilation Abnormalities

Individuals with ST repolarization changes, including classic ST depression with hyperventilation prior to treadmill testing, can have abnormal exercise-induced ST-segment changes without CAD. Such changes are unusual and have rarely been responsible for false-positive tests.[118] Orthostatic and hyperventilation changes have been associated with the mitral valve prolapse syndrome, vasoregulatory asthenia and vasoregulatory abnormalities. When they do occur with exercise-induced changes, the interpretation of ischemia should be avoided and the clinician must rely on other parameters to make a diagnosis. Prolonged hyperventilation should be avoided because it can induce ECG abnormalities and arrhythmia in both normals and patients with heart disease. The associated tachycardia can even precipitate angina in patients with obstructive coronary disease. Shorter periods of hyperventilation (<30 seconds) may be used to identify a small percentage of those

with "false-positive" abnormal exercise-induced ST responses.[119]

Other Causes

Individuals with the left ventricular hypertrophy and strain pattern on their resting ECG are at high risk for CAD, but the ST ischemic response is less specific in them. This may be due to an imbalance between the supply and demand of the hypertrophied muscle. Healthy individuals with the WPW syndrome can have exercise-induced ST-segment depression. Some individuals with pre-excitation, a short PR interval, and a normal QRS complex may have a false-positive exercise test. Patients with the mitral valve prolapse have been reported to have abnormal exercise tests but normal coronary angiograms.

Persons with hypertension or an excessive double product (SBP × HR) during exercise could hypothetically have a physiologic imbalance between myocardial oxygen supply and demand. However, an excessive number of false positives were not found in one reported population of mild hypertensives. Barnard et al[120] demonstrated that a sudden high workload of treadmill exercise can yield ST-segment depression in healthy individuals on this basis. Foster et al[121] could not reproduce the ST-segment depression with sudden strenuous bicycle exercise even though EF dropped in their normal subjects. A recorder with an inadequate frequency response can either artifactually induce ST-segment depression in normal subjects or show upsloping depression when horizontal depression is actually present. Use of the proper equipment should avoid this type of distortion. In conclusion, the conditions discussed above can be avoided and should not be the major causes of false-positive responses in a good exercise laboratory. The most common cause of a false-positive test should be the normal variant in a patient who has a physiologic ST-segment vector that is similar to that produced by ischemia. It is interesting to hypothesize that a genomic variation might be responsible for this response.

ST Shift Location and Ischemia

Validating the localization of ischemia with coronary angiography has several limitations. First, collaterals may adequately perfuse areas of the heart served by an obstructed artery. Second, coronary angiography cannot quantify the degree to which an infarcted area of the heart remains ischemic. Finally, the validity of relating anatomic lesions visualized at rest to exercise-induced changes in the ECG both only inferring ischemia is questionable. These limitations partially explain the difficulty correlating ECG alterations with the specific number or location of coronary angiographic obstructions. Precise localization of critical ischemia has assumed more than academic interest, with coronary interventions so widely available. Localization could help to direct surgical intervention to the site of jeopardized myocardium and/or the source of angina pectoris.

Abouantoun et al[122] studied 54 patients with stable CHD, all having exercise-induced perfusion defects. Their exercise ECG test results were compared to their nuclear images and also to 14 low-risk normal subjects. Exercise data was analyzed for spatial ST-vector shifts using a computer program in order to most accurately classify ST-segment depression and elevation. None of the ischemic sites or angiographic diseased areas could be specifically identified by exercise-induced ST-vector shifts.

Fuchs et al[123] evaluated the 12-lead ECG for localizing the site of CAD in 134 patients with angiographically documented single-vessel coronary disease. They reviewed 10 years of cardiac catheterization at John Hopkins Hospital to select these patients who had ECGs recorded during MI, spontaneous rest angina, and/or treadmill exercise. Q-wave location correctly identified the location of the coronary lesion in 98% of the cases, ST elevation in 91%, T-wave inversion in 84%, and ST depression in only 60%. No response could separate right from left circumflex CAD. ST-segment elevation was recorded in 20 of the 56 patients who underwent exercise testing. All 56 had angina during the test. An association was found only between elevation in limb lead III and right CAD.

Simoons et al[47] studied the exercise-induced spatial ST-vector shifts 30 and 80 msec after QRS-end in 34 patients who had coronary angiography and nuclear perfusion exercise scans because of clinically important chest pain. Twenty-two had significant coronary artery obstructions and 12 had normal angiograms. Four of these "normals" (33%) had abnormal exercise tests as well as chest pain. They found that in patients with exercise thallium ischemia defects, the ST vectors were posteriorly oriented in 15 of 22 and anteriorly oriented in 9 of 12 of those without ischemia defects. However, they could find no systematic difference

in the ST-vector direction of patients with anteroseptal, compared to patients with posterolateral, perfusion defects. These studies have been corroborated by the excellent angiographic study by Mark et al from Duke (see earlier description of this study).

Localized transmural ischemia results in generalized subendocardial ischemia that slows electrical conduction, changing the action potentials, as is seen in MI. The ST changes registered during exercise are partially dependent upon the location of scar tissue. ST-segment elevation or depression, or various combinations of ST-segment shifts, do not localize ischemia to myocardial areas or the arteries inferred by these areas. For instance, ST-segment depression in II and AV_F do not necessarily mean that there is inferior ischemia (or right CAD) nor does ST depression in V_5 mean that there is lateral ischemia (or left CAD).

T-WAVE ALTERNANS

Definition/History

T-wave alternans (TWA), a beat-to-beat fluctuation in the amplitude or shape of the T wave, has been noted since the early days of electrocardiography.[124] Ever since its early description TWA has been associated with pathologic findings, including autonomic imbalance,[125] electrolyte abnormalities,[126,127] coronary spasm,[128,129] and sudden death.[130] The earliest laboratory studies noted it to be a feature of myocardial ischemia[131,132] and later studies focused on its relationship to arrhythmias and arrhythmic risk.[133,134] Although the exact cause of TWA remains elusive, it is thought to correlate with cardiac events, and hence is a subject of great interest among investigators.

Physiology

Despite a lack of complete understanding of the physiological basis of TWA, there are several hypotheses to explain the ventricular repolarization and the beat-to-beat pattern. The T wave is a symbol of transmural dispersion of repolarization which results from differences in the size, duration, and shape of the phase 3 plateau cellular action potentials.[135-137] This dispersion of repolarization can be explained by alterations in cellular calcium,[138] inhibition of adenosine triphosphate production,[139] and/or impairment of connexins (membrane ion channel proteins that control conduction).[140] TWA results from changes in the electrical conduction pattern of the myocardium between consecutive beats. These alterations in repolarization or cellular action potentials can be represented by alternating action potential amplitudes or alternating changes in the T-wave spatial direction (or angle) of repolarization or both.

Heterogeneities of repolarization can cause spatially discordant alternans which can be amplified and form a substrate for re-entrant excitation.[141] Although TWA appears to be a possible cause of arrhythmias, it may alternatively just be a reflection of arrhythmogenic substrate. In response to ischemia, action potential duration differences occur in an alternating beat-to-beat pattern and with spatial heterogeneity.[142] Scars, premature ventricular contractions (PVCs), or sympathetic stimulation can also result in alternans.

Animal Studies Linking TWA to Arrhythmias

Several animal studies have been conducted to address the physiologic basis of TWA. In a canine model of experimental MI, Rosenbaum et al[143] studied the beat-to-beat variability in local activation time during sustained monomorphic ventricular tachycardia (VT) and during ventricular pacing and sinus rhythm as controls. The mean variability of local activation time during VT was much higher (3.2 msec) compared to ventricular pacing (0.2 msec) and sinus rhythm (0.7 msec). In addition, oscillations in local activation time manifested alternans-type periodicity. Since beat-to-beat variability and activation-time alternans are common during sustained monomorphic VT and are negligible during sinus rhythm or ventricular pacing, they may be intrinsic to reentry.

Other animal studies have established a mechanism linking TWA to the pathogenesis of sudden cardiac death (SCD). Surface ECGs from guinea pig hearts during pacing with simultaneously recorded action potentials demonstrated discordant alternans of the repolarization phase of the action potential above a critical threshold heart rate (about 200 bpm).[144] Membrane repolarization alternated with the depolarization

between neighboring cells, creating large spatial gradients of repolarization. In the presence of discordant alternans, a small acceleration of the pacing cycle length produced unidirectional block of an impulse propagating against steep gradients of repolarization leading to re-entry which initiated VF.

Methodology

The multiple methods which are available for measuring TWA differ significantly because they focus on different etiologies of TWA. TWA can be due to either alternating beat-to-beat changes in action potential amplitudes of T waves or alternating beat-to-beat changes in the T-wave spatial direction (known as T-wave "wobble").[145] For the former, signal-averaged ECG are used to average the ECG complexes and T-wave amplitudes, and the standard deviation of the waveforms is the marker of the beat-to-beat variability. For the latter, T-wave spatial angle is interpreted as alternations in T-wave amplitude when it is measured in one lead rather than spatially.[146] Three-dimensional leads can also be used, and the actual T-wave spatial vector amplitude derived and measured.

Since macroscopic or visible alternations of T waves are rare, specialized technology has been developed to detect subtle microvolt differences. The first studies used vectorcardiographic leads (orthogonal leads and body surface maps including 12-lead ECGs) to measure the variability of the T-wave spatial angle or amplitude.[147,148] This technology was easily applied during exercise using standard signal-averaging techniques, focusing on diagnosing ischemia. Other studies used fast Fourier transform spectral analysis to indirectly calculate the power spectra of beat-to-beat fluctuations in the T-wave amplitude using the vector magnitude from three-dimensional ECG leads over 128 consecutive beats.[149] Modified moving average is a newer technique that uses a nonspectral method and avoids the need to increase and stabilize heart rate and enables TWA measurement from an ambulatory ECG.[150] A stream of digitized beats is divided into odd and even bins, and each bin is averaged creating odd- and even-beat amplitude averages, which are then subtracted to give the TWA.

Mathematical algorithms such as autocorrelation,[151] auto-regression,[152] and complex demodulation[153] are applied to decrease background noise and measure the alternans ratio (the extent to which the measured alternans exceeds noise) and convey the statistical degree of confidence in the alternans measurement. Sophisticated noise reduction techniques combined with commercially available analytic tools allow measurement of microvolt TWA during routine exercise testing.[154] This advancement is important because TWA often only appears at heart rates above 90 bpm.

TWA Detection: Exercise or Atrial Pacing?

Exercise or atrial pacing is often used to increase the heart rate sufficiently for TWA to be detected. A study of 30 patients with a history of ventricular tachyarrhythmias was performed to compare the two methods.[155] Heart rate thresholds for the onset of TWA were comparable between submaximal exercise (100 ± 14 bpm) and atrial pacing (97 ± 9 bpm). The concordance rate for the presence or absence of TWA using the two techniques was 84%. Although both methods to increase heart rate appear to provide similar results, there is evidence that exercise is better for prognostication.[156]

Clinical Studies

There has been considerable interest in using TWA as a noninvasive test for susceptibility to ventricular arrhythmias and SCD. TWA has been found prospectively in patients referred for diagnostic EPS to be a significant and independent predictor of inducibility of ventricular arrhythmias (RR = 5).[157] Further, in this study arrhythmia-free survival at 20 months was significantly lower among the patients with TWA (19%) than in those without TWA (94%). Similarly, in a smaller study of patients undergoing EPS, the accuracy of TWA in predicting inducibility of ventricular arrhythmias was 84%, and the accuracy of TWA testing in predicting arrhythmia-free survival was 86%.[158]

Gold et al[159] reported on a larger prospective multicenter trial of 313 patients undergoing EPS.[159] Kaplan-Meier survival analysis of the primary endpoint of SCD, sustained VT, VF, or appropriate automatic implantable cardioverter defibrillator therapy showed that TWA predicted events with a relative risk of 11. Meanwhile, EPS had a relative risk of 7 and SAECG had a relative risk of 5. Multivariate analysis identified only TWA and EPS as independent predictors of events.

Cardiomyopathy Patients

Ischemic and nonischemic cardiomyopathy patients are thought to be distinct populations and have often been evaluated separately. In an interesting study of 104 nonischemic cardiomyopathy patients undergoing TWA exercise testing, multivariate Cox hazard analysis revealed that TWA with an onset heart rate of 100 bpm or less and LVEF were independent predictors of arrhythmic events.[160] Hohnloser et al[161] reported a prospective study of dilated cardiomyopathy patients in which, among several potential predictors, microvolt TWA was a significant univariate predictor of VT and was the only significant independent predictor in multivariate Cox regression analysis.

Klingenheben et al[162] found that in patients with congestive heart failure and no history of sustained ventricular arrhythmias, those with negative TWA testing had no ventricular arrhythmic events in the follow-up period. Among tested parameters, only TWA was a significant and independent predictor of arrhythmic events.

Coronary Disease Patients

Patients with CAD and decreased LVEF are known to be at increased risk of ventricular arrhythmias and SCD. In the MADIT II trial of prophylactic implantation of a defibrillator, a mortality benefit was seen among patients with a previous MI and an LVEF of 30% or less. As mentioned previously, it would be useful to have criteria to identify which of the many patients who fulfill these criteria are at highest risk. Ikeda et al[163] prospectively assessed prognostic predictors in 102 post-MI patients and found that of the 15% that had symptomatic sustained VT or VF, the event rates were significantly higher in patients with TWA, late potentials, or an abnormal EF. The sensitivity and negative predictive value of TWA in predicting arrhythmic event were 93% and 98%, respectively. However, its positive predictive value was only 28%.

In a prospective study evaluating several ECG and echocardiographic features to predict mortality in post-MI patients, incomplete TWA test (the inability to perform exercise test or reach the required target heart rate of 105 bpm) was the most significant predictor of cardiac death in multivariate analysis (relative risk of 11).[162] However, sustained TWA during the predischarge exercise test after acute MI did not indicate increased risk for mortality.

It has been suggested that TWA should only be used in the absence of QRS prolongation due to the study by Rashba et al[165] investigating the effect of QRS prolongation on the utility of TWA for risk stratification. In patients with CAD and LVEF of 40% or less referred for EPS, TWA and QRS prolongation were both significant and independent predictors of arrhythmic events. TWA was a highly significant predictor of events in patients with a normal QRS duration (hazard ratio 6) but not patients with QRS prolongation.

In a retrospective analysis of MADIT, 129 patients were identified as having microvolt TWA assessed.[166] In patients that were negative for TWA, there was no cardiac arrest or SCD in follow-up, compared with an event rate of 15.6% among the rest. While the authors concluded that TWA testing could help identify patients who are at low risk of ventricular tachyarrhythmias, reviewers have suggested that we still need a randomized trial comparing MADIT II post-MI patients with and without TWA testing.[167]

Summary

TWA has been incorporated as a noninvasive test into exercise testing protocols or during cardiac pacing. The pathophysiologic mechanism may involve cellular calcium transients, which can be caused by ischemia, that result in alternating changes in action potential durations. It is uncertain whether these changes, and TWA, are the byproduct or the cause of an arrhythmogenic substrate. Furthermore, TWA on surface ECG may reflect actual differences in action potential amplitude or may be due to alternating changes in T-wave spatial direction. The methods (electrode system and measurement algorithms) to record these two phenomena differ. Heart rate is also an important consideration, as increases in rate seem to be necessary to induce TWA. As there is uncertainty in what is actually being measured, the optimal testing technique remains undefined.

Not only is there variability in the measurement definitions of TWA in the clinical studies, the evidence for TWA testing is limited. For patients referred for EPS, TWA seems to be predictive of greater inducibility of ventricular arrhythmias and less arrhythmia-free survival. In patients with dilated cardiomyopathy, TWA appears to be predictive of ventricular arrhythmias. In ischemic cardiomyopathy patients, the reported accuracy of TWA testing is mixed.

The broad use of TWA testing is not supported by the prospective outcome trials to date. Future research should center on using an optimal testing approach in appropriately designed outcomes trials.

SUBJECTIVE RESPONSES

Careful observation of the patient's appearance is necessary for the safe performance of an exercise test and is helpful in the clinical assessment of a patient. Patients who exaggerate their limitations or symptoms and those unwilling to cooperate are usually easy to identify. A drop in skin temperature during exercise can indicate an inadequate cardiac output with secondary vasoconstriction and can be an indication for not encouraging a patient to a higher workload. Neurological manifestations, such as lightheadedness or vertigo, can also be indications of an inadequate cardiac output.

Findings on physical examination can be helpful, but their sensitivity and specificity have not been demonstrated. Gallop sounds, a mitral regurgitant murmur, or a precordial bulge could be due to left ventricular dysfunction. An S3 can sometimes be heard normally after exercise, but a new S4 brought out by exercise has been said to be specific for CHD. The physical findings of congestive heart failure, including rales and neck vein distention, should be encountered rarely in patients referred for exercise testing. However, some exercise testing laboratories use the sitting position for the recovery period to avoid problems with the patient who develops orthopnea. It is preferable to have patients lie supine after exercise testing and allow those who develop orthopnea to sit up. In addition, allowing the patient to sit up can lessen severe angina or ominous dysrhythmias following exercise. Attempts to make the findings of the physical examination less subjective include the use of phonocardiography, apexcardiography, and cardiokymography. Left ventricular ejection time can be determined by the ear densitigram and its first derivative more easily than by trying to obtain a carotid pulse tracing.

Chest Pain

The reproduction of chest pain during the test is very important to classify and report. While nonspecific chest pain is of importance to recognize, true angina pectoris has diagnostic and prognostic importance. The Duke Treadmill angina score should always be recorded as part of the test (Table 6-12).

Typical angina pectoris is a pressure, tightness, and/or pain located substernally. It can radiate or be centered in the neck or down the left arm. Some patients have a shortness of breath that has been called an "angina equivalent" but this is not true angina. Patients can describe an angina that comes on at low levels of exercise and goes away as they warm up and progress to higher work levels (walk-through or warm-up angina). Some patients get angina in the recovery phase, usually within 5 minutes. Angina is not pinpoint, pleuritic, knife-like, or palpable. The exercise test is an important opportunity to reproduce the patient's symptoms and determine if they are really having angina pectoris or a nonspecific chest pain.

Weiner et al[168] reported 281 consecutive patients studied with treadmill testing and coronary angiography. They were grouped according to the following responses: (l) 76 patients with ST-segment depression and treadmill test-induced chest pain, (2) 85 patients with ST-segment depression and no chest pain, (3) 40 patients with treadmill test induced-chest pain who had no ST-segment changes, and (4) 80 patients with neither chest pain nor ST-segment changes. They found that 91% of the first group, 65% of the second group, 72% of the third group, and only 35% of the fourth group had significant angiographically determined CAD. Cole and Ellestad[169] followed 95 patients with abnormal treadmill tests. At 5 years of follow-up, the incidence of CAD was 73% in those with both chest pain and an abnormal ST-segment response compared with 43% in those who only had an abnormal ST-segment response. Mortality was also twice as high in those with both ST-segment changes and chest pain induced by the treadmill test.

A fascinating study from Norway has added additional importance to angina and exercise testing. During 1972–1975, 2014 apparently healthy men aged 40 to 59 years underwent an examination program including history, clinical examination, exercise ECG, and the WHO angina questionnaire.[170] Sixty-eight had possible angina and 115 were excluded because they had definite angina or abnormal exercise ECGs. At 26 years, men with possible angina had a cardiovascular mortality of 25% (17/68) versus 14% (252/1831) among men without angina. They also had a higher incidence of cardiac events. Multivariate analysis including risk factors showed that possible angina was an independent risk factor (two times relative risk). This study demonstrates that men with possible angina, even with a normal exercise test, have a greater risk of CHD. Note that the exercise test did not bring on the angina in these men with a positive angina history.

The results of these studies suggest that ischemic chest pain induced by the exercise test predicts the presence of CAD as well as ST-segment depression, and when they occur together, they are even more predictive of CAD than either is alone. It is important though, that a careful description of the pain be obtained from the patient to ascertain that it is typical rather than atypical angina or non-ischemic chest pain.

EVIDENCE BASIS FOR EXERCISE TEST–INDUCED SILENT ISCHEMIA

There are two clinical settings in which evidence exists regarding the significance of silent ischemia (SI) during exercise testing: (1) screening studies of asymptomatic individuals and (2) exercise testing as part of the workup of patients with known or suspected coronary disease.

In each setting, those without diabetes (A) and those with diabetes (B) will be considered separately because of the clinical impression that they are more likely to have SI.[171] This evidence-based review will close with a subsection (#3) considering the evidence for this impression.

Screening Studies with Follow-up Not Considering Diabetic Status

Unfortunately the first screening studies of exercise testing in asymptomatic individuals included angina as a cardiac disease endpoint.[172-176]

TABLE 6–12. The duke treadmill angina score	
Score	Definition
0	No angina
1	Angina occurred
2	Angina was the reason for stopping the test

This led to a bias for individuals with abnormal tests to subsequently report chest pain diagnosed as angina. When only hard endpoints (death or MI) were used, as in the reports from MRFIT,[177] Lipid Research Clinics,[178] Indiana State Police[179] or the Seattle Heart Watch,[180] the results suggested that ST depression had a lower predictive value than initially thought. Asymptomatic abnormal ST depression could only identify one third of the patients with hard events and 95% of abnormal ST responders were false positives; that is, they did not die or have an MI. While the predictive value of an abnormal ST response was as high as 50% in the early studies, in the studies using appropriate endpoints, only 5% of the abnormal responders developed CHD over the follow-up period. Thus, more than 90% of the abnormal responders were false positives. Some of the abnormal responders have coronary disease that has yet to manifest itself, but angiographic studies have validated this high false-positive rate when using the exercise test in asymptomatic populations.[181] It is unlikely that the false positives have other forms of heart disease since the Coronary Artery Surgery Study documented that they have a good prognosis.[182] In a second Lipid Research Clinics study, only asymptomatic individuals with elevated cholesterols were considered, and yet only a 6% positive prediction value was found (i.e., only 6 out of 100 with ST depression went on the have CAD events).[183]

From the Cooper Clinic comes the largest study of the exercise test to predict death from CHD and death from any cause in a population of asymptomatic men.[184] It was a prospective study performed between 1970 and 1989, with an average follow-up of 8.4 years. There were 25,927 healthy men, 20 to 82 years of age at baseline (mean 43 years) who were free of cardiovascular disease and evaluated in a preventive medicine clinic. During follow-up there were 612 deaths from all causes and 158 deaths from CHD. The sensitivity of an abnormal exercise test to predict coronary death was 61%. The age-adjusted relative risk of an abnormal exercise test for CHD death was 21 times in those with no risk factors, 27 times in those with one risk factor, 54 times in those with two risk factors, and 80 times in those with three or more factors. This elegant study supports the incredible risk generated by SI as found in earlier studies.

Please refer to the chapter on screening for a more complete discussion of this issue.

Screening Studies with Follow-up Considering Diabetic Status

The seminal study performed by Gerson et al[185] is the only appropriate screening study in diabetics with follow-up. To identify predictors of asymptomatic CAD, they performed noninvasive screening of 110 insulin-requiring diabetic patients with a normal resting ECG. At entry, their mean age was 35 years and mean duration of insulin use was 19 years. Screening included history and physical examination, exercise ECG, echocardiography, and blood testing. Approximately a quarter had abnormal ST depression or an inadequate heart rate response, but these responses were not separated. During 8 years follow-up, 14 developed clinical evidence of CAD consisting of acute MI, SCD, or anginal chest pain confirmed by angiography. Only three of these patients had ST depression during the exercise test. Age, maximal heart rate, and retinal neovascularization were variables univariately predictive of subsequent clinical coronary disease. According to multivariate analysis, the treadmill heart rate was the single most important predictor of subsequent development of clinical coronary disease. Chronotropic incompetence identified each patient in whom CAD developed within 4 years after entry testing but was only 43% sensitive at 8 years with a specificity of 77%. More studies of similar design are needed in other groups of diabetics using risk factors and diabetic complications to increase the pretest probability of coronary disease. Unfortunately, these investigators mixed the criteria for an abnormal test (both heart rate and ST criteria were applied) so that test characteristics could not be determined. It is apparent though that exercise-induced ST depression had a low sensitivity (21%) with only 3 of the 14 patients with endpoints identified.

We found only four studies which considered a truly asymptomatic diabetic population and screened them for cardiovascular disease. Koistinen[186] found 29% of diabetics and 5% of controls had ischemic results in one or more noninvasive tests, while Gerson et al[185] found that a quarter of 110 asymptomatic, insulin-requiring diabetic patients had abnormal ST depression or an inadequate heart rate response. Janand-Delenne et al[187] found 16% of noninvasive tests to be positive in 203 patients screened for 1 year with exercise ECG and nuclear perfusion, followed-up with coronary angiography. Angiographically significant (>50% stenosis) disease was found in 9.3%. Finally, May et al[188] found the prevalence of SI to be 13.5% in a randomly chosen diabetic population.

Exercise Test-Induced Silent Ischemia in Patients with Known or Suspected Coronary Disease

Prognosis of Silent Ischemia during Exercise Testing, Not Considering Diabetic Status

To evaluate the significance of SI during exercise testing, data were analyzed from 2982 patients from the Coronary Artery Surgery Study registry who underwent coronary angiography and exercise testing and were followed up for 7 years.[189,190] Four hundred twenty-four patients had ischemic ST depression without angina, 232 had angina but no ischemic ST depression, 456 had both ischemic ST depression and angina, and 471 had neither ischemic ST depression nor angina. The 7-year survival rates were similar for patients in all groups (77%), except for patients without ST depression or angina who did better (88%).

Using the Duke database, Mark et al[191] evaluated the clinical correlates and long-term prognostic significance of SI during exercise. They analyzed 1698 consecutive symptomatic patients with CAD, who had both treadmill testing and cardiac catheterization. Compared with symptomatic ischemia, SI indicated a subgroup of patients who had a less aggressive anginal course, less CAD and a better prognosis.

Dagenais et al[192] reported 6-year cumulative survival in 298 moderately treated patients with exercise-induced ST-segment depression equal or greater than 2 mm. In those with silent myocardial ischemia, survival was 85%, whereas it was significantly lower (80%) in those with angina pectoris. Patients with silent myocardial ischemia reached a greater heart rate and higher MET level than those with painful ischemia. Cumulative survival was very much related to the MET level achieved. Those who reached 10 METs had very few deaths while those with less than 5 METs had approximately a 50% survival.

Casella et al[193] examined the prognostic significance of silent myocardial ischemia detected on exercise treadmill testing in stable patients with previous MI in an attempt to clarify the degree of concern physicians should have for this patient population. Seven hundred sixty-six stable patients with a remote history of MI (3 years) underwent exercise testing and were followed for 7 years. There was no significant difference in the primary endpoint of cardiac death or nonfatal reinfarction between patients with silent and painful ischemia; however, when unstable angina and revascularization procedures were included in the analysis, patients with symptomatic ischemia had a higher incidence of events. The average annual mortality rate was only 1.2% in patients with SI.

Angiographic Studies of Silent Ischemia without Consideration of Diabetic Status

Visser et al[194] from the Netherlands studied 280 patients with anginal complaints, without prior MI and with a positive exercise test. Miranda et al[195] performed a retrospective analysis of 416 male veterans referred for exercise testing who were selected for cardiac catheterization. Falcone et al[196] compared the clinical and angiographic characteristics of 269 patients who complained of chest pain during an exercise test with those of 204 who developed silent myocardial ischemia. In these studies encompassing almost 1000 patients, a consistent finding was that patients with symptomatic ischemia had a higher prevalence of severe angiographic coronary disease than did patients with SI.

Conclusion of the Follow-up and Angiographic Studies

From these follow-up and angiographic studies we could conclude that silent myocardial ischemia during treadmill testing in patients without their diabetic status being considered does not predict increased risk for death. The concern that patients with silent myocardial ischemia were at higher risk than their peers with angina because of failure of their warning mechanism was not substantiated. However, these are patients who presented for testing with chest pain symptoms and either did or did not manifest this pain during the treadmill test. Thus, their ischemia was not always silent or asymptomatic but its symptomatic presentation was the reason they underwent testing.

Do Diabetics Have a Higher Prevalence of Silent Ischemia During Treadmill Testing than Nondiabetics?

Silent Ischemia More Common in Diabetics

Nesto et al[197] studied 50 patients with diabetes and 50 patients without diabetes, selected consecutively following ischemia on exercise thallium scintigraphy. Their purpose was to evaluate angina as a marker for exertional ischemia. The two groups had similar clinical characteristics, treadmill test results, and extent of infarction and ischemia, but only 14 patients with diabetes compared with 34 patients without diabetes had angina during exertional ischemia. In diabetic patients the extent of retinopathy, nephropathy, or peripheral neuropathy was similar in patients with and without angina. These authors found angina to be an unreliable index of myocardial ischemia in diabetic patients and felt that periodic objective assessment of the extent of ischemia was warranted. A similar study, but with angiographic endpoints, found diabetics receiving insulin or with retinopathy to have twice the prevalence of SI than nondiabetics[198], and two studies found diabetics with neuropathy to have more SI than nondiabetics.[199,200]

One hundred and fourteen diabetic patients with percutaneous coronary intervention followed by a nuclear perfusion scan were followed up for 2 years for cardiac events.[201] After percutaneous coronary intervention, these now asymptomatic diabetic patients had a high frequency of persistent SI, which was associated with a high risk for repeat interventional procedure, although no increase in major cardiac events was observed.

In the Detection of Ischemia in Asymptomatic Diabetics study, 1123 patients with type 2 diabetes, aged 50 to 75 years, with no known or suspected CAD, were randomly assigned to either stress testing and 5-year clinical follow-up or to follow-up only.[202] The prevalence of ischemia in 522 patients randomized to stress testing was assessed by adenosine myocardial perfusion imaging. A total of 113 patients (22%) had SI, including 83 with regional myocardial perfusion abnormalities and 30 with normal perfusion but other abnormalities (i.e., adenosine-induced ST-segment depression, ventricular dilation, or rest ventricular dysfunction). Moderate or large perfusion defects were present in 33 patients. The strongest predictors for abnormal tests were abnormal Valsalva (six times odds ratio), male sex (3 times), and diabetes duration (5 times). These investigators concluded that silent myocardial ischemia occurs in greater than one in five asymptomatic patients with type 2 diabetes. Traditional and emerging cardiac risk factors were not associated with abnormal stress tests, although cardiac autonomic dysfunction was a strong predictor of ischemia. While suggesting a high prevalence of SI in diabetics, there was no comparison with nondiabetics using the same techniques.

Silent Ischemia Not More Common in Diabetics

In a landmark Danish study, the prevalence of ischemia was compared in diabetics and nondiabetics.[203] A random sample of 120 users of insulin and 120 users of oral hypoglycemic agents aged 40 to 75 years, living in Denmark, were asked to participate. Abnormal ST depression on either exercise or Holter was considered indicative of myocardial ischemia. Angina pectoris was considered present if the Rose questionnaire was positive, or chest pain accompanied ECG evidence of ischemia. The observed prevalence of SI in diabetics was 13.5% and was no different in matched controls. No association was found between SI and gender or diabetes type. Hypertension was highly predictive of SI in the diabetic subjects but other variables did not have a predictive value. In this population-based study of SI in diabetes, the frequency of SI did not differ significantly between diabetics and nondiabetics.

An analysis was performed to determine whether diabetic patients with coronary disease enrolled in the Asymptomatic Cardiac Ischemia Pilot had more episodes of asymptomatic ischemia during exercise testing and Holter monitoring than nondiabetic patients.[204] Angiographic findings and the prevalence and magnitude of ischemia during the qualifying Holter and exercise study were compared by the presence and absence of diabetes mellitus in 558 randomized Asymptomatic Cardiac Ischemia Pilot patients. Seventy-seven patients had a history of diabetes and were taking oral hypoglycemics or insulin.

Multivessel disease (87% versus 74%) was more frequent in the diabetics. The percentages of patients without angina during the exercise test were similar in the diabetic and nondiabetic groups (36% and 39%, respectively). Time to onset of 1-mm ST-segment depression and time to onset of angina were similar in both groups. The percentages of patients with only asymptomatic ST-segment depression during the Holter were similar in the diabetic and nondiabetic groups (94% versus 88%, respectively). However, total ischemic time, ischemic time per episode, and the maximum depth of ST-segment depression tended to be less in the diabetic group. Unlike the previous study, entry into the Asymptomatic Cardiac Ischemia Pilot study required a cardiac event so the subjects were not truly asymptomatic.

Falcone et al[205] recruited a total of 618 patients with CAD: 309 were consecutive diabetic patients and 309 were age- and gender-matched nondiabetic patients. Myocardial ischemia was evaluated both during daily life and exercise testing. Angina pectoris during daily life was more frequent in diabetic than in nondiabetic patients (80% versus 74%). The anginal pain intensity either during daily life or acute MI, the prevalence of a previous MI, the extent of CAD, and exercise parameters were similar in diabetics and nondiabetics. SI during exercise occurred in 179 (58%) diabetics and in 197 (64%) nondiabetics. Both diabetics and nondiabetics with silent exertional myocardial ischemia differed from symptomatic subjects in higher heart rate, systolic blood pressure, METs and maximum ST-segment depression at peak exercise. The prevalence of silent myocardial ischemia during exercise was similar in diabetic and nondiabetic CAD patients, as has been our experience with exercise testing in veterans.[206]

Conclusions Regarding Silent Ischemia

In patients with stable CAD who have not suffered a recent MI, SI on exercise testing does not identify a high-risk population and actually predicts a better outcome than symptomatic ischemia. In this instance it may be appropriate that "only the squeaky wheel gets the grease"; that only those patients with angina and exercise-induced ST depression should be considered for interventions.[207] Furthermore, the evidence base for the common clinical axiom that diabetics have a higher prevalence of SI is far from conclusive.

INTERPRETATION OF EXERCISE TEST-INDUCED ARRHYTHMIAS (ETIA)

Definition and Historical Perspective

It has been recommended that exercise testing be used as a noninvasive method for exposing cardiac arrhythmias, particularly when symptoms are brought on by exercise.[208] The information obtained can complement information obtained from ambulatory monitoring and electrophysiologic testing.[209] We discuss this here since the data so far indicates the safety of ETIA, except in certain high-risk situations (i.e., cardiomyopathy and valvular patients, when exercise test-induced ST elevation occurs), the fact that their diagnostic and prognostic characteristics are weak, and perhaps that they only have long-term significance. Couplets, or nonsustained ventricular tachycardia (NSVT), occur during exercise or recovery in up to a third of patients tested, and even in patients with known heart disease, there is a small risk of inducing sustained VT or VF during exercise. In patients in whom arrhythmias are known to be induced by exercise, exercise testing is an excellent method by which the effectiveness of antiarrhythmic drug treatment can be assessed, bearing in mind that certain antiarrhythmic drugs are known to be associated with ETIVT.[210-213]

Poor exercise capacity and exercise-induced cardiac ischemia are the strongest predictors of mortality while the prognostic significance of exercise-induced arrhythmias (ETIA) remains unclear.[214] Some studies suggest that exercise test-induced ventricular arrhythmias (ETIVA) confer a poor prognosis [215-217] and others contest this.[218-220] Less data is available regarding exercise test-induced supraventricular arrhythmias (ETISVA). The clinical significance of ETIVA in those without documented cardiovascular disease presents another dilemma. Although a recent study found that healthy volunteers with ETIVA had increased mortality,[221] earlier studies did not produce similar results.[222,223] It is unclear if the prognosis associated with ETIVA differs based on the presence of cardiovascular disease, ischemic changes during exercise, and/or the presence of PVCs at rest (i.e., an indicator of the arrhythmic substrate).

Physiologic and Pathophysiologic Basis

Exercise produces a number of important physiologic changes, namely the activation of the sympathetic nervous system and an increase in the availability of circulating catecholamines, which can predispose to arrhythmias.[224–226] These changes interact with the three major mechanisms involved in the generation of arrhythmias: enhanced automaticity, triggered automaticity, and re-entry. Other potential proarrhythmic mechanisms include electrolyte shifts, baroreceptor activation, myocardial stretch, and ischemia.[227,228] Atrial arrhythmias may reflect underlying left atrial enlargement and ventricular dysfunction.

In arterial blood, vigorous exercise can double the plasma potassium, decrease pH, and raise catecholamines more than 10-fold. If any of these changes are experienced at rest, there is an increased risk of arrhythmia and cardiac arrest, yet in exercise they are usually well tolerated.[229] It has been postulated that the heart may be protected from exercise induced-chemical stress by an antiarrhythmic interaction between these chemical changes. Catecholamines can offset the harmful cardiac effects of hyperkalemia and acidosis and improve action potential characteristics in potassium-depolarized ventricular myocytes. This results from an increase in the inward calcium current modulated by both adrenergic and nonadrenergic hormones.

Conversely, hyperkalemia decreases the incidence of norepinephrine-induced arrhythmias. The efficacy of the mutual antagonism is reduced when the combination of acidosis, hyperkalemia, and high levels of norepinephrine are superimposed on a heart with regional ischemia or a small infarct. However, the heart may be at greatest risk in the postexercise period, when plasma potassium is low and the adrenergic tone is high. Most dangerous ETIA occur at this time and they can be lessened or avoided by cool-down activities. Abnormal regulation of electrolyte and cardiac sympathovagal balance in recovery most likely increases the susceptibility to arrhythmias, particularly when ischemia is present.

Any alteration in the delicate chemical balance and natural pathophysiologic response to exercise may also contribute to cardiac arrhythmias. Recent studies have linked certain antiarrhythmic drugs with ETIVT.[210–213] Ranger et al[230] hypothesized that the sinus tachycardia seen during exercise may enhance flecainide-induced conduction slowing by increasing use-dependent sodium channel blockade, thereby facilitating the occurrence of ventricular reentry.[230] Their study found that the best predictor of further exercise-induced QRS slowing was the change in QRS duration produced by flecainide at rest.

Other studies have delineated varying electrical patterns that may predispose patients to exercise-induced ventricular arrhythmias. A Dutch group studied the initiating mechanisms of ETIVT in 6000 patients.[231] One percent had 194 episodes of VT during the test. Forty-two percent of these occurred during exercise and 58% during recovery. Two different initiating patterns were observed prior to VT: a short-long-short sequence of R-R intervals (28%) or a regular RR pattern (63%).

In addition to a regular RR pattern, one of the forms of the long QT syndrome (LQTS) has also been linked to exercise-induced sudden death.[232] The gene KCNQ1 (formerly called KVLQT1) is a Shaker-like voltage-gated potassium channel gene responsible for the LQT1 subtype of LQTS. In general, heterozygous mutations in KCNQ1 cause Romano-Ward syndrome (LQT1 only), while homozygous mutations cause Jervell and Lange-Nielsen Syndrome (LQT1 and deafness). The majority of these mutations are missense mutations. However, other types of mutations, such as deletions, frame-shifts, and splice-donor errors, have also been reported. The combination of normal and mutant KCNQ1 alpha-subunits has been found to form abnormal IKs channels, hence mutations associated with the KCNQ1 gene are also believed to act mainly through a dominant-negative mechanism or loss of function mechanism.[233]

Paavonen et al[234] studied the effects of mental and physical stress on LQTS patients.[234] During exercise, the corresponding QT adaptation to exercise stress was more pronounced in healthy controls (−47 msec) than in LQT1 (−38 msec) or LQT2 patients (−38 ms). During exercise, changes in serum potassium concentrations were correlated to changes in QT intervals in controls, but not in LQTS patients.

Familial catecholaminergic polymorphic VT is a rare arrhythmogenic disease manifesting with exercise- or stress-induced ventricular arrhythmias, syncope, and even sudden death. Catecholaminergic polymorphic VT is inherited as an autosomal dominant or autosomal recessive trait, usually with high penetrance.[235] The clinical, structural, and ECG findings in this disorder have been characterized by use of genome-wide linkage analysis, mapping the disease-causing gene to chromosome 1q42–q43. Mutations of the cardiac ryanodine receptor gene (RyR2) have been demonstrated to underlie this life-threatening disease. In addition, RyR2 mutations were identified in patients affected with a variant form of arrhythmogenic right ventricular dysplasia 2, a phenotypically distinct disease entity. Identification of the causal mutations has enabled molecular diagnosis in the affected families, which is of major importance in identifying individuals at risk of an arrhythmia. Recently, several groups have delineated the functional effects of the RyR2 mutations associated with Catecholaminergic polymorphic VT and arrhythmogenic right ventricular dysplasia 2. The results are slightly contradictory, and further studies are thus needed to clarify the exact molecular mechanisms leading to arrhythmia induction.

Methodology

Arrhythmia Detection Technology

The reported studies have used a number of different technologies to record and diagnose arrhythmias occurring in association with exercise testing. The earliest studies simply relied on physicians and/or technicians to recognize arrhythmias appearing on the monitor and/or recorded on the ECG output. This was dependent upon the skill and attention of the observer to note the arrhythmia and record it by manually initiating an ECG recording. As the exercise devices became more sophisticated, they incorporated software algorithms that detected arrhythmias and automatically initiated an ECG recording. The noise associated with exercise represented "a challenge to these algorithms frequently triggering them. Therefore, in most clinical settings they are disabled to prevent wastage of ECG paper.

Because of the exercise environment, algorithms developed for monitoring patients in the hospital or during ambulatory ECG recordings could not easily be implemented or relied upon. A Holter technique that has been enabled in some commercially available exercise systems provides total disclosure of all ECG complexes. Noise can make the recognition of arrhythmias difficult even when using these types of printouts. More recently exercise systems have included the capacity to record all ECG data during and after

exercise. These stored, digitized signals can be subjected to sophisticated software techniques off-line, employing noise reduction algorithms and Holter-like ECG analysis.

Definition

Study design and the means by which ETIA have been captured have differed significantly enough that it has been difficult to come to a consensus regarding prevalence rates, much less extrapolating prognostic information from data available. Clearly, the methods of recording and capturing PVCs greatly affect the prevalence data and as technology advances, the multitude of options available for data collection may make standardization even more difficult. Even in studies where data has been obtained using similar equipment setups, there have been discrepancies in categorizing and defining the information acquired. These discrepancies often stem from basic controversy in deciding what data should be labeled as an exercise-induced ventricular arrhythmia. This inconsistency in the definition of ETIA has played a large role in limiting not only data collection, but also the prognostic value of much of the information available. Studies have used varying criteria to define ETIA, with some studies considering ETIA to be present if any PVC or PAC was recorded during exercise. Furthermore, runs defined as VT or supraventricular tachycardia (SVT) have varied from three to more than three. One approach has been to consider a certain threshold of complexes per minute or an absolute number of ectopy per minute.

The prevalence of ETIVA has been shown to be more reproducible on future exercise tests if frequent or complex PVCs are used as markers for ETIVA, as compared to occasional PVCs.[239] In addition, others have documented an increased risk of mortality in those with frequent or complex PVCs during exercise compared to those with only occasional PVCs.[215,221]

The problems with defining ETIVA do not lie solely in differentiating how many PVCs occur, but also include issues such as the time frame and pattern in which they occur. In addition to examining ventricular arrhythmias during the actual exercise period, data observed prior to the test and in the cool-down period should be considered, and also how the timing impacts their occurrence. Furthermore, whether or not one does a cool-down walk after exercise can affect the appearance of ectopy. To complicate things further, data has also been extrapolated from studies examining the prognostic importance of resting PVCs immediately prior to testing (i.e., the arrhythmic substrate).

Population Selection

Multiple factors have been shown to be associated with the prevalence of ETIVA. The problem lies in elucidating the exact relationship between these factors and ETIVA, and explaining their prognostic significance. In the past, many studies attempted to clarify the relationship between ETIVA and factors such as age, sex, arrhythmic substrate and presence of cardiac disease, but conflicts remain. Analysis of these studies suggests that the inconsistencies between them may be secondary to differences in patient selection, data stratification, and study design.

Studies have focused on particular healthy populations such as aviators and policeman, and others have targeted random samples of such with or without screening for baseline heart disease (e.g., Framingham). Other studies have targeted patients referred for exercise testing for clinical reasons, including those known to have arrhythmias. Certainly, different prevalences of ETIVA can be expected from these different populations.

Age. Many studies demonstrated a direct relationship between age and the prevalence of ETIVA.[236] In 1984, Fleg and Lakatta[236] assessed the prevalence of ETIVT in 597 males and 325 female volunteers, between 21 and 96 years of age. All subjects were healthy volunteers without any evidence of CAD. Of the 1.1% with identifiable ETIA, only one was younger than 65 years. In other studies, the incidence of ETIVA and increasing age was not shown to be congruent. During serial maximal treadmill testing on 543 male volunteers, the prevalence of ETIVA was 30% to 36% in men aged 25 to 34 years, 32% to 38% in those aged 35 to 44 years, and 36% to 42% in those aged 45 to 54 years. These differences were not statistically significant.[243] As the relationship between ETIVA and age becomes more clearly identified, it would be useful to categorize data into age-specific subsets and determine if the prevalence of ETIVA at a younger age carries more prognostic significance than that in the elderly. This was confirmed in studies from USAFSAM in healthy aviators. What remains unresolved is whether this is due to aging itself, alterations in sympathetic tone or the diseases that accrue with aging. We reported similar results in the USAF (Tables 6-13 and 6-14).

TABLE 6–13. Number and percentage of subjects with other than single or occasional PVCS

Age	Number	Percent
20–29	24	6.6
30–39	52	7.6
40–53	78	13.1

*Froelicher et al, AGARD Study, $n = 1640$ healthy aviators.

Ischemia. In addition to stratifying the patient population based on age, studies have also examined ETIVA as it relates to a patient's risk for myocardial ischemia. Since arrhythmias are a part of acute coronary occlusion and acute coronary syndromes, particularly MI, it seems reasonable to expect this association during exercise. Some studies have suggested an association of ETIVA with exercise-induced ischemia[217,237]; however, other studies refute these results.[218,220,221,238,239] It does seem apparent that ETIVA are more common in patients with CAD. In 2002, Elhendy et al[255] evaluated the relationship between ETIVA and myocardial wall motion abnormalities during exercise echocardiography. The study included 1460 patients with intermediate pretest probability of CAD. ETIVA occurred in 146 (10%) of patients evaluated. Compared to those without ETIVA, patients with documented ETIVA had a greater prevalence of abnormal exercise echocardiographic findings and ischemia on exercise echocardiography, greater increase in wall motion score index with exercise, and a greater percentage of abnormal segments with exercise. Similar conclusions were reached by McHenry et al[238] in their evaluation of 482 patients with and without CAD. During exercise testing up to a heart rate of 130 bpm, 27% of patients with angiographic CAD experienced ETIVA, compared to only 9% of patients with normal angiograms. Patients with three-vessel CAD and left ventricular wall motion abnormalities were found to have a significantly greater prevalence of ETIVA. Data from other

TABLE 6–14. Number and percentage of subjects with "OMINOUS" patterns of PVC occurrence

Age	Number	Percent
20–29	3	0.8%
30–39	7	1.0%
40–53	21	3.5%

*Froelicher et al, AGARD Study, $n = 1640$ healthy aviators.

studies have not been in complete accordance. Casella et al[220] tested 777 consecutive patients and found that although patients with ETIVA were older, with higher blood pressures and double product, the prevalence of exercise-induced ischemia was the same as in those without ETIVA.

In general during exercise, transmural ischemia associated with ST-segment elevation is arrhythmogenic, while subendocardial ischemia associated with ST depression is not. Detry et al[240] reported six patients without MI specifically referred to them for spontaneous angina known to be associated with ST elevation. During exercise testing, five of them exhibited elevation, three of whom developed VT and one whom developed VF. We have subsequently seen one such patient who developed ST elevation and then VT (20 beats) at maximal exercise.

Gender. Bias in many of the previously reported series has also limited their external validity. Few studies have been able to compare ETIVA data from both male and female subjects, and those that have, report disparate findings. The Framingham study reported that while asymptomatic males with frequent or complex PVCs on ambulatory ECG were at increased risk of mortality, asymptomatic females were not.[241] Jouven et al.[221] found ETIVA to be predictive of mortality only when male populations were considered.

Reproducibility

The issue of reproducibility has complicated the defining of the prognostic significance of ETIVA as it relates to outcomes. In 1989, Saini et al[242] evaluated the reproducibility of ETIA by performing repeat treadmill tests on 28 patients referred for evaluation of ventricular arrhythmia. In half of these subjects the clinical arrhythmia was sustained VT or VF. The prevalence rates of arrhythmia were greater than 80% and did not significantly differ between test 1 and test 2. Excluding infrequent single ventricular premature complexes, the reproducibility of a test with positive outcome was 76%. Thus, it appears that ETISVA are very reproducible in patients known to have serious arrhythmias.

In a study performed by Faris et al[243] in 1976, two serial maximal treadmill exercise tests were performed in a study population of 543 male Indian State policemen at an average interval of 3 years. Four hundred sixty-two subjects were clinically free of cardiovascular disease, and

81 had definite or suspected cardiovascular disease. The prevalence of ETISVA during the first test was 30% in men aged 25 to 34 years, 32% in those aged 35 to 44 years, and 36% in those aged 45 to 54 years. The group with definite or suspected cardiovascular disease had a greater prevalence of ETISVA than normal subjects during both tests, but the prevalence rate with repeat testing remained constant. The occurrence of ETIVA was reproducible in individual subjects during the second test in 55% of 25 to 34 year olds, 58% of 35 to 44 year olds, and 62% of 45 to 54 year olds. Thus, it was concluded that individual reproducibility in two consecutive tests was only slightly greater than reproducibility by chance alone. The group with known or suspected cardiovascular disease did demonstrate a trend toward greater reproducibility with repeat testing, although ETIVA were not reproducible by type or complexity. It must be concluded that the marked variability of ETIVA during repeat maximal exercise testing in a clinically normal population appears to negate the usefulness of this finding during a single test as a marker of future cardiovascular disease. However, subjects whose arrhythmias are reproducible may form a group more likely to develop clinical cardiovascular disease in long-term follow-up studies.

Prevalence of Exercise-Induced Ventricular Tachycardia (ETIVT)

Three studies considering the safety of exercise testing reported the occurrence of VT during the test specifically. Condini et al[244] described 47 patients with ETIVT occurring during exercise testing (a prevalence of 0.8% in 5730 treadmill tests). Forty of the 47 patients had heart disease, mostly CAD. VT was brief and self-terminated in all but one instance. Milanes et al[245] reported a 4.0% prevalence of VT in 900 treadmill tests performed in patients with CAD compared to 0.07% prevalence in 1700 tests among patients without CAD. Of note, 79% of patients with VF or VT had an abnormal ST response as well. In 2000, Fujiwara et al[246] examined the conditions surrounding the onset of VT and VF following the completion of exercise testing. From a database of 7594 patients, 60 patients (0.8%) were identified as having had ETIVT during treadmill testing. In the recovery period, within 2 minutes after exercise, nine patients experienced VT (four sustained).

Follow-Up Issues

Completeness and length of follow-up are both very important since some of the studies suggest that the risk of EIVA appear later (>10 years) rather than early. This makes studying EIVA more difficult, since the longer the follow up the greater the risk of losing patients to follow-up. It is also important to consider comorbidities, particularly cigarette smoking and lung disease because they appear to associate with EIVA and affect outcomes. Endpoints that have been used include all-cause mortality, cardiovascular death, sudden death, MI, as well as surrogate endpoints, including nuclear studies and angiography. The choice of endpoints greatly affects the results as well as the clinical utility of the results. To the clinician wishing to make an intervention that could improve outcome, the prediction of sudden or cardiovascular death or the converse of infarct-free survival is important. Therefore, studies using other endpoints are somewhat irrelevant.

Clinical Prognostic Studies

Exercise Test-Induced Supraventricular Arrhythmias

Few studies have evaluated if ETISVA (i.e., supraventricular or atrial arrhythmias during exercise testing) are predictive of an increased risk of cardiac events and death. Atrial arrhythmias may reflect underlying left atrial enlargement and ventricular dysfunction, prognostic of mortality. The following two studies were the only recent studies we could find on this subject.

Bunch et al[247] performed exercise echocardiography in 5375 patients (age 61 ± 12 years) with known or suspected CAD. An abnormal result was defined as exercise-induced atrial fibrillation (AF)/atrial flutter, SVT, or atrial ectopy. A total of 311 (5.8%) patients died (132 [2.5%] from cardiac causes) over a period of 3 years. In addition, 193 (3.6%) patients experienced a MI and 531 (9.9%) patients required revascularization. During exercise testing, 1272 (24%) patients developed atrial ectopy, 185 (3.4%) developed SVT, and 43 (0.8%) developed AF. The 5-year cardiac death rate was not statistically different between groups (under 4% with no deaths in the AF group). The 5-year rate of MI was significantly different between groups being highest in the AF group (9%) and with none in the SVT group. The 5-year rate of revascularization between groups was not significantly different (less than 15%). A composite of all 5-year adverse endpoints was similar between groups (about 25%). In stepwise multivariate analysis, ETISVA were not predictive of any endpoint when taking into account traditional clinical variables and exercise test results.

The prevalence, characteristics, and prognostic significance of ETISVA were examined in 843 male and 540 female asymptomatic volunteers aged 20 to 94 years from the Baltimore Longitudinal Study of Aging who underwent exercise testing a mean of 2.3 times between 1977 and 1991.[248] ETISVA occurred during at least one test in 51 men (6.0%) and 34 women (6.3%). The 85 subjects with ETISVA were significantly older than the 1298 free from this arrhythmia (66 versus 50 years of age). The prevalence of ETISVA increased with age in men ($P < 0.001$) but not in women. Most of the 141 discrete episodes of ETISVA were paroxysmal SVT (PSVT), with heart rates varying from 105 to 290 bpm. Nearly half of ETISVA occurred at peak effort. Coronary risk factors, echocardiographic left atrial size, and the prevalence of exercise-induced ischemic ST-segment depression (11% versus 13%) were similar in 85 subjects with ETISVA and 170 control subjects matched for age and sex. During follow-up, eight subjects (10%), but only three controls (2%), developed AF or PSVT a mean of 6 years (range 2 to 12) after their index exercise test. Six subjects developed AF; in four of these six the arrhythmia was sustained. In two subjects, paroxysmal AF was observed on ambulatory 24-hour ECG, recorded because of palpitations. Among the 1360 subjects for whom follow-up information was available, the relative risk of developing lone AF during follow-up in those subjects with exercise-induced SVT was eight times. Thus, exercise-induced SVT does not appear to be a marker for latent heart disease but 10% of those with exercise-induced SVT and only 2% of controls developed spontaneous AF or PSVT during the follow-up period.

These two studies lead us to the conclusion that ETISVA are relatively rare, compared to ventricular arrhythmias, and appear to be benign except for their association with AF.

Exercise Test-Induced Ventricular Arrhythmias

In examining patients without any prior evidence of CAD, most recent studies suggest that ETIVA are associated with increased cardiovascular morbidity or mortality while the earlier studies are mixed (Table 6-15a). In 1989, Busby et al[249] studied

TABLE 6–15a.   The demographics of the populations in major studies of exercise test-induced arrhythmias

Study	Year	Sample size	Population	Age (years)	Gender (% female)	Rest/Pretest PVCS or arrhythmias considered?*	History of arrhythmias considered?
Clinical Population, PVC Studies:							
Partington et al, Am Heart J, Beckerman, ANIE, LB and PA VAHCS	2004	6,213	Patients referred for clinical reasons	59 ± 11	0	Not excluded, considered	Not excluded, ignored
Frolkis et al, NEJM, Cleveland Clinic	2003	29,244	Referred patients without heart failure, valve disease, or arrhythmia	56 ± 11	30	Excluded	Excluded
Elhendy et al, Am J Cardiol, Mayo Clinic, Rochester, Minnesota	2002	1,460	Patients with intermediate pretest probability of CAD, no hx MI/CABG, no arrythmia hx	64 ± 10	41	Not excluded, ignored	Excluded
Schweikert et al, Am J Cardiol, Cleveland Clinic Foundation	1999	2,743 with perfusion scan, 424 with coronary angio	Adults without heart failure or known PVCs at rest; no hx invasive cardiac procedures	62 ± 10	30	Excluded, ignored	Severe cases excluded
Casella et al, Int J Cardiol, Ospedale Maggiore, Bologna, Italy	1993	777	Consecutive stable out-patients 1 year post-Q-wave MI	57 ± 9	9	Not excluded, ignored	Not excluded, ignored
Marieb et al, Am J Cardiol, University of Virginia School of Medicine	1990	383	Patients with chest pain, cath and perfusion scan	58 ± 10	15	Not excluded, ignored	Not excluded, ignored
Nair et al, Am J Cardiol, Creighton University School of Medicine, Nebraska	1984	186	Patients with CAD by coronary angio (excluding CHF, PVCs, other ECG abnormalities); many had MI	59 ± 9	16	Excluded, ignored	Excluded
Nair et al, J Am Coll Cardiol, Creighton University School of Medicine, Nebraska	1983	280	Patients referred for chest pain, no MI or PVCs at rest	Men: 55 ± 9 women: 53 ± 9	30	Excluded	Excluded
Califf et al, JACC, Duke University Medical Center	1983	1,293	Medically treated patients with cardiac cath; if evaluated for VAs or CHF excluded; 620 patients had CAD	48	?	Not excluded, considered	Excluded

continued

TABLE 6–15a. The demographics of the populations in major studies of exercise test-induced arrhythmias—cont'd

Study	Year	Sample size	Population	Age (years)	Gender (% female)	Rest/Pretest PVCS or arrhythmias considered?*	History of arrhythmias considered?
Sami et al, Am J Cardiol, Stanford University, Montreal Heart Institute, Mayo Clinic, University of Washington	1984	1,486	Coronary Artery Surgery Study registry with angiographic CAD	50 ± 10	20	Not excluded, ignored	Not excluded, ignored
Weiner et al, Am J Cardiol, Boston University Medical Center	1984	446 (group 1 with arrhythmias and group 2 without)	Consecutive series of patients with cath	53 ± 7	22	Not excluded, considered (5% with rest PVCs)	Not excluded, ignored
Udall et al, Circulation, Long Beach and UCI Medical Center	1977	6,500	Patients referred for clinical reasons	?	20	Not excluded, considered	Not excluded, ignored
Clinical Population, Heart Failure Patients:							
O'Neill, JACC, Cleveland Clinic	2004	2,123	Left ventricular EF ≤35%	54 ± 12	25	Considered	Considered
Healthy Population, PVC Studies:							
Morshedi-Meibodi et al, Circulation, Framingham Heart Study	2004	2,885	Healthy individuals screened to exclude heart disease (n = 542)	43 ± 10	52	Not excluded, ignored	Excluded
Jouven et al, NEJM Paris Prospective Study	2000	6,101	Asymptomatic men without CVD employed by the Paris Civil Service	42-53	0	Not excluded, considered	Polymorphic PVCs excluded
Busby et al, J Am Coll Cardiol, Baltimore, Maryland	1989	1,160	Asymptomatic volunteer participants screened for cardiac disease	21-96	35	Not excluded, considered (9/40 had resting PVCs)	Excluded (major abnormalities)
Froelicher et al, Am J Cardiol, USAFSAM	1974	1,390	USAF aircrewmen referred for evaluation	38 (20-54)	0	Not excluded, ignored	Not excluded, ignored
Ventricular Tachycardia Studies:							
Tamakoshi et al, J Cardiol, Cardiovascular Institute Hospital Tokyo	2002	25,075	Healthy patients without hx PVC/VT	53 ± 9	44	Not excluded, ignored	Excluded
Yang et al, Arch Intern Med, LBVAHCS	1991	3,351	Veterans	60 ± 9 (21-88)	3	Not excluded, ignored	Not excluded, considered (reason for exercise test)
Fleg et al, Am J Cardiol, Baltimore	1984	922	Healthy volunteers without CAD	54 ± 16 (21-96)	35.2	Not excluded, ignored	Not excluded, ignored

| Detry et al, Catholic Hosp Brussels, Belgium | 1981 | 7,500 | Patients referred for clinical reasons | ? | ? | Not excluded (26 patients had PVCs at rest, 6 had hx VT), considered | Not excluded, ignored |
| Codini et al, Cathet Cardiovasc Diagn | 1981 | 5,730 (47 had VT and composed the study group) | Consecutive patients, 40 with heart disease | 57 ± 11 (32–76) | 13 | Not excluded, considered (resting PVCs in 10 patients) | Not excluded, ignored |

*Rest/Pretest PVCs refer to those PVCs/arrhythmias recorded directly prior to exercise testing.

Hx arrythmias refer to a medical history of resting PVCs or arrhythmias.

"Not excluded" indicates that a study ignores (does not mention) rest/pretest PVCs or hx arrhythmias, and does not consider them in the analysis.

TABLE 6–15b. The methodologies used in the major studies of exercise test-induced arrhythmias

Study	Exercise test	Method	Definition	Categorization**	Endpoints	Follow-up (years)
Clinical Population, PVC Studies:						
Partington et al, Am Heart J, Beckerman, ANIE, LB and PA VAHCS	Symptom-limited ramp treadmill	All tests coded by MDs/RNP during test, over read by authors	Frequent PVCs = >10% of QRS complexes during any 30 sec, or ≥ 3 consecutive PVCs during exercise or recovery	During exercise or recovery	All-cause mortality (1,256 total deaths, 550 CV deaths, CV mortality in later paper)	6 ± 4
Frolkis et al, NEJM, Cleveland Clinic	Symptom-limited treadmill	ECG images and arrhythmias "prospectively recorded"	Frequent = ≥ 7 PVCs/min, bi/trigeminy, couplets/ triplets, VT/VF. Classified according to Lown	During each stage of exercise, during recovery, during exercise and recovery	All-cause mortality (1,862 deaths)	5.3
Elhendy et al, Am J Cardiol, Mayo Clinic, Rochester, Minnesota	Symptom-limited treadmill, Bruce protocol in 91%, more gradual protocol in remainder	ECG	Classified as complex (couplets, bi/trigeminy, or multiform), frequent (>5 PVCs/min), NSVT (≥3 PVCs during episodes <30 sec), VT, or VF	At rest, during exercise or recovery	Cardiac death and nonfatal MI (36 patients)	2.7
Schweikert et al, Am J Cardiol, Cleveland Clinic Foundation	Symptom-limited Bruce protocol treadmill	ST segments collected and entered online	Significant ETIVA = frequent or complex ventricular activity (>7 PVCs/min, couplets, triplets, bi/ trigeminy), NSVT = ≥3 PVCs of <30 sec duration, or VT or VF	During exercise, final stages of exercise	All-cause mortality	2
Casella et al, Int J Cardiol, Ospedale Maggiore, Bologna, Italy	Symptom-limited Bruce protocol treadmill	12-lead ECG continuously monitored	Any PVC, not detected at rest but observed during exercise, categorized into simple (≤2 Lown) versus complex (≥3 Lown) ETIVAs	At rest, during exercise and recovery	All-cause mortality (24 deaths, 5 had ETIVAs)	2
Marieb et al, Am J Cardiol, University of Virginia School of Medicine	Symptom-limited exercise test	12-lead ECG continuously monitored, technicians recorded arrhythmias detected on monitor	Any PVCs not noted at rest, but observed during exercise or recovery; classified as rare (<5) or frequent (>5), multiform PVCs, couplets, VT (≥3 PVCs), and VF	At rest, each minute of exercise, and after exercise	CV death (41 deaths), 9 MIs, 39 CABG 1, 2, 3, and 5 min	4–8
Nair et al, Am J Cardiol, Creighton University School of Medicine, Nebraska	Symptom-limited Bruce protocol treadmill	12-lead ECG recorded and continuously monitored during and for ≥6 min after exercise	Complex ETIVA = pairs or runs, multiform, or ≥10/min	Supine and standing, end each 3-min exercise stage, max and each min recovery	CV death (8 deaths) and sudden death (4 deaths)	4 ± 1

Nair et al, J Am Coll Cardiol, Creighton University School of Medicine, Nebraska	Bruce protocol treadmill	12-lead ECG continuously monitored during and for ≥6 min after exercise; all PVCs recorded and counted	Complex ETIVA = pairs or runs, multiform, or frequency >10/min	Supine and standing, end each 3-min exercise stage, max and each min recovery	Coronary events (1 CABG and ETIVAs, 6 w/o CABG with ETIVAs, 5 with CABG w/o ETIVAs, and 12 w/o ETIVAs or CABG)	4 ± 2
Califf, et al, JACC, Duke University Medical Center	Treadmill	Samples of each arrhythmia recorded on ≥4 leads of 12-lead ECG	Simple VAs = ≥1 PVC; VAs further categorized into paired complexes (2 consecutive PVCs) and VT (≥3 PVCs)	2 min pre, during and for 8 min after testing	CV death	3
Sami et al, Am J Cardiol, Stanford University, Montreal Heart Institute, Mayo Clinic, University of Washington	Bruce protocol	12-lead ECG continuously monitored	ETIVA = PVCs during exercise or recovery, provided a 3 min control pre-exercise test showed no PVCs	At rest, every 3 min during exercise, at peak and each minute recovery	Death from any cause, cardiac death, and cardiac event	4.3
Weiner et al, Am J Cardiol, Boston University Medical Center	Bruce protocol graded treadmill	12-lead ECG continuously monitored on a 3-channel oscilloscope; all PVCs recorded	Complex PVCs = pairs or runs, multiform, or >20 beats/min	At rest, during exercise, during recovery	Total cardiac mortality (6 deaths in group 1 and 23 in group 2)	5.3
Udall et al, Circulation, Long Beach and UCI Medical Center	Ellestad max protocol treadmill	ECG	"Ominous" PVCs = multiform, bigeminal, repetitive and VT	At rest, during exercise (increased/ decreased PVCs during exercise), during recovery	Coronary events (MI, angina, or cardiac death)	5

Clinical Population, Heart Failure Patients:

O'Neill, JACC, Cleveland Clinic	Symptom-limited—cardio-pulmonary treadmill testing	Systematic ECG data during rest, exercise, and recovery	Severe PVCs = ventricular triplets, sustained/ nonsustained VT, ventricular flutter, polymorphic VT or VF	Rest, exercise and recovery	All-cause mortality, with censoring for interval cardiac transplantation	3

Healthy Population, PVC Studies:

Morshedi-Meibodi et al, Circulation, Framingham Heart Study	Symptom-limited/ submax bike/treadmill	Digital computer system used, arrhythmias identified by technician and verified by cardiologist	ETIVAs = PVCs/min of exercise (mean = 0.22/min exercise) frequent ETIVAs = above the median	During each stage of exercise (submax up to 85% age predicted) and during recovery	CV events (142 events [MI, ACS, CV death]), all-cause mortality (171 deaths)	15
Jouven et al NEJM Paris Prospective Study	Bicycle (>3 successive workloads and max duration of 10 max	ECG continuously monitored	Frequent PVCs = ≥2 PVCs, making up >10% of all ventricular depolarizations on any 30-sec ECG	Before exercise, during exercise, and during recovery	Death from CV, fatal MI, sudden death	23

continued

TABLE 6–15b. The methodologies used in the major studies of exercise test-induced arrhythmias—*cont'd*

Study	Exercise test	Method	Definition	Categorization**	Endpoints	Follow-up (years)
Busby et al, J Am Coll Cardiol, Baltimore, Maryland	Symptom-limited max Balke treadmill (done an average of 2.4×)	ECGs; aVF, V1, and V4 continuously monitored by oscilloscope and audible cardiotachometer; analog recordings for playback	Complex ETIVAs = frequent or repetitive PVCs, frequent = ≥10% of the beats/min, and repetitive = salvos of ≥3 at ≥100 bpm; complex ETIVA characterized by their time of first occurrence	Before exercise (supine, sitting and after HV and standing), during exercise, ≥6 min into recovery	All-cause death and cardiac events	6 ± 3
Froelicher et al, Am J Cardiol, USAFSAM	Symptom-limited Balke protocol treadmill	Continuous ECG strips reviewed on microfilm	Ominous ETIVA = frequent PVCs at/near max or 3 consecutive PVCs/VT any time, frequent PVCs = ≥10 PVCs out of any 50 beats with other PVCs that increased with exercise or 3 in a row	During the control period (supine and standing), during and after exercise	Angina, MI, CV death	6.3
Ventricular Tachycardia (VT) Studies:						
Tamakoshi et al, J Cardiol, Cardiovascular Institute Hospital Tokyo	Max bicycle/ treadmill	Reviewed	NSVT = ≥8 PVCs at >100 beats/min	During exercise and recovery	0.08% Angiographic findings (6 patients had ischemia, 2 had cardiomyopathy, 5 had other CV disease	No follow-up; cross sectional retrospective study
Yang et al, Arch Intern Med, LBVAHCS	Symptom-limited Balke treadmill	3 leads (II, V2, V5) continuously monitored during exercise; recorder automatically printed out any ectopic beats	NSVT = ≥3 consecutive PVCs, VT = >30 sec or requiring intervention	During exercise and recovery	Death from CV (1 death), sudden death (1 death)	2
Fleg et al, Am J Cardiol, Baltimore	Modified Balke max treadmill	Leads I, aVF, V5 screen and audibly monitored/FM tape storage; 12-lead ECG last 15 sec each exercise stage	VT = ≥3 consecutive PVCs	During exercise and recovery	Heart disease, syncope, sudden death	2

Detry et al, Catholic Hosp Brussels, Belgium	Max symptom-limited bicycle (20 watts and increased 20 watts every min)	ECG	VT = ≥4 consecutive PVCs (sustained VT = >20 consecutive beats or recurring VT; single short run VT = 4-12 consecutive PVCs)	During exercise	Cardiac death (10 sudden deaths and 1 operative death, 91% had CAD)	2.6
Codini et al, Cathet Cardiovasc Diagn	Bruce or modified Bruce protocol treadmill	12-lead ECG screen monitored; 24 patients Holtered	VT defined as a run of ≥3 PVCs in a row	At rest, during exercise, during 10-min recovery, during exercise and recovery	Cardiac disease	no follow-up

**Categorization refers to the time periods into which ECG recording was classified.

1160 subjects between the ages of 21 to 96 years who underwent treadmill testing an average of 2.4 times. Eighty (6.9%) developed frequent (>10% of beats in any 1 minute) or repetitive (more than three beats in a row) PVCs on at least one of these tests. Only age appeared to distinguish those with ETIVA, but in these predominantly older, asymptomatic individuals without apparent heart disease, ETIVA did not appear to predict increased cardiac morbidity or mortality.

A 6-year follow-up study of 1390 male USAF aircrewmen referred to the USAF School of Aerospace Medicine was reported in 1974.[250] The ECG strips were continuously recorded and stored on 8-mm microfilm, which was replayed by a trained observer, and the arrhythmias were recorded retrospectively. Specifically regarding arrhythmias, ominous treadmill-induced arrhythmias were defined as: frequent PVCs at near-maximal or maximal exercise, or three consecutive PVCs or more occurring at any time.[251] Frequent PVCs were defined as 10 or more PVCs out of any 50 consecutive beats. Ominous arrhythmias were noted in 2.1% of this apparently healthy, select population. Coronary heart disease (CHD) was defined as onset of angina pectoris, MI, or cardiovascular death. The risk of developing CHD over the follow-up period with these arrhythmias was three times greater than in those who did not develop ominous arrhythmias.

In 2000, Jouven et al[221] evaluated 6101 asymptomatic French men between the ages of 42 to 53 years who were free of clinically detectable cardiovascular disease. Patients underwent exercise testing and were monitored for the presence of two or more consecutive PVCs. In their multivariate model, adjustments were made for age, body-mass index, heart rate at rest, systolic blood pressure, tobacco use, level of physical activity, diabetes, cholesterol, and PVCs before exercise and during recovery from exercise. The subjects were followed for 23 years for cardiovascular death. They concluded that frequent PVCs (a run of two or more making up 10% of any 30 seconds) during exercise in men without detectable cardiovascular disease is associated with a long-term increase in cardiovascular mortality.[221]

Califf et al[252] at DUKE studied the prognostic value of ETIVA in 1293 consecutive nonsurgically treated patients.[252] They defined simple ventricular arrhythmias as at least one PVC, but without paired complexes or VT. In the 236 patients with these simple ventricular arrhythmias, there was indeed a higher prevalence of significant CAD (57% versus 44%), three-vessel disease (31% versus

17%), and abnormal left ventricular function (43% versus 24%) than in those patients without any ventricular arrhythmias. Patients with paired complexes or VT had an even higher prevalence of significant CAD (75%), three-vessel disease (39%), and abnormal left ventricular function (54%). In the 620 patients with significant CAD, patients with paired complexes or VT had a lower 3-year survival rate (75%) than did patients with simple ventricular arrhythmia (83%) and patients with no ventricular arrhythmia (90%).

At our Veterans Affairs Medical Center, Partington et al concluded that the presence of ETIVA is predictive of mortality.[253] In a retrospective analysis of 6213 consecutive males that were referred for exercise tests, exercise test responses and all-cause mortality were examined after a mean follow-up of 6 ± 4 years. In this study, ETIVA were defined as frequent PVCs constituting greater than 10% of all ventricular depolarizations during any 30-second ECG recording, or a run of 3 or more consecutive PVCs during exercise or recovery. During the analysis, it was discovered that a total of 1256 patients (20%) died during follow-up. ETIVA occurred in 503 patients (8%); the prevalence of ETIVA increased in older patients and in those with cardiopulmonary disease, resting PVCs, and ischemia during exercise. ETIVA were associated with mortality irrespective of the presence of cardiopulmonary disease or exercise-induced ischemia. In those without cardiopulmonary disease, mortality differed more so later in follow-up than earlier. In those without resting PVCs, ETIVA were also predictive of mortality, but in those with resting PVCs, poorer prognosis was not worsened by the presence of ETIVA. We concluded that exercise-induced ischemia does not affect the prognostic value of ETIVA, whereas the arrhythmic substrate does, and furthermore that ETIVA and resting PVCs are both independent predictors of mortality after consideration of other clinical and exercise-test variables. A redo of this data set was performed when cardiovascular mortality became available.[254] From this subsequent analysis, we concluded that ETIVA are independent predictors of cardiovascular mortality after adjusting for other clinical and exercise test variables; combination with resting PVCs carries the highest risk.

In 2002, Elhendy et al[255] assessed the relationship between ETIVA and exercise echocardiography in patients with suspected CAD. Their study included 1460 patients (mean age 64 ± 10 years; 867 men) with intermediate pretest probability of CAD and no history of MI or revascularization.

ETIVA occurred in 146 patients (10%). Compared with patients without ventricular arrhythmias, those with ventricular arrhythmias had a greater prevalence of abnormal exercise echocardiographic findings. During 2.7 years follow-up, cardiac death and nonfatal MI occurred in 36 patients. Following a multivariate analysis of combined clinical and exercise stress test variables, the authors concluded that independent predictors of cardiac events were ETIVA and maximal heart rate.

The Framingham Offspring Study participants (1397 men; mean age, 43 years), who were free of cardiovascular disease and who underwent a routine exercise test, were recently reported. ETIVA were noted in 792 participants (27%) using an off-line Holter-type analysis computer system (median, 0.22 PVCs per minute of exercise).[256] Logistic regression was used to evaluate predictors of ETIVA. Cox models were used to examine the relations of infrequent (less than or equal to median) and frequent (greater than median) versus no ETIVA to incidence of hard CHD event (recognized MI, coronary insufficiency, or CHD death) and all-cause mortality, adjusting for vascular risk factors and exercise variables. Age and male sex were key correlates of ETIVA. During follow-up (mean, 15 years), 142 (113 men) had a first hard CHD event and 171 participants (109 men) died. ETIVA were not associated with hard CHD events but were associated with increased all-cause mortality rates (multivariable-adjusted hazards ratio, 1.9, 95% CI, 1.2 to 2.8 for infrequent, and 1.7, 95% CI, 1.2 to 2.5 for frequent ETIVA versus none). The relations of ETIVA to mortality risk were not influenced by ETIVA grade, presence of recovery ETIVA, left ventricular dysfunction, or an ischemic ST-segment response. In this large, community-based sample of asymptomatic individuals, ETIVA were associated with up to a greater than two times increased risk of all-cause mortality at a much lower threshold than previously reported. Surprisingly, the risk is not found isolated to those with cardiovascular endpoints, making the mechanism unsettled.

Researchers at Cleveland Clinic reported 29,244 patients (56 years of age; 70% men) who had been referred for exercise testing without chronic heart failure, valve disease, or arrhythmia.[257] ETIVA were defined by the presence of seven or more PVCs per minute, ventricular bigeminy or trigeminy, ventricular couplets or triplets, VT, or VF. ETIVA occurred only during exercise in 945 patients (3%), only during recovery in 589 (2%), and during both exercise and recovery in 491 (2%). There were 1862 deaths during a mean of 5.3 years of follow-up.

ETIVA during exercise predicted an increased risk of death (5-year death rate, 9%, versus 5% among patients without ETIVA; hazard ratio 1.8), but ETIVA during recovery was a stronger predictor (11% versus 5%; hazard ratio 2.4). After propensity matching for confounding variables, ETIVA during recovery predicted an increased risk of death (adjusted hazard ratio, 1.5), but ETIVA did not.

In 1984, Sami et al[258] performed a retrospective study to examine the significance of ETIVA in patients with stable CAD from the Coronary Artery Surgery Study. The population included 1486 patients selected from 1975 to 1979, followed for an average of 4.3 years. Patients with CAD and ETIVA had similar clinical and angiographic characteristics, as compared to those with CAD without ETIVA. The only difference discovered was the average ejection fraction (EF), which was 50% for those with ETIVA and 64% for those without any PVCs. The 5-year event-free survival was not influenced by the presence of ETIVA in this study. Using a stepwise Cox regression analysis, the authors concluded that only the number of coronary arteries diseased and the EF were associated with cardiac events.[258] Similar conclusions were drawn by Weiner et al[259] and Nair et al[260] in two separate studies that same year. Weiner et al[259] investigated ETIVA in a consecutive series of 446 patients who underwent treadmill testing and cardiac catheterization. The prevalence of ETIVA was found to be 19% in the total group but increased to 30% in the 120 patients with 3-vessel or left main CAD. Patients with ETIVA also were more likely to have ST depression and abnormal LV function. Despite these findings, at 5-year follow-up, ETIVA were not associated with increased cardiac mortality.[259] In a small study by Nair et al[260], frequent or complex exercise-induced PVCs were not shown to predict 4-year mortality in patients with CAD.[260] Schweikert et al also reported that in patients with documented CAD and no prior history of severe ventricular ectopy at rest, exercise-induced frequent or complex PVCs were not predictive of 2-year mortality.

Even in patients with a documented MI, studies have refuted the proposed relationship between ETIVA and increased risk of cardiovascular death. In 1993, Casella et al[220] reported 777 consecutive patients who underwent a treadmill test at least a year following an MI. The 228 patients who experienced ETIVA were older, had higher blood pressures, and peak exercise rate pressures. No difference was found in the prevalence of exercise-induced ischemia. Furthermore, in 2 years of follow-up, of the 24 deaths, only five were in patients with ETIVA, whereas 19 were in patients without.

In 1990, Marieb et al[261] analyzed the significance of ETIVA in 383 patients who had undergone both exercise perfusion testing and cardiac catheterization. Two hundred twenty-one patients (58%) had no ETIVA while 162 (42%) did. There was no difference between patients with and without ETIVA in terms of previous MI, fixed perfusion defects, number of diseased vessels, and resting EF. In contrast, ischemia (perfusion defect or ST depression) was more likely to be seen in patients with ETIVA. In an 8-year follow-up, patients with ETIVA were shown to be more likely to have cardiac events, although it is unclear if any of these events led to increased mortality.

Exercise Test-Induced Ventricular Tachycardia

In a retrospective review of 3351 veterans who had undergone routine clinical exercise testing, we identified 55 patients with ETIVT.[262] NSVT was defined as greater or equal to three consecutive ventricular premature beats. Sustained VT was defined as VT longer than 30 seconds or requiring intervention. Fifty patients had NSVT during exercise testing and one of these patients died due to congestive heart failure during the follow-up period. Five patients had sustained VT during exercise testing and one died suddenly 7 months after the test. VT was reproduced in only two of the 29 patients who underwent repeat exercise testing. Mean follow-up was 2 years. Of the 50 episodes of NSVT, 26 episodes occurred during exercise and 24 occurred in recovery; only 10 occurred at peak exercise and led to cessation of the exercise test. Five patients had exercise-induced sustained VT; two patients had their bouts of VT during exercise and three during recovery. Of these five patients, only two patients required intervention: one was given lidocaine intravenously and one was cardioverted because of hypotension. The only other episode of serious ventricular arrhythmia to occur in this time period occurred in a patient without prior cardiac history who developed VF during exercise, which required electrical defibrillation. Of the 55 patients with ETIVT, 45 had clinical evidence of CAD; this included 19 with a prior MI, five patients who had undergone percutaneous transluminal coronary angioplasty, and nine patients with prior coronary artery bypass surgery. Two patients had cardiomyopathy and three patients had valvular heart disease. Five patients had no clinical evidence of heart disease.

Our major findings were that the occurrence of nonsustained ETIVT during routine treadmill testing is not associated with complications during testing or with increased cardiovascular mortality within 2 years after testing. In our study, the prevalence and reproducibility of ETIVT were both low (1.2% and 6.9%, respectively), despite a high prevalence of structural heart disease (mostly CAD) in the study population. The annual mortality among patients with ETIVT was 1.7% compared to 2.4% (171 deaths in 3351 patients) in the study population. Thus, ETIVT during treadmill testing did not portend a worsened prognosis, even among our patients with CAD. This statement cannot be extended to the five patients with sustained VT, because of their small number and because they were treated.

In general during exercise, transmural ischemia associated with ST-segment elevation is arrhythmogenic, while subendocardial ischemia associated with ST depression is not. In our study, none of the patients with nonsustained VT had ST elevation with their exercise test and 20 had abnormal ST depression. Of the five patients with sustained VT, none had ST elevation and two patients had abnormal ST depression prior to the onset of VT. Detry et al[263] reported six patients without MI, specifically referred to them for spontaneous angina, known to be associated with ST elevation. During exercise testing, five of them exhibited elevation, three of whom developed VT and one who developed VE. We have subsequently seen one such patient who developed ST elevation and then VT (20 beats) at maximal exercise.

Complications during exercise testing were reviewed in 25,075 consecutive patients, 14,037 men and 11,038 women, who underwent a total of 47,656 maximal treadmill or bicycle exercise tests between April 1985 and March 1999.[264] The mean age of the patients was 53 ± 9 years. NSVT was defined as eight or more consecutive ventricular ectopic beats at more than 100 bpm. Patients undergoing exercise testing to evaluate the efficacy of pharmacotherapy for VT were excluded. The major reasons for the exercise test were chest pain (27%) and screening (20%). Twenty patients (0.08%) had ETIVT. Six patients had ischemic heart disease, two had cardiomyopathy, five had other cardiac diseases, and seven patients showed no clinical evidence of heart disease. VT was documented at heart rates of more than 80% of predicted maximal heart rate in 12 of the 20 patients.

Detry et al[265] observed six cases of VF and 40 cases of VT in 7500 consecutive maximal exercise tests (0.6%); 13 patients had a sustained VT and 27 patients had a single short run of VT. No patient died immediately but 11 patients died during the follow-up. The prognosis was determined by the underlying disease (most often CAD) and the type of arrhythmia. The 5-year survival rate was 84% in patients with a short run of VT and only 43% in patients with VF or sustained VT.

Fleg and Lakatta[236] analyzed data from the Baltimore Longitudinal study on Aging to evaluate the prognostic impact of ETIVT. Of 597 male and 325 female volunteers between the ages of 21 to 96 years, 10 subjects (7 men and 3 women) with EITVT (three PVCs in a row) were identified, representing 1.1% of those tested; only one was younger than 65 years. All episodes of VT were asymptomatic and nonsustained. In 9 of 10 subjects, VT developed at or near peak exercise. The longest run of VT was six beats; multiple runs of VT were present in four subjects. Two subjects had exercise-induced ST-segment depression, but subsequent exercise thallium results were negative in each. Compared with a group of age- and sex-matched control subjects, those with asymptomatic, NSVT displayed no difference in exercise duration, maximal heart rate, or the prevalence of coronary risk factors of exercise-induced ischemia, as measured by the ECG and thallium perfusion. Over a mean follow-up period of 2 years, no subject developed symptoms of heart disease or experienced syncope or sudden death. ETIVT in apparently healthy subjects occurred mainly in the elderly, was limited to short, asymptomatic runs of three to six beats usually near peak exercise, and did not predict increased cardiovascular morbidity or mortality rates over a 2-year follow-up.

The finding in all of these studies is summarized in Table 6-15c, Results obtained and its analyses are given in Table 6-16.

ETIVA in Hypertrophic Cardiomyopathy

In addition to the research examining the prognostic value of ETIVA in patients with CAD, studies have also explored the implications of ETIVA in patients with other cardiac disorders such as hypertrophic cardiomyopathy (HCM). It had been proposed that NSVT is only of prognostic importance in patients with HCM when repetitive, prolonged, or associated with symptoms. In 2003, Monserrat et al[266] examined the characteristics of NSVT episodes during Holter monitoring in patients with HCM in an attempt to determine their relationship to age and prognosis. The study

included 531 patients with HCM (323 male, 39 ± 15 years). All underwent ambulatory ECG monitoring (41 ± 11 hours). They discovered that a total of 104 patients (19.6%) had NSVT and that the proportion of patients with NSVT increased with age ($P = 0.008$). Maximum left ventricular wall thickness and left atrial size were greater in patients with NSVT. Mean follow-up for this study was 70 ± 40 months. Sixty-eight patients died, 32 from SCD. Twenty-one patients received an implantable cardioverter defibrillator. There were four appropriate implantable cardioverter defibrillator discharges. In patients equal to or less than 30 years (but not more than 30), 5-year freedom from sudden death was lower in those with NSVT (77.6% [95% confidence interval (CI): 59.8 to 95.4] versus 94.1% [95% CI: 90.2 to 98.0]; $P = 0.003$). There was no relation between the duration, frequency, or rate of NSVT runs and prognosis at any age. The odds ratio of sudden death in patients equal to or less than 30 years of age with NSVT was 4.4 (95% CI: 1.5 to 12; $P = 0.006$) compared with 2.2 (95% CI: 0.8 to 6; $P = 0.1$) in patients more than 30 years of age. It appears that NSVT is associated with a substantial increase in sudden death risk in young patients with HCM, although a relation between the frequency, duration, and rate of NSVT episodes could not be demonstrated.

Exercise Testing to Evaluate ST Depression during SVT

Petsas et al[267] studied 16 patients who had manifested ST-segment depression during episodes of PSVT with exercise testing in order to detect CAD and MI. No ST-segment depression was observed during exercise testing in 15 of the 16 patients tested. Paroxysms of SVT associated with ST-segment depression occurred during exercise testing in three cases. The ST-segment depression was immediately apparent, remained constant throughout the SVT, and was almost instantly abolished following conversion to sinus rhythm. Patients with heart rates greater than 250 bpm during PSVT had marked ST-segment depression associated with the tachycardia. These results suggest that CAD and myocardial ischemia are not involved in the genesis of ST-segment depression during PSVT. Tachycardia per se may be the cause of ST-segment depression by altering the slope of phase 2 of the ventricular action potential. Retrograde atrial activation may also induce ST-segment shifts in some of the cases.

TABLE 6–15c.   The results of the major studies of exercise test-induced arrhythmias

Study	Prevalence	More ETIVA with ischemia/ST depression?	Risk of hazard	Conclusion
Clinical Population, PVC Studies:				
Partington et al, Am Heart J, Beckerman, ANIE, LB and PA VAHCS	8% (n = 503)	Yes (patients with ETIVAs with higher prevalence EI ischemia)	HR = 2	Rest/ETIVAs both predict CV mortality EI-ischemia no effect on prognostic value of ETIVAs/arrhythmic substrate does ETIVAs predict mortality in those with or w/o disease
Frolkis et al, NEJM, Cleveland Clinic	3% (2% during recovery, 2% exercise and recovery)	Yes (higher prevalence ischemia for those with recovery PVCs)	HR = 1.5 during recovery	ETIVAs in recovery, but not exercise, associated with increased risk of death
Elhendy et al, Am J Cardiol, Mayo Clinic, Rochester, Minnesota	10% (n = 146)	Yes	2.5 × (1–6)	ETIVAs predict cardiac death/nonfatal MI in suspected CAD. Independent predictors of cardiac events were ETIVAs and MaxHR
Schweikert et al, Am J Cardiol, Cleveland Clinic Foundation	5% (n = 128), 10% (n = 42 angio cohort)	No	HR = 0 (for short-term mortality)	ETIVAs associated with perfusion defects but not angiographic severity/short-term mortality
Casella et al, Int J Cardiol, Ospedale Maggiore, Bologna, Italy	29% (n = 228)	No	RR = 0	In patients with coronary disease or MI, ETIVAs w/o prognostic power
Marieb et al, Am J Cardiol, University of Virginia School of Medicine	42% (n = 162)	Yes (patients with ETIVAs more likely to have ST-segment depression)	2× risk univariately (weakly significant in Cox model)	ETIVAs predicted CV death/events. ETIVA patients did not differ (MI, perfusion defects, EF, diseased vessels)
Nair et al, Am J Cardiol, Creighton University School of Medicine, Nebraska	2% (n = 3)	Ignored	RR = 0	ETIVAs more likely with EI ischemia ETIVAs did not predict sudden death or 4-year mortality in patients with CAD
Nair et al, J Am Coll Cardiol, Creighton University School of Medicine, Nebraska	27% (n = 76)	Ignored	1.25× risk for those with ETIVAs or surgery, no increased risk for those with both surgery and ETIVAs	ETIVAs has lower predictive value for significant CAD than ST segment depression ETIVA site of origin not helpful
Califf et al, JACC, Duke University Medical Center	23% prevalence in CAD patients, 7% in those with normal coronary arteries	Ignored	2.5× for severe, 1.7× for simple	Higher prevalence of CAD Left ventricular dysfunction in patients with paired complexes and VT
Sami et al, Am J Cardiol, Stanford University, Montreal Heart Institute, Mayo Clinic, University of Washington	10%	Ignored	RR = 0	Only the number of coronary arteries diseased and the EF were associated with cardiac events
Weiner et al, Am J Cardiol, Boston University Medical Center	19% (30% in the 120 patients with 3-vessel/LM CAD)	Yes (patients with ETIVAs more likely to have severe ischemia)	1.4×	In asymptomatic persons w/o CAD, ETIVAs not predictive ETIVA associated with exercise-induced

Udall et al, Circulation, Long Beach and UCI Medical Center	20% (n = 1,327)	Not mentioned	3.8× for PVCs alone, 6.7× for ischemic ST changes and PVCs	ischemia, but not increased cardiac mortality PVCs suggested heart disease when they increased with exercise. Patients with PVCs plus ischemic ST changes had higher risk coronary events than those with either alone

Clinical Population, Heart Failure Patients:

O'Neill, JACC, Cleveland Clinic	140 (7%) had severe ventricular ectopy during recovery	Not mentioned	Severe PVCs during recovery with adjusted HR 1.5	Adjusting for PVCs at rest and during exercise, VO$_2$ max, and other potential confounders, severe PVCs during recovery predictive of death (adjusted HR 1.5), PVCs during exercise not predictive

Healthy Population, PVC Studies:

Morshedi-Meibodi et al, Circulation, Framingham Heart Study	27% (n = 792)	No	Greater than 2× adjusted risk for all-cause mortality but not CV endpoints	ETIVAs were associated with increased risk of death (but not CV events or ischemic ST-segment response) at much lower threshold than previously reported
Jouven et al, NEJM Paris Prospective Study	6% (0.8% before exercise, 2.3% during exercise, 2.9% during recovery)	Not clarified	RR = 2.7 (1.8–4.0)	ETIVA during exercise associated with risk of CV death, but frequent PVCs before exercise and infrequent PVCs were not. ETIVA during recovery associated with non-CV death.
Busby et al, J Am Coll Cardiol, Baltimore, Maryland	7% (frequent or repetitive PVCs)	No	RR = 0	Risk similar to ST depression ETIVA did not predict increased cardiac morbidity/mortality and not associated with EI ischemia. ETIVA increased with age
Froelicher et al, Am J Cardiol, USAFSAM	2% with ominous ETIVA	Not mentioned	3×	ETIVA had a low predictive value for CV events but significant risk

Ventricular Tachycardia (VT) Studies:

Tamakoshi et al, J Cardiol, Cardiovascular Institute Hospital Tokyo	1% with 7% reproducible; sustained VT = 5/55 patients	Yes	VT more common in cardiomyopathy	VT at elevated HR in 12 of the 20 patients
Yang et al, Arch Intern Med, LBVAHCS	1.10%	No (those with VT w/o increased prevalence of ischemic response)	RR = 0	Ischemia is more likely with ETIVT, but ETIVT does not increase risk of mortality
Fleg et al, Am J Cardiol, Baltimore	0.6% (40 with VT/6 with VF)	Yes (SVT and VF associated with ST depression)	RR = 0	Asymptomatic nonsustained VT at peak exercise w/o risk
Detry et al, Catholic Hosp Brussels, Belgium			No risk for short run VT, 3.6× risk for sustained VT or VF	Sustained ETIVT is associated with poor prognosis compared to short-run VT
Codini et al, Cathet Cardiovasc Diagn	0.08%	Yes (44/47 with VT had ischemic ST changes)	No follow-up	ETIVT rare in heart disease patients >45 years

TABLE 6–16. Analysis of 22 clinical prognostic studies of ventricular ectopy during exercise testing

Populations	Results	Number of studies	Does ischemia predict ETIVA? (when considered)	Is ventricular ectopy predictive of mortality? (Number of studies)		
				rest	exercise	recovery
Clinical population	Referred for symptoms	8	5 out of 6	1	5	1
	Known CAD	7	2 out of 3	0	2	1
Healthy population	Asymptomatic	5	1 out of 4	0	1	0
	Screening Study for Employment	2	Not evaluated	0	2	1

This table demonstrates that the majority of clinical studies of exercise testing and arrhythmias have included populations with clinical indications for exercise testing. In these populations, those with symptoms were more likely to have exercise-induced ventricular ectopy, which was predictive of mortality. In addition, ischemia was correlated with exercise-induced ventricular arrhythmias. However, given the limited number of studies and absence of follow-up and assessment of ischemia in some reports, the data remain inconclusive.

ETIVA, exercise test induced ventricular arrhythmias. Modified from Beckerman J, Wu T, Jones S, Froelicher VF: Exercise test-induced arrhythmias. Prog Cardiovasc Dis 2005;47:285-305.

OBSERVER AGREEMENT IN INTERPRETATION

The complexity of not only the human body, but also the human mind, has created in medicine measurements, that when applied to medical diagnosis, lead to observations with large variability, that is, ST-segment displacement. The inherent subjective nature of these medical observations requires questioning of the results of most diagnostic methods-not only in regard to accuracy or validity but also agreement (among different interpreters for a given test). Attempts at describing or assessing agreement have been complex and variable as evidenced in the literature by the numerous terms used: agreement, variability, consistency, within-observer correlation coefficients of disagreement, and many others. Agreement has two subgroupings: intraobserver, referring to agreement of the individual observer with himself on two separate occasions, and interobserver, referring to agreement among two or more individuals.

Blackburn[268] had 14 observers (from seven separate institutions) interpret 38 individual exercise ECG tests as to normal, abnormal, or borderline. Five readers repeated the readings. In only nine of the 38 (24%) exercise ECGs was there complete agreement among the 14 readers and only 22 ECGs (58%) were read in agreement. This low value may be due to the fact that Blackburn's study did not allow a dichotomous decision because there was the third interpretation of borderline. In terms of intraobserver agreement there was a wide range from 58% to 92% and an average still less than ours for a dichotomous decision. Blackburn attributed this wide variation in both inter- and intraobserver agreement to: (1) the absence of defined criteria, (2) technical problems such as noise, and (3) differences in opinion as to ST-segment upsloping. Strict criteria such as the Minnesota code and computer analysis have been recommended as a means to increase agreement in electrocardiography.

Reproducibility of Treadmill Test Responses

Sullivan et al[269] studied 14 male patients with exercise test-induced angina and ST segment-depression with treadmill testing on three consecutive days to evaluate the reproducibility of certain treadmill variables. Computerized ST-segment analysis and expired gas analysis, including anaerobic threshold, were evaluated for reproducibility using an intraclass correlation coefficient analysis. The intraclass correlation coefficient is a generalization of the Pearson product-moment correlation that is not affected by the addition or multiplication of a given number of observations and provides a better indication of reproducibility than does the coefficient of variation. Oxygen uptake had a higher reliability coefficient ($r = 0.88$) and a smaller 90% confidence interval when compared to treadmill time ($r = 0.70$) consistent with a better correlation. The double product and heart rate were highly reproducible ($r = 0.90$ and $r = 0.94$, respectively). In addition, the 90% confidence interval for both double product and heart rate was small. The ST60 displacement in lead X and the lead of greatest displacement were very reproducible ($r = 0.83$).

Measured oxygen uptake displayed better reproducibility than treadmill time at peak exercise, the onset of angina, and the gas exchange anaerobic threshold. The double product, heart rate, and ST-segment displacement in lead X were found to be reproducible at peak exercise, the onset of angina, and the gas exchange anaerobic threshold. Gas exchange analysis provided accurate physiological determinants of exercise capacity in patients with angina pectoris. Noninvasive estimates of myocardial oxygen demand and ischemia were reproducibly determined. These findings are summarized in Table 6-17.

SUMMARY

The interpretation of the exercise test requires understanding exercise physiology and pathophysiology as well as expertise in electrocardiography. One should not assume that all medical professionals can adequately interpret an exercise test. Certification is extremely important now that this technology is rapidly spreading beyond the subspecialty of Cardiology. Training and experience are required as they are in other diagnostic procedures. For these reasons, the American College of Physicians and American College of Cardiology, and the American Heart Association have published guidelines on clinical competence for physicians performing exercise testing.[270-272]

All the results of the test must be considered. Attempts should be made to make the interpretation reliable by using good methods and following the above suggestions. When properly interpreted, the exercise test is one of the most important diagnostic and clinically helpful tests in medicine. Observer agreement is best when using dichotomous interpretations, and worst (most variable) when using more complex descriptions, such as are involved in specifying location or overlapping areas. Several possible modes for improvement include: (1) simple dichotomous decisions, (2) standardized report forms, (3) multiple observers or one very experienced reader, (4) multiple blinded or unbiased interpretations, and (5) computer analysis. Computer analysis of the exercise ECG and measurement of gas exchange variables can be highly reproducible. However, as long as human judgment with all its complexities remains the basis for the final interpretation, there will always be some variation and the human element will always be needed in medical diagnosis.

ST-segment depression is a representation of global subendocardial ischemia, with a direction determined largely by the placement of the heart in the chest. ST depression does not localize coronary artery lesions. ST depression in the inferior leads (II, AV_F) is most often due to the atrial repolarization wave which begins in the PR segment and can extend to the beginning of the ST segment. Severe transmural ischemia, resulting in wall motion abnormalities, causes a shift of the vector in the direction of the wall motion abnormality. However, pre-existing areas of wall motion abnormality (i.e., scar) usually indicated by a Q wave, also cause such a shift resulting in ST elevation without ischemia being present. When the resting ECG shows Q-waves of an old MI, ST elevation is due to ischemia or wall motion abnormalities or both, whereas accompanying ST depression can be due to a second area of ischemia or reciprocal changes. When the resting ECG is normal, however, ST elevation is due to severe ischemia (spasm or a critical lesion), though accompanying

TABLE 6-17. Mean ± Standard deviation of exercise test variables at maximal angina-limited exercise

Variable	Mean and standard deviation			Intraclass correlation coefficient		
	Day 1	Day 2	Day 3	ANOVA $p < 0.05^*$	R	90% Confidence Interval
Time (sec)	503 ± 72	516 ± 85	526 ± 66	0.35	0.70	0.48–0.86
VO_2	1.56 ± 0.29	1.55 ± 0.33	1.56 ± 0.29	0.99	0.88	0.76–0.95
Double product $\times 10^3$	18.9	19.6	18.9			
Heart rate (beats/min)	111 ± 19	112 ± 20	110 ± 17	0.66	0.94	0.88–0.97
ST_{60} X (mV)	-0.14 ± 0.11	-0.14 ± 0.10	-0.14 ± 0.10	0.99	0.83	0.63–0.92
ST_{60} GD (mV)	-0.19 ± 0.08	-0.17 ± 0.11	-0.20 ± 0.09	0.17	0.82	0.60–0.92

$^*p > 0.05$ would indicate a significant change over three testing periods.

ANOVA, analysis-of-variance model to determine time trends; GD, lead of greatest ST-segment depression; ST_{60}, ST-segment depression at 60 msec after QRS end; VO_2, volume of oxygen; X, lead X.

Based on data from Sullivan M, Genter F, Roberts M, et al: The reproducibility of hemodynamic, electrocardiographic, and gas exchange data during treadmill exercise in patients with stable angina pectoris. Chest 1984;86:375-382.

ST depression is reciprocal. Such ST elevation is uncommon, very arrhythmogenic and it localizes. Exercise-induced ST depression loses its diagnostic power in patients with LBBB, WPW, electronic pacemakers, intraventricular conduction delay with inverted T waves, and in patients with more than 1 mm of resting ST depression.

Exercise-induced R- and S-wave amplitude changes do not correlate with changes in left ventricular volume, EF, or ischemia. The consensus of many studies is that such changes do not have diagnostic value. ST-segment depression limited to the recovery period does not generally represent a "false positive" response. Inclusion of analysis during this time period increases the diagnostic yield of the exercise test. Performing exercise ECG analysis in conjunction with nuclear imaging or performing a cool-down walk can falsely lower the sensitivity of the exercise ECG, since they obscure ST-segment changes occurring in recovery. Other criteria including downsloping ST changes in recovery and prolongation of depression can improve test performance.

The evidence base for an exaggerated concern with silent ischemia (SI) is scant. Patients with SI (painless ST depression) usually have milder forms of coronary disease and a better prognosis. The evidence base for SI being more prevalent in diabetics is not as convincing as one would think, given its widespread clinical acceptance. Many physicians feel that treadmill testing should be used for routine screening of diabetics.

TWA, a beat-to-beat fluctuation in the amplitude or shape of the T wave, has been associated with pathologic findings, including autonomic imbalance, electrolyte abnormalities, coronary spasm, and sudden death. The earliest laboratory studies noted it to be a feature of myocardial ischemia, and later studies focused on its relationship to arrhythmias and arrhythmic risk. Although the exact cause of TWA remains elusive, it is thought to correlate with cardiac events, and hence is a subject of great interest among investigators. It was hoped that this technology could help physicians decide who really needs implantable cardioverter defibrillators but it has yet to fulfill this promise.

As with resting ventricular arrhythmias, exercise-induced ventricular arrhythmia have an independent association with death in most patients with coronary disease and in asymptomatic individuals. The risk may be more delayed (more than 6 years) than that associated with ST depression. Non-sustained ventricular tachycardia is uncommon during routine clinical treadmill testing and is usually well tolerated. In patients with a history of syncope, sudden death, physical exam revealing a large heart, murmurs, ECG showing prolonged QT, pre-excitation, Q waves, and chronic heart failure, ETIVA are more worrisome, but when seen in other patients, one must not behave like one does in a CCU. The two available studies support the conclusion that exercise test-induced supraventricular arrhythmias are relatively rare compared to ventricular arrhythmias and appear to be benign, except for their association with the development of AF in the future.

REFERENCES

1. Einthoven W: Weiteres uber das elektrokardiogramm. Arch fd ges Physiol 1908;122:517.
2. Simonson E: Electrocardiographic stress tolerance tests. Prog Cardiovasc Dis 1970;13:269-292.
3. Blomqvist G: The Frank lead exercise electrocardiogram. Acta Med Scand 1965;178:1-98.
4. Rautaharju PM, Punsar S, Blackburn H, et al: Waveform patterns in frank-lead rest and exercise electrocardiograms of healthy elderly men. Circulation 1973;48:541-548.
5. Simoons ML, Hugenholtz PG: Gradual changes of ECG waveform during and after exercise in normal subjects. Circulation 1975; 52:570-577.
6. Wolthuis RA, Froelicher VF, Hopkirk A, et al: Normal electrocardiographic waveform characteristics during treadmill exercise testing. Circulation 1979;60:1028-1035.
7. Coester N, Elliott JC, Luft UC: Plasma electrolytes, pH, and ECG during and after exhaustive exercise. J Appl Physiol 1973;34:677-682.
8. Wilkerson JE, Horvath SM, Gutin B, et al: Plasma electrolyte content and concentration during treadmill exercise in humans. J Appl Physiol 1982;53:1529-1539.
9. Grant SM, Green HJ, Phillips SM, et al: Fluid and electrolyte hormonal responses to exercise and acute plasma volume expansion. J Appl Physiol 1996;81:2386-2392.
10. Nordsborg N, Bangsbo J, Pilegaard H: Effect of high-intensity training on exercise-induced gene expression specific to ion homeostasis and metabolism. J Appl Physiol 2003;95:1201-1206. Epub 2003 May 23.
11. McKenna MJ: Effects of training on potassium homeostasis during exercise. J Mol Cell Cardiol 1995;27:941-949.
12. Morales-Ballejo H, Greenberg P, Ellestad M, et al: Septal Q wave in exercise testing: Angiographic correlation. Am J Cardiol 1981; 48:247-253.
13. Kentala E, Luurela O: Response of R wave amplitude to posterior changes and to exercise. Ann Clin Res 1975;7:258-263.
14. Bonoris PE, Greenberg PS, Christison GW, et al: Evaluation of R wave amplitude changes versus ST segment depression in stress testing. Circulation 1978;57:904-910.
15. Uhl GS, Hopkirk AC: Analysis of exercise-induced R wave amplitude changes in detection of coronary artery disease in asymptomatic men with left bundle branch block. Am J Cardiol 1979;44:1247-1250.
16. Yiannikas J, Marcomichelakis J, Taggart P, et al: Analysis of exercise induced changes in R wave amplitude in asymptomatic men with electrocardiographic ST-T changes at rest. Am J Cardiol 1981;47:238-243.
17. Greenberg PS, Ellestad MH, Berg R, et al: Correlation of R wave and EF changes with upright bicycle stress testing. Circulation 1980;62:111-200.
18. Baron DW, Lisley C, Sheiban I, et al: R-wave amplitude during exercise: Relation to left ventricular function coronary artery disease. Br Heart J 1980;44:512-517.
19. De Feyter PJ, Jong JP, Roos et al JP: Diagnostic incapacity of exercise-induced QRS wave amplitude changes to detect coronary artery disease and left ventricular dysfunction. Eur Heart J 1982;3:9-16.

20. Battler A, Froelicher VF, Slutsky R, et al: Relationship of QRS amplitude changes during exercise to left ventricular function and volumes and the diagnosis of coronary artery disease. Circulation 1979;60:1004-1013.

21. Luwaert R, Cosyns J, Rousseau M, et al: Reassessment of the relation between QRS forces to the orthogonal electrocardiogram and left ventricular ejection fraction. Eur Heart J 1983;4:103-109.

22. Brody DA: A theoretical analysis of intracavitary blood mass influence on the heart-lead relationship. Circ Res 1956;54:731-738.

23. Levken J, Chatterjee K, Tyberg JV, et al: Influence of left ventricular dimensions on endocardial and epicardial QRS amplitude and ST segment elevations during acute myocardial ischemia. Circulation 1980;61:679-689.

24. Deanfield JE, Davies G, Mongiadi F, et al: Factors influencing R wave amplitude in patients with ischaemic heart disease. Br Heart J 1983;49:8-14.

25. David D, Naito M, Michelson E, et al: Intramyocardial conduction: A major determinant of R wave amplitude during acute myocardial ischemia. Circulation 1982;65:161-167.

26. Myers J, Ahnve S, Froelicher V, Sullivan M: Spatial R wave amplitude during exercise: Relation with left ventricular ischemia and function. J Am Coll Cardiol 1985;6:603-608.

27. Gerson MC, Morris SN, McHenry PL: Relation of exercise induced physiologic ST segment depression to R wave amplitude in normal subjects. Am J Cardiol 1980;46:778-782.

28. Kodama K, Hiasa G, Ohtsuka T, et al: Transient U wave inversion during treadmill exercise testing in patients with left anterior descending coronary artery disease. Angiology 2000;51:581-589.

29. Hayat NH, Salman H, Daimee MA, Thomas CS: Abolition of exercise induced positive U-wave after coronary angioplasty: Clinical implication. Int J Cardiol 2000;73:267-272.

30. Miwa K, Igawa A, Nakagawa K, et al: Exercise-induced negative U waves in precordial leads as a marker of viable myocardium in patients with recent anterior myocardial infarction. Int J Cardiol 2000;73:149-156.

31. Miwa K, Nakagawa K, Hirai T, Inoue H: Exercise-induced U-wave alterations as a marker of well-developed and well-functioning collateral vessels in patients with effort angina. J Am Coll Cardiol 2000;35:757-763.

32. Mirvis DM, Ramanathan KB, Wilson JL: Regional blood flow correlates of ST segment depression in tachycardia-induced myocardial ischemia. Circulation 1986;2:363-373.

33. Prinzmetal M, Kennamer R, Merliss R, et al: Angina pectoris. I.A variant form of angina pectoris; preliminary report. Am J Med 1959;27:375-388.

34. Endo M, Kanda I, Hosoda: Prinzmetal's variant form of angina pectoris. Re-evaluation of mechanisms. Circulation 1975;52:33-37.

35. Shubrooks SJ, Bete JM, Hutter AM: Variant angina pectoris: Clinical and anatomic spectrum and results of coronary bypass surgery. Am J Cardiol 1975;36:142-147.

36. Higgins CB, Wexler L, Silverman JF, Schroeder JS: Clinical and arteriographic features of Prinzmetal's variant angina: Documentation of etiologic factors. Am J Cardiol 1976;37:831-839.

37. Maseri A, Severi S, DeNes M: Variant angina: One aspect of continuous spectrum of vasospastic myocardial ischemia Pathogenetic mechanisms, estimated incidence and clinical and coronary arteriographic findings in 138 patients. Am J Cardiol 1978;42:1019-1035.

38. Weiner DA, Schick EC Jr., Hood WB Jr., Ryan TJ: ST segment elevation during recovery from exercise. A new manifestation of Prinzmetal's variant angina. Chest 1978;74:133-138.

39. Oliva PB, Potts DE, Pluss G: Coronary arterial spasm in Prinzmetal angina: Documentation by coronary angiography. New Engl J Med 1973;288:745-748.

40. Maseri A, Mimmo R, Chiecia S, et al: Coronary artery spasm as a cause of acute myocardial ischemia in man. Chest 1975;68:625-633.

41. Schroeder JS, Bolen JL, Quint RA, et al: Provocation of coronary spasm with ergonovine maleate. New test with results in 57 patients undergoing coronary arteriography. Am J Cardiol 1977;40:487-491.

42. Bory M, Pierron F, Panagides D, et al: Coronary artery spasm in patients with normal or near normal coronary arteries: Long-term follow-up of 277 patients. Eur Heart J 1996;17:1015-1021.

43. Fortuin NJ, Friesinger GC: Exercise-induced S-T segment elevation: Clinical, electrocardiographic and arteriographic studies in twelve patients. Am J Med 1970;49:459-464.

44. Hegge FN, Tuna N, Burchell HB: Coronary arteriographic findings in patients with axis shifts or S-T-segment elevations on exercise testing. Am Heart J 1973;86:603-615.

45. Chahine RA, Raizner AE, Ishimori T: The clinical significance of exercise-induced ST-segment elevation. Circulation 1976;54:209-213.

46. Manvi KN, Ellestad MH: Elevated ST segments with exercise in ventricular aneurysm. J Electrocardiol 1972;5:317-323.

47. Simoons M, Withagen A, Vinke R, et al: St-vector orientation and location of myocardial perfusion defects during exercise. Nuklearmedizin 1978;17:154-156.

48. Sriwattanakomen S, Ticzon AR, Zubritzky SA, et al: ST segment elevation during exercise: Electrocardiographic and arteriographic correlation in 38 patients. Am J Cardiol 1980;45:762-768.

49. Longhurst JC, Kraus WL: Exercise-induced ST elevation in patients without myocardial infarction. Circulation 1979;60:616-629.

50. Dunn RF, Freedman B, Kelly DT, et al: Exercise-induced ST-segment elevation in leads V1 or AVL. A predictor of anterior myocardial ischemia and left anterior descending coronary artery disease. Circulation 1981;63:1357-1363.

51. Braat SH, Kingma H, Brugada P, Wellens HJJ: Value of lead V4R in exercise testing to predict proximal stenosis of the right coronary artery. J Am Coll Cardiol 1985;5:1308-1311.

52. Mark DB, Hlatky MA, Lee KL, et al: Localizing coronary artery obstructions with the exercise treadmill test. Ann Intern Med 1987;106:53-55.

53. Waters DD, Chaitman BR, Bourassa MG, Tubau JF: Clinical and angiographic correlates of exercise-induced ST-segment elevation. Increased detection with multiple ECG leads. Circulation 1980;61:286-296.

54. Bruce RA, Gey GO Jr., Cooper MN, et al: Seattle Heart Watch: Initial clinical, circulatory and electrocardiographic response to maximal exercise. Am J Cardiol 1974;33:459-469.

55. Bruce RA, Fisher LD: Unusual prognostic significance of exercise-induced ST elevation in coronary patients. J Electrocardiol 1987;20(suppl)84-88.

56. De Feyter PJ, Majid PA, Van Eenige MJ, et al: Clinical significance of exercise-induced ST segment elevation. Br Heart J 1981;46:84-92.

57. Bruce RA, Fisher LD, Pettinger M, et al: ST segment elevation with exercise: A marker for poor ventricular function and poor prognosis. Coronary Artery Surgery Study (CASS) confirmation of Seattle Heart Watch results. Circulation 1988;4:897-905.

58. Hegge FN, Tuna N, Burchell HB: Coronary arteriographic findings in patients with axis shifts or S-T-segment elevations on exercise-stress testing. Am Heart J 1973;5:603-615.

59. Lahiri A, Subramanian B, Miller-Craig M, et al: Exercise-induced ST-segment elevation in variant angina. Am J Cardiol 1980;45:887-894.

60. Caplin JL, Banim SO: Chest pain and electrocardiographic ST-segment elevation occurring in the recovery phase after exercise in a patient with normal coronary arteries. Clin Cardiol 1985;8:228-229.

61. Hill JA, Conti CR, Feldman RL, Pepine CJ: Coronary artery spasm and its relationship to exercise in patients without severe coronary obstructive disease. Clin Cardiol 1988;11:489-494.

62. Fox KM, Jonathan A, England D, Selwyn AP: Significance of exercise-induced ST-segment elevation in patients with previous myocardial infarction. Am J Cardiol 1982;49:933.

63. Gewirtz H, Sullivan M, O'Reilly G, et al: Role of myocardial ischemia in the genesis of exercise-induced S-T segment elevation in previous anterior myocardial infarction. Am J Cardiol 1983;51:1289-1293.

64. Stiles GL, Rosati RA, Wallace AG: Clinical relevance of exercise-induced S-T segment elevation. Am J Cardiol 1980;46:931-936.

65. Shimokawa H, Matsuguchi T, Koiwaya Y, et al: Variable exercise capacity in variant angina and greater exertional thallium-201 myocardial defect during vasospastic ischemic ST segment elevation than with ST depression. Am Heart J 1982;103:142-145.

66. Arora R, Ioachim L, Matza D, Horowitz SF: The role of ischemia and ventricular asynergy in the genesis of exercise-induced ST elevation. Clin Cardiol 1988;11:127-131.

67. Nobel RJ, Rothbaum DA, Knoebel SB, et al: Normalization of abnormal T waves in ischemia. Arch Intern Med 1976;136:391-395.

68. Sweet RL, Sheffield LT: Myocardial infarction after exercise-induced electrocardiographic changes in a patient with variant angina pectoris. Am J Cardiol 1974;33:813-817.

69. Lavie CJ, Oh JK, Mankin HT, et al: Significance of T-wave pseudo-normalization during exercise. A radionuclide angiographic study. Chest 1988;94:512-516.

70. McHenry PL, Morris SN: Exercise electrocardiography—current state of the art. In Schlant RC, Hurst JW (eds): Advances in Electrocardiography, vol 2. New York, Grune & Stratton, 1976, pp.265-304.

71. Maseri A, Severi S, De Nes M, et al: "Variant" angina: One aspect of a continuous spectrum of vasospastic myocardial ischemia. Am J Cardiol 1978;42:1019-1025.

72. Detrano R, Janosi A, Lyons KP, et al: Factors affecting sensitivity and specificity of a diagnostic test: The exercise thallium scintigram. Am J Med 1988;84:699-710.

73. Gutman RA, Bruce R: Delay of ST depression after maximal exercise by walking for 2 minutes. Circulation 1970;42:229-233.

74. Gibbons L, Blair SN, Kohl HW, Cooper K: The safety of maximal exercise testing. Circulation 1989;80:846-852.

75. Lachterman B, Lehmann KG, Abrahamson D, Froelicher VF: "Recovery only" ST-segment depression and the predictive accuracy of the exercise test. Ann Intern Med 1990;112(1):11-16.

76. Karnegis JN, Matts J, Tuna N, et al: Comparison of exercise-positive with recovery-positive treadmill graded exercise tests. Am J Cardiol 1987;60:544-547.

77. Savage MP, Squires LS, Hopkins JT, et al: Usefulness of ST-segment depression as a sign of coronary artery disease when confined to the post exercise recovery period. Am J Cardiol 1987;60:1405-1406.

78. Froelicher VF, Thompson AJ, Longo MR, et al: Value of exercise testing for screening asymptomatic men for latent coronary artery disease. Prog Cardiovasc Dis 1976;18:265-276.

79. Ellestad M: Stress Testing. Principles and Practice, 3rd edn. Philadelphia, F.A. Davis, 1986.

80. Rywik TM, Zink RC, Gittings NS, et al: Independent prognostic significance of ischemic ST-segment response limited to recovery from treadmill exercise in asymptomatic subjects. Circulation 1998;97:2117-2122.

81. Lanza GA, Mustilli M, Sestito A, et al: Diagnostic and prognostic value of ST segment depression limited to the recovery phase of exercise stress test. Heart 2004;90:1417-1421.

82. Berman, JA, Wynne J, Mellis G, Cohn PF: Improving diagnostic accuracy of the exercise test by combining R wave changes with duration of ST segment depression in a simplified index. Am Heart J 1983;105:60-66.

83. Froelicher VF, Myers J, Follansbee WP, Labovitz AJ: Exercise and the Heart. St. Louis, Mosby, 1993, pp. 48-69.

84. Hollenberg M, Mateo GO, Massie BM, et al: Influence of R wave amplitude on exercise-induced ST depression: Need for a "gain factor" correction when interpreting stress electrocardiograms. Am J Cardiol 1985;56:13-17.

85. Hakki A, Iskandrian AS, Kutalek S, et al: R wave amplitude: A new determinant of failure of patients with coronary heart disease to manifest ST segment depression during exercise. J Am Coll Cardiol 1984;3:1155-1160.

86. Jaffe MD: Effect of oestrogens on postexercise electrocardiogram. Br Heart J 1976;38:1299-1303.

87. James FW, Chung EK (eds): Exercise ECG Test in children. In Exercise Electrocardiography: A Practical Approach, 2nd ed. Baltimore, Williams and Wilkins, 1983, p. 132.

88. Sundqvist K, Atterhog JH, Jogestrand T: Effect of digoxin on the electrocardiogram at rest and during exercise in healthy subjects. Am J Cardiol 1986;57:661-665.

89. Sundqvist K, Jogestrand T, Nowak J: The effect of digoxin on the electrocardiogram of healthy middle-aged and elderly patients at rest and during exercise—A comparison with the ECG reaction induced by myocardial ischemia. J Electrocardiol 2002;35:213-217.

90. Tonkon MJ, Lee G, DeMaria AN, et al: Effects of digitalis on the exercise electrocardiogram in normal adult subjects. Chest 1977;72:714-718.

91. Sketch MH, Moss AN, Butler ML, et al: Digoxin-induced positive exercise tests: Their clinical and prognostic significance. Am J Cardiol 1981;48:655-659.

92. LeWinter M, Crawford M, O'Rourke R, Karliner J: The effects of oral propanolol, digoxin and combined therapy on the resting and exercise ECG. Am Heart J 1977;93:202-209.

93. Whinnery JE, Froelicher VF, Stuart AJ: The electrocardiographic response to maximal treadmill exercise in asymptomatic men with left bundle branch block. Am Heart J 1977;94:316-324.

94. Ibrahim NS, Selvester RS, Hagar JM, Ellestad MH: Detecting exercise-induced ischemia in left bundle branch block using the electrocardiogram. Am J Cardiol 1998;82:832-835.

95. Vasey CG, O'Donnell J, Morris SN, McHenry P: Exercise-induced left bundle branch block and its relation to coronary artery disease. Am J Cardiol 1985;56:892-895.

96. Grady TA, Chiu AC, Snader CE, et al: Prognostic significance of exercise-induced left bundle-branch block. JAMA 1998;279:153-156.

97. Whinnery JE, Froelicher VF, Stuart AJ: The electrocardiographic response to maximal treadmill exercise in asymptomatic men with right branch bundle block. Chest 1977;71:335.

98. Wolff L, Parkinson J, White P: Bundle branch block with short PR interval in healthy young people prone to paroxysmal tachycardia. Am Heart J 1930;5:685-704.

99. Gazes PC: False positive exercise test in the presence of the Wolff-Parkinson-White syndrome. Am J Cardiol 1969;78:13-15.

100. Poyatos ME, Suarez L, Lerman J, et al: Exercise testing and thallium-201 myocardial perfusion scintigraphy in the clinical evaluation of patients with Wolff Parkinson White syndrome. J Electrocardiol 1986;19:319-326.

101. Jezior MR, Kent SM, Atwood JE: Exercise testing in Wolff-Parkinson-White syndrome: Case reports with ECG and literature review. Chest 2005;127:1454-1457.

102. Strasberg B, Ashley WW, Wyndham CRC, et al: Treadmill exercise testing in the Wolff-Parkinson-White Syndrome. Am J Cardiol 1980;45:742-747.

103. Paquet N, Verreault J, Lepage S, et al: False-positive thallium study in Wolff-Parkinson-White syndrome. Can J Cardiol 1996;12:499-502.

104. Archer S, Gornick C, Grund F, et al: Exercise thallium testing in ventricular preexcitation. Am J Cardiol 1987;59:1103-1106.

105. Tawarahara K, Kurata C, Taguchi T, et al: Exercise testing and thallium-201 emission computed tomographic in patients with intraventricular conduction disturbances. Am J Cardiol 1992;69:97-102.

106. Pattoneri P, Astorri E, Calbiani B, et al: Thallium-201 myocardial scintigraphy in patients with Wolff-Parkinson-White syndrome. Minerva Cardioangiol 2003;51:87-93.

107. Greenland P, Kauffman R, Weir KE: Profound exercise-induced ST segment depression in patients with Wolff-Parkinson-White syndrome and normal coronary arteriograms. Thorax 1980;35:559-605.

108. Rosenbaum MB, Blanco H, Elizari MV, et al: Electrotonic modulation of the T wave and cardiac memory. Am J Cardiol 1982;50:213-222.

109. Sharma AD, Yee R, Guiraudon G, et al: Sensitivity and specificity of invasive and noninvasive testing for risk of sudden death in Wolff-Parkinson-White syndrome. J Am Coll Cardiol 1987;10:373-381.

110. Daubert C, Ollitrault J, Descaves C, et al: Failure of the exercise test to predict the anterograde refractory period of the accessory pathway in Wolff-Parkinson-White syndrome. PACE 1988;11:1130-1138.

111. Lévy S, Broustet JP: Exercise testing in the Wolff-Parkinson-White syndrome (letter). Am J Cardiol 1981;48:976-977.

112. Klein GJ, Bashore TM, Sellers TD, et al: Ventricular fibrillation in the Wolff-Parkinson-White syndrome. N Engl J Med 1979;301:1980-1985.

113. Gaita F, Giustetto C, Riccardi R, et al: Exercise and pharmacologic tests as methods to identify patients with Wolff-Parkinson-White syndrome at risk of sudden death. Am J Cardiol 1989;64:487-490.

114. Pappone C, Santinelli V, Rosanio S, et al: Usefulness of invasive electrophysiologic testing to stratify the risk of arrhythmic events in asymptomatic patients with Wolff-Parkinson-White pattern. J Am Coll Cardiol 2003;41:239-244.

115. Riff DP, Carleton RA: Effect of exercise on the atrial recovery wave. Am Heart J 1971;82:759-763.

116. Sapin PM, Koch G, Blauwet MB, et al: Identification of false positive exercise tests with use of electrocardiographic criteria: A possible role for atrial repolarization waves. J Am Coll Cardiol 1991;18:127-135.

117. Myrianthefs MM, Nicolaides EP, Pitiris D, et al: False positive ST-segment depression during exercise in subjects with short PR segment and angiographically normal coronaries: Correlation with exercise-induced ST depression in subjects with normal PR and normal coronaries. J Electrocardiol 1998;31:203-208.

118. McHenry PL, Cogan OJ, Elliott WC, Knoebel SB: False positive ECG response to exercise secondary to hyperventilation: Cineangiographic correlation. Am Heart J 1970;79:683-687.

119. McHenry PL, Richmond HW, Weisenberger BL, et al: Evaluation of abnormal exercise electrocardiogram in apparently healthy subjects: Labile repolarization (ST-T) abnormalities as a cause of false positive responses. Am J Cardiol 1981;47:1152-1160.

120. Barnard R, MacAlpin R, Kattus A, Buckberg G: Ischemic response to sudden strenuous exercise in healthy men. Circulation 1973; 48:936-942.

121. Foster C, Dymond DS, Carpenter J, Schmidt DH: Effect of warm-up on left ventricular response to sudden strenuous exercise. J Appl Physiol 1982;53:380-383.

122. Abouantoun S, Ahnve S, Savvides M, et al: Can areas of myocardial ischemia be localized by the exercise electrocardiogram? A correlative study with thallium-201 scintigraphy. Am Heart J 1984;108:933-941.

123. Fuchs RM, Achuff SC, Grunwald L, et al: Electrocardiographic localization of coronary artery narrowings: Studies during myocardial ischemia and infarction in patients with one-vessel disease. Circulation 1982;66:1168-1175.

124. Lewis T: Notes upon alternation of the heart. Q J Med 1910;4: 141-144.

125. Schwartz PJ, Malliani A: Electrical alternation of the T-wave: Clinical and experimental evidence of its relationship with the sympathetic nervous system and with the long Q-T syndrome. Am Heart J 1975;89:45-50.

126. Shimoni Z, Flatau E, Schiller D, et al: Electrical alternans of giant U waves with multiple electrolyte deficits. Am J Cardiol 1984;54: 920-921.

127. Reddy CV, Kiok JP, Khan RG, El-Sherif H: Repolarization alternans associated with alcoholism and hypomagnesia. Am J Cardiol 1984;53:390-391.

128. Cheng TC: Electrical alternans: An association with coronary artery spasm. Arch Intern Med 1983;143:1052-1053.

129. Kleinfeld MJ, Rozanski JJ: Alternans of the ST segment in Prinzmetal's angina. Circulation 1977;55:574-577.

130. Raeder EA, Rosenbaum DS, Bhasin R, Cohen RJ: Alternating morphology of the QRST complex preceding sudden death. N Engl J Med 1992;326:271-272.

131. Smith JM, Clancy EA, Valeri CR, et al: Electrical alternans and cardiac electrical instability. Circulation 1988;77:110-121.

132. Joyal M, Feldman RL, Pepine CJ: ST-segment alternans during percutaneous transluminal coronary angioplasty. Am J Cardiol 1984;54:915-916.

133. Salerno JA, Previtali M, Panciroli C, et al: Ventricular arrhythmias during acute myocardial ischaemia in man: The role and significance of R-ST-T alternans and the prevention of ischaemic sudden death by medical treatment. Eur Heart J 1986;7(suppl A):63-75.

134. Adam DR, Smith JM, Akselrod S, et al: Fluctuations in T-wave morphology and susceptibility to ventricular fibrillation. J Electrocardiol 1984;17:209-218.

135. Yan GX, Lankipalli RS, Burke JF, et al: Ventricular repolarization components on the electrocardiogram: Cellular basis and clinical significance. J Am Coll Cardiol 2003;42:401-409.

136. Yan GX, Martin J: Electrocardiographic T wave: A symbol of transmural dispersion of repolarization in the ventricles. J Cardiovasc Electrophysiol 2003;14:639-640.

137. Chinushi M, Kozhevnikov D, Caref EB, et al: Mechanism of discordant T wave alternans in the in vivo heart. J Cardiovasc Electrophysiol 2003;14:632-638.

138. Choi BR, Salama G: Simultaneous maps of optical action potentials and calcium transients in guinea-pig hearts: Mechanisms underlying concordant alternans. J Physiol 2000;529(Pt 1):171-188.

139. Huser J, Wang YG, Sheehan KA, et al: Functional coupling between glycolysis and excitation-contraction coupling underlies alternans in cat heart cells. J Physiol 2000;524(Pt 3):795-806.

140. Pastore JM, Rosenbaum DS: Role of structural barriers in the mechanism of alternans-induced reentry. Circ Res 2000;87: 1157-1163.

141. Walker ML, Rosenbaum DS: Repolarization alternans: Implications for the mechanism and prevention of sudden cardiac death. Cardiovasc Res 2003;57:599-614.

142. Clusin W: Calcium and cardiac arrhythmias: DADs, EADs, and alternans. Crit Rev Clin Lab Sci 2003;40:337-375.

143. Rosenbaum DS, Wilber DJ, Smith JM, et al: Local activation variability during monomorphic ventricular tachycardia in the dog. Cardiovasc Res 1992;26:237-243.

144. Pastore JM, Girouard SD, Laurita KR, et al: Mechanism linking T-wave alternans to the genesis of cardiac fibrillation. Circulation 1999;99:1385-1394.

145. Sanz E, Steger JP, Thie W: Cardiogoniometry. Clin Cardiol 1983; 6:199-206.

146. Hunt AC: T Wave Alternans in high arrhythmic risk patients: Analysis in time and frequency domains: A pilot study. BMC Cardiovasc Disord 2002;2:6.

147. Saner H, Baur HR, Sanz E, Gurtner HP: Cardiogoniometry: A new noninvasive method for detection of ischemic heart disease. Clin Cardiol 1983;6:207-210.

148. Meier A, Hoflin F, Herrmann HJ, et al: Comparative diagnostic value of a new computerized vectorcardiographic method (cardiogoniometry) and other noninvasive tests in medically treated patients with chest pain. Clin Cardiol 1987;10:311-316.

149. Smith JM, Clancy EA, Valeri CR, et al: Electrical alternans and cardiac electrical instability. Circulation 1988;77:110-121.

150. Nearing BD, Verrier RL: Modified moving average analysis of T-wave alternans to predict ventricular fibrillation with high accuracy. J Appl Physiol 2002;92:541-549.

151. Zareba W, Moss AJ, le Cessie S, Hall WJ: T wave alternans in idiopathic long QT syndrome. J Am Coll Cardiol 1994;23:1541-1546.

152. Zareba W, Moss AJ, le Cessie S, et al: Risk of cardiac events in family members of patients with long QT syndrome. J Am Coll Cardiol 1995;26:1685-1691.

153. Nearing BD, Huang AH, Verrier RL: Dynamic tracking of cardiac vulnerability by complex demodulation of the T wave. Science 1991;252:437-440.

154. Bloomfield DM, Hohnloser SH, Cohen RJ: Interpretation and classification of microvolt T wave alternans tests. J Cardiovasc Electrophysiol 2002;13:502-512.

155. Hohnloser SH, Klingenheben T, Zabel M, et al: T wave alternans during exercise and atrial pacing in humans. J Cardiovasc Electrophysiol 1997;8:987-993.

156. Rashba EJ, Osman AF, MacMurdy K, et al: Exercise is superior to pacing for T wave alternans measurement in subjects with chronic coronary artery disease and left ventricular dysfunction. J Cardiovasc Electrophysiol 2002;13:845-850.

157. Rosenbaum DS, Jackson LE, Smith JM, et al: Electrical alternans and vulnerability to ventricular arrhythmias. N Engl J Med 1994;330:235-241.

158. Armoundas AA, Rosenbaum DS, Ruskin JN, et al: Prognostic significance of electrical alternans versus signal averaged electrocardiography in predicting the outcome of electrophysiological testing and arrhythmia-free survival. Heart 1998;80:251-256.

159. Gold MR, Bloomfield DM, Anderson KP, et al: A comparison of T-wave alternans, signal averaged electrocardiography and programmed ventricular stimulation for arrhythmia risk stratification. J Am Coll Cardiol 2000;36:2254-2256.

160. Kitamura H, Ohnishi Y, Okajima K, et al: Onset heart rate of microvolt-level T-wave alternans provides clinical and prognostic value in nonischemic dilated cardiomyopathy. J Am Coll Cardiol 2002;39:295-300.

161. Hohnloser SH, Klingenheben T, Bloomfield D, et al: Usefulness of microvolt T-wave alternans for prediction of ventricular tachyarrhythmic events in patients with dilated cardiomyopathy: Results from a prospective observational study. J Am Coll Cardiol 2003;41:2220-2224.

162. Klingenheben T, Zabel M, D'Agostino RB, et al: Predictive value of T-wave alternans for arrhythmic events in patients with congestive heart failure. Lancet 2000;356:651-652.

163. Ikeda T, Sakata T, Takami M, et al: Combined assessment of T-wave alternans and late potentials used to predict arrhythmic events after myocardial infarction: A prospective study. J Am Coll Cardiol 2000;35:722-730.

164. Tapanainen JM, Still AM, Airaksinen KE, Huikuri HV: Prognostic significance of risk stratifiers of mortality, including T wave

alternans, after acute myocardial infarction: Results of a prospective follow-up study. J Cardiovasc Electrophysiol 2001;12:645-652.

165. Rashba EJ, Osman AF, MacMurdy K, et al: Influence of QRS duration on the prognostic value of T wave alternans. J Cardiovasc Electrophysiol 2002;13:770-775.

166. Hohnloser SH, Ikeda T, Bloomfield DM, et al: T-wave alternans negative coronary patients with low ejection and benefit from defibrillator implantation. Lancet 2003;362:125-126.

167. Francis DP, Salukhe TV: Who needs a defibrillator after myocardial infarction? Lancet 2003;362:91-92.

168. Weiner DA, McCabe C, Hueter DC, et al: The predictive value of anginal chest pain as an indicator of coronary disease during exercise testing. Am Heart J. 1978;96:458-462.

169. Cole JP, Ellestad MH: Significance of chest pain during treadmill exercise: Correlation with coronary events. Am J Cardiol 1978; 41:227-232.

170. Bodegard J, Erikssen G, Bjornholt JV, et al: Possible angina detected by the WHO angina questionnaire in apparently healthy men with a normal exercise ECG: Coronary heart disease or not? A 26 year follow up study. Heart 2004;90:627-632.

171. Scheidt-Nave C, Barrett-Connor E, Wingard DL: Resting electrocardiographic abnormalities suggestive of asymptomatic ischemic heart disease associated with non-insulin-dependent diabetes mellitus in a defined population. Circulation 1990;81:899-906.

172. Bruce RA, McDonough JR: Stress testing in screening for cardiovascular disease. Bull NY Acad Med 1969;45:1288-1295.

173. Aronow WS, Cassidy J: Five year follow-up of double Master's test, maximal treadmill stress test, and resting and postexercise apexcardiogram in asymptomatic persons. Circulation 1975;52: 616-622.

174. Froelicher VF, Thomas M, Pillow C, et al: An epidemiological study of asymptomatic men screened with exercise testing for latent coronary heart disease. Am J Cardiol 1975;34:770-779.

175. Allen WH, Aronow WS, Goodman P, Stinson P: Five-year follow-up of maximal treadmill stress test in asymptomatic men and women. Circulation 1980;62:522-531.

176. Manca C, Barilli AL, Dei Cas L, et al: Multivariate analysis of exercise ST depression and coronary risk factors in asymptomatic men. Eur Heart J 1982;3:2-8.

177. Rautaharju PM, Prineas RJ, Eifler WJ, et al: Prognostic value of exercise electrocardiogram in men at high risk of future coronary heart disease: Multiple risk factor intervention trial experience. J Am Coll Cardiol 1986;8:1-10.

178. Gordon DL, Ekelund LG, Karon JM, et al: Predictive value of the exercise tolerance test for mortality in North American men: The Lipid Research Clinics Mortality Follow-Up Study. Circulation 1986;74:252-261.

179. McHenry PL, O'Donnell J, Morris SN, Jordan JJ: The abnormal exercise electrocardiogram in apparently healthy men: A predictor of angina pectoris as an initial coronary event during long-term follow-up. Circulation 1984;70:547-551.

180. Bruce RA, Fisher LD, Hossack KF: Validation of exercise-enhanced risk assessment of coronary heart disease events: Longitudinal changes in incidence in Seattle community practice. J Am Coll Cardiol 1985;5:875-881.

181. Froelicher VF, Thompson AJ, Wolthuis R, et al: Angiographic findings in asymptomatic aircrewmen with electrocardiographic abnormalities. Am J Cardiol 1977;39:32-39.

182. Kemp HG, Kronmal RA, Vlietstra RE, Frye RL: Seven year survival of patients with normal and near normal coronary arteriograms: A CASS registry study. J Am Coll Cardiol 1986;7:479-483.

183. Ekelund LG, Suchindran CM, McMahon RP, et al: Coronary heart disease morbidity and mortality in hypercholesterolemic men predicted from an exercise test: The Lipid Research Clinics Coronary Primary Prevention Trial. J Am Coll Cardiol 1989;14: 556-563.

184. Gibbons LW, Mitchell TL, Wei M, et al: Maximal exercise test as a predictor of risk for mortality from coronary heart disease in asymptomatic men. Am J Cardiol 2000;86:53-58.

185. Gerson MC, Khoury JC, Hertzberg VS, et al: Prediction of coronary artery disease in a population of insulin-requiring diabetic patients: Results of an 8-year follow-up study. Am Heart J 1988; 116:820-826.

186. Koistinen MJ: Prevalence of asymptomatic myocardial ischaemia in diabetic subjects. BMJ 1990;301:92-95.

187. Janand-Delenne B, Savin B, Habib G, et al: Silent myocardial ischemia in patients with diabetes: Who to screen. Diabetes Care 1999;22:1396-1400.

188. May O, Arildsen H, Damsgaard EM, Mickley H: Prevalence and prediction of silent ischaemia in diabetes mellitus: A population-based study. Cardiovasc Res 1997;34:241-247.

189. Weiner DA, Ryan TJ, McCabe CH, et al: Significance of silent myocardial ischemia during exercise testing in patients with coronary artery disease. Am J Cardiol 1987;59:725-729.

190. Weiner DA, Ryan TJ, McCabe CH, et al: Risk of developing an acute myocardial infarction or sudden coronary death in patients with exercise-induced silent myocardial ischemia. A report from the Coronary Artery Surgery Study (CASS) Registry. Am J Cardiol 1988;62:1155-1158.

191. Mark DB, Hlatky MA, Califf RM, et al: Painless exercise ST deviation on the treadmill: Long-term prognosis. J Am Coll Cardiol 1989;14:885-892.

192. Dagenais GR, Rouleau JR, Hochart P, et al: Survival with painless strongly positive exercise ECG. Am J Cardiol 1988;62:892-895.

193. Casella G, Pavesi P, diNiro M, et al: Long-term prognosis of painless exercise induced ischemia in stable patients with previous MI. Am Heart J 1998;136:894-904.

194. Visser FC, van Leeuwen FT, Cernohorsky B, et al: Silent versus symptomatic myocardial ischemia during exercise testing: A comparison with coronary angiographic findings. Int J Cardiol 1990; 27:71-78.

195. Miranda C, Lehmann K, Lachterman B, et al: Comparison of silent and symptomatic ischemia during exercise testing in men. Ann Intern Med 1991;114:649-656.

196. Falcone C, de Servi S, Poma E, et al: Clinical significance of exercise-induced silent myocardial ischemia in patients with coronary artery disease. J Am Coll Cardiol 1987;9:295-299.

197. Nesto RW, Phillips RT, Kett KG, et al: Angina and exertional myocardial ischemia in diabetic and nondiabetic patients: Assessment by exercise thallium scintigraphy. Ann Intern Med 1988;108:170-175.

198. Naka M, Hiramatsu K, Aizawa T, et al: Silent myocardial ischemia in patients with non-insulin-dependent diabetes mellitus as judged by treadmill exercise testing and coronary angiography. Am Heart J 1992;123:46-53.

199. Hikita H, Kurita A, Takase B, et al: Usefulness of plasma beta-endorphin level, pain threshold and autonomic function in assessing silent myocardial ischemia in patients with and without diabetes mellitus. Am J Cardiol 1993;72:140-143.

200. Marchant B, Umachandran V, Stevenson R, et al: Silent myocardial ischemia: Role of subclinical neuropathy in patients with and without diabetes. J Am Coll Cardiol 1993;22:1433-1437.

201. L'Huillier I, Cottin Y, Touzery C: Predictive value of myocardial tomoscintigraphy in asymptomatic diabetic patients after percutaneous coronary intervention. Int J Cardiol. 2003;90:165-173.

202. Wackers FJ, Young LH, Inzucchi SE, et al: Detection of silent myocardial ischemia in asymptomatic diabetic subjects: The DIAD study. Diabetes Care 2004;27:1954-1961.

203. May O, Arildsen H, Damsgaard EM, Mickley H: Prevalence and prediction of silent ischaemia in diabetes mellitus: A population-based study. Cardiovasc Res 1997;34:241-247.

204. Caracciolo EA, Chaitman BR, Forman SA, et al: Diabetics with coronary disease have a prevalence of asymptomatic ischemia during exercise treadmill testing and ambulatory ischemia monitoring similar to that of nondiabetic patients. An ACIP database study. Circulation 1996;93:2097-2105.

205. Falcone C, Nespoli L, Geroldi D, et al: Silent myocardial ischemia in diabetic and nondiabetic patients with coronary artery disease. Int J Cardiol 2003;90:219-227.

206. Lee DP, Fearon WF, Froelicher VF: Clinical utility of the exercise ECG in patients with diabetes and chest pain. Chest 2001;119:1576-1581.

207. Fearon W, Voodi L, Atwood J, Froelicher V: The prognostic significance of silent ischemia detected by treadmill testing. Am Heart J 1998;136:759-761.

208. Candinas RA, Podrid PJ: Evaluation of cardiac arrhythmias by exercise testing. Herz 1990;15:21-27.

209. Kafka W, Petri H, Rudolph W: Exercise testing in the assessment of ventricular arrhythmias Herz 1982;7:140-149.

210. Hoffmann A, Wenk M, Follath F: Exercise-induced ventricular tachycardia as a manifestation of flecainide toxicity. Int J Cardiol 1986;11:353-355.

211. Anastasiou-Nana MI, Anderson JL, Stewart JR, et al: Occurrence of exercise-induced and spontaneous wide complex tachycardia during therapy with flecainide for complex ventricular arrhythmias: A probable proarrhythmic effect. Am Heart J 1987;113: 1071-1077.
212. Gosselink AT, Crijns HJ, Wiesfeld AC, Lie KI: Exercise-induced ventricular tachycardia: A rare manifestation of digitalis. Clin Cardiol 1993;16:270-272.
213. Nazari J, Bauman J, Pham T, et al: Exercise induced fatal sinusoidal ventricular tachycardia secondary to moricizine. PACE 1992;15(10 Pt 1):1421-1424.
214. Gibbons RJ, Balady GJ, Bricker JT, et al: ACC/AHA 2002 guideline update for exercise testing: A report of the American College of Cardiology/American Heart Association Task Force on Practice Guidelines (Committee on Exercise Testing). Circulation 2002;106:1883-1892. Full text available at: www.acc.org/clinical/guidelines/exercise/dirIndex.htm
215. Udall JA, Ellestad MH: Predictive implications of ventricular premature contractions associated with treadmill stress testing. Circulation 1977;56:985-989.
216. Califf RM, McKinnes RA, McNeer R, et al: Prognostic value of ventricular arrhythmias associated with treadmill testing in patients studied with cardiac catheterization for suspected ischemic heart disease. J Am Coll Cardiol 1983;2:1060-1067.
217. Marieb MA, Beller GA, Gibson RS, et al: Clinical relevance of exercise-induced ventricular arrhythmias in suspected coronary artery disease. Am J Cardiol 1990;66:172-178.
218. Schweikert RA, Pashkow FJ, Snader CE, et al: Association of exercise-induced ventricular ectopic activity with thallium myocardial perfusion and angiographic coronary artery disease in stable, low-risk populations. Am J Cardiol 1999;83:530-534.
219. Sami M, Chaitman B, Fisher L, et al: Significance of exercise-induced ventricular arrhythmia in stable coronary artery disease: A coronary artery surgery study project. Am J Cardiol 1984;54:1182-1188.
220. Casella G, Pavesi PC, Sangiorgio P, et al: Exercise-induced ventricular arrhythmias in patients with healed myocardial infarction. Int J Cardiol 1993;40:229-235.
221. Jouven X, Zureik M, Desnos M, et al: Long-term outcome in asymptomatic men with exercise-induced premature ventricular depolarizations. N Engl J Med 2000;343:826-833.
222. Busby MJ, Shefrin EA, Fleg JL: Prevalence and long-term significance of exercise-induced frequent or repetitive ventricular ectopic beats in apparently healthy volunteers. J Am Coll Cardiol 1989;14:1659-1665.
223. Froelicher VF, Thomas MM, Pillow C, et al: Epidemiologic study of asymptomatic men screened by maximal treadmill testing for latent coronary artery disease. Am J Cardiol 1974;34:770-776.
224. Billman GE, Schwartz PJ, Gagnol JP, Stone HL: The cardiac response to submaximal exercise in dogs susceptible to sudden cardiac death. J Appl Physiol 1985;59:890-897.
225. Friedwald, VE, Spence DW: Sudden death associated with exercise: The risk-benefit issue. Am J Cardiol 1990;66:183-188.
226. Verrier RL, Lown B: Behavorial stress and cardiac arrhythmias. Annu Rev Physiol 1984;46:155-176.
227. Gettes LS: Electrolyte abnormalities underlying lethal and ventricular arrhythmias. Circulation 1992;85(suppl):170-176.
228. Schwartz PJ, Billman GE, Stone HL: Autonomic mechanisms in VF due to acute myocardial ischemia during exercise in dogs with healed myocardial infarction: An experimental model for sudden cardiac death. Circulation 1984;69:790-800.
229. Paterson DJ: Antiarrhythmic mechanisms during exercise. Exercise disturbs cardiac sympathovagal and ionic balance. J Appl Physiol 1996;80:1853-1862.
230. Ranger S, Talajic M, Lemery R: Amplification of flecainide-induced ventricular conduction slowing by exercise. A potentially significant clinical consequence of use-dependent sodium channel blockade. Circulation 1989;79:1000-1006.
231. Tuininga YS, Crijns HJ, Wiesfeld AC, et al: Electrocardiographic patterns relative to initiating mechanisms of exercise-induced ventricular tachycardia. Am Heart J 1993;126:359-367.
232. Kaufman ES, Priori SG, Napolitano C, et al: Electrocardiographic prediction of abnormal genotype in congenital long QT syndrome: Experience in 101 related family members. J Cardiovasc Electrophysiol 2001;12:455-461.
233. Herbert E, Trusz-Gluza M, Moric E, et al: KCNQ1 gene mutations and the respective genotype-phenotype correlations in the long QT syndrome. Med Sci Monit 2002;8:RA240-248.
234. Paavonen KJ, Swan H, Piippo K, et al: K. Response of the QT interval to mental and physical stress in types LQT1 and LQT2 of the long QT syndrome. Heart 2001;86:39-44.
235. Laitinen PJ, Swan H, Piippo K, et al: Genes, exercise and sudden death: Molecular basis of familial catecholaminergic polymorphic ventricular tachycardia. Ann Med 2004;36(suppl 1):81-86.
236. Fleg JL, Lakatta EG: Prevalence and prognosis of exercise-induced nonsustained ventricular tachycardia in apparently healthy volunteers. Am J Cardiol 1984;54:762-764.
237. Weiner DA, Levine SR, Klein MD, Ryan TJ: Ventricular arrhythmias during exercise testing: Mechanism, response to coronary bypass surgery, and prognostic significance. Am J Cardiol 1984;53:1553-1557.
238. McHenry PL, Morris SN, Kavalier M, Jordan JW: Comparative study of exercise-induced ventricular arrhythmias in normal subjects and patients with documented coronary artery disease. Am J Cardiol 1976;37:609-616.
239. DeBusk RF, Davidson DM, Houston N, Fitzgerald J: Serial ambulatory electrocardiography and treadmill exercise testing after uncomplicated myocardial infarction. Am J Cardiol 1980;45:547-554.
240. Detry JR, Mengeot P, Ronsseau MF, et al: Maximal exercise testing in patients with spontaneous angina pectoris associated with transient ST segment elevation: Risks and electrocardiographic findings. Br Heart J 1975;37:897-905.
241. Bikkina M, Larson M, Levy D: Prognostic implications of asymptomatic ventricular arrhythmias: The Framingham Heart Study. Ann Intern Med 1992;117:990-996.
242. Saini V, Graboys TB, Towne V, Lown B: Reproducibility of exercise-induced ventricular arrhythmia in patients undergoing evaluation for malignant ventricular arrhythmia. Am J Cardiol 1989;63:697-701.
243. Faris JV, McHenry PL, Jordan JW, Morris SN: Prevalence and reproducibility of exercise-induced ventricular arrhythmias during maximal exercise testing in normal men. Am J Cardiol 1976;37:617-622.
244. Condini M, Sommerfeldt L, Eybel C, Messer J: Clinical significance and characteristics of exercise-induced ventricular tachycardia. Cathet Cardiovasc Diagn 1981;7:227-234.
245. Milanes J, Romero M, Hultgren, et al: Exercise tests and ventricular tachycardia. West J Med 1986;145:473-476.
246. Fujiwara M, Asakuma S, Ohhira A, et al: Clinical characteristics of ventricular tachycardia and ventricular fibrillation in exercise stress testing. J Cardiol 2000;36:397-404.
247. Bunch TJ, Chandrasekaran K, Gersh BJ, et al: The prognostic significance of exercise-induced atrial arrhythmias. J Am Coll Cardiol 2004;43:1236-1240.
248. Maurer MS, Shefrin EA, Fleg JL: Prevalence and prognostic significance of exercise-induced supraventricular tachycardia in apparently healthy volunteers. Am J Cardiol 1995;75:788-792.
249. Busby MJ, Shefrin EA, Fleg JL: Prevalence and long-term significance of exercise-induced frequent or repetitive ventricular ectopic beats in apparently healthy volunteers. J Am Coll Cardiol 1989;14:1659-1665.
250. Froelicher VF, Thomas M, Pillow C, et al: An epidemiological study of asymptomatic men screened with exercise testing for latent coronary heart disease. Am J Cardiol 1974;34:770-776.
251. Froelicher VF, Thompson AJ, Longo M, et al: The value of exercise testing for screening asymptomatic men for latent CAD. Prog Cardiovasc Dis 1976;18:265-276.
252. Califf RM, McKinnis RA, McNeer M, et al: Prognostic value of ventricular arrhythmias associated with treadmill exercise testing in patients studied with cardiac catheterization for suspected ischemic heart disease. J Am Coll Cardiol 1983;2:1060-1067.
253. Partington S, Myers J, Cho S, et al: Prevalence and prognostic value of exercise-induced ventricular arrhythmias. Am Heart J 2003;145:139-146.
254. Beckerman J, Mathur A, Stahr S, et al: Exercise-induced ventricular arrhythmias and cardiovascular death. Ann Noninvasive Electrocardiol 2005;10:47-52.
255. Elhendy A, Chandrasekaran K, Gersh BJ, et al: Functional and prognostic significance of exercise-induced ventricular arrhythmias

in patients with suspected coronary artery disease. Am J Cardiol 2002;90:95-100.

256. Morshedi-Meibodi A, Evans JC, Levy D, et al: Clinical correlates and prognostic significance of exercise-induced ventricular premature beats in the community: The Framingham Heart Study. Circulation 2004;109:2417-2422. Epub 2004 May 17.

257. Frolkis JP, Pothier CE, Blackstone EH, Lauer MS: Frequent ventricular ectopy after exercise as a predictor of death. N Engl J Med 2003;348:781-790.

258. Sami M, Chaitman B, Fisher L, Holmes D, et al: Significance of exercise-induced ventricular arrhythmia in stable coronary artery disease: A coronary artery surgery study project. Am J Cardiol 1984;54:1182-1188.

259. Weiner DA, Levine SR, Klein MD, Ryan TJ: Ventricular arrhythmias during exercise testing: Mechanism, response to coronary bypass surgery and prognostic significance. Am J Cardiol 1984;53:1553-1557.

260. Nair CK, Thomson W, Aronow WS, et al: Prognostic significance of exercise-induced complex ventricular arrhythmias in coronary artery disease with normal and abnormal left ventricular ejection fraction. Am J Cardiol 1984;54:1136-1138.

261. Marieb MA, Beller GA, Gibson RS, et al: Clinical relevance of exercise-induced ventricular arrhythmias in suspected coronary artery disease. Am J Cardiol 1990;66:172-178.

262. Yang JC, Wesley RC, Froelicher VF: Ventricular tachycardia during routine treadmill testing. Risk and prognosis. Arch Int Med 1991;151:349-353.

263. Detry JM, Mengeot P, Ronsseau MF, et al: Maximal exercise testing in patients with spontaneous angina pectoris associated with transient ST segment elevation: Risks and electrocardiographic findings. Br Heart J 1975;37:897-905.

264. Tamakoshi K, Fukuda E, Tajima A, et al: Prevalence and clinical background of exercise-induced ventricular tachycardia during exercise testing. J Cardiol 2002;39:205-212.

265. Detry JM, Abouantoun S, Wyns W: Incidence and prognostic implications of severe ventricular arrhythmias during maximal exercise testing. Cardiology 1981;68(suppl 2):35-43.

266. Monserrat L, Elliott PM, Gimeno JR, et al: Non-sustained ventricular tachycardia in hypertrophic cardiomyopathy: An independent marker of sudden death risk in young patients. J Am Coll Cardiol 2003;42:873-879.

267. Petsas AA, Anastassiades LC, Antonopoulos AG: Exercise testing for assessment of the significance of ST segment depression observed during episodes of paroxysmal supraventricular tachycardia. Eur Heart J 1990;11:974-979.

268. Blackburn H and the Technical Group on Exercise ECG: The exercise electrocardiogram: differences in interpretation. Am J Cardiol 1968;21:871-880.

269. Sullivan M, Genter F, Savvides M, et al: The reproducibility of hemodynamic, electrocardiographic, and gas exchange data during treadmill exercise in patients with stable angina pectoris. Chest 1984;86:375-382.

270. Schlant RC, Friesinger GC, Leonard JL: Clinical competence in exercise testing. Circulation 1990;5:1884-1888.

271. COCATS Guidelines: Guidelines for training in adult cardiovascular medicine. Core Cardiology Training Symposium, June 27-28, 1994. American College of Cardiology [see comments]. J Am Coll Cardiol 1995;25:1-34

272. Schlant RC, Friesinger GC, Leonard JJ, Clinical competence in exercise testing. A statement for physicians from the ACP/ACC/AHA Task Force on Clinical Privileges in Cardiology. J Am Coll Cardiol 1990;16:1061-1065.

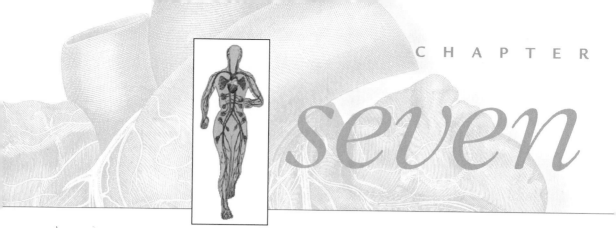

seven

Diagnostic Application of Exercise Testing

INTRODUCTION

Exercise can be considered the true test of the heart because it is the most common everyday stress that humans undertake. The exercise test is the most practical and useful procedure in the clinical evaluation of cardiovascular status. The common clinical applications of exercise testing to be discussed in this book are listed in Table 7-1. In a sense, the human genome has been selected out to perform exercise. Five applications that require extensive review: diagnostic exercise testing, prognostic exercise testing, exercise testing of patients who had a previous myocardial infarction (MI) and chronic heart failure, and screening of apparently healthy individuals will be covered in separate chapters. More specific uses, some of which will be discussed in another chapter, are listed in Table 7-2.

This chapter focuses on the most common use of the exercise test: to diagnosis coronary artery disease (CAD) in patients presenting with symptoms of ischemic CAD. The most common clinical presentation of CAD is angina pectoris and the latest guideline for evaluation of such patients still calls for the standard exercise ECG test as the first test.[1]

DIAGNOSTIC TEST PERFORMANCE DEFINITIONS

Sensitivity and specificity are the terms used to define how reliably a test distinguishes diseased from nondiseased individuals. They are parameters of the accuracy of a diagnostic test. Sensitivity is the percentage of times that a test gives an abnormal ("positive") result when those with the disease are tested. Specificity is the percentage of times that a test gives a normal ("negative") result when those without the disease are tested. This is quite different from the colloquial use of the word specific.

The eponyms SnNout and SpPin can help to remember the performance of a test with high values of either sensitivity or specificity. When a test has a very high sensitivity a Negative test rules out the diagnosis (SnNout); when a test has a very high specificity, a Positive test rules in the diagnosis (SpPin).

Two problems with determining specificity are including sufficient normal individuals and the definition of normal individuals. They should not be low-risk individuals, but instead patients without clinically meaningful angiographic disease as confirmed by catheterization. The inclusion of low–risk, normal individuals represents limited challenge, which invalidates evaluation of test performance. The decline of specificity in other forms of exercise testing may well be due to pretest and post-test reference bias.[2]

The method of calculating these terms is shown in Table 7-3.

Cutpoint or Discriminate Value

A basic step in applying any testing procedure for the separation of normal individuals from patients

TABLE 7–1.   The five most common clinical applications of exercise test

To make the diagnosis of coronary artery disease
To estimate prognosis in heart disease in general
Management of congestive heart failure patients (new)
Treatment/intervention evaluation
Exercise capacity determination

TABLE 7–2.   Additional applications of excercise test

After myocardial infarction (totally changed by current
  interventions)
Screening (to be readdressed because of recent studies)
Cardiac rehabilitation
Exercise prescription
Arrhythmia evaluation
Intermittent claudication
Preoperative evaluation

TABLE 7–3.   Definitions and calculation of the terms used to quantify the discriminatory characteristics of a test

$\text{Sensitivity} = (TP/TP + FN) \times 100$ $\text{Specificity} = (TN/FP + TN) \times 100$

where

TP = those with abnormal test and disease (true positives)
TN = those with a normal test and no disease (true negatives)
FP = those with an abnormal test but no disease (false positives)
FN = those with a normal test but disease (false negatives)

$$TP + TN + FP + FN = \text{total population}$$

+ Likelihood ratio = ratio that a positive response is likely to have disease versus a negative response:

$$\frac{\text{sensitivity}}{1 - \text{specificity}}$$

– Likelihood ratio = ratio that a negative response is not likely to have disease versus a positive response:

$$\frac{1 - \text{sensitivity}}{\text{specificity}}$$

$$P(CAD) = \text{probability of CAD} = \frac{TcP + FN}{\text{total population}}$$

$$P(\text{no CAD}) = 1 - P(\text{no CAD}) = \frac{TN + FP}{\text{total population}}$$

PV+ = percentage of those with an abnormal (positive) test result who have disease
PV– = percentage of those with a negative test that do not have disease
Predictive accuracy = percentage of correct classifications, both positive and negative
ROC = range of characteristics curve; plot of sensitivity versus specificity for the range of
    measurement cutpoints

$$\text{Predictive value of an abnormal test (PV+)} = \frac{TP}{TP + FP} \times 100$$

or

$$\text{Sensitivity} \times \frac{P(CAD) +}{\text{Sensitivity} \times P(CAD)} \ (1 - \text{Specificity})[1 - P(CAD)]$$

$$\text{Predictive accuracy} = \frac{TP + TN}{TP + TN + FP + FN} \times 100$$

or

$$[\text{Sensitivity} \times P(CAD)] + [\text{Specificity} \times [1 - P(CAD)]]$$

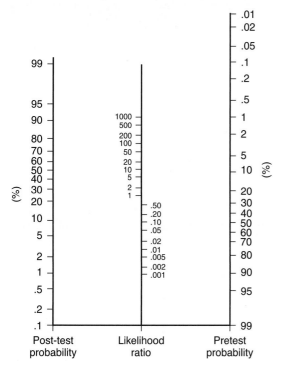

Nomogram for Bayes theorem

■ FIGURE 7–4

A simple nomogram with information presented in likehood ratios that avoids the need for calculations.

By analyzing the statements in the equations on the left side, it can be seen that they are equivalent to the numerators and denominators in the brackets on the right.

The LR is an indicator of the diagnosticity of a test; the higher it is, the greater the diagnostic impact of the test. Using conventional techniques of analyzing ST-segment depression with a cutpoint of 0.1 mV, the maximal or near-maximal exercise test has a sensitivity of approximately 50% and a specificity of 85%. Therefore, the LR for an abnormal test result equals:

$$\text{Positive likelihood ratio (+LR)} = \frac{0.50}{1 - 0.85} = 3.3$$

while for a test with a 70% sensitivity and a 90% specificity the +LR is 7, and the likelihood ratio for a normal test result equals:

$$\text{Negative likelihood ratio (-LR)} = \frac{0.85}{1 - 0.50} = 1.7$$

while for a test with a 70% sensitivity and a 90% specificity the −LR is 3.

Bayes' Theorem may be expressed in the following fashion:
Post-test odds of disease = Pretest odds of disease
× LR of the results

The clinician often makes this calculation intuitively when he suspects as a false result the abnormal exercise test of a 30-year-old woman with chest pain (low prior odds or probability). The same abnormal response would be accepted as a true result in a 60-year-old man with angina who had a previous MI (high prior odds or probability). Examples of these calculations for different test characteristics are provided in Tables 7-5 and 7-6.

Angiographic studies have been used to investigate the prevalence of significant CAD in patients with different chest pain syndromes. Because chest pain is the presenting complaint in the majority of patients referred for a diagnostic exercise test, the nature of the pain would seem a practical basis for estimating the prior probability of CAD. Approximately 90% of the middle-aged male patients in developed countries with true angina pectoris have been found to have angiographically significant coronary disease. Similarly, in patients presenting with atypical angina pectoris, approximately 50% have been found to have angiographically significant coronary disease.

and the test result really affects the outcome. The pretest probability is the basis for incorporating the test result. You can use the pretest probability from the study as a guide, especially if the patients were randomly selected from a defined group or a consecutive series and the clinical setting was similar to yours. Even then, the findings from the patient must be taken into account.

The probability of a test result being true can be shown as the *likelihood ratio*, which is the ratio of true results to false results.

In the case of an abnormal test result, the positive LR equals:
Percent with disease with abnormal test (or sensitivity)

Percent without disease with abnormal test (or 1 − specificity)

In the case of a normal test result, the negative LR equals:
Percent without disease with normal test (or specificity)

Percent with disease with normal test (or 1 − sensitivity)

TABLE 7–5. Calculation of probability for coronary artery disease in a test with 70% sensitivity and 90% specificity

Pretest odds for chest pain symptoms	Likelihood ratio normal test	Likelihood ratio abnormal test	Post-test odds	Post-test probability
Angina		×7	63 (9 × 7):1	63/64 = 98%
9:1	×3		9:3 (3 × 1)	9/12 = 75%
Atypical Angina		×7	7:1	7/8 = 88%
1:1				
	×3		1:3	1/4 = 25%
Nonanginal pain		×7	7:9	7/16 = 44%
1:9	×3		1:27 (3 × 9)	1/28 = 4%
Asymptomatic		×7	7:19	7/26 = 27%
1:19	×3		1:57 (3 × 19)	1/58 = 2%

TABLE 7–6. Calculation of probability for coronary artery disease in a test with 50% sensitivity and 85% specificity

Pretest odds for chest pain symptoms	Likelihood ratio normal test	Likelihood ratio abnormal test	Post-test odds	Post-test probability
Angina		×3.3	30 (9 × 3.3):1	30/31 = 98%
9:1	×1.7		9:1.7 (1.7 × 1)	9/10.7 = 82%
Atypical Angina		×3.3	3.3:1	3.3/4.3 = 76%
1:1				
	×1.7		1:1.7	1/2.7 = 38%
Nonanginal pain		×3.3	3.3:9	3.3/12.3 = 27%
1:9	×1.7		1:27(1.7 × 9)	1/16.3 = 6%
Asymptomatic		×3.3	3.3:19	3.3/26 = 15%
1:19	×1.7		1:32.3(1.7 × 19)	1/33.3 = 3%

Atypical angina refers to pain that has an unusual location, prolonged duration, or inconsistent precipitating factors or that is unresponsive to nitroglycerin. Table 7-7 demonstrates the estimation of the probability of CAD in such patients. Although this can be simplified for the target age range, it is probably more appropriate to consider a wider age range as illustrated in the table. As mentioned before, patients in the intermediate risk group are the most appropriate for diagnostic testing with the standard exercise ECG test or, for that matter, any of the available tests.

TABLE 7–7. Probability of coronary artery disease in middle-aged males or postmenopausal (without estrogen replacement therapy) females pre/post any noninvasive test

Chest pain character	Pretest	Postabnormal test	Postnormal test
Typical angina	90%	98%	75–80%
Atypical angina	50%	75–90%	25–40%
Non-anginal pain	10%	25–45%	4–6%
No chest pain	2%	6–15%	<1–3%

The 50-year-old male patient with typical angina pectoris has a 90% probability, or 9:1 chance, of having significant CAD. An abnormal exercise test increases these odds rather impressively but this change in odds represents a relatively small increase in the probability of disease from 90% to 98%. Because such a patient still has a high probability of disease after a negative test, coronary angiography may yet be required to definitely rule out coronary disease. The greatest diagnostic impact of such a circumstance would be in patients with atypical angina. An abnormal test result would increase the odds from 1:1 to 4:1, the probability of disease to 80%, and for practical purposes, establish the diagnosis. With a normal test, the probability of coronary disease would be reduced.

An important fact when using the Bayes theorem is that sensitivity and specificity depend on the variables that determine the pretest probability. For example, if the pretest probability is determined using knowledge of the patient's gender, then the theorem will not be completely valid if the specificity of the test depends on gender, as many investigators have found to be the case for exercise testing. Likewise, if the pretest probability is based on the character of the chest pain reported, then any dependence of specificity on this symptom will invalidate the application of the theorem. Since there is evidence that exercise test results (ST depression) are more sensitive in patients with typical angina pectoris, this would appear to invalidate the theorem's application. Actually, this problem is not as serious as one might imagine as long as the number of variables determining the pretest probability is relatively small. Caution is needed when attempting to apply the theorem to the results of tests and populations of patients that are very different from those used to determine sensitivity and specificity, as large errors in post-test probabilities can result.

DIAGNOSTIC ENDPOINTS

Symptoms, History, or Findings, Possibly Due to Coronary Artery Disease

The flow diagram (Fig. 7-5) illustrates the clinical logic for the diagnosis of CAD. Though the exercise test can be used to evaluate other disease processes, all of the available publications regarding diagnosis have addressed the issue of coronary disease. In fact, though a logical thought process can lead to performing exercise tests for diagnosing other situations, studies have only evaluated test performance in patients with chest pain.

Diagnosis of Coronary Artery Disease

To evaluate a test for a disease, one must demonstrate how well the test distinguishes between those individuals with and without the disease. Evaluation of exercise testing as a diagnostic test for CAD depends on the population tested, which must be divided into those with and without CAD by independent techniques. Coronary angiography and clinical follow-up for coronary events are two methods of separating a population into those with and without coronary disease. Surrogates for CAD, such as other test results or therapeutic interventions, are not valid ways to discriminate those with and without disease for the purpose of evaluating a diagnostic procedure. One must also be clear regarding whether the test is diagnosing ischemia or CAD. Although the contrary is rarely true, CAD can be present and not cause ischemia.

In fact, MIs or unstable angina can occur in patients with subcritical lesions because of spasm or thrombus. These lesions rarely cause death or major myocardial damage, but they are responsible for a portion of the morbidity of coronary disease. The mechanism is thought to be plaque rupture or fracturing which release thrombogenic material to the arterial surface. Neither the exercise test nor any other noninvasive tests available at this time can identify patients with subclinical atherosclerotic lesions; the tests should be able to recognize myocardial ischemia, however, due to flow-limiting lesions.

The mechanisms to explain the clinical impact of atherosclerosis has evolved over time and currently includes a classification of acute coronary syndromes. The current conceptualization has its stages defined by the status of the resting ST segments, chest pain presentation, and troponin levels. Treatment is determined by the stage and is based on the mechanism thought to be associated with it. The following figures (Figs. 7-6 to 7-8) summarize these concepts.

Limitations of Coronary Angiography

Studies comparing angiographic and pathologic findings have demonstrated that coronary angiography usually underestimate the pathologic severity of CAD. Coronary angiography can be interpreted as normal when severe CAD is present. This can be due to total cut-off of an artery at its origin, by diffuse atherosclerotic narrowing of an artery, and by failure to use axial views to visualize proximal left coronary artery lesions. Another limitation of coronary angiography involves the rare instance when coronary artery spasm is the cause of ischemia but is missed because it is transient. Coronary spasm is rare during exercise and is usually associated with ST elevation. In addition, coronary angiographic interpretation is subject to observer variability. Digital methods of quantifying coronary lesions or estimating luminal dimensions have added visual estimates of coronary occlusion and flow wires can assess the physiological significance of obstructions.

Coronary Reserve

One study using Doppler flow techniques and videodensitometric techniques showed a wide discrepancy between angiographic lesions and coronary flow reserve. To determine the accuracy of the exercise electrocardiography in detecting a physiologically significant coronary stenosis, Wilson et al[4]

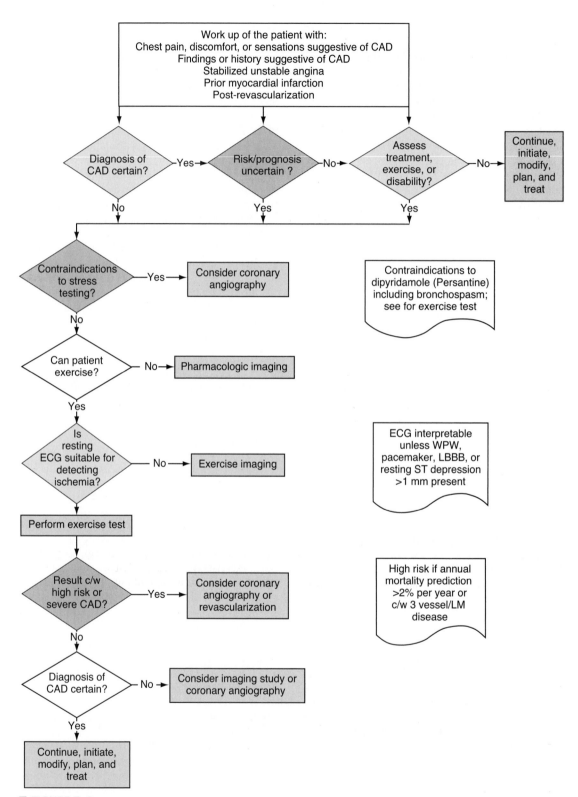

■ FIGURE 7–5

Flow diagram illustrating the clinical logic for the diagnosis of coronary artery disease (from the ACC/AHA exercise test guidelines).

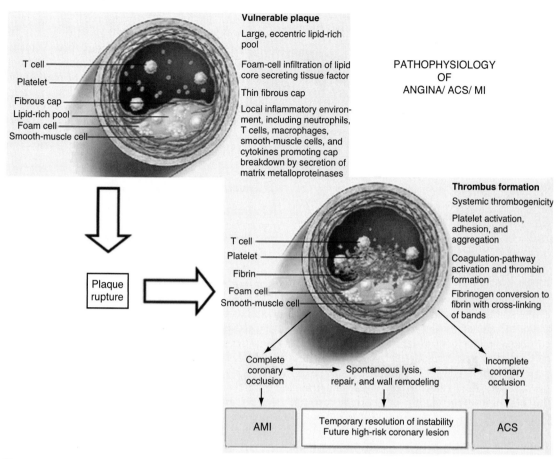

Vulnerable plaque

Large, eccentric lipid-rich pool

Foam-cell infiltration of lipid core secreting tissue factor

Thin fibrous cap

Local inflammatory environment, including neutrophils, T cells, macrophages, smooth-muscle cells, and cytokines promoting cap breakdown by secretion of matrix metalloproteinases

T cell
Platelet
Fibrous cap
Lipid-rich pool
Foam cell
Smooth-muscle cell

PATHOPHYSIOLOGY
OF
ANGINA/ ACS/ MI

Plaque rupture

T cell
Platelet
Fibrin
Foam cell
Smooth-muscle cell

Thrombus formation

Systemic thrombogenicity

Platelet activation, adhesion, and aggregation

Coagulation-pathway activation and thrombin formation

Fibrinogen conversion to fibrin with cross-linking of bands

Complete coronary occlusion

Spontaneous lysis, repair, and wall remodeling

Incomplete coronary occlusion

AMI

Temporary resolution of instability
Future high-risk coronary lesion

ACS

■ **FIGURE 7–6**
Pathophysiology of angina, acute coronary syndrome (ACS), and myocardial infarction (MI).

studied 40 patients with one-vessel, one-lesion CAD, a normal resting ECG, and no hypertrophy or prior infarction. Each patient underwent exercise electrocardiography that was interpreted as abnormal if the ST segment developed 0.1-mV or greater depression. The physiologic significance of each coronary stenosis was assessed by measuring of coronary flow reserve (peak divided by resting blood flow velocity) in the stenotic artery using a Doppler catheter and intracoronary papaverine. The percent diameter and percent area stenosis produced by each lesion were determined using quantitative angiography. Of the 17 patients with reduced coronary flow reserve in the stenotic artery, 14 had an abnormal exercise ECG (sensitivity of 82%). Conversely, 20 of 23 patients with normal coronary flow reserves had normal exercise tests (specificity of 87%). The exercise ECG was abnormal in each of 11 patients with markedly reduced coronary flow reserve and in three of

six patients with moderately reduced reserve. The products of systolic blood pressure and heart rate at peak exercise were significantly correlated with coronary reserve in patients with truly abnormal exercise tests. In comparison, the sensitivity (61%) and specificity (73%) of exercise electrocardiography in detecting a 60% or greater diameter stenosis was significantly lower. Exercise electrocardiography, therefore, was a good predictor of the physiologic significance (assessed by coronary flow reserve) of a coronary stenosis but less so for angiographically classified disease. This seminal study was validated by the following large, multicenter European study.

A total of 225 patients with one-vessel disease were studied before percutaneous transluminal coronary angioplasty and at 6 months follow-up.[5] Exercise electrocardiography was performed to document presence ($n = 157$) or absence ($n = 138$) of an ST-segment shift (≥ 0.1 mV). Intracoronary

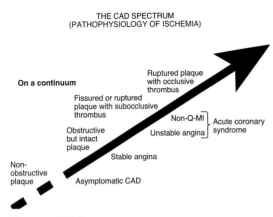

THE CAD SPECTRUM
(PATHOPHYSIOLOGY OF ISCHEMIA)

Ruptured plaque
with occlusive
thrombus

On a continuum

Fissured or ruptured
plaque with subocclusive
thrombus

Non-Q-MI ⎤ Acute coronary
Unstable angina ⎦ syndrome

Obstructive
but intact
plaque

Stable angina

Non-
obstructive
plaque

Asymptomatic CAD

■ **FIGURE 7–7**
The coronary artery disease spectrum (pathophysiology of ischemia).

blood flow velocity analysis was performed to determine the proximal/distal flow velocity ratio, the distal diastolic/systolic flow velocity ratio and coronary flow velocity reserve. ROC curves were calculated to assess the predictive value of these variables compared with the exercise test. The distal coronary flow velocity reserve demonstrated the best linear correlation for both percentage diameter stenosis and minimum lumen diameter ($r = 0.67$ and $r = 0.66$), compared to the diastolic/systolic flow velocity ratio ($r = 0.19$ and $r = 0.14$) and the proximal/distal flow velocity ratio (not significant). The areas under the curve were roughly 0.83 for diameter stenosis, minimum lumen diameter, and coronary flow velocity reserve. Logistic regression analysis revealed that the percentage diameter stenosis or minimum lumen diameter

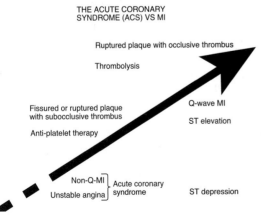

THE ACUTE CORONARY
SYNDROME (ACS) VS MI

Ruptured plaque with occlusive thrombus

Thrombolysis

Fissured or ruptured plaque
with subocclusive thrombus

Q-wave MI

ST elevation

Anti-platelet therapy

Non-Q-MI ⎤ Acute coronary
Unstable angina ⎦ syndrome

ST depression

■ **FIGURE 7–8**
The acute coronary syndrome compared to myocardial infarction.

and coronary flow velocity reserve were independent predictors for the result of ECG testing. It appeared that the distal coronary flow velocity reserve was the best intracoronary Doppler parameter for evaluation of coronary narrowing. Angiographic estimates of coronary lesion severity and distal coronary flow velocity reserve were both good, but surprisingly independent, predictors for the assessment of functional severity of coronary stenosis.

Coronary Collateral Vessels

The influence of coronary collateral circulation on exercise test results was studied by Pellinen et al[6] in a random sample of 286 patients with angiographically documented CAD. Collateral vessels increased in all three main coronary arteries in proportion to the grade of luminal obstruction. The highest prevalence of collaterals occurred in stenosis of the right coronary artery (60%), followed by the left descending artery (45%); they occurred least in the left circumflex artery (21%). The frequency of intra-arterial collateral circulation was 42%, 11%, and 12%, respectively. In triple-vessel disease, exercise capacity was greater when collateral arteries to the left anterior descending were not jeopardized than when jeopardized. Collateral vessels had no obvious influence on exercise-induced ST depression.

Limitations of Other End Points

There are some important limitations of using clinical events and pathologic endpoints to separate CAD patients and disease-free groups. Coronary disease events and symptoms can be due to relatively minor lesions. Hemorrhage into nonobstructive plaques or thrombosis due to unstable plaques can cause symptoms or even death. Spasm has been demonstrated to occur proximal to relatively minor lesions. Pathologic studies have shown that approximately 7% of people dying from a clinically diagnosed MI have insignificant or no coronary atheroma. Coronary angiographic studies have shown that some patients with classic angina pectoris and MI can have normal coronary angiograms. In spite of these limitations, coronary angiography and the observation of clinical symptoms or coronary events are at present the most practical endpoints that distinguish between those with and without CAD. Surrogates for CAD, such as other test results or therapeutic interventions, are not valid ways to discriminate those with and without disease for the purpose of evaluating a diagnostic procedure. In addition, it must be declared whether the test is diagnosing ischemia or CAD. Though ischemia is usually in proportion to angiographic coronary disease, they are not equivalent, as demonstrated by the coronary flow studies. Clearly, exercise-induced ST changes are associated with ischemia rather than being an indicator of coronary anatomy.

ECG TEST CRITERIA

The standard criterion for an abnormal ECG response is horizontal or downward sloping ST-segment depression of 0.1 mV or more for 80 msec. It appears to be due to generalized subendocardial ischemia. A "steal" phenomenon is likely from ischemic areas because of the effect of extensive collateralization in the subendocardium. ST depression does not localize the area of ischemia, as does ST elevation or help to indicate which coronary artery is occluded. The normal ST-segment vector response to tachycardia, and to exercise, is a shift rightward and upward. The degree of this shift appears to have a fair amount of biologic variation. Most normal individuals will have early repolarization at rest, which will shift to the isoelectric PR-segment line in the inferior, lateral, and anterior leads with exercise. This shift can be further influenced by ischemia and myocardial scars. When the later portions of the ST segment are affected, flattening or downward depression can be recorded. Both local effects and the direction of the spatial changes during repolarization cause the ST segment to have a different appearance at the many surface sites that can be monitored. The more leads with these apparent ischemic shifts, the more severe the disease.

The probability and severity of CAD are directly related to the amount of J-junction depression and are inversely related to the slope of the ST segment. Downsloping ST-segment depression is more serious than is horizontal depression, and both are more serious than upsloping depression. However, patients with upsloping ST-segment depression, especially when the slope is less than 1 mV/sec, probably are at increased risk. If a slowly ascending slope is utilized as a criterion for abnormal, the specificity of exercise testing will be decreased (more false positives), although the test may become more sensitive. One electrode can show upsloping ST depression, while an adjacent electrode shows horizontal or downsloping depression.

If an apparently borderline ST segment with an inadequate slope is recorded in a single precordial lead in a patient highly suspected of having CAD, multiple precordial leads should be scanned before the exercise test is called normal. An upsloping depressed ST segment may be the precursor to abnormal ST-segment depression in the recovery period or at higher heart rates during greater work loads.

ST-Segment Interpretation Issues

Leads in Which ST Depression Occurs

Blackburn and Katigbak[7] studied 100 consecutive patients and found that lead V_5 alone detected 89% of ischemic ST-segment responses. Miller et al[8] evaluated 44 consecutive patients who had both abnormal exercise tests and perfusion defects. Thirty patients (68%) had ST-segment changes in the inferior leads, but all of these patients had concomitant ST-segment changes in leads V_4 and/or V_5 as well, leading to the conclusion that monitoring of the inferior leads rarely provides additional diagnostic information. Mason et al[9] found that in 67 patients with angina who underwent exercise testing, 19 of them showed an abnormal ECG response in one lead only (a total of seven leads were monitored) and of these only two were isolated to lead II alone. Sketch et al[10] studied 203 men with both exercise testing and coronary angiography and found that lead II had a sensitivity of only 34%. In evaluating body surface potential distributions in 50 subjects with normal baseline ECGs, of which 25 had documented CAD, Simoons and Block[11] concluded that a single bipolar V_5 lead was adequate to diagnose ischemia in patients without a prior MI and a normal ECG at rest. Miranda et al[12] found exercise-induced ST-segment depression in inferior limb leads to be a poor marker for CAD in and of itself. Precordial lead V_5 alone consistently outperformed the inferior lead, and the combination of leads V_5 with II, because lead II had such a high false-positive rate. Miranda et al[12] had seven patients manifest ST-segment depression in lead II only, without concomitant changes in lead V_5, and only three of these responses were true positives. A Finnish group compared the diagnostic characteristics of the individual exercise ECG leads.[13] The lead system used was the Mason-Likar modification of the standard 12-lead system, and exercise tests were performed on a bicycle ergometer. Leads I, $-aV_R$, V_4, V_5, and V_6 had the greatest diagnostic value.

These studies are all supportive of the concept that exercise-induced ST-segment depression in lead V_5 is an excellent marker for coronary disease and that any inferior lead provides little additional diagnostic information. This is consistent with the fact that ST depression is a global subendocardial phenomenon that is directed down the long axis of the ventricle towards V_5. The vector can be shifted if there is inferior or posterior infarction resulting in inferior or anterior lead depression.

Riff and Carleton[14] studied patients in atrioventricular dissociation and demonstrated that atrial repolarization can cause J-point depression in the inferior leads, and this may produce the false-positive responses. It should be remembered that even though the inferior lead ST-segment depression is not a reliable, independent marker for the diagnosis of CAD, it is helpful in diagnosing severe ischemia, as multiple lead involvement has been associated with multivessel[15] and left main CAD.[16] However, concomitant exercise-induced inferior lead ST-segment depression may be an indicator of multivessel ischemia, but it does not localize right coronary involvement.[17] In patients without prior MI and with normal resting ECG, precordial lead V_5 alone is a reliable marker for CAD, and the monitoring of inferior limb leads adds little additional diagnostic information. Exercise-induced ST-segment depression confined to the inferior leads is of little value for the identification of coronary disease.

Upsloping ST Depression

Downsloping ST-segment depression is more serious than is horizontal depression, and both are more serious than upsloping depression. However, patients with upsloping ST-segment depression, especially when the slope is less than 1 mV/sec, have an increased probability of coronary disease. If a slowly ascending slope is utilized as a criterion for abnormal, the specificity of exercise testing will be decreased (more false positives), although the test becomes more sensitive. One electrode can show upsloping ST-depression while an adjacent electrode shows horizontal or downsloping depression.

ST Elevation

Early repolarization is a common resting pattern of ST elevation that occurs in normal individuals. Exercise induced ST segment elevation is always considered from the baseline ST level. ST elevation is relatively common after a Q wave infarction but ST elevation in leads without Q waves only occurs in one out of a thousand patients seen in a typical exercise lab.[17-23] ST elevation on a normal ECG (other than in AV_R or V_1) represents transmural ischemia (caused by spasm or a critical lesion), is very rare (0.1% in a clinical lab) and in contrast to ST depression, elevation is very arrhythmogenic and localizes the ischemia. When it occurs in V_2 to V_4 the left anterior descending is involved, in the lateral leads the left circumflex and diagonals are involved, and in II, III, and aV_F the right coronary artery is involved. This phenomenon appears to be 100% specific but is not very sensitive. When the resting ECG shows Q waves of an old MI, ST elevation is due to wall motion abnormalities and a large area of infarction, whereas accompanying ST depression can be due to a second area of ischemia or reciprocal changes.

R-Wave Changes

Multitudes of factors affect the R-wave amplitude response to exercise[24] and the response does not have diagnostic significance.[25,26] R-wave amplitude typically increases from rest to submaximal exercise, perhaps to a heart rate of 130 beats per minute, then decreases to a minimum at maximal exercise.[27] If objective or subjective symptoms or signs limited a patient, the R-wave amplitude would increase from rest to such an endpoint. Such patients may be demonstrating a normal R-wave response but can be classified "abnormal" because of a submaximal effort. Exercise-induced changes in R-wave amplitude have no independent predictive power but are associated with CAD because such patients are often tested only to a submaximal level and an R wave decrease normally occurs at maximal exercise. Adjusting the amount of ST-segment depression by the R-wave height showed no improvement in the diagnostic value of exercise-induced ST depression.

ST-Segment Depression Late into Recovery

Although previous studies have not specifically evaluated patients with resting ST-segment depression with the criterion of ST-segment depression late into recovery, data have been presented supporting a correlation between prolonged ST-segment depression during recovery and severe CAD. Goldschlager et al[28] noted that patients with rapid normalization of their ST-segments during recovery had a 58% prevalence of two- or three-vessel CAD, and that patients who had ischemic changes persisting 8 minutes or more into recovery had a 67% prevalence of three-vessel or left main disease. Callaham and co-workers studied 290 patients and noted that prolonged ST-segment depression during recovery was a highly specific marker for proximal left anterior descending, multivessel, and left main coronary disease.[29]

Downsloping ST-Segment Depression During Recovery

Goldschlager et al[28] studied 330 patients with both exercise testing and coronary angiography and found seventy-six patients to have a non-upsloping ST-segment depression confined to the recovery period. Of these 76 patients, 47 (62%) developed downsloping depression during recovery, and only one of these patients was a false-positive finding.

INFLUENCE OF OTHER FACTORS ON TEST PERFORMANCE

Medications

Drugs and resting ECG abnormalities can affect the results of exercise testing. The meta-analysis and the previously mentioned study addressed these issues, but other studies will also be discussed here.

Digoxin

A study by Meyers et al[30] demonstrated a decreased diagnostic accuracy of exercise testing in patients on digoxin. This is in agreement with observations made by Tonkon et al,[31] who studied 15 normal subjects who underwent exercise testing before and after the administration of digoxin[31] Fourteen subjects developed 0.1 to 0.5 mm of ST-segment depression with exercise, but the ST segments normalized at maximal stress and remained normal throughout recovery. Sketch et al[32] studied 98 healthy males, aged 22 to 70 years, who were administered digoxin at 0.25 mg per day for 14 days and then underwent daily exercise testing until it was interpreted as normal. Twenty-four subjects had an abnormal ST-response to exercise, and in 20 of them the ST-segment depression resolved less than 4 minutes into recovery. Sundqvist et al[33] studied 11 healthy people on digoxin with a mean age of 28 years with bicycle ergometry. Six subjects developed ST-segment depression that resolved quickly upon cessation of exercise and was not present in the first 2 minutes of recovery. Some subjects, though, apparently redeveloped ST-segment depression later in recovery, and this was different from the typical ischemic response.

Digoxin has been shown to produce abnormal ST depression in response to exercise in from 25% to 40% of apparently healthy individuals.[34] The prevalence of abnormal responses is directly related to age, and there is some evidence to believe that digoxin can uncover subclinical coronary disease. The meta-analysis shows that the diagnostic characteristics of the exercise ECG are not affected sufficiently enough to negate the exercise test as the first test in the patient receiving digoxin and with possible coronary disease. Although patients must be off the medication for at least 2 weeks for its effect to be gone, it is not necessary to do so prior to diagnostic testing.[33] The reason for which digoxin is administered can affect test interpretation. However, the most common response to testing is a negative response, and this still has an important impact because sensitivity is not altered by digoxin.

Beta Blockers

Herbert et al[35] have demonstrated how the ST-segment response and diagnostic testing are affected by beta-blocker therapy. In their sample of 200 middle-aged men referred for exercise testing to evaluate possible or definite CAD, no differences were found in test performance with the use of classical ST criteria or the ST/HR index. In spite of the marked effect of beta-blockers on maximal exercise heart rate, with patients subgrouped according to beta-blocker administration as initiated by their referring physician, no differences in test performance were found. Therefore, for routine exercise testing in the clinical setting it appears unnecessary for physicians to accept the risk of stopping beta-blockers before testing when a patient is showing possible symptoms of ischemia.

Exercise test results are often considered "inadequate" or "nondiagnostic" in patients taking beta-blockers, and in patients who do not achieve 85% of their age-predicted maximal heart rate. Therefore, we assessed the diagnostic characteristics of the exercise test in patients who fail to reach conventional target heart rates and in patients on beta-blockers.[36] The results of exercise tests and coronary angiography performed to evaluate chest pain in 1282 male patients without a prior history of MI, coronary revascularization, diagnostic Q wave on the baseline ECG, or previous cardiac catheterization were analyzed with respect to beta-blocker exposure and failure to reach 85%

age-predicted maximal heart rate. Sensitivity, specificity, and predictive accuracy of exercise testing, as well as area under the curve (AUC) for the receiver operating characteristic (ROC) plots were calculated for these subgroups with use of coronary angiography as the reference. The angiographic criterion for significant CAD was 50% narrowing or more in one or more major coronary arteries. The population was divided into four exclusive groups on the basis of whether they reached their target heart rates and whether they were receiving beta-blockers. Forty percent to 60% of this clinical population failed to reach target heart rate, of which 24% ($n = 303$) were receiving beta-blockers and 40% ($n = 518$) were not. The group of patients who reached target heart rate and were not taking beta-blockers was taken as the reference group ($n = 409$). The group of patients who were supposedly beta-blocked, but who reached the target heart rate ($n = 52$), had hemodynamic and test characteristics similar to those of the reference group and most likely were not taking their beta-blockers or were not adequately dosed. The prevalence of angiographic coronary disease was significantly higher in the two groups failing to reach target heart rate, both in the presence and absence of beta-blockers, compared with the reference group (68% and 64%, respectively, versus 49%). Although the areas under the curve of the ROC curves for ST depression of the groups failing to reach target heart rate were not significantly different from the reference group, the predictive accuracy and sensitivity were significantly lower for 1 mm of ST depression in the beta-blocked group who did not reach target heart rate (predictive accuracy of 56% versus 67%, sensitivity of 44% versus 58%). *The only way to maintain sensitivity with the standard exercise test in the beta-blocker group, who failed to reach target heart rate, was to use a treadmill score or 0.5-mm ST depression as the criterion for abnormal.* Thus, we found the sensitivity and predictive accuracy of standard ST criteria for exercise-induced ST depression significantly decreased in male patients taking beta-blockers and do not reach target heart rate. In those who fail to reach target heart rate and are not beta-blocked, sensitivity and predictive accuracy were maintained.

Other Medications

Various medications can affect test performance by altering the hemodynamic response of blood pressure, including antihypertensives and vasodilators. Acute administration of nitrates can attenuate the angina and ST depression associated with myocardial ischemia. Flecainide has been associated with exercise-induced ventricular tachycardia.[37,38] Anecdotal reports of the effects of other medications are unsubstantiated.

Effect of Baseline ECG Abnormalities

Left Bundle Branch Block

Exercise-induced ST depression usually occurs with left bundle branch block (LBBB) and has no association with ischemia.[39] Exercise-induced ST depression of even up to 1 cm can occur in healthy normal subjects. Ellestad's group studied ECG changes during exercise in 41 patients with LBBB.[40] Seven were nonischemic and 34 had coronary artery obstruction. ST depression equaling 0.5 mm or more from baseline, when measured at the J point in leads II and AV_F (p = 0.004), and an increase of R-wave amplitude in lead II (p = 0.05) significantly identified ischemia. A German group published a case report and review of the literature. They performed perfusion scans three times in a 55-year-old woman with LBBB who was free of angiographic evidence of left anterior descending disease.[41] The first scan was performed with technitium Tc-99m sestamibi after submaximal bicycle exercise and revealed a septal perfusion deficit as has previously been reported. This deficit could not be reproduced in the following examinations after pharmacological stress testing with dipyridamole using both thallous Tl-201 and chloride technicium Tc-99m sestamibi. Perfusion at rest assessed with thallous chloride Tl-201 was normal in all studies. They concluded that pharmacologic stress testing with dipyridamole is preferable in patients with LBBB because septal defects are common with exercise.

Exercise-Induced Left Bundle Branch Block

From their exercise testing experience at Mayo Clinic, Grady et al[42] estimated a 0.5% prevalence of the development of transient LBBB during exercise. They performed a matched control cohort study to determine whether exercise-induced LBBB is an independent predictor of mortality and cardiac morbidity. Seventy cases of exercise-induced LBBB were identified and matched with 70 controls based on age, test date, sex, prior history of CAD, hypertension, diabetes, smoking, and beta-blocker use. A total of 37 events (28 events from the exercise-induced LBBB cases and nine from the control cohort) occurred in 25 patients (17 exercise-induced LBBB patients and eight control patients) during a mean follow-up period of 3.7 years. There were seven deaths, of which five occurred among patients with exercise-induced LBBB. Exercise-induced LBBB independently was associated with a three times higher risk of death and major cardiac events. They did not reproduce the finding from the Krannert Institute that suggested CAD was more likely if the LBBB occurred below a heart rate of 125 beats per minute.

A review of the English and French language literature regarding intermittent exercise-induced LBBB published from January 1985 to January 1996 was carried out.[43] Exercise-induced LBBB was reported in association with and without structural heart disease. Pooled mortality in the group with structural heart disease was 2.7% per year and 0.2% per year when no structural heart disease was identified. Noninvasive testing appears to have limited ability to detect or exclude CAD in this group.

Right Bundle Branch Block

Exercise-induced ST depression usually occurs with right bundle branch block in the anterior chest leads (V_1 to V_3) and has no association with ischemia.[44] However, when ST depression occurs in the left chest leads (V_5,V_6) or inferior (II, AV_F) leads, it has test characteristics similar to those of a normal resting ECG.

Left Ventricular Hypertrophy with Strain

This ECG abnormality is associated with a decreased specificity of exercise testing but the sensitivity is unaffected or increased. Therefore, a standard exercise ECG test could be the first test, with referrals for other tests indicated only in those patients with an abnormal result.

Resting ST Depression

Resting ST-segment depression has been identified as a marker for adverse cardiac events in patients with and without known CAD.[45-49] Miranda et al[50] performed a retrospective study of 223 patients without clinical or ECG evidence of prior MI. Excluded were women, patients with resting ECGs showing LBBB or left ventricular hypertrophy (LVH) and those on digoxin or with valvular or congenital heart disease. Ten percent of patients had persistent resting ST-segment depression and nearly twice the prevalence of severe coronary disease

(30%) than those without resting ST-segment depression (16%). The criterion of 2 mm of additional exercise-induced ST-segment depression or downsloping depression of 1 mm or more in recovery was a particularly useful marker for the diagnosis of any coronary disease (likelihood ratio 3.4, sensitivity 67% and specificity 80%).

One Additional Millimeter Depression with Baseline ST Depression

Kansal et al[51] evaluated 37 patients with chest pain and resting ST-segment depression of 0.5 mm or more (not due to LVH or drugs) with exercise testing and coronary angiography; patients with Q waves were not excluded. An additional 1 mm of ST-segment depression during exercise was found to be 92% sensitive and 75% specific for the diagnosis of at least one significant coronary artery obstruction. Harris et al[52] studied 80 patients with at least 0.5 millimeters of resting horizontal ST-segment depression and/or T-wave inversion with exercise testing and coronary angiography. Patients with diagnostic Q waves, conduction defects, LVH, and those on digoxin were excluded. They found a sensitivity of 75% for an additional 1 mm of ST-segment depression for the diagnosis of CAD, but the specificity was only 53%. Other studies have found decreased sensitivity and specificity in patients with resting ST-segment depression.[30,53] However, these studies included bundle branch blocks, previous infarction, "nonspecific" ST-T changes, such as T-wave inversions and/or flattening, and they did not isolate LVH and resting ST-segment depression groups.

The three studies that considered isolated resting ST depression and the meta-analysis support the conclusion that additional exercise-induced ST-segment depression in the patient with resting ST-segment depression represents a sensitive indicator of CAD. The meta-analysis was reprocessed considering the status of digoxin, resting ST depression and LVH as exclusion criteria in the 58 studies that excluded patients with an MI. Only those that included at least 100 patients and provided patient numbers, as well as both sensitivity and specificity, were considered in the average. Those studies with less than 100 patients were averaged together as "other" studies. Although the specificity is lowered in certain groups, the sensitivity is unaffected so the standard exercise test is still the first test option. If the standard exercise test is negative, CAD is unlikely, but if an abnormal response is obtained then further testing is indicated. Resting ST-segment depression is a marker for a higher prevalence and severity of CAD and is associated with a poor prognosis; standard exercise testing continues to be diagnostically useful in these patients. The published data appear to contain few patients with major resting ST depression (>1 mm); thus exercise testing is unlikely to provide important diagnostic information in such patients, and exercise-imaging modalities are preferred for them.

Clinical Factors

Gender

There has been controversy regarding the use of the standard exercise ECG test in women. In fact, some experts have recommended that only imaging techniques be used for testing women because of the impression that the standard exercise ECG did not perform as well in them as it did in men. The recent ACC/AHA guidelines reviewed this subject in detail and came to another conclusion, which was based on evidence obtained from meta-analysis, focusing on 15 studies that considered only women. These latter studies are based on the standard exercise test, with the gold standard being coronary angiography.

The recent guidelines have definitely stated that exercise testing for the diagnosis of significant obstructive coronary disease in adult patients, including women, with symptoms or other clinical findings suggestive of CAD is a class I indication (i.e., definitely indicated). The statement reads that adult male or female patients with an intermediate pretest probability of coronary disease (the intermediate probability based on gender, age, and chest pain symptoms) is a definite indication for the standard exercise test. Women in intermediate classification are those who are 30 to 59 years of age with typical or definite angina pectoris, those who are 30 to 69 years of age with atypical or probable angina pectoris, and those who are 60 to 68 years of age with nonanginal chest pain (see Table 7-13).

Numerous studies have now shown that equations or scores based on multivariable statistical analysis enable prediction of prognosis and improve the diagnostic characteristics of the exercise test. Equations, which consider hemodynamic and clinical variables, enable a better diagnosis of CAD in both men and women. Studies have shown that if estrogen status is considered, the diagnostic characteristics can be very much improved in women. In general, what this means is that women who

are premenstrual or are receiving estrogen can obtain the same result from these equations if the exercise ST response is not considered. The Duke Treadmill score has been validated in both genders as well.

Pretest Selection in Women. There is some concern that ischemic symptoms are gender-specific. Although typical angina is as meaningful in women over 60 as in men, the clinical diagnosis of coronary disease in women may be more difficult. For instance, in the CASS study, 50% of women with angina who were less than 65 years of age had normal coronary angiograms as compared to 10% of men. There are interesting test selection biases that are operative in women as well. Women undergo fewer tests and procedures than men do, and they are usually performed later in the course of their disease. This pattern has been studied for exercise testing in Olmstead County, Minn, and has been documented specifically for this form of testing as well.[54] In addition, there are gender-specific differences in the standard exercise test. From the Bayesian standpoint, the low prevalence of CAD in women presents a difficult situation for noninvasive testing unless pretest probability is considered. Gender-specific ST responses are operating since adolescent girls have a higher rate of abnormal ST responses than do boys.[55] This is not just due to estrogen, since estrogen did not increase the rate of abnormal exercise tests in men. It has been hypothesized that estrogen functions similar to digoxin, since it has a comparable chemical structure. In addition, the exercise hemodynamic responses are gender-specific, with women usually having lower maximal heart rates and ventilatory oxygen consumption.

At Cleveland Clinic, post-test sex differences were examined in diagnostic evaluation after exercise testing according to a broader endpoint than just coronary angiography alone.[56] The design was a cohort analytic study with a 90-day follow-up. Patients included consecutive adults (1023 men and 579 women) with chest pain but no documented coronary disease who were referred for symptom-limited treadmill testing without adjunctive imaging; none had undergone prior invasive cardiac procedures. Main outcome measures included (1) performance of any subsequent diagnostic study (invasive or noninvasive) and (2) performance of coronary angiography as the next diagnostic study. During follow-up, 89 (8.7%) men and 48 (8.3%) women underwent a second diagnostic study (odds ratio [OR] of 1), whereas

64 (6.3%) men and 21 (3.6%) women went straight to coronary angiography (OR 0.56; $P = 0.02$). In multivariable logistic regression analyses, which considered baseline clinical characteristics, the ST-segment response, and other prognostically important exercise responses, women tended to be less likely than men to be referred to any second test (adjusted OR 0.70) and were markedly and significantly less likely to be referred straight to coronary angiography. After exercise treadmill testing, women were only slightly less likely than men to be referred for subsequent diagnostic testing; they were, however, much less likely to be referred straight to coronary angiography as opposed to another noninvasive study.

One can argue that the standard exercise is perfectly suited for the women that should be tested. Because sensitivity and specificity are affected by referral bias, the studies with the higher prevalence of abnormal test responses are not representative of the real world and should not be used to assess the accuracy of the test in women (or men for that matter). For women, the important test characteristic is specificity, not sensitivity. In women with a low probability of disease, the high specificity guarantees a high rate of true negative responses and the low prevalence guarantees a small number of false negatives (despite the low sensitivity). This means that the negative predictive value (TN/TN + FN) is high for women with a low pretest probability. Although the positive predictive value for women with a low pretest probability is poor, the frequency of abnormal exercise tests in low probability women is low (10% to 15% in the unbiased group). In addition, the actual unbiased prevalence of CAD in low-probability women is lower (5% to 7% estimated by algorithm) than from biased data (15%). Therefore, given a specificity of 85% to 90%, a pretest probability of 5% to 7%, and an abnormal test prevalence of 10% to 15%, the predictive value of a negative test in an unbiased group of low pretest probability women is in the 90% range.

Summary of the Guidelines Regarding Women

The summary from the guidelines are well stated: concern about false-positive ST responses may be addressed by careful assessment of post-test probability and selective use of stress imaging test before proceeding to angiography. Although the optimal strategy for circumventing false-positive test results for the diagnosis of coronary disease in women remains to be defined, there is currently insufficient data to justify routine stress imaging test as the initial test in coronary disease in women.

Diabetics

Lee et al[57] performed a retrospective analysis of standard exercise test results in 1282 male patients without prior MI, who had undergone coronary angiography and were being evaluated for possible CAD at two Veterans Administration institutions. In patients with diabetes, 38% had an abnormal exercise test result, and the prevalence of angiographic CAD was 69%; the sensitivity of the exercise test was 47%, and specificity was 81%. In patients without diabetes, 38% had an abnormal exercise test result, and the prevalence of angiographic CAD was 58%; the sensitivity of the exercise test was 52%, and specificity was 80%. The ROC curves were also similar in both diabetic and nondiabetic patients (0.67 and 0.68, respectively). In both groups, nearly half of the abnormal ST responses occurred without angina (i.e., silent ischemia). These data demonstrate that the standard exercise test has similar diagnostic characteristics in diabetic as in nondiabetic patients.

Elderly

In our lab, Lai et al[58] considered both death and angiographic endpoints in the elderly. In the angiographic subset (elderly, $n = 405$; younger, $n = 809$), the prevalence of angiographic disease was significantly higher in the elderly (72% versus 53%). Patients with CAD in both age groups had a significantly higher prevalence of hypercholesterolemia, typical angina, and abnormal exercise tests. They were also significantly older than patients without CAD. Elderly patients with CAD were more likely to have hypertension. Patients below the age of 65 with CAD had about 1.7 MET lower exercise capacity than those without CAD. Of those below 65 years of age, 33% had abnormal exercise tests, and in those above 65, 49% had abnormal exercise tests compared to 21% and 33%, respectively, in the total population, consistent with work-up bias (i.e., angiograms were more likely in those with abnormal studies).

There were no significant differences in test characteristics for the standard criterion of 1 mm of ST depression (predictive accuracy of 59% for the elderly and 65% for the younger group, sensitivity of 55% for the elderly and 47% for the younger group). The AUC of the ROC curves for ST depression, the Duke Treadmill Score (DTS), and a previously validated diagnostic score (Veterans affairs/University of West Virginia angiographic score, VA/UWV) were compared. The z-score was calculated to compare the ability to discriminate between the age groups and then for the scores compared to the ST measurements alone. For the younger group, the AUC of the ROC plot for the ST response alone, DTS and VA/UWV score were 0.67, 0.72, and 0.79, respectively. For the elderly population, the AUC of the ROC plot for the ST response alone, DTS and VA/UWV score were 0.66, 0.72, and 0.75, respectively. These were not significantly different between the age groups. In those less than 65 years of age, AUC for VA/UWV score was significantly greater than the ST response alone and DTS, but both scores were significantly better than the ST measurements alone. For the elderly, only the AUC for VA/UWV score was significantly greater than that of ST response alone.

Major Depressive Disorder (MDD)

Since many key symptoms of major depressive disorder (MDD), such as reduced interest in daily activities, lack of energy, and fatigue, affect exercise performance and the detection of ischemia in patients with MDD, Lavoie et al performed the following study.[59] They screened 1367 consecutive patients referred for exercise testing with a questionnaire assessing depression. A total of 183 patients (13%) met diagnostic criteria for MDD. Patients with MDD achieved a significantly lower maximal heart rate, less METs, and spent less time exercising compared with patients without depression. There were no differences in rates of SPECT ischemia in patients with (40%) versus patients without MDD; however, rates of ECG ischemia were significantly lower (30%) in patients with than in patients without MDD (48%).

CLINICAL META-ANALYSIS OF EXERCISE TESTING STUDIES

Focusing on the clinical and test methodological issues, Gianrossi et al[60] investigated the variability of the reported diagnostic accuracy of the exercise ECG by applying meta-analysis. One hundred forty-seven consecutively published reports, involving 24,074 patients who underwent both coronary angiography and exercise testing, were summarized and the results entered into a computer spreadsheet. Details regarding population characteristics and methods were entered including publication year, number of ECG leads, exercise protocol, pre-exercise hyperventilation, definition of an abnormal ST response, exclusion of certain subgroups, and blinding of test interpretation. Wide variability in sensitivity and specificity was found (the mean sensitivity was 68% with a range of 23% to 100% and a standard deviation of 16%; the mean specificity was 77% with a range of 17% to 100% and a standard deviation 17%). The median predictive accuracy (percentage of total true calls) was approximately 73%.

Sensitivity was found to be significantly and independently related to four study characteristics:

1. The method of dealing with equivocal or nondiagnostic tests: sensitivity decreased when "nondiagnostic" tests were considered normal.
2. Comparison with a "better" test (i.e., nuclear perfusion or echocardiography): the sensitivity of the exercise ECG was lower when the study compared it with another testing method being reported as "superior."
3. Exclusion of patients on digitalis: exclusion of patients taking digitalis was associated with a greater sensitivity.
4. Publication year: an increase in sensitivity and decrease in specificity were noted over the years the exercise test was gathered (more work-up bias). This may be due to the fact that as clinicians become more familiar with a test and increasingly trust its results, they allow its results to influence the decision to perform angiography. However, since the 1980s there has been a reversal with less work-up bias probably due to the effect of percutaneous transluminal coronary angioplasty (i.e., more patients undergo catheterization).

Specificity was found to be significantly and independently related to four variables:

1. Treatment of upsloping ST depression: when upsloping ST depression was classified as abnormal, specificity was lowered significantly, (73% versus 80%).
2. Exclusion/inclusion of subjects with prior infarction: the exclusion of patients with prior MI was associated with a decreased specificity.
3. Exclusion/inclusion of patients with LBBB: the specificity increased when patients with LBBB were excluded.

4. Pre-exercise hyperventilation: the use of pre-exercise hyperventilation was associated with a decreased specificity.

Stepwise linear regression explained less than 35% of the variance in sensitivities and specificities reported in the 147 publications. This wide variability in the reported accuracy of the exercise ECG is not explained by the information available in the published reports. This could be explained by unsuspected technical, methodological, or clinical variables that affect test performance. However, it is more likely that the authors of the 147 reports did not disclose important information and/or did not consider the key points that are known to effect test performance when performing and analyzing their studies.

This wide variability in test performance makes it important that clinicians apply rigorous control of the methods they use for testing and analysis. Individuals with truly nondiagnostic or equivocal tests should be retested or offered other testing methods, and ST-segment analysis should not be used to make a diagnosis in patients with marked degrees of resting ST depression or with LBBB or Wolff-Parkinson-White Syndrome. Upsloping ST depression should be considered borderline or negative and hyperventilation should not be performed prior to testing.

Results of Meta-Analysis in Studies That Correctly Removed MI Patients

To more accurately portray the performance of the exercise test, only the results in 41 studies out of the original 147 were considered. These 41 studies removed patients with a prior MI from this meta-analysis, fulfilling one of the criteria for evaluating a diagnostic test, and provided all of the numbers for calculating test performance. These 41 studies, including nearly 10,000 patients, demonstrated *a lower mean sensitivity of 68% and a lower mean specificity of 74%; this also means that there is a lower predictive accuracy of 71%.* Notice that the predictive accuracy has the least variation. In several studies where work-up bias has been lessened, fulfilling the other major criteria, the *sensitivity is approximately 50% and the specificity 90% with the predictive accuracy staying at 70%.*[61] *This demonstrates that the key feature of the standard exercise ECG test for clinical utility is its high specificity and that the low sensitivity of the ST response is problematic.*

Effects of Digoxin, LVH, and Resting ST Depression from the Meta-Analysis

For resolving the issues of LVH, resting ST depression, and digoxin, the studies were organized as follows. Of the appropriate studies, only those that provided sensitivity, specificity, total patient numbers, and included more than 100 patients were considered. Regarding the effect of resting ECG abnormalities, the studies that included patients with LVH had a mean sensitivity of 68% and a mean specificity of 69%, and the studies that excluded them had a mean sensitivity of 72% and a mean specificity of 77%. Studies that included patients with resting ST depression had a mean sensitivity of 69% and a mean specificity of 70%, and studies that excluded them had a mean sensitivity of 67%, and a mean specificity 84%. Regarding the effect of digoxin, the studies that included patients receiving digoxin had a mean sensitivity of 68% and a mean specificity of 74%, and the studies that excluded them had a mean sensitivity of 72% and a mean specificity of 69%. Comparing these results with the average sensitivity of 67% and specificity of 72% for all 58 studies, as well as to the study pairs with and without the feature, it was found that all of these situations lower specificity and predictive accuracy. However, this effect is not sufficient to negate the utility of the standard exercise ECG for diagnosis in these patients. This is particularly the case for the most common response, which is a negative test, since specificity is not altered. The *box* below presents these results.

These conclusions were based on evidence obtained from recalculation of the meta-analysis performed by Detrano et al. Of the 150 plus studies that were included in this meta-analysis, four included only women and these studies had a mean sensitivity of 75% and a mean specificity of 75%. In comparison, there were seven studies that included only men with a mean sensitivity of 67% and a mean specificity of 79%. These numbers were not statistically different.

Women in the Meta-Analysis

We recalculated the data from this meta-analysis as well as data from the table in the guidelines that included 15 studies that only tested women (Table 7-8). These 15 studies were listed in the guidelines and included 2787 women. The mean

Grouping	No. of Studies	No. of Patients	Sensitivity	Specificity	Predictive Accuracy
Meta-analysis of standard ET	147	24,047	68%	77%	73%
==> Meta-analysis without MI	58	11,691	67%	72%	69%
==> Meta-analysis with resting ST depression	22	9153	69%	70%	69%
==> Meta-analysis without resting ST depression	3	840	67%	84%	75%
==> Meta-analysis with digoxin	15	6338	68%	74%	71%
==> Meta-analysis without digoxin	9	3548	72%	69%	70%
==> Meta-analysis with LVH	15	8016	68%	69%	68%
==> Meta-analysis without LVH	10	1977	72%	77%	74%

LVH, left ventricular hypertrophy; MI, myocardial infarction.

sensitivity was 65% and the mean specificity was 68%. When sensitivity and specificity were plotted against the percentage of women in each group that had an abnormal exercise test, an interesting relationship became apparent (Fig. 7-9). Sensitivity was lower and specificity was higher in the studies that had the lowest percentage of women with an abnormal exercise test. In other words, using the percentage of abnormal tests as a rough indicator of the degree of work-up bias showed that studies with the least work-up bias had the lowest

sensitivity and highest specificity. This finding is consistent with studies from the VA and West Virginia University that have reduced work-up bias by protocol.

The rationale for this is as follows: the studies evaluating the exercise test were done as part of clinical practice. The degree of work-up bias depends upon how physicians make clinical decisions at the institutions that the studies were performed. For instance, if the exercise test is used as a gatekeeper, then patients with an abnormal ST

TABLE 7–8.   Test characteristics of exercise electrocardiogram in women

Author	Year of study	Number of patients	Mean age	Any CAD (%)	MV CAD (%)	ABNL st depr (%)	Sensitivity (%)	Specificity (%)
Guiteras	1972	112	49	12	37.5	38	79	66
Linhart	1974	98	46	24.5	na	34	71	78
Sketch	1975	56	50	17.9	na	27	50	78
Barolsky	1979	92	50	32.6	16	41	60	68
Weiner	1979	580	na	29.1	16	48	76	64
Isley	1982	62	51	43.5	27	44	67	74
Hung	1984	92	51	30.4	16	51	75	59
Hlatky	1984	613	na	31.6	na	na	57	86
Melin	1985	93	51	25.8	20	30	58	80
Robert	1991	135	53	41.5	29	37	68	48
Chae	1993	114	na	62.3	na	54	66	60
Williams	1995	118	60	47.1	19	57	67	51
Marwick	1995	118	60	40.7	17	58	77	56
Morise	1995	264	56	30.7	27	33	46	74
Morise	1995	288	57	36.8	26	36	55	74

Abnl ST Depr = abnormal criteria for ST depression; any CAD = significant angiographic obstruction; MV CAD = multivessel coronary angiographic obstruction; na = not available.

response and low exercise capacities are going to be selected for cardiac catheterization, and others excluded. At another institution, where the exercise test is not as important in the decision-making process, or where the study designers specifically tried to reduce work-up bias (i.e., had patients presenting with symptoms undergo both studies regardless of their results), there would be less work-up bias. Thus, graphing the percentage of abnormal exercise tests in a study against sensitivity and specificity is a valid way of evaluating the relationship of test characteristics relative to work-up bias. Since this relationship was first detected in the studies of women, it was important to determine if this relationship also existed for men. We recalculated the data from the meta-analysis, so that we could plot the sensitivity and specificity versus the percentage of abnormal exercise tests. The same relationship existed in the 41 studies that largely consisted of men. Figure 7-10 is a box plot based on these data. The data from the women are based on the 15 studies that only tested women. The data from the men are from the studies that were largely based on men, although they had a varying percentage of women in them, usually 25% or less. As you can see from the box plots, there is no significant difference in the sensitivity or specificity in the studies between men and women. However, notice that there is a slightly lower percentage of abnormal exercise test responses in the women's studies, which means that the specificity should be higher and the sensitivity lower in the women studies, but they are not. This suggests that specificity is a little bit lower in women, but not enough to negate the exercise test as the first diagnostic test in women.

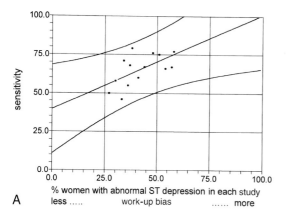

A

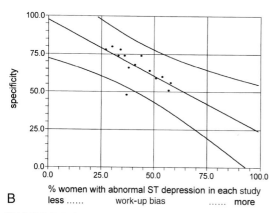

B

■ **FIGURE 7–9**

Plots of the sensitivity *(A)* and specificity *(B)* of the exercise ECG compared to rates of abnormal ST depression in the 15 angiographic studies of women. When sensitivity and specificity are plotted against the percentage of women in each group that had an abnormal exercise test, an interesting relationship is apparent. Sensitivity was lower and specificity was higher in the studies that had the lowest percentage of women with an abnormal exercise test. In other words, using the percentage of abnormal tests as a rough indicator of the degree of work bias showed that studies with the least work-up bias had the lowest sensitivity and the highest specificity.

METHODOLOGICAL STANDARDS FOR STUDIES TO DETERMINE THE PERFORMANCE OF A DIAGNOSTIC TEST

In order to determine why the diagnostic characteristics of the exercise test for CAD varied so much from study to study, Philbrick et al[62] undertook a methodological review of 33 studies comprising 7501 patients who had undergone both exercise tests and coronary angiography. These studies were published between 1976 and 1979 and had to include at least 50 patients. Seven methodologic standards were declared necessary:

1. adequate identification of the groups selected for study.
2. adequate variety of anatomic lesions.
3. adequate analysis for relevant chest pain syndromes.
4. avoidance of a limited challenge group.
5. avoidance of work-up bias.
6. avoidance of diagnostic review bias (the result of the exercise test is allowed to influence the interpretation of the coronary angiogram)

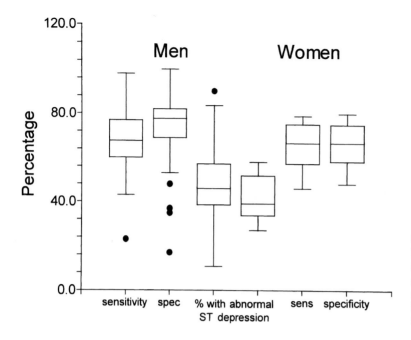

■ **FIGURE 7-10**
Box plots of the results of the angiographic correlative studies in men and women. The box plots show no significant difference in the sensitivity or specificity in the studies between men and women.

7. avoidance of test review bias (occurring when the result of the coronary angiogram is allowed to influence the interpretation of the exercise test)

Of these seven methodology standards for research design, only the requirement for an adequate variety of anatomic lesions received general compliance. Less than half of the studies complied with any of the remaining six standards: adequate identification of the groups selected for study; adequate analysis for relevant chest pain syndromes; avoidance of a limited challenge group; and avoidance of bias due to work-up, diagnostic review or test review. Only one study met as many as five of the seven standards.

The failure of the studies to fulfill the criteria help explain the wide range of sensitivity (35% to 88%) and specificity (41% to 100%) found for exercise testing. The variations could not be attributed to the usual explanations: definition of anatomic abnormality, exercise test technique, or definition of an abnormal test. Determining the true value of exercise testing requires methodological improvements in patient selection, data collection, and data analysis. Another important consideration is the exclusion of patients who had MI. These patients most often have obstructive CAD and should not be included in diagnostic studies of any type of CAD but can be included when evaluating disease severity.

Reid et al[63] updated these criteria for "methodological standards" for diagnostic tests in 1995. Their purpose in refining these standards was to improve patient care, reduce healthcare costs, improve the quality of diagnostic test information, and eliminate useless tests or testing methodologies. The seven standards are listed below:

Standard 1: Spectrum Composition.
a. Exclusion of patients who had had a prior MI or previous coronary artery bypass surgery
b. Adequate variety of anatomic lesions
c. Adequate analysis for relevant chest pain symptoms
d. Avoidance of limited challenge

Standard 2: Analysis of Pertinent Subgroups. Gender consideration is essential since the prevalence of disease is different in men and women and perhaps even the presentation of chest pain. Estrogen status is perhaps a more correct way to deal with this issue.

Standard 3: Avoidance of Work-Up Bias. After an exercise test or a nuclear perfusion test, patients with positive results for ischemia (chest pain, ST depression), rather than negative results, are preferentially referred for coronary angiography. In addition, patients with a high exercise capacity are usually not referred for catheterization, while those with a poor exercise capacity are referred. This causes the prevalence of disease in study populations to be higher than in clinical practice. Also, the coefficients for these variables will have different weights when chosen in mathematical models.

Standard 4: Avoidance of Diagnostic Review Bias. Observers without prior knowledge of the exercise test should interpret the angiograms in order to fulfill this standard.

Standard 5: Precision of results for test accuracy. Standard errors or confidence intervals for sensitivity or specificity or for ROC curve areas should be provided.

Standard 6: Presentation of Indeterminate Test Results. Exercise tests that do not achieve a certain age-predicted maximal heart rate have been declared indeterminate in some studies, but often it is not clear how indeterminate tests were dealt with in other studies. A test can have only limited value if a sizable percentage of patients tested must go on to other tests. If indeterminate results are included but considered negative, specificity is artifactually increased and sensitivity decreased. The reverse occurs if indeterminate results are classified as positive results. Therefore, no tests should be eliminated for analysis by calling them indeterminate.

Standard 7: Test Reproducibility (Validation). Although most studies include sensitivity, specificity, or the error rate of their models, these test characteristics are related to disease prevalence and other population characteristics. Validation studies should be carried out to evaluate the portability of the results to other populations. The performance of the test should be documented in an independent testing group (i.e., by splitting the population into a training and test set) or by using the Jack-knife method in the entire population. ROC curves and the AUC are important to report for comparison purposes. Although the scores or models may be reproducible in their discriminating capabilities, a more recent concern has been the issue of calibration. That is, a score could be portable to other populations and discriminate as reflected by a good ROC curve area, but the estimated probability could be displaced from the real probability (e.g., the score could estimate a probability of 50% when it actually is 75%).

Guyatt's Criteria for Judging Studies Evaluating Diagnostic Tests

Guyatt recommends that certain criteria must be applied to judge the credibility and applicability of the results of studies evaluating diagnostic tests.[64] First, the evaluation must include clearly defined comparison groups, at least one of which is free of the disease of interest. The studies should include consecutive patients or randomly selected patients for whom the diagnosis is in doubt. Any diagnostic test appears to function well if obviously normal subjects are compared with those who obviously have the disease in question (limited challenge). In most cases we do not need sophisticated testing to differentiate the normal population from the sick. Rather, the clinician is interested in examining patients who are suspected, but not known, to have the disease of interest and in differentiating those who do have the disease from those who do not. If the patients enrolled in the study do not represent this "diagnostic dilemma" group, the test may perform well in the study, but not in clinical practice. Another problem is including patients who most certainly have the disease (i.e., post-MI patients) in this diagnostic sample. They may be included in studies to predict disease severity but should not be included in studies attempting to distinguish those with disease from those without disease.

The second "believability" criterion requires an independent, "blind" comparison of the test with the performance of a "gold" standard. The "gold" standard really should measure a clinically important state. For example, for CAD, an invasive test, such as catheterization, is used as the gold standard rather than symptoms of chest pain alone. The gold standard result should not be available to those interpreting the test. In addition, if the gold standard requires subjective interpretation (as would be the case even for coronary angiography), the interpreter should not know the test result. Blinding the interpreters of the test to the gold standard and vice versa minimizes the risk of bias.

If these two criteria are met, the study can be used as a basis for performance of the test in clinical practice. To apply the test properly to patients, the following must be considered. Most tests merely indicate an increase or decrease in the probability of disease. To apply imperfect tests appropriately, you must estimate the probability of disease before the test is done ("pretest probability"), then revise this probability according to the test result ("post-test probability").

Conclusions Regarding Standards Criteria

Most of the diagnostic test standards, such as blinding of test interpreters, exclusion of patients with prior MIs, and classification, of chest pain are very logical and easy to appreciate. The two subtle standards that are least understood but effect test performance drastically and are most commonly not fulfilled are *limited challenge* and *work-up bias*. Therefore, these two standards will be discussed further. Limited challenge actually could be justified as the first step of looking at a new measurement or test. An investigator may choose both healthy and sick people and test them using the new measurement to see if they respond differently. If no difference was noted, then further investigation would not be indicated. Such a subject choice favors the measurement but its true test is in consecutive patients presenting for evaluation. A measurement or test may function well to separate the extremes but fail in a clinical situation. Work-up bias just means that the decision of who undergoes catheterization is made by the physician using the test and his/her clinical acumen, and so the patients in the study are different from patients presenting for evaluation before this selection process occurs. This can only be avoided by having patients agree to both procedures prior to any testing.

Populations chosen for test evaluation that fail to avoid limited challenge will result in predictive accuracies and ROC curves greater than those truly associated with the test measurement. Although this is not the case for populations with work-up bias, the calibration of the measurement cutpoints can be affected. That is, a score or ST measurement can have a different sensitivity and specificity for a particular cutpoint when work-up bias is present.

Limited Challenge

Limited challenge means that rather than studying the test in consecutive patients, a group of healthy or least diseased patients are compared to patients who have severe disease (Fig. 7-11). This is only appropriate as the first step in evaluating a new test or measurement and is not appropriate for evaluating or demonstrating true test characteristics. Actual test characteristics are only defined in consecutive patients with the complaint that requires testing (i.e., chest pain). Such patients are the only patients who should be included in a study to determine test-discriminating characteristics. When the healthy or least diseased are studied, the specificity of the test should be very high, usually greater than 90%. When the most diseased are studied, the sensitivity should be very high, often 90% or more. Even when ROC curves are calculated from results from these two disparate groups, a relatively large area will be

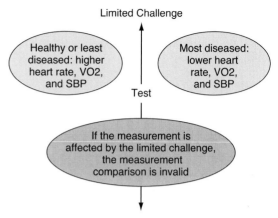

■ FIGURE 7–11

"Limited challenge" means that rather than studying the test in consecutive patients, a group of healthy or least diseased patients are compared to patients who have severe disease.

obtained. It is only when the test or measurement is applied in consecutive patients with a complaint that requires testing that we see the actual test characteristics. Usually the sensitivity and specificity are much lower.

An argument could be made that limited challenge does not matter if only certain measurements are being compared. However, limited challenge can cause differences in other factors that cause the measurements to be different. For instance, heart rate, systolic blood pressure, and exercise capacity are markedly different in healthy subjects compared to those with severe disease (Fig. 7-11). The discriminatory capacity of any ST measurement divided by heart rate (i.e., ST/HR index) is exaggerated when compared in samples with limited challenge.

Work-Up Bias

Another problem with most of the studies has been failure to limit work-up bias. Consider Figure 7-12: patients with chest pain being seen in a physician's office are in the left upper circle. Normal clinical practice then results in an exercise test being done, and only certain patients being selected for further work-up. Cardiac catheterization would be chosen particularly for those with a low exercise capacity and an abnormal ST response. Others might also be catheterized but the population will be selected to favor these responses of low exercise capacity and abnormal ST. Patients excluded from cardiac catheterization after the exercise test will be those with a high exercise capacity and a normal ST response. Others might

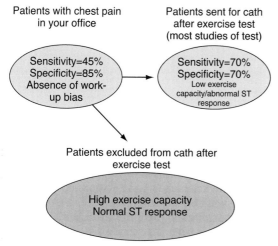

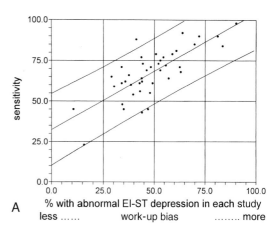

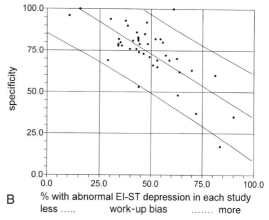

FIGURE 7–12

A problem with most of the studies has been failure to limit work-up bias. Patients with chest pain being seen in the physician's office are in the left upper circle. Normal clinical practice then results in an exercise test being done and only certain patients being selected for further work-up. Cardiac catheterization would be chosen particularly for those with a low exercise capacity and an abnormal ST response.

FIGURE 7–13

The relationship between sensitivity *(A)* and specificity *(B)* with the percent of abnormal tests in each of the 50 studies. There is a good correlation between the percent of abnormal tests and specificity and sensitivity. Specificity is higher with less work-up bias, and sensitivity is lower.

also be excluded but in the majority, but these characteristics of high exercise capacity and normal ST will predominate. Figure 7-13 shows the results. Most of the studies that have looked at the characteristics of the exercise test, using the gold standard of cardiac catheterization, had work-up bias. Sensitivity usually is about 70% and specificity is about 70% in such populations. What we would really like to know is how the test functions in the population of patients who present to the office in the upper left circle. In the few studies that have limited work-up bias by protocol or have had a lower degree of work-up bias because of clinical practice (where the exercise test is largely ignored) showed different test characteristics: the sensitivity is roughly 40% and the specificity is 85%. These are the characteristics of test performance in the typical office setting.

The meta-analysis of 50 studies that have performed tests with angiographic correlates have been reanalyzed considering the percent of abnormal exercise-induced ST-segment depression in each study. One assumes that there is less work-up bias the lower the percentage of patients with an abnormal exercise test and more work-up bias in those with a higher percentage of abnormal exercise tests. As seen in Figure 7-13 there is a correlation between the percent of abnormal tests and specificity and sensitivity. Specificity is higher with less work-up bias and sensitivity is lower. This is

consistent with the studies that have removed work-up bias by protocol.

The rationale for this is as follows: the studies evaluating the exercise test were done as part of clinical practice. The degree of work-up bias depends upon how the physicians make clinical decisions at the institutions where the studies were performed. For instance, if the exercise test is used as a gatekeeper, then patients with an abnormal ST response and low exercise capacity are going to be selected for the cardiac catheterization, and others excluded. At another institution where the exercise test is not as important in the decision-making process, or where the study designers specifically tried to reduce work-up bias (i.e., had patients presenting with symptoms undergo both studies regardless of their results), there would be less work-up bias. Thus, graphing the percentage of abnormal exercise tests in a study against sensitivity and specificity is a valid way of evaluating the relationship of test characteristics relative to work-up bias.

It could be argued that the clinician does not want to insist everyone undergoes cardiac catheterization. That is not the point, however, for performing studies to demonstrate how well a test can be expected to function for the clinician. The point is that to determine the actual test characteristics, a study protocol must be followed to catheterize and exercise-test all patients presenting with chest pain. Then the practicing physician can tell from the study how the test performs in his or her office practice, and thus make better decisions as to who would need further evaluation.

In summary, work-up bias is when not all patients seen with chest pain and undergoing exercise tests undergo a cardiac catheterization, because of clinical judgement. Excluded by work-up bias are those with high exercise capacity and normal ST responses for the most part. Patients with low exercise capacity and abnormal ST responses are selected for further study. Although this is not 100% in any of the studies, tendencies for this to occur vary from study to study, and that is why different test performance characteristics have been obtained with the exercise test. In the studies that have removed work-up bias by protocol, these differences are very clearly seen. As you can see in the Table 7-9, approximately 12,000 patients were included in the 58 studies with varying degrees of work-up bias. The mean sensitivity was 67% and mean specificity 72%. The two studies that have removed work-up bias by protocol included 2000 patients and showed considerably different test characteristics.

MULTIVARIABLE TECHNIQUES TO DIAGNOSE ANGIOGRAPHICALLY DETERMINED CORONARY DISEASE

Since the seminal work of Ellestad et al[65] demonstrated that the accuracy of the test could be improved by combining other clinical and exercise parameters along with the ST responses, many clinical investigators have published studies proposing multivariable equations to enhance the accuracy of the standard exercise test. Nonetheless, the clinical implementation of the exercise test still concentrates on the ST response because the clinician

TABLE 7–9. The effect of work-up bias on the standard exercise ECG test

Studies	Number of patients	Sensitivity	Specificity
58 with work-up bias	12,000	67%	72%
2 without work-up bias	2,000	45%	90%

remains uncertain of which equations and variables to apply and how to include them in prediction.

Studies utilizing modern statistical techniques have demonstrated that combinations of clinical and exercise test variables could more accurately predict the probability of angiographic CAD than the standard ST depression criteria. Although the statistical models proposed have proven to be superior, the available equations have differed as to the variables and coefficients chosen. Furthermore, the definitions and criteria for variables or angiographic interpretation have not been standardized. For instance, hypercholesterolemia has been defined as "yes" or "no" with different levels, while other studies have considered the actual cholesterol level but not indicated whether or not this was a treated or untreated value. The angiographic interpretation criteria have varied from 50% to 80% luminal narrowing, and severe disease has been defined as more than one-diseased vessel or as triple-vessel disease. In addition, the available equations were usually derived in study populations with a higher prevalence of disease than seen in clinical settings because of work-up bias. For these reasons, the discriminating power of these equations remains controversial and their usage limited. Unfortunately, these uncertainties exist at a time when managed care providers are trying to apply cost-containment algorithms to healthcare.[66]

Over a 15-year period from 1980 through 1995, there were 30 articles published that used multivariable statistical analysis for the diagnosis of the presence of any or of severe angiographically determined CAD.[67] Since some did both, there were 24 studies that predicted presence of angiographic CAD and 13 studies that predicted disease extent or severe angiographically determined CAD.

In 16 of the 24 studies predicting the presence of angiographic disease, patients with prior MI were excluded as they should be, and in five studies they were improperly included. In the remaining three studies, exclusions were unclear. In 16 studies that excluded patients with MI, it was defined by history in six, by ECG findings in one and by either criterion in five. In the remaining five studies the criteria for MI exclusion were unclear. Ten of the 24 studies clearly excluded patients with previous coronary artery bypass surgery or prior percutaneous coronary intervention, while in the remainder exclusions were unclear. The definition of significant coronary angiographic stenosis ranged from 50% to 80%, and in one study a coronary angiographic score was used instead. The prevalence of angiographic disease ranged from 30% to 78%. The percentages of patients with one-, two- and three-vessel disease were provided in only 13 of the 24 studies.

Statistical Techniques

Multivariable analysis is a statistical technique that seeks to separate subjects into different groups on the basis of measured variables.[68] Clinical investigators have commonly used two types of analysis: discriminate function and logistic regression analysis. Logistic regression has been preferred since it models the relationship to a sigmoid curve (which often is the mathematical relationship between a risk variable and an outcome) and its output is between zero and one (i.e., from zero to 100% probability of the predicted outcome). The appropriate values are inserted into the following logistic regression formula to calculate an estimate of the probability for angiographic coronary disease:

$$\text{Probability (0 to 1) of disease} = 1/(1 + e^{-(a + bx + cy \ldots)})$$

where a = intercept, b and c are coefficients, x and y are variable values.

Thus, the output of a discriminate function prediction equation is a unitless numerical score, whereas a logistic regression equation provides an actual probability.

Fifteen of the 30 studies applied discriminate function analysis and the other 15 studies applied logistic regression analysis. In most studies, the groups to be separated were formed by the classification of presence or severity of coronary disease. The variables found to have discriminating power (consisting of clinical information and treadmill responses) were combined to form an algorithm for estimating the probability of CAD.

In 13 studies applying an incremental approach simulating clinical practice, pre-exercise and post-exercise test predictive models was developed

separately. Therefore, the discriminating power of clinical variables was evaluated separately from exercise test variables. The remaining 17 studies did not take an incremental approach, but combined clinical variables with exercise test variables. Consequently, the discriminating power of clinical variables was underestimated, because exercise test variables generally have stronger discriminating power than clinical variables. Some have suggested that the incremental approach, which takes advantage of the information content available from the basic history and physical exam, is more logical. The logic is based on the fact that 80% of diagnoses in patient evaluations are made by the medical history and that the results so obtained should be used to decide what further testing is required.[69] On the other hand, some would argue that the discriminating power of the test results are especially required when less experienced clinicians are performing the patient evaluations (i.e., they do not know how to take a history to distinguish angina from noncardiac chest pain).

Not all of the publications of the reviewed studies included the equations derived from the multivariable analyses they performed; these equations are critical to the validation of their findings.[70] The equations developed in the studies were available for 16 of the 24 studies predicting disease presence.

Comparison of Clinical and Exercise Test Variables

Table 7-10 lists and counts the predictors of disease presence in 24 studies that considered exercise test and clinical variables to predict presence of any angiographic disease. Thirty equations were created but not all of the models were given all of the variables for consideration. The denominator is the number of equations that considered the variable and the numerators are the numbers of equations that chose the specific variable to be significant.

The discriminating power of the variables listed in Table 7-10 that appear in more than 50% of the equations can be assumed as occurring more than by chance. However, the predictive power of other variables remains undecided. The differences in the variables chosen for predicting presence and severity of coronary disease are discussed in Chapter 8. The reasons why the variables had different results in many of the studies remains uncertain but the following sections discuss possible explanations.

TABLE 7–10. Clinical and exercise test variables considered in studies using multivariable statistical techniques to predict the presence of angiographically determined coronary artery disease

Clinical variables	Number of studies/number of equations*	Significant predictor
Gender	20/20	100%
Chest pain	17/18	94%
Age	19/27	70%
Elevated cholesterol	8/13	62%
Diabetes mellitus	6/14	43%
History of smoking	4/12	33%
Abnormal resting ECG	4/17	24%
Hypertension	1/8	13%
Family history of CAD	0/7	0%
Exercise test variables	**Number of studies/number of equations***	**Significant predictor**
ST-segment slope	14/22	64%
ST-segment depression	17/28	61%
Maximal heart rate	16/28	57%
Exercise capacity	11/24	46%
Exercise-induced angina	11/26	42%
Double product	2/13	15%
Maximal systolic BP	1/12	8%

*The denominator is the number of published equations that considered the variable as a candidate for consideration and the numerator is the number of studies that found the variable to be an independently significant predictor.

Differences in Definitions Applied for Variables

The way in which many of the clinical risk predictors were defined or classified differed in many of the studies. For example, smoking history was classified as current smoking, history of smoking, or both. In all four studies where smoking was classified by history, it was not a good predictor. Furthermore, the classification of current smoking was not detailed; for instance, how many packs per day or how many years a person smoked or which type of smoking (pipe, cigar, or cigarette).

Diabetes was classified by history in most studies but how it was diagnosed was usually not declared. Medications required, including insulin, were not routinely reported. In addition, no study considered the control status of blood sugar concentration or the degree of diabetic complications.

Exercise-induced chest pain was a good predictor of disease presence in all three studies where angina was rated from moderate to severe chest pain. On the contrary, this variable was not a good predictor of disease presence in 9 of the 14 studies where angina was classified as only "yes" or "no." Clearly the severity and length of time since it first occurred have potential for better discriminating ability. Clearly, how a variable is defined can determine how predictive the variable will be.

Differences in the Degree of Work-Up Bias

A problem with these exercise test-angiographic correlation studies has been the failure to remove work-up bias. Physicians selected patients in studies for angiography and others were excluded. This selection process results in patients with abnormal tests (i.e., with exercise-induced chest pain or ST depression) being more likely to be chosen, while patients with high exercise capacities would be excluded from such studies, resulting in a relatively higher prevalence of disease than seen in a clinic population. Prior prediction equations, scores, and heart rate adjustment schema were derived from populations with extensive work-up bias and are less applicable to unselected patients who present to their physician with chest pain.

Effect of Prevalence of a Characteristic

Prevalence in this discussion relates to the difference of frequency in the clinical variables and their impact on prediction. Diabetes was classified by history in seven studies. All three studies in which the prevalence of diabetes was greater than

19% demonstrated that diabetes was a good predictor. In contrast, in four studies where the frequency of diabetes was less than 16%, diabetes was not a good predictor. The same phenomenon occurred with hypercholesterolemia. In all four studies in which the mean serum cholesterol concentration was more than 240 mg/dl, hypercholesterolemia was a good predictor.

Whether a variable is shown to be a good predictor or not may depend on the frequency of the abnormal characteristic in the population being studied. Analytic results based upon a group with a low frequency of the characteristic should be interpreted with caution.

Interactions between Variables

Morise et al[74] demonstrated that when serum cholesterol concentration was included in the model, smoking lost its significance as a predictor of disease presence and extent. In four of the nine studies where smoking was not a significant predictor, serum cholesterol was included into the model. In contrast, the Goldman study demonstrated that smoking was still a significant predictor even though hypercholesterolemia was included in the model. In the latter study, smoking was strictly classified as at least 1/2 pack per day in the past 5 years and the frequency of smoking was very high (65%). Morise et al[74] also demonstrated that maximal heart rate became more significant as a predictor when exercise capacity was not entered into the model.

Therefore, analyses should consider potential interactions between variables. These interactions need not necessarily be consistent with intuition, as previously unknown interactions may be overlooked. Multivariable analytic tools should have enough flexibility to handle an infinite variety of potential interactions.

Effect of Drug Administration

Beta-blockers have a profound effect upon exercise test responses. These agents generally keep maximal heart rate under 120 beats per minute, they can mask angina yet worsen ST depression, and they can lower the BP response. In 8 of the 22 studies that considered maximal heart rate for the presence of disease, patients taking beta-blockers were included. In five of these eight studies maximal heart rate was a good predictor. In only three of

the eight studies the percentages were described separately in patients with and without angiographic CAD. In two of these studies the percentages of patients with angiographic CAD taking beta-blockers were twice as high as those for patients without angiographically determined CAD (55% versus 29%, 47% versus 15%, respectively). In the remaining one study the percentage of patients taking beta-blockers was similar between the two groups; however, the percentage of patients with CAD taking calcium channel blockers was two times higher than that in patients without angiographically determined CAD (45% versus 19%). Therefore, in the studies which included patients taking beta-blockers or calcium channel blockers, the medications might be selected as predictive variables because the patients with angiographically determined CAD would be given these medications more frequently than the patients without disease. Separate analysis of those not receiving these drugs or incorporation of a variable that accounts for these drugs should be considered.

Over-Fitting

The risk estimates may be unreliable if the multivariable data contain too few outcome events relative to the number of independent variables. In general, the results of models having fewer than 10 outcome events per independent variable are thought to have questionable accuracy. This criterion was not satisfied in only 1 of 24 studies for disease presence and in 3 of 13 studies for disease extent. When the number of variables exceeds the 1 per 10 event or outcome (abnormal angiogram) rule, combining variables into scores or composite variables should be considered.

Missing Data

In several studies reviewed, the investigators included patients who had missing data. If a complete data set cannot be included for all patients in a training population, the model generated will not include the entire population. This can greatly reduce the population size. Therefore, some investigators designed their models to handle missing data. Detrano et al[75] computed many equations to deal with patients with different combinations of the 13 variables that were found to be good predictors. They then classified all test patients with the equation that fit the variables available for each of them individually. Morise et al[74] developed two equations, one for patients whose serum cholesterol level was known and another for patients for whom it was not known. Morise et al[74] also presented two different equations, one for interpretable and the other for uninterpretable resting ECGs. Another approach to handling missing data of the continuous type is to insert the average value in the data set for that variable (i.e., if a cholesterol value is missing for a patient, insert the average value found in the population).

Calibration

Although the discriminating power of the equations may persist when they are applied to another population, the calibration can be off.[71] For instance, an equation may predict a 50% chance of coronary disease in one population for certain patient characteristics and a 70% chance in another. In addition, one equation may predict an 80% probability for disease in a specific patient, whereas another equation predicts a 50% probability for the same patient even though both equations can discriminate equally between those with and without CAD in various populations. Calibration remains a difficult problem to understand and to resolve. In order to enhance calibration, investigators have suggested that calibration be corrected by the disease prevalence in the clinical population in which the equation is applied.[72] This is not a practical solution since most clinicians do not know the disease prevalence in their exercise laboratory and even if they did, it could change from month to month. Morise et al[73] have proposed some brilliant techniques for adjusting calibration based on the frequency of abnormal responses and other population characteristics that are related to prevalence of disease.

Gender Differences

For predicting the presence of disease, age and chest pain were good predictors in both genders. ST-segment depression, ST-segment slope, exercise-induced angina, and maximal heart rate were good predictors in males; however, these variables were not good predictors or had relatively lower discriminating power in females. On the other hand, hypertension, family history of CAD, maximal systolic blood pressure, double product, and exercise capacity were not good predictors in both genders. The discriminating powers of smoking history, diabetes mellitus, and cholesterol were controversial because their classification was varied and the number of studies considering these variables was small, especially in females.

Robert et al[76] assessed whether the diagnostic value of exercise testing could be enhanced in women by using multivariate analysis of exercise data.[76] Between 1978 and 1984, 135 infarct-free women underwent exercise testing and coronary angiography in Brussels. Significant CAD was present in 41% of the patients. In this first group, maximal exercise variables were submitted to a stepwise logistic analysis. Work load, heart rate, and ST_{60} in lead X were selected to build a diagnostic model. The model was tested in a second group of 115 catheterized women (significant CAD in 47%) and of 76 volunteers. They compared their model with conventional analysis of the exercise ECG, with ST changes adjusted for heart rate, and with a previously described analysis. In both groups, sensitivity was better with the present model (66% and 70%) than by conventional (68% and 59%) and by the previously described analysis (57% and 44%) without a loss of specificity (85% and 93%). ROC curves showed also a better diagnostic accuracy with the present model. They concluded that in women, logistic analysis of exercise variables improves the diagnostic value of exercise testing. Unfortunately, they did not consider estrogen status.

Considering the extent of disease, there were only three equations developed for females. Age, chest pain, ST-segment depression, and ST-segment slope were good predictors. In comparison, smoking history, hypertension, family history of CAD, exercise-induced angina, maximal heart rate, maximal systolic blood pressure, and exercise capacity were not good predictors. The discriminating power of diabetes mellitus, cholesterol, resting ECG, change in systolic blood pressure, and double product remain undetermined.

Recommendations for Defining Clinical Variables

In our recommendations, the clinical variables are ranked according to their relative importance as demonstrated by the percentages of the studies in which they were chosen as listed above.

1. *Gender:* This variable has so much interaction with both other clinical and exercise responses

that it may be better to derive two equations, a separate one for men and women. Morise et al[77] demonstrated that estrogen status was an independent predictor of disease presence when used either in a separate equation for women or in a combined equation that also included gender. In this latter case, both gender and estrogen status were independent predictors. Consideration of estrogen and/or menopausal status and their interactions with gender allow for a single equation to be used for both men and women.

2. *Chest pain symptoms:* The presenting symptoms are extremely important and should be classified by their nature prior to antianginal therapy. There appears to be little difference between the classification according to the Coronary Artery Surgery Study (none, noncardiac, probable, definite) or Diamond (none, noncardiac, atypical, typical). In order to incorporate each of these approaches into an equation in the simplest manner, most have used a symptom score, e.g., 1 to 4, for each subcategory. However, this imparts a quantitative value to one form of chest symptom over another that may not accurately reflect the relative value of each. Consideration of the individual characteristics that contribute to these symptom categories, such as exertional quality or relief by rest or nitroglycerin, should be explored. Length of time of the symptoms should also be considered, especially concerning disease extent.

3. *Age:* This variable is so important that some would recommend that it be forced into all prediction equations even if it is not chosen. It should be used as a continuous variable rather than age grouping.

4. *Cholesterol:* Patients can be coded as having hypercholesterolemia if they have a history of being told by their physician that they have elevated serum cholesterol or are on cholesterol-lowering treatment. Given that the cutpoint for separating a normal from an abnormal cholesterol level is a moving target, defining an abnormal level as above 220 mg/dl, for example, is arbitrary and is not recommended. Serum cholesterol levels can be entered as a continuous variable but it should be declared whether the level was taken during therapy or not. This is especially important since the statins have become available. Incorporation of HDL cholesterol, such as in the total cholesterol/HDL ratio, is encouraged.

5. *Diabetes mellitus:* Diabetes has been classified by simple history, by the use of insulin or other hypoglycemic, or by a fasting serum glucose concentration of more than 120 to 140 mg/dl. Either a separate consideration of the different forms of diabetic therapy or a classification as "1" for oral hypoglycemics only and "2" for insulin should be considered.

6. *Smoking:* Smoking history can be defined as current smoking, a history of present or past smoking, or by considering the duration and amount of smoking (e.g., packs per year). Both a classification of yes/no for current smoking as well as packs per year is recommended.

7. *Resting ST-segment abnormalities:* There are several different ways this variable can be defined: dichotomously as resting ST abnormalities (with criteria) or as ST depression greater than 0.5 mm or continuously giving the specific magnitude of ST depression.

8. *Hypertension:* Patients can be classified as hypertensive if they have a simple history of hypertension associated with treatment. Given the variability and the response to therapy of resting systolic blood pressure, we cannot recommend this variable. Consideration of the duration and severity of hypertension such as evidence of end-organ damage, for example left ventricular hypertrophy, should be given.

9. *Family history of coronary artery disease:* This variable should be defined as having a cardiac event (infarction, angioplasty, bypass, sudden death) in a first-degree relative under age 55 years for men and 65 years for women.

Other Considerations

History of Myocardial Infarction

Although MI was an exclusion criterion in most of the diagnostic studies, it was improperly considered in several of them. Although it makes little sense to consider it in studies dealing with diagnosis, there is some justification for considering this variable in studies dealing with disease severity. Due to the inaccuracy of historical data, exclusion should be based on objective measures such as diagnostic criteria for Q waves.

Medication Status

Ideally, beta-blockers and digitalis should be exclusion criteria if not withheld in sufficient time prior to testing. Digitalis affects the ST segments and is also a marker for patients with heart failure and atrial fibrillation. Beta-blockers are used for treating angina and are effective in lessening symptoms. They lower the heart rate response to exercise and decrease exercise capacity in normal individuals and increase it in patients with angina.

Summary of Multivariate Diagnostic Prediction Studies

These studies consistently demonstrate that the multivariable equations outperform simple ST diagnostic criteria. These equations generally provide an ROC area of 0.8. Whether they will function accurately in a clinic or office practice is uncertain because work-up bias will never be totally removed. This selection process results in patients with abnormal ST responses and/or chest pain being more likely chosen, whereas patients with high exercise capacities would be excluded from such studies, resulting in a relatively higher prevalence of disease than seen in a clinic population. Thus, the coefficients for METs and ST depression are probably not totally appropriate. Another limitation of the early equations was their complexity. However, a computer program can make the use of the complex equations transparent. In addition, while the discriminating power of the equations may persist when they are applied to another population, the calibration can be off.[78] For instance, the equation may predict a 50% chance of coronary disease given a set of variables in one population and a 70% chance in another population with the same variables.

Managed care and capitation require that tests be utilized only when they can accurately and reliably identify which patients need medications, counseling, further evaluation, or intervention. The add-ons to the standard exercise ECG test (nuclear perfusion scanning and echocardiography) require expensive equipment and personnel, and their incremental value is currently being evaluated. Since general practitioners are to function as gatekeepers and decide which patients must be referred to the cardiologist, they will need to use the basic tools they have available (i.e., history, physical exam, and the exercise test) in an optimal fashion. The newer generation of multivariable equations hopefully is robust and portable, and will empower the clinician to assure the cardiac patient access to appropriate cardiologic care.

EXERCISE TEST SCORES

A variety of statistical tools are available to create diagnostic and prognostic scores and the use of exercise testing scores has been well studied, as the applicability and reliability of scores is key to their optimal use.[79] The ACC/AHA guidelines suggest the use of scores to enhance the predictive ability of exercise tests.

Statistical Techniques to Develop Scores

When developing a score or prediction rule, investigators consider variables that they believe may predict the occurrence of an outcome and then make use of those variables which are found to have discriminating power.[80] The standard approach for creating an exercise test score is to use a combination of clinical information and exercise test results to form an algorithm for estimating the probability of disease. Although many mathematical techniques are available for demonstrating what variables are predictive as well as their relative predictive power, logistic regression is preferred since it models the relationship to a sigmoid curve (the most common mathematical relationship between a probability variable and an outcome) and its output is between zero and one (i.e., from 0% to 100% probability of the predicted outcome).

Application of Scores

The ability of any score or measurement to diagnose a disease depends upon how much the score differs among those with and without the disease.[81] Figure 7-14 shows the application of a simple treadmill score to an actual population of over 1000 male veterans who underwent both exercise testing and coronary angiography. Unfortunately, there is a great deal of overlap in scores between patients with and without CAD. Using a cutpoint of 50 may be a practical choice to separate patients but will not absolutely classify those with and without disease. The better the test or measurement, the further apart the curves of the measurement and the less they overlap.

Score Evaluation

The accuracy of a model to separate patients with and without a certain disease or outcome

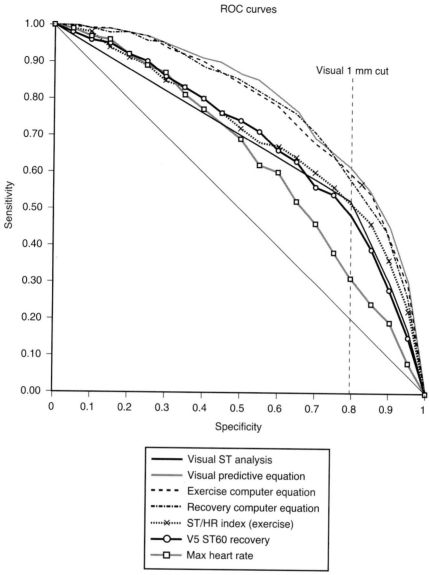

FIGURE 7–14

The probabilities generated using the models were plotted as ROC curves. There was a significant improvement in the ROC areas for each of the models compared to the visual analysis or to one of the best computer measurements. In addition, sensitivities for the models at a specificity comparable to visual criteria of 1mm (80%) were obtained from the ROC curves and tabulated. ROC curves of the three prediction equations, visual analysis, and the best computerized measurements from exercise and recovery are shown. For reference, a straight line is drawn representing no discrimination, and the ROC curve for maximal heart rate (area = 0.63) is plotted to demonstrate its relative symmetry compared to the ROC curves based on ECG variables. A vertical line is drawn through the ROC curves, representing the point where specificity is 80%, which matches visual analysis. The curves are asymmetrical at the end where specificity is high, demonstrating that sensitivities can differ around the region where the exercise test normally functions even when there are small or no differences between ROC curve areas. In addition, because of the fewer ST points measured by physicians (rounding off to 0.5 mm) as compared with computer measurements, the area formed by visual analysis is always less than computer measurements, putting the visual analysis at a disadvantage.

is assessed by evaluating the ROC curve. An ROC curve is a plot of the sensitivity and specificity for the full range of cutpoints (criteria for abnormal) for a test measurement or the value of a score. The shape of the curve shows the trade-offs between sensitivity and specificity produced at different cutoff criteria, with specificity and sensitivity being inversely related. The AUC of the ROC curve ranges from 0 to 1, with 0.5 corresponding to no discrimination (i.e., random performance), 1.0 to perfect discrimination, and values less than 0.5 to worse-than-random performance. Figure 7-2 is an ROC plot of the simple treadmill score ranging from 0 to 100 with two other cutpoints, 40 and 60 as illustrated. These cutpoints could be appropriate for particular purposes of the test; i.e., the higher cutpoint of 60 would be useful for screening healthy people where a high specificity is needed, while the lower cutpoint of 40 would be well suited for ruling out ischemia after presentation to an emergency department for chest pain, where high sensitivity is required. Plotting ROC curves for different diagnostic techniques or scores allows their discriminatory or diagnostic value to be compared. Figure 7-14 illustrates a comparison of the diagnostic characteristics of a pretest clinical score, visual ST analysis alone, computerized ST analysis, and the simple treadmill score. Comparison of the ROC curves clearly shows that the treadmill test adds to the discriminatory value of clinical data.[82]

Pretest Scores

The exercise ECG test is the recommended test for diagnosing CAD in patients at intermediate probability for CAD. In the ACC/AHA exercise test guidelines, the Diamond-Forrester tabular method is used to determine pretest probability with consideration of age, gender, and chest pain characteristics. The intermediate pretest probability category was assigned a class I indication, whereas the low and high pretest probability were assigned class IIb indications for exercise testing. The Morise score for categorizing patients as to pretest probability of angiographic disease (Fig. 7-15) appears superior to the tabular method.[83]

Failure to Assimilate Scores into Practice

Many investigators have proposed multivariable scores combining clinical and exercise parameters,

Variable	Circle response	Sum
Age	Men<40, Women<50 = 3	
	Men 40–55, Women 50–65 = 6	
	Men>55, Women>65 = 9	
Estrogen status	Positive = –3	
	Negative = +3	
Hypercholesterolemia?	Yes = 1	
HBP?	Yes = 1	
Smoking?	Yes = 1	
	Total score:	

Choose only one per group

≤8 low probability

9–15 = intermediate probability

≥16 high probability

FIGURE 7-15

Calculation of the simple pretest clinical score for angiographic coronary disease. Choose only one per group.

in addition to the ST responses, to enhance the accuracy of the standard exercise test.[67] Age, gender, chest pain, elevated cholesterol, ST-segment slope and depression, and maximum heart rate were the variables chosen as significant predictors in more than half of the studies. As presented above, statistical techniques which combine the patient's medical history, chest pain, hemodynamic data, exercise capacity, and exercise ECG response have been proven to be better predictors for CAD than a single ECG criterion like ST-segment depression. However, despite the validation of logistic equations (i.e., predictive scores) in large patient samples,[74,75] the methodology has not been widely disseminated.

Clinicians remain skeptical regarding the applicability of logistic equations to clinical practice. The variability in disease prevalence among populations with suspected CAD, the lack of standards for defining and capturing clinical data needed for calculation of probability scores, and the lack of an efficient mechanism for calculation of scores remain. These factors make diagnostic techniques with radioisotope imaging or echocardiography more attractive and more immediately relevant for decisions regarding individual patients. Although the continuing development of expert systems may remove the impediment of the physician needing to calculate the score, other concerns remain. These concerns include differences in disease prevalence and severity, definition of discriminate variables, missing data, as well as angiographic and exercise testing methodology. These factors could affect the portability of these equations to other populations and thus limit their dissemination in clinical practice.[84]

Management Strategy Using Scores

Exercise test scores can also assist in managing patients with possible CAD by placing them into three categories of risk rather than just dichotomizing them as positive or negative. Low-risk patients can be treated safely with medical management of coronary risk factors and watchful waiting prior to further testing. High-risk patients should be considered candidates for more aggressive management that may include cardiac catheterization. In patients with an intermediate-probability treadmill score, myocardial perfusion imaging and other tests are of value for further risk stratification.

Consensus of Scores

A consensus approach was developed for the purpose of increasing accuracy and making the diagnostic scores broadly applicable to different populations.[85] NASA uses the same approach to calculate spacecraft trajectories, applying several equations and then using the ones that agree. Three validated scores with established thresholds were used. If a patient showed high probability in at least two of the three equations, then he or she was considered high-risk; similarly, if a low probability was found in at least two of three equations he or she was considered low-risk. All others were considered to be of intermediate-risk. Since the patients in the intermediate group were sent for further testing and would eventually be

correctly classified, both the sensitivity and specificity of the consensus approach was greater than 90%. Although too complex for practical use by clinicians, computers can automatically apply the consensus approach as part of an exercise test report.

"Simplified" Score Derivation

Simplified scores derived from multivariable equations have been developed to determine the probability of disease and prognosis. All variables are coded with the same number of intervals so that the coefficients will be proportional. For instance, if 5 is the chosen interval, dichotomous variables are 0 if not present and 5 if present. Continuous variables like age and maximum heart rate are coded in five groups associated with increasing prevalence of disease. The relative importance of the selected variables is obvious and the healthcare provider merely compiles the variables in the score, multiples by the appropriate number and then adds up the products. Calculation of the "simple" exercise test score can be done using Figure 7-16[86] for men and Figure 7-17[87] for women.

Predictive Accuracy

Some test results are dichotomous (normal versus abnormal, positive versus negative) rather than continuous like a score; perfusion defects and wall motion abnormalities are examples.

Variable	Circle response	Sum
Maximal heart rate	Less than 100 bpm = 30	
	100 to 129 bpm = 24	
	130 to 159 bpm = 18	
	160 to 189 bpm = 12	
	190 to 220 bpm = 6	
Exercise ST depression	1–2mm = 15	
	>2mm = 25	
Age	>55 yrs = 20	
	40 to 55 yrs = 12	
Angina history	Definite/typical = 5	
	Probable/atypical = 3	
	Non-cardiac pain = 1	
Hypercholesterolemia?	Yes = 5	
Diabetes?	Yes = 5	
Exercise test	Occurred = 3	
induced Angina	Reason for stopping = 5	
	Total score:	

MALES

Choose only one per group

<40 = low probability

40–60 = intermediate probability

>60 = high probability

FIGURE 7–16

Calculation of the "simple" exercise test score for men. Choose only one per group.

Variable	Circle response	Sum
Maximal heart rate	Less than 100 bpm = 20	
	100 to 129 bpm = 16	
	130 to 159 bpm = 12	
	160 to 189 bpm = 8	
	190 to 220 bpm = 4	
Exercise ST depression	1–2mm = 6	
	>2mm = 10	
Age	>65 yrs = 25	
	50 to 65 yrs = 15	
Angina history	Definite/typical = 10	
	Probable/atypical = 6	
	Non-cardiac pain = 2	
Smoking?	Yes = 10	
Diabetes?	Yes = 10	
Exercise test	Occurred = 9	
induced Angina	Reason for stopping = 15	
Estrogen status	Positive = −5, negative = 5	

WOMEN

Choose only one per group

<37 = low probability

37–57 = intermediate probability

>57 = high probability

FIGURE 7–17

Calculation of the "simple" exercise test score for women. Choose only one per group.

Predictive accuracy (true positives plus true negatives divided by the total population studied) can be used to compare dichotomous test results. Any score can also be dealt with as a dichotomous variable by choosing a cutpoint. An advantage of predictive accuracy is that it provides an estimate of the number of patients correctly classified by the test out of 100 tested. The disadvantage of predictive accuracy is that it is much more dependent on disease prevalence than ROC curves. Therefore, when predictive accuracy is used to compare tests, populations with roughly the same prevalence of disease should be considered. Table 7-11 summarizes the predictive accuracy of the major diagnostic tests that are currently available for CAD.[88]

Scores Compared to Physicians

If physicians can estimate the probability of CAD and prognosis as well as the scores, there is no reason to add this complexity to test interpretation. Two early studies compared a prediction equation with clinicians. A computer algorithm for estimating probabilities of any significant coronary obstruction and triple-vessel/left main obstruction was derived, validated, and compared with the assessments of clinician cardiologists.[75] The algorithm performed at least as well as the clinicians when the latter knew the identity of the patients whose angiograms they had decided to perform. The clinicians were more accurate when they did not know the identity of the subjects but worked from tabulated objective data. It appeared that referral and societal value-induced bias affected physician judgment in assessing disease probability. The authors concluded that the application of expert systems or consultation with cardiologists not directly involved with patient management might assist in more rational assessments and decision-making. In the second seminal study, Hlatky et al[89] attempted to validate two available methods of probability calculation by comparing their diagnostic accuracy with that of cardiologists. Ninety-one cardiologists evaluated the clinical summaries of eight randomly selected patients. For each patient, the cardiologist assessed the probability of coronary heart disease after reviewing the clinical history, physical examination, and laboratory data, including an exercise test. The probability of coronary disease was also obtained for each patient using identical information from: (1) a published table of data based on age, sex, symptoms, and degree of ST-segment

Grouping	Number of studies	Total number of patients	Sensitivity	Specificity	Predictive accuracy	Medcare (rvus)
Meta analysis of standard exercise test using ST criteria alone	147	24,047	68%	77%	73%	1.8 million
Meta analysis without MI	58	11,691	67%	72%	69%	(3.3 rvu)
Meta analysis with reduced work-up bias	3	>1000	50%	90%	69%	
Meta-analysis of multivariable equations with standard exercise testing	24	11,788			80%	
Simple score	2					
Consensus	1	2000	85%	92%	88%	
Cardiokymography	1	617	71%	88%	79%	
Electron beam computed tomography	4	1631	90%	45%	68%	
Nuclear perfusion imaging	59	6038	85%	85%	85%	900,000
SPECT nuclear imaging without MI	27	2136	86%	62%	74%	(18 rvu + cost of isotope)
Persantine nuclear perfusion	11		85%	91%	87%	
Exercise ECHO	58	5000	84%	75%	80%	200,000
Exercise ECHO without MI	24	2109	87%	84%	85%	
Dobutamine ECHO	5		88%	84%	86%	(8 rvu + cost of doppler)

ECHO, echocardiography; MI, myocardial infarction.
The characteristics of the different tests can be compared because the prevalence of angiographic disease in the studies averaged at 50% (i.e., pretest probabilities were equal).

change during exercise; and (2) the Cadenza software using the age, sex, risk factors, resting ECG, and multiple exercise measurements. With the coronary angiogram as the gold standard, average diagnostic accuracy was best for the Cadenza computer program.

After carefully reading these two papers, we used our database to compare exercise test scores and ST measurements with a physician's estimation of the probability of the presence and severity of angiographically determined CAD and the risk of death.[90,91] A clinical exercise test was performed and an angiographic database was used to print patient summaries and treadmill reports. The clinical/treadmill test reports were sent to expert cardiologists and to two other groups, including randomly selected cardiologists and internists. They classified the patients summarized in the reports as having a high, low, or intermediate probability for the presence of any and also severe angiographically determined CAD using a numerical probability from 0% to 100%. The Social Security Death Index was used to determine survival status of the patients. Twenty-six percent of the patients had severe angiographically determined CAD, and the annual mortality rate of the population was 2%. Forty-five expert cardiologists returned estimates on 473 patients, 37 randomly chosen practicing cardiologists returned estimates on 202 patients, 29 randomly chosen practicing internists returned estimates on 162 patients, 13 academic cardiologists returned estimates on 145 patients, and 27 academic internists returned estimates on 272 patients. When probability estimates for presence of CAD were compared, the scores were superior in all physician groups (0.76 AUC of the ROC curve to 0.70 for experts, 0.73 to 0.58 for cardiologists, and 0.76 to 0.61 for internists). Using a probability cutpoint of greater than 70% for abnormal, predictive accuracy was 69% for scores compared with 64% for experts, 63% to 62% for cardiologists, and 70% to 57% for internists. When probability estimates for presence and severity of angiographically determined CAD were compared, in general, the treadmill scores and ST analysis were superior to that of physicians' at predicting severe angiographically determined CAD. When prognosis was estimated, treadmill prognostic scores did as well as expert cardiologists and better than most other physician groups.

This demonstrated that by using simple clinical and exercise test variables, we could improve on the standard use of ECG criteria during exercise testing for diagnosing CAD. Using the consensus approach divided the test set into populations with low, intermediate and high risk for CAD. Since the patients in the intermediate group would be sent for further testing and would eventually be correctly classified, the sensitivity of the consensus approach was 94% and the specificity was 92%. This consensus approach controls for varying disease prevalence, missing data, inconsistency in variable definition, and varying angiographic criterion for stenosis severity. The percent of correct diagnoses increased from the 70% for standard exercise ECG analysis and the 80% for multivariable predictive equations to greater than 90% correct diagnoses for the consensus approach.

The consensus approach has made population-specific logistic regression equations portable to other populations. Excellent diagnostic characteristics can be obtained using simple data and measurements. The consensus approach is best applied by utilizing a programmable calculator or a computer program (such as EXTRA) to simplify the process of calculating the probability of CAD using the three equations.

OUR STUDIES

Quantitating Exercise Testing and Angiography (QUEXTA)

QUEXTA was performed to compare the diagnostic utility of scores, measurements, and equations with that of visual ST-segment measurements in patients with reduced work-up bias.[92] Included were 814 consecutive male patients who presented with angina pectoris and agreed to undergo both exercise testing and coronary angiography. Digital ECG recorders and angiographic calipers were used for testing at each site, and test results were sent to core laboratories. Although 25% of patients had previously had testing, work-up bias was reduced, as shown by comparison with a pilot study group. This reduction resulted in a sensitivity of 45% and a specificity of 85% for visual analysis. Computerized measurements and visual analysis had similar diagnostic power. Equations incorporating non-ECG variables and either visual or computerized ST-segment measurement had similar discrimination and were superior to single ST-segment measurements. These equations correctly classified five more patients of every 100 tested (areas under the ROC curve, 0.80 for equations and 0.68 for visual analysis) in this population with a 50% prevalence of disease. It is the only one of the 150 studies evaluating the diagnostic characteristics of the exercise test to lessen work-up bias by having a protocol where patients presenting with chest pain agreed to have both procedures.

Long Beach—Palo Alto—Hungarian Multivariable Prediction Study

We performed a study to determine if computerized exercise ECG measurements could replace visual exercise ECG measurements and improve upon the discriminating power obtained from prediction equations for diagnosing angiographically determined CAD.[82] A secondary objective was to demonstrate the effects of medication status and resting ECG abnormalities on the diagnostic characteristics of the equations. It was based on a retrospective analysis of consecutive patients referred for evaluation of chest pain at two university-affiliated Veteran's Affairs Medical Centers and the Hungarian Heart Institute who underwent both exercise testing with digital recording of their exercise ECGs and coronary angiography. There were 1384 consecutive male patients, without a prior MI and who had complete data, who underwent exercise tests between 1987 and 1995. Patients with previous cardiac surgery, valvular heart disease, LBBB, or Wolff-Parkinson-White syndrome on their resting ECG were excluded from the study. Patients with a previous MI by history or by diagnostic Q wave were excluded from the diagnostic subgroup, leaving a target population of 1384 patients. Prior cardiac surgery was the predominant reason for exclusion of patients who underwent exercise testing during this time period.

The clinical variables considered were obtained from the initial history using computerized forms.[93,94] Angina during testing was classified according to the Duke Exercise Angina Index (DAP = 2 if angina required stopping the test, 1 if angina occurred during or after exercise testing, and 0 for no angina).[95] No test was classified as indeterminate,[96] medications were not withheld, and no maximal heart rate targets were applied.[97] Although all the exercise tests were performed, analyzed, and reported as per standard protocol and by utilizing a computerized database (EXTRA), the cardiac catheterization was consistent with clinical practice at each institution, and results were abstracted from clinical reports. All exercise ECG analysis and comparisons were performed blinded from clinical and angiographic results.

Three logistic regression models were developed using clinical, hemodynamic, and non-ECG variables. Then one model added visual ST measurement, a second added the best ST measurement in recovery, and the third added the best computerized ST measurement at maximal exercise. The measurements and the models were then tested in the three subpopulations, each with a different prevalence of coronary disease and a different rate of abnormal exercise tests. The results in the three subpopulations were then used to demonstrate how the prediction equations should function in different types of office practice.

The performance of visual and computerized exercise ECG measurements and the models were also assessed considering medication status and the resting ECG. The resting ECG was classified by visual criteria and also by the computer ST measurements made at rest.

Prediction Equation Development

The following three sets of intercepts, variables, and their coefficients were developed using stepwise logistic regression:

1. Prediction model equation considering visually measured ST depression:

$$0.35 + 0.05 * age - 0.3 * chest\ pain + 0.6 *$$
$$elevated\ cholesterol + 0.4 * diabetes - 0.02 *$$
$$maximal\ heart\ rate + 0.3 * DAP + 0.7 * visual$$
$$ST\ depression$$

2. Prediction model equation using the best computer measurement during recovery:

$$- 1.34 + 0.05 * age - 0.3 * chest\ pain\ symptom$$
$$+ 0.6 * elevated\ cholesterol + 0.4 * diabetes -$$
$$0.012 * maximal\ heart\ rate + 0.5 * DAP - 5.7 *$$
$$ST_{60}\ V_5\ 3.5\ min\ recovery$$

3. Prediction model equation using the best computer measurement during exercise:

$$- 3.42 + 0.6 * age - 0.3 * chest\ pain\ symptom +$$
$$0.6 * elevated\ cholesterol + 0.4 * diabetes + 0.45$$
$$* DAP - 0.50 * (ST/HR\ index * 1000)$$

Variable definitions for calculations:
Chest pain symptoms from 1 [typical] to 4 [none], DAP: 2 = angina major reason for stopping, 1 = exercise induced angina, 0 = no angina.

ST: Maximal visual ST depression in exercise or during recovery. ST was recorded in millimeters if ST depression was at least 0.5-mm horizontal or downsloping or at least 2-mm upsloping.

ST_{60} in V_5 at 3 minutes in recovery in negative millivolts.

The appropriate values are inserted into the following logistic regression formula to calculate an estimate of the probability for angiographically determined CAD:

$$\text{Probability } (0 \text{ to } 1) = 1/(1 + e^{-(a + bx + cy...)})$$

where a is the intercept, b and c are coefficients, x and y are variable values.

Prediction Equation Performance and Validation

The models were developed considering the fact that some clinicians prefer to use a maximal exercise ST measurement rather than one from recovery. For the recovery ST measurement to have the same diagnostic characteristics as it did in our study, exercise must be stopped abruptly (no cool-down walk performed) and the patient placed supine postexercise. The probabilities generated using the models were plotted as ROC curves (see Fig. 7-14) and the areas calculated (Table 7-12). There was a significant improvement in the ROC areas for each of the models when compared to the visual analysis or one of the best computer measurements. In addition, sensitivities for the models at a specificity comparable to visual criteria of 1mm (80%) were obtained from the ROC curves and tabulated. Predictive accuracy was also calculated since it represents the percentage of patients correctly classified and is a more practical measure for comparing the discriminating methods. As can be seen in Table 7-12, all three models provided similar discriminating capability and were superior to solitary ST measurements made either visually or by computer. In addition, the cutpoints

of the predicted probabilities to match the specificity of visual analysis were 0.67, 0.65, and 0.64 for the three equations. Thus, for comparison purposes, a predicted probability for coronary disease of 0.65 is a cutpoint associated with a specificity of 80% comparable to visual analysis.

Effect of Medications and Resting ECG Abnormalities

Beta-blocker administration did not affect the diagnostic characteristics of the standard visual criteria. Although digoxin lowered the specificity of the test, it was only administered to a small number of patients. LVH and resting ST depression had a similar association with a lowered specificity. T-wave inversion had a trend toward similar changes but did not affect test characteristics as much. The exclusion of all patients with resting ECG abnormalities as well as digoxin use significantly lowered sensitivity and raised specificity. The computer classification of resting ST depression confirmed the visual classification results by obtaining nearly the same sensitivity and specificity.

Population and Prevalence Effects

The percentage of patients with angiographically determined coronary occlusions of 50% or more ranged from 35% in the Hungarians to 60% of the veterans from Palo Alto and 80% in the veterans from Long Beach. Exercise test hemodynamic responses had no significant population differences after age adjustment. The cutpoints were chosen to match the specificity obtained with visual analysis (i.e., 80%). For instance, the amplitude of V_5 ST_{60} depression in recovery that had a specificity of 80% in the PAHCS patients was −0.06 mV, and the probability generated by the equation using visual

TABLE 7–12.   Comparison of three predictive equations (pe) with reference to visual analysis and the single best computer measurement (st$_{60}$ v$_5$ recovery)

	Cutpoint	Sensitivity	Specificity	Predictive accuracy	ROC area
Visual ST	1 mm	52%	79%	63%	0.67
V_5 ST_{60} 3.5 min of recovery	−0.054 mV	49%	80%	61%	0.68
PE with visual ST	0.67	61%	80%	69%	0.79
PE with recovery V_5 ST_{60} (comp)	0.65	59%	80%	68%	0.77
PE with exercise ST/HR index (comp)	0.64	59%	80%	68%	0.77

Note that the cutpoint for calculated probability of coronary artery disease averages out to be 0.65 to match the specificity obtained with simple visual analysis. PE, Predictive equation.

criteria was 64%, giving rise to an 80% specificity. Test characteristics were relatively constant over the three populations.

This comparison permitted us to estimate the effect of CAD prevalence, percentage of abnormal treadmill tests, and the varying degrees of work-up bias in the three populations on the calibration of the cutpoints of the probability scores from the models. These results suggest that the clinician should use the computed probability of coronary disease of 65% or greater as a cutpoint. This is associated with an odds of disease of three times that if the probability is less than 65%. The prediction equation cutpoint of 65% is associated with a greater OR than that of an abnormal ST response (3× versus 1.7×). In addition, the prediction equations discriminate in the patients with resting ST depression classified by computer measurement.

Effect of Medication Status and the Resting ECG

Beta-blocker administration did not affect the diagnostic characteristics of the standard visual criteria, in agreement with previous findings.[35] Digoxin lowered the specificity but it was only administered to a small number of patients. It was not clear why it was administered to many of the patients and the reason or condition for which it was prescribed could affect the ST response. LVH and visually classified resting ST depression had a similar association, with a lowered specificity, also in agreement with previous findings.[50] T-wave inversion had a trend toward similar changes but did not affect test characteristics as much. The exclusion of all patients with resting ECG abnormalities as well as those taking digoxin significantly lowered sensitivity and raised specificity. This is the first study that utilized computer classification of resting ST depression to confirm the visual classification by obtaining nearly the same sensitivity and specificity with both methods.

Multivariable Prediction of Any Coronary Artery Disease

Consistent with prior studies, age, hypercholesterolemia, maximal heart rate, and exercise-induced ST depression were significant predictors of CAD. This study differed in that patients with diabetes and angina induced by the exercise test were selected. The failure of METs to be chosen could be due to work-up bias or estimation of METs with both ergometer and treadmill. Somewhat surprising was the fact that even by forcing into the

prediction model ST measurements from both exercise and recovery, slope and depression, or multiple leads, the ROC areas could not be improved beyond those obtained with the equations listed above.

The choice of a probability level from the prediction equations has always been problematic due to population differences that result in miscalibration of the probabilities. Analysis of the subpopulations supports the recommendation that a probability cutpoint of 65% will function well in a population similar to that presenting to a practitioner. The equations also improved the diagnostic characteristics of the test in the patients with resting repolarization abnormalities, who are frequently referred to imaging modalities.

OTHER SCORING METHODS

Bayesian versus Multivariate Diagnostic Techniques

To compare the relative accuracy of Bayesian versus discriminant function, Detrano et al[98] analyzed 303 subjects referred for coronary angiography who also had exercise testing, perfusion imaging, and cine fluoroscopy. Angiographically significant disease was defined as one with at least greater than 50% occlusion of a major vessel. Four calculations were done: (1) Bayesian analysis using literature estimates of pretest probabilities, sensitivities, and specificities was applied to the clinical and test data of a randomly selected subgroup (group I, 151 patients) to calculate post-test probabilities; (2) Bayesian analysis using literature estimates of pretest probabilities (but with sensitivities and specificities derived from the remaining 152 subjects [group II]) was applied to group I data to estimate post-test probabilities; (3) a discriminant function with logistic regression coefficients derived from the clinical and test variables of group II was used to calculate post-test probabilities of group I; and (4) a discriminant function derived with the use of test results from group II and pretest probabilities from the literature was used to calculate post-test probabilities of group I. ROC curve analysis showed that all four calculations could equivalently rank the disease probabilities for our patients.

These results suggest that data-based discriminant functions are more accurate than literature-based Bayesian analysis, assuming independence in predicting coronary disease based on clinical and noninvasive test results. The accuracy of the Bayesian method is degraded by the assumption of independence and perhaps more importantly by the use of sensitivities and specificities derived from other patient populations with different testing protocols.[99,100]

Although a test may not have an important impact on disease probability in a patient, the test can be used for other purposes, such as demonstrating the severity or prognosis of a disease or the result of a therapeutic intervention. In addition, any test only gives a probability statement and how this impacts on an individual patient is greatly dependent upon the physicians' clinical judgment.

The Duke Score

The Duke treadmill score (DTS) is a composite index that was designed to provide survival estimates based on results from the exercise test. To calculate the score, five times the amount of ST-segment depression and four times the chest pain score (2 points if chest pain was the reason the test was stopped, 1 if angina occurred) is subtracted from METs. To test its potential usefulness for providing diagnostic estimates, Duke researchers used a logistic regression model to predict significant ($\geq 75\%$ stenosis) and severe (three-vessel or left main) CAD.[101] After adjustment for baseline clinical risk, the DTS was effectively diagnostic for significant and severe CAD. For low-risk patients (score $\geq +5$), 60% had no coronary stenosis and 16% had single-vessel stenosis. By comparison, 74% of high-risk patients (score < -11) had three-vessel or left main coronary disease. Five-year mortality was 3%, 10%, and 35% for low-, moderate-, and high-risk DTS groups. The AUC of the ROC curves for predicting significant CAD was 0.70 for ST deviation alone, 0.76 for the score alone, and 0.91 for the score plus clinical history prediction. It appears that the DTS provides accurate diagnostic and prognostic information for the evaluation of symptomatic patients evaluated for clinically suspected ischemic heart disease.

COMPARISON WITH OTHER DIAGNOSTIC TESTS

Nuclear Perfusion Scanning and Echocardiography

Investigators from UCSF reviewed the contemporary literature to compare the diagnostic performance of exercise echocardiography (ECHO) and exercise nuclear perfusion scanning (NUC) in the diagnosis of CAD.[102] These included studies published between January 1990 and October 1997 identified from MEDLINE search, bibliographies of reviews and original articles, and suggestions from experts in each area. Articles were included if they discussed exercise ECHO and/or exercise NUC imaging with thallium or sestamibi for detection and/or evaluation of CAD, if data on coronary angiography were presented as the reference test, and if the absolute numbers of true-positive, false-negative, true-negative, and false-positive observations were available or derivable from the data presented. Studies performed exclusively in patients after MI, after percutaneous transluminal coronary angioplasty, after coronary artery bypass grafting, or with recent unstable coronary syndromes were excluded. Two reviewers used a standardized spreadsheet to independently extract clinical variables, technical factors, and test performance. Discrepancies were resolved by consensus. Forty-four articles met inclusion criteria: 24 reported exercise ECHO results in 2637 patients with a weighted mean age of 59 years, 69% were men, 66% had CAD, and 20% had prior MI; 27 reported exercise SPECT in 3237 patients, 70% were men, 78% had CAD, and 33% had prior MI. In pooled data weighted by the sample size of each study, exercise ECHO had a sensitivity of 85% (95% CI, 83% to 87%) with a specificity of 77% (95% CI, 74% to 80%). Exercise NUC yielded a similar sensitivity of 87% (95% CI, 86% to 88%) but a lower specificity of 64% (95% CI, 60% to 68%). In a summary ROC model comparing exercise ECHO performance to exercise NUC, exercise ECHO was associated with significantly better discriminatory power when adjusted for age, publication year, and a setting including known CAD for NUC studies. In models comparing the discriminatory abilities of exercise ECHO and exercise NUC versus exercise testing without imaging, both ECHO and NUC performed significantly better than the exercise ECG.

A similar meta-analysis from DUKE of the diagnostic characteristics of exercise ECHO, which considered 58 studies performed over 15 years, has been reported in abstract form. The average sensitivity was 84% and the specificity was 75%. An earlier meta-analysis considering 59 studies of thallium perfusion obtained a mean sensitivity of 85% and a specificity of 85%,[103] suggesting that the newer SPECT technique has degraded the discriminating characteristics of perfusion imaging. The contemporary studies, however, agree that exercise ECHO (specificity of 84%) has better specificity than SPECT (specificity of 62%) but not the exercise ECG (specificity of 90%). Thus, a positive response with the exercise ECG test is more likely to rule in disease than a positive response with the other two tests.

Cardiokymography

A multicenter study has demonstrated the diagnostic accuracy of cardiokymography (CKG) recorded 2 to 3 minutes after exercise in 617 patients undergoing cardiac catheterization.[104] Of these patients, 29% had prior MI. There were 12 participating centers using a standardized protocol. Adequate CKG tracings, which were obtained in 82% of patients, were dependent on the skill of the operator and on certain patient characteristics. Of the 327 patients without prior MI who had technically adequate CKG and electrocardiographic tracings, 166 (51%) had coronary disease. Both the sensitivity and specificity of CKG (71% and 88%, respectively) were significantly greater than the values for the exercise ECG (61% and 76%, respectively). CAD and multivessel disease were present in 98% and 68%, respectively, of the 70 patients with both abnormal CKG and ECG results, and in 15% and 5%, respectively, of the 132 patients with normal results on both studies. The CKG was most helpful in those patients in whom the posttest probability of coronary disease was between 21% and 72% after the exercise ECG. In these patients, an abnormal concordantly positive CKG result increased the probability of coronary disease to between 67% and 100%, whereas a normal response decreased it to between 12% and 15%. In the subgroup of 102 patients undergoing concomitant exercise thallium testing, the sensitivity and specificity for the thallium perfusion imaging (81% and 80%, respectively) were similar to the values for CKG (72% and 84%, respectively).

To determine which subgroup of patients derive the most benefit from testing, they categorized the chest pain of the 327 patients who did not have a prior MI and were undergoing testing for the purpose of diagnosis into four symptom groups:

1. Typical angina: A history of typical angina pectoris in men was very predictive of both CAD (85%) and multivessel disease (51%). An abnormal exercise ECG increased the probability of coronary disease to 94%. In these patients, an abnormal CKG only slightly increased the probability of coronary disease (to 95%), whereas a normal

CKG was still associated with a high probability.
2. Atypical angina: 51% of these men and 33% of these women had CAD. An abnormal exercise ECG increased the probability of coronary disease to 90% in men and to 86% in women, while a negative result was associated with a probability of 27% in men and 25% in women. A normal exercise ECG in patients with atypical angina was still associated with a 37% probability of coronary disease in men and a 20% probability in women. In these patients, when the CKG was normal, the probability of coronary disease (15% in men and 12% in women) and of multivessel disease (5% in men and 3% in women) was very low.
3. Nonischemic chest pain: Of 43 patients, 24% had coronary disease and 7% had multivessel disease. An abnormal ST response resulted in a 45% probability of coronary disease, while a negative ECG result was associated with a 17% probability. In the 14 patients with an abnormal exercise ECG, a positive CKG response increased the probability of coronary disease to 80%. In the 30 patients with negative ECG, a negative CKG response, which was present in 26 patients, lowered the probability to 8% and none had multivessel disease.
4. Asymptomatic: This group had too few individuals for analysis.

This study confirmed that CKG performed during exercise testing improves the diagnostic accuracy of the ECG response and is a cost-effective indicator of myocardial ischemia. Unfortunately, this device is no longer available commercially. The technical skills and need for breath-holding after exercise were impediments in the widespread acceptance of this procedure, but failure to obtain generalized reimbursement is the more likely explanation. Several German companies have resolved some of the difficulties by signal averaging and using multiple transducers.

A total of 171 consecutive patients were examined with the newly developed German CKG device capable of recording signal-averaged precordial impulses during supine bicycle exercise in combination with exercise ECG.[105] All patients had undergone coronary angiography within the past 3 months. ECG criteria for CAD was typical ST depression; CKG criteria for ischemia was late or holosystolic bulging (type 2 or type 3).

Eight patients were excluded because of inadequate quality of their CKG-recording. There were 163 patients (144 men and 19 women, mean age 55 years) in the study. The overall sensitivity of the exercise CKG for a significant stenosis was 61%, the specificity was 77%, and almost the same results were obtained with the ECG. The combination of CKG and ECG testing improved overall sensitivity to 89%, specificity 59%. Combined CKG-ECG testing was superior to exercise ECG alone, particularly in patients with stenoses in the left anterior descending coronary artery. The device used has not become commercially available.

Biomarkers

The latest add-on to exercise testing in an attempt to improve its characteristics are biomarkers. The first and most logical biomarker evaluated to detect ischemia brought about by exercise was troponin. Unfortunately, it has been shown that even in patients who develop ischemia during exercise testing, serum elevations in cardiac-specific troponins do not occur, demonstrating that myocardial damage does not occur.[106,107] B-type natriuretic peptide (BNP) which is released by myocardial stretching also appears to be released by myocardial hypoxia. Armed with this knowledge, investigators have reported the following studies.

Foote et al[108] examined the effect of exercise-induced ischemia on levels of BNP and its inactive N-terminal fragment (NT-pro-BNP) to determine whether measurement of these peptides could improve the diagnostic accuracy of exercise testing. A total of 74 patients with known CAD, normal left ventricular function, and normal resting levels of NT-pro-BNP and BNP referred for exercise testing with radionuclide imaging, and 21 healthy volunteers, were enrolled. Blood was drawn before and after maximal exercise and analyzed for NT-pro-BNP and BNP. Of the patients with CAD, 40 had ischemia on perfusion images and 34 did not. Median postexercise increases in NT-pro-BNP and BNP (DeltaNT-pro-BNP and DeltaBNP) were approximately fourfold higher in the ischemic group than in the nonischemic group. In volunteers, median DeltaNT-pro-BNP was almost identical to that of the nonischemic patient group. At equal specificity to ST depression (60%), the sensitivities of DeltaNT-pro-BNP and DeltaBNP for detecting ischemia were 90% and 80%, respectively; in contrast, the sensitivity of the exercise ECG was 38%.

Thus, measurement of exercise-induced increases in BNPs doubled the sensitivity of the exercise test for detecting ischemia with no loss of specificity.

Sabatine et al[109] reported the effect of transient myocardial ischemia on circulating natriuretic peptide levels. BNP, its N-terminal fragment (NT-pro-BNP), and N-terminal fragment of atrial natriuretic peptide pro-hormone (NT-pro-ANP) levels were measured in 112 patients before, immediately after, and 4 hours after exercise testing with nuclear perfusion imaging. Baseline levels of BNP were associated with the subsequent severity of perfusion defects, with median levels of 43, 62, and 101 pg/ml in patients with none, mild-to-moderate, and severe inducible ischemia, respectively. Immediately after exercise, the median increase in BNP was 14 pg/ml in patients with mild-to-moderate ischemia and 24 pg/ml in those with severe ischemia. In contrast, BNP levels only rose by 2.3 pg/ml in those who did not develop ischemia. A similar relationship was seen between baseline NT-pro-BNP levels and inducible ischemia, but the changes in response to ischemia were less pronounced. NT-pro-BNP levels rose with exercise in both ischemic and nonischemic patients. When added to traditional clinical predictors of ischemia, a postexercise test BNP equaling 80 pg/ml or more remained a strong and independent predictor of inducible myocardial ischemia (OR 3). Thus, exercise testing was associated with an immediate rise in circulating BNP levels, and the magnitude of rise was proportional to the severity of ischemia. Furthermore, baseline differences in BNP were noted proportional to the level of ischemia induced by the test.

The point-of-contact analysis techniques available for these assays involves a hand-held battery-powered unit that uses a replaceable cartridge. Finger stick blood samples are adequate for analyses and the results are available immediately. If validated using appropriate study design (similar to QUEXTA), biomarker measurements could greatly improve the standard office/clinic exercise test.

Electron Beam Computed Tomography

One hundred sixty men and women with coronary disease aged 45 to 62 years (138 had obstructive CAD and 22 had normal coronary arteries) and 56 age-matched healthy control subjects underwent double-helix CT.[110] Double-helix CT findings indicated that calcification was significantly more prevalent in patients with CAD (>83%) than in patients with normal coronary arteries (27%) or in healthy control subjects (34%). Sensitivity in detecting obstructive CAD was high (91%); however, specificity was low (52%) because of calcification in nonobstructive lesions.

Using the volume mode of electron beam computed tomography (EBCT), 251 consecutive patients who underwent elective coronary angiography because of suspected CAD disease had their results compared with those of ECG and nuclear perfusion tests.[111] Calcification was first noted in women in the 4th decade of life, approximately 10 years later than its occurrence in men. Nine percent of patients with significant stenoses had no calcification. A cut-off calcification score for prediction of significant stenosis, determined by ROC curve analysis, showed high sensitivity (≥0.77) and specificity (0.86) in all study patients; sensitivity was similarly high even in older patients (≥70 years) and was enhanced in middle-aged patients (40 to ≤60 years).

A multicenter investigational study studied the relative prognostic value of coronary calcific deposits and coronary angiographic findings for predicting coronary heart disease-related events in patients referred for angiography.[112] Four hundred ninety-one symptomatic patients underwent coronary angiography and EBCT at five different centers between 1989 and 1993. A cardiologist with no knowledge of the coronary angiographic and clinical data interpreted the EBCTs. ROC curves were constructed to determine the relation between EBCT and coronary angiographic findings. The AUC of the ROC curve was 0.75 for the coronary calcium score, indicating moderate discriminatory power for this score for predicting angiographic findings. In this group, sensitivity of any detectable calcification by EBCT as an indicator of significant stenosis (>50% narrowing) was 92% and specificity 43%. When these CT images were reinterpreted in a blinded and standardized manner, however, specificity was only 31%.

In another multicenter study[113] of 710 enrolled patients, 427 had significant angiographic disease, and coronary calcification was detected in 404, yielding a sensitivity of 95%. Of the 23 patients without calcification, 83% had single-vessel disease on angiography. Of the 283 patients without angiographically significant disease, 124 had negative EBCT studies for a specificity of 44%.

Thus, three of the four studies demonstrated a high sensitivity and a low specificity with a predictive accuracy of about 68%. Although adjusting the cutpoint for calcium density can alter the sensitivity and specificity, the EBCT is not diagnostically superior for angiographically significant CAD compared to the standard exercise test.

THE ACC/AHA GUIDELINES FOR DIAGNOSTIC USE OF THE STANDARD EXERCISE TEST

The task force to establish guidelines for the use of exercise testing has met and produced guidelines in 1986, 1997, and 2002. The 1997 publication had some dramatic changes from the first publication, including the recommendation that the standard exercise test be the first diagnostic procedure in women and in most patients with resting ECG abnormalities, rather than performing imaging studies. The 2002 update added two items to class I indications. The following is a synopsis of these evidence-based guidelines.

Class I (Definitely Appropriate)

Conditions for which there is evidence and/or general agreement that the standard exercise test is useful and helpful for the diagnosis of CAD.

1. Adult male or female patients (including those with complete right bundle branch block or with <1mm of resting ST depression) with an *intermediate pretest probability* (Table 7-13) of CAD based on gender, age, and symptoms (specific exceptions are noted under class II and III, discussed in the following sections).
2. Patients with suspected or known CAD, previously evaluated, now presenting with significant change in clinical status.
3. Low-risk unstable angina (USA) patients 8 to 12 hours after presentation who have been free of active ischemic or chronic heart failure symptoms (level of evidence: B).
4. Intermediate-risk USA patients 2 to 3 days after presentation who have been free of active ischemic or chronic heart failure symptoms (level of evidence: B).

Class IIa (Probably Appropriate). Conditions for which there is conflicting evidence and/or a divergence of opinion that the standard exercise test is useful and helpful for diagnosis but the weight of evidence for usefulness or efficacy is in favor of the exercise test.

1. Intermediate-risk USA patients who have initial cardiac markers that are normal,

TABLE 7–13.   Pretest probability of coronary artery disease by symptoms, gender, and age

Age	Gender	Typical/definite angina pectoris	Atypical/probable angina pectoris	Nonanginal chest pain	Asymptomatic
30–39	Males	Intermediate	Intermediate	Low (<10%)	Very low (<5%)
	Females	Intermediate	Very low (<5%)	Very low	Very low
40–49	Males	High	Intermediate	Intermediate	Low
	Females	Intermediate	Low	Very low	Very low
50–59	Males	High (>90%)	Intermediate	Intermediate	Low
	Females	Intermediate	Intermediate	Low	Very low
60–69	Males	High	Intermediate	Intermediate	Low
	Females	High	Intermediate	Intermediate	Low

High = >90% Intermediate = 10–90% Low = <10% Very low = <5%
There is no data for patients younger than 30 or older than 69 but it can be assumed that coronary artery disease prevalence is directly related to age.

unchanged repeat ECG, cardiac markers that are normal for up to 12 hours, and no other evidence of ischemia (level of evidence: B).
2. Patients with vasospastic angina (see Chapter 6, page 12)

Class IIb (Maybe Appropriate). Conditions for which there is conflicting evidence and/or a divergence of opinion that the standard exercise test is useful and helpful *for the diagnosis of CAD* but the usefulness/efficacy is less well established.

1. Patients taking digoxin with less than 1mm of baseline ST depression.
2. Patients with the following ECG abnormalities:

- Wolff-Parkinson-White syndrome
- Electronic pacing
- 1 mm or less ST depression
- Complete LBBB or any intraventricular conduction delay of greater than 120 msec

3. Patients with stable clinical course who undergo periodic monitoring to guide therapy.
4. Patients with a low pretest probability of CAD by age, symptoms, and gender.

Class III (Not Appropriate). Conditions for which there is evidence and/or general agreement that the standard exercise test is not useful or helpful for the diagnosis of CAD, and in some cases may be harmful.

1. The use of ST segment response for the diagnosis of CAD in patients who demonstrate the following baseline ECG abnormalities:

- Pre-excitation (Wolff-Parkinson-White) syndrome

- Electronically paced ventricular rhythm;
- More than 1mm of resting ST depression;
- Complete LBBB (see Chapter 6, page 25)

2. Patients with comorbidities likely to limit life expectancy and candidacy for interventions
3. High-risk USA patients (level of evidence: C)

IMMEDIATE MANAGEMENT OF ACUTE CORONARY SYNDROME (ACS) PATIENTS

The exercise test has been recommended as part of the diagnostic work-up of selected patients with ACS. The 2002 guidelines list the following:

Recommendations

Class I

1. The history, physical examination, 12-lead ECG, and initial cardiac marker tests should be integrated to assign patients with chest pain into 1 of 4 categories: a noncardiac diagnosis, chronic stable angina, possible ACS, and definite ACS. (level of evidence: C)
2. Patients with definite or possible ACS, but whose initial 12-lead ECG and cardiac marker levels are normal, should be observed in a facility with cardiac monitoring (e.g., chest pain unit), and a repeat ECG and cardiac marker measurement should be obtained 6 to 12 hours after the onset of symptoms. (level of evidence: B)
3. *Patients in whom ischemic heart disease is present or suspected, if the follow-up 12-lead ECG and cardiac marker measurements*

are normal, a stress test (exercise or pharmacological) to provoke ischemia may be performed in the Emergency Department- (ED), in a chest pain unit, or on an outpatient basis shortly after discharge. Low-risk patients with a negative stress test can be managed as outpatients. (level of evidence: C)

4. Patients with definite ACS and ongoing pain, positive cardiac markers, new ST-segment deviations, new deep T-wave inversions, hemodynamic abnormalities, or a positive stress test should be admitted to the hospital for further management. (level of evidence: C)

5. Patients with possible ACS and negative cardiac markers who are unable to exercise or who have an abnormal resting ECG should undergo a pharmacological stress test. (level of evidence: B)

6. Patients with definite ACS and ST-segment elevation should be evaluated for immediate reperfusion therapy. (level of evidence: A)

By integrating information from the history, physical examination, 12-lead ECG, and initial cardiac marker tests, clinicians can assign patients into 1 of 4 categories: noncardiac diagnosis, chronic stable angina, possible ACS, and definite ACS (Fig. 7-18).

Patients who arrive at a medical facility in a pain-free state, have unchanged or normal ECGs, are hemodynamically stable, and do not have elevated cardiac markers represent more of a diagnostic than an urgent therapeutic challenge. Evaluation begins in these patients by obtaining information from the history, physical examination, and ECG (Tables 7-14 and 7-15), which can be used to confirm or reject the diagnosis of USA or non-ST elevation MI.

Patients with a low likelihood of CAD should be evaluated for other causes of the presentation, including musculoskeletal pain; gastrointestinal disorders, such as esophageal spasm, gastritis, peptic ulcer disease, or cholecystitis; intrathoracic disease, such as pneumonia, pleurisy, pneumothorax, or pericarditis; and neuropsychiatric disease, such as hyperventilation or panic disorder. Patients who are found to have evidence of one of these alternative diagnoses should be excluded from management with these guidelines and referred for appropriate follow-up care. Reassurance should be balanced with instructions to return for further evaluation if symptoms worsen or if the patient fails to respond to symptomatic treatment.

Chronic stable angina may also be diagnosed in this setting, and patients with this diagnosis should be managed according to the ACC/AHA/ACP-ASIM Guidelines for the Management of Patients With Chronic Stable Angina.[114]

Patients with possible ACS (B3 and D1) are candidates for additional observation in a specialized facility (e.g., chest pain unit) (E1). Patients with definite ACS (B4) are triaged based on the pattern of the 12-lead ECG. Patients with ST-segment elevation (C3) are evaluated for immediate reperfusion therapy (D3) and managed according to the ACC/AHA Guidelines for the Management of Patients With Acute Myocardial Infarction, whereas those without ST-segment elevation (C2) are either managed by additional observation (E1) or admitted to the hospital (H3). Patients with low-risk ACS (see Table 7-14) without transient ST-segment depressions of greater than or equal to 0.05 mV and/or T-wave inversions of greater than or equal to 0.2 mV, *without* positive cardiac markers, and without a positive stress test (H1) may be discharged and treated as outpatients (I1).

Chest Pain Units

To facilitate a more definitive evaluation while avoiding the unnecessary hospital admission of patients with possible ACS (B3) and low-risk ACS (F1), and the inappropriate discharge of patients with active myocardial ischemia without ST-segment elevation (C2), special units have been devised that are variously referred to as "chest pain units" and "short-stay ED coronary care units." Personnel in these units use critical pathways or protocols designed to arrive at a decision about the presence or absence of myocardial ischemia and, if present, to characterize it further as USA or non-ST elevation MI and to define the optimal next step in the care of the patient (e.g., admission, acute intervention).[115] The goal is to arrive at such a decision after a finite amount of time, which usually is between 6 and 12 hours but may extend up to 24 hours depending on the policies in individual hospitals. Although chest pain units are useful, other appropriate observation areas in which patients with chest pain can be evaluated may be used as well.

The physical location of the chest pain unit or site where patients with chest pain are observed is variable, ranging from a specifically designated area of the ED to a separate unit with the appropriate equipment.[116] Similarly, the chest pain unit may be administratively a part of the ED and staffed by emergency physicians or may be administered and

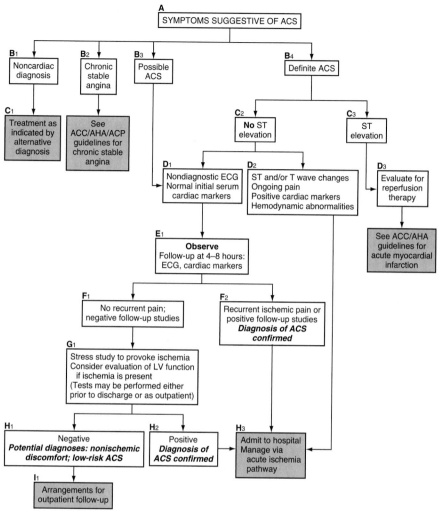

A
SYMPTOMS SUGGESTIVE OF ACS

B₁ Noncardiac diagnosis

B₂ Chronic stable angina

B₃ Possible ACS

B₄ Definite ACS

C₁ Treatment as indicated by alternative diagnosis

See ACC/AHA/ACP guidelines for chronic stable angina

C₂ **No** ST elevation

C₃ ST elevation

D₁ Nondiagnostic ECG Normal initial serum cardiac markers

D₂ ST and/or T wave changes Ongoing pain Positive cardiac markers Hemodynamic abnormalities

D₃ Evaluate for reperfusion therapy

See ACC/AHA guidelines for acute myocardial infarction

E₁ **Observe** Follow-up at 4–8 hours: ECG, cardiac markers

F₁ No recurrent pain; negative follow-up studies

F₂ Recurrent ischemic pain or positive follow-up studies *Diagnosis of ACS confirmed*

G₁ Stress study to provoke ischemia Consider evaluation of LV function if ischemia is present (Tests may be performed either prior to discharge or as outpatient)

H₁ Negative *Potential diagnoses: nonischemic discomfort; low-risk ACS*

H₂ Positive *Diagnosis of ACS confirmed*

H₃ Admit to hospital Manage via acute ischemia pathway

I₁ Arrangements for outpatient follow-up

■ **FIGURE 7–18**
ACC/AHA flow diagram for the management of patients with ACS.

staffed separately. Suggestions for the design of chest pain units have been presented by several authoritative bodies and generally include provisions for continuous monitoring of the patient's ECG, ready availability of cardiac resuscitation equipment and medications, and appropriate staffing with nurses and physicians. Given the evolving nature of the field and the recent introduction of chest pain units into clinical medicine, the American College of Emergency Physicians (ACEP) has published guidelines that recommend a program for the continuous monitoring of outcomes of patients evaluated in such units as well as the impact on hospital resources.[117] A Consensus Panel statement from ACEP emphasized that chest

pain units should be considered one part of a multifaceted program that also includes efforts to minimize patient delays in seeking medical care and delays in the ED itself.

Several groups have studied the impact of chest pain units on the care of patients with chest pain who present to the ED. It has been reported, both from studies with historical controls and from randomized trials, that the use of chest pain units is cost saving compared with an in-hospital evaluation to "rule-out MI."[118,119]

A common clinical practice is to minimize the chance of "missing" an MI in a patient with chest discomfort by admitting to the hospital *all* patients with suspected ACS and by obtaining serial

TABLE 7–14.   Likelihood that signs and symptoms represent an acute coronary syndrome secondary to coronary artery disease (CAD)

Feature	High likelihood _any of the following features:_	Intermediate likelihood _absence of high-likelihood features and presence of any of the following features:_	Low likelihood _absence of high- or intermediate-likelihood features but may have:_
History	Chest or left arm pain or discomfort as chief symptom reproducing prior documented angina Known history of CAD, including MI	Chest or left arm pain or discomfort as chief symptom Age >70 years Male sex Diabetes mellitus	Probable ischemic symptoms in absence of any of the intermediate likelihood characteristics Recent cocaine use
Examination	Transient MR, hypotension, diaphoresis, pulmonary edema, or rales	Extracardiac vascular disease	Chest discomfort reproduced by palpation
ECG	New, or presumably new, transient ST-segment deviation ($\geq$0.05 mV) or T-wave inversion ($\geq$0.2 mV) with symptoms	Fixed Q waves Abnormal ST segments or T waves not documented to be new	T-wave flattening or inversion in leads with dominant R waves Normal ECG
Cardiac markers	Elevated cardiac TnI, TnT, or CK-MB	Normal	Normal

From Braunwald E, Mark DB, Jones RH, et al: Unstable angina: Diagnosis and management. Rockville, MD, Agency for Health Care Policy and Research and the National Heart, Lung, and Blood Institute, US Public Health Service, US Department of Health and Human Services; 1994; AHCPR Publication No. 94-0602.

12-lead ECGs and biochemical cardiac marker measurements to either exclude or confirm the diagnosis of MI. Such a practice typically results in a low percentage of admitted patients actually being confirmed to have an MI. Given the inverse relationship between the percentage of patients with a "rule-out MI evaluation" and the "MI miss rate," the potential cost savings of a chest pain unit varies depending on the practice pattern for the disposition of chest pain patients at individual hospitals. Hospitals with a high admission rate of low-risk patients to "rule-out MI" (70% to 80%) will experience the largest cost savings by implementing a chest pain unit approach but will have the smallest impact on the number of missed MI patients. In contrast, hospitals with relatively low admission rates of such patients (30% to 40%) will experience greater improvements in the quality of care because fewer MI patients will be missed but will have a smaller impact on costs because of the low baseline admission rate.

Potential Expansion of the Use of Chest Pain Units for Intermediate-Risk Patients

Farkouh et al[120] extended the use of a chest pain unit in a separate portion of the ED to include patients at an intermediate risk of adverse clinical outcome based on the previously published Agency for Health Care Policy and Research guidelines for the management of USA (see Table 7-14). They reported a 46% reduction in the ultimate need for hospital admission in intermediate-risk patients after a median stay of 9.2 hours in the chest pain unit. Extension of the use of chest pain units to intermediate-risk patients in an effort to reduce inpatient costs is facilitated by making available diagnostic testing modalities, such as treadmill testing and stress imaging (ECHO or NUC), 7 days a week.[121]

Triage of Patients

Patients with chest discomfort for whom a specific diagnosis cannot be made after a review of the history, physical examination, initial 12-lead ECG, and biochemical cardiac marker data should undergo a more definitive evaluation. Several categories of patients should be considered according to the algorithm shown in Figure 7-18:

- Patients with possible ACS (B3) are those who had a recent episode of chest discomfort at rest, not entirely typical of ischemia, but are pain free when initially evaluated, have a normal or unchanged ECG, and have no elevations of cardiac markers.
- Patients with a recent episode of typical ischemic discomfort that either is of new onset or severe or exhibits an accelerating

TABLE 7–15.   Short-term risk of death or nonfatal myocardial infarction (MI) in patients with unstable angina (ua)*

Feature	High risk *at least one of the following features must be present:*	Intermediate risk *no high-risk feature but must have one of the following features:*	Low risk *no high- or intermediate-risk feature but may have any of the following features:*
History	Accelerating tempo of ischemic symptoms in preceding 48 hr	Prior MI, peripheral or cerebrovascular disease, or CABG, prior aspirin use	
Character of pain	Prolonged ongoing (>20 min) rest pain	Prolonged (>20 min) rest angina, now resolved, with moderate or high likelihood of CAD Rest angina (<20 min) or relieved with rest or sublingual NTG	New-onset or progressive CCS Class III or IV angina in the past 2 weeks without prolonged (>20 min) rest pain but with moderate or high likelihood of CAD (see Table 7-14)
Clinical findings	Pulmonary edema, most likely due to ischemia New or worsening MR murmur S_3 or new/worsening rales Hypotension, bradycardia, tachycardia Age >75 years	Age >70 years	
ECG	Angina at rest with transient ST-segment changes >0.05 mV Bundle branch block, new or presumed new Sustained ventricular tachycardia	T-wave inversions >0.2 mV Pathological Q waves	Normal or unchanged ECG during an episode of chest discomfort
Cardiac markers	Elevated (e.g., TnT or TnI >0.1 ng/mL)	Slightly elevated (e.g., TnT >0.01 but <0.1 ng/mL)	Normal

*Estimation of the short-term risks of death and nonfatal cardiac ischemic events in UA is a complex multivariable problem that cannot be fully specified in a table such as this; therefore, this table is meant to offer general guidance and illustration rather than rigid algorithms. CABG, coronary artery bypass graft; CAD, coronary artery disease; CCS, Canadian Cardiovascular Society; NTG, nitroglycerin.
From AHCPR Clinical Practice Guideline No. 10, Unstable Angina: Diagnosis and Management, May 1994. Braunwald E, Mark DB, Jones RH, et al: Unstable angina: Diagnosis and management. Rockville, MD, Agency for Health Care Policy and Research and the National Heart, Lung, and Blood Institute, US Public Health Service, US Department of Health and Human Services; 1994; AHCPR Publication No. 94-0602.

pattern of previous stable angina (especially if it has occurred at rest or is within 2 weeks of a previously documented MI) should initially be considered to have a "definite ACS" (B4). However, such patients may be at a low risk if their ECG obtained at presentation has no diagnostic abnormalities and the initial serum cardiac markers (especially cardiac-specific troponins) are normal (C2 and D1). As indicated in the algorithm, patients with either "possible ACS" (B3) or "definite ACS" (B4), but with nondiagnostic ECG and normal initial cardiac markers (D1), are candidates for additional observation in the ED or in a specialized area such as a chest pain unit (E1). In contrast, patients who present without ST-segment elevation but have features indicative of active ischemia (ongoing pain, ST-segment and/or T-wave changes,

positive cardiac markers, or hemodynamic instability) (D2) should be admitted to the hospital (H3).

Discharge from ED or Chest Pain Unit

The initial assessment of whether a patient has USA or non-ST elevation MI and which triage option is most suitable generally should be made immediately on the patient's arrival at a medical facility. Rapid assessment of a patient's candidacy for additional observation can be accomplished based on the status of the symptoms, ECG findings, and serum cardiac marker measurements. Patients who experience recurrent ischemic discomfort, evolve abnormalities on a follow-up 12-lead ECG or cardiac marker measurements, or develop hemodynamic abnormalities, such as new or worsening congestive heart failure (CHF) (D2), should be admitted to the hospital (H3).

Patients who are pain free, have either a normal or nondiagnostic ECG or one that is unchanged from previous tracings, and have a normal set of initial cardiac marker measurements are candidates for further evaluation to screen for nonischemic discomfort (B1) versus a low-risk ACS (D1). If the patient is low risk and does not experience any further ischemic discomfort and a follow-up 12-lead ECG and cardiac marker measurements after 6 to 8 hours of observation are normal (F1), the patient may be considered for an early stress test to provoke ischemia (G1). This test can be performed before the discharge and should be supervised by an experienced physician. Alternatively, the patient may be discharged and return for a stress test as an outpatient within 3 days. The exact nature of the stress test may vary depending on the patient's ability to exercise on either a treadmill or bicycle and the local expertise in a given hospital setting (e.g., availability of different testing modalities at different times of the day or different days of the week). Patients who are capable of exercise and are free of confounding features on the baseline ECG, such as bundle branch block, LVH, or paced rhythms, can be evaluated with routine symptom-limited conventional exercise stress testing. Patients who are incapable of exercise or who have an uninterpretable baseline ECG should be considered for pharmacological stress testing with either nuclear perfusion imaging or two-dimensional ECHO. Because left ventricular function is so integrally related to prognosis and heavily affects therapeutic options, strong consideration should be given to the assessment of left ventricular function with ECHO or radionuclide ventriculography in patients with documented ischemia. In sites at which stress tests are not available, low-risk patients may be discharged and the test scheduled within 3 days.

Patients who develop recurrent pain during observation or in whom the follow-up studies (12-lead ECG, cardiac markers) show new abnormalities (F2) should be admitted to the hospital (H3).

Because continuity of care is important in the overall management of patients with a chest pain syndrome, the patient's primary physician (if not involved in the care of the patient during the initial episode) should be notified of the results of the evaluation and should receive a copy of the relevant test results. Patients with a noncardiac diagnosis and those with low risk or possible ACS with a negative stress test should be counseled to make an appointment with their primary care physician as outpatients for further investigation into the cause of their symptoms (I1). They should be seen by a physician within 72 hours of discharge from the ED or chest pain unit.

Patients with possible ACS (B3) and those with a definite ACS but a nondiagnostic ECG and normal biochemical cardiac markers when they are initially seen (D1) at institutions without a chest pain unit (or equivalent facility), should be admitted to an inpatient unit. The inpatient unit to which such patients are to be admitted should have the same provisions for continuous ECG monitoring, availability of resuscitation equipment, and staffing arrangements as described earlier for the design of chest pain units.

Studies published since the guidelines include the excellent review from the Davis Group[122] and the following. At Mayo Clinic a study was performed to assess the outcome of patients discharged with a diagnosis of chest pain of undetermined origin and to identify predisposing factors for further cardiac events.[123] Patient records from 1985 through 1992 were reviewed for the occurrence of adverse cardiac events and subsequent ED visits for recurrent chest pain within 12 months of discharge. Associations between patient characteristics and an adverse cardiac event were evaluated univariately and summarized by using odds ratios (ORs). Long-term mortality was also determined. Among 1973 admitted ED patients with chest pain, 230 were given a diagnosis of chest pain of undetermined origin. Ten (4.4%) of 230 patients experienced an adverse cardiac event. Factors significantly associated with an adverse cardiac event included an abnormal ECG on admission (OR 10×), pre-existing diabetes mellitus (OR 7×), and pre-existing CAD (OR 28×). Thirty-three (14%) patients returned to the ED within 12 months of discharge; five patients were given a diagnosis of a cardiac condition, and five were given a diagnosis of a gastrointestinal condition. In long-term follow-up, 46 patients died, with a mean time of 6.1 years from hospital discharge to death due to any cause and an estimated 5-year survival of 91.4%. They found that patients discharged from the hospital with a diagnosis of chest pain of undetermined origin, those with an initial abnormal ECG, pre-existing diabetes, or pre-existing CAD are at higher risk of a subsequent adverse cardiac event. In the absence of such factors, cardiac outcome is excellent.

The belief that chest pain relief with nitroglycerin indicates the presence of active CAD is common and often used in the ED.[124] To define the diagnostic and prognostic value of chest pain relief with nitroglycerin, a prospective observational cohort study was performed in an urban community teaching hospital. There were 459 consecutive patients with chest pain admitted through the ED who received nitroglycerin from emergency services personnel or an ED nurse. Follow-up was obtained by telephone contact at 4 months. Chest pain relief was defined as a decrease of at least 50% in patients' self-reported pain within 5 minutes of the initial dose of sublingual or spray nitroglycerin. Active CAD was defined as any elevated serum enzyme level, coronary angiography demonstrating a 70% or greater stenosis, or a positive exercise test result. Nitroglycerin relieved chest pain in 39% of patients (181 of 459). In patients with active CAD as the likely cause of their chest pain, 35% (49 of 141) had chest pain relief with nitroglycerin. In contrast, in patients without CAD, 41% (113 of 275) had chest pain relief ($P > 0.2$). Four-month clinical outcomes were similar in patients with or without chest pain relief with nitroglycerin ($P > 0.2$). These data suggest that, in a general population admitted for chest pain, relief of pain after nitroglycerin treatment does not predict active CAD and should not be used to guide diagnosis.

A Spanish group reported 701 consecutive patients evaluated by clinical history (chest pain score and risk factors), ECG, troponin I, and early (< 24 hours) exercise testing in low-risk patients ($n = 165$) in the ED.[125] A composite endpoint (recurrent USA, acute MI, or cardiac death) was recorded during hospital stay or in ambulatory care settings for patients discharged after early exercise testing and occurred in 122 patients (17%). Multivariate analysis identified the following predictors: chest pain score equaling 11 points or more (OR = 2×), age equal to or greater than 68 (OR 2×), insulin-dependent diabetes mellitus (OR 2×), a history of coronary surgery (OR 3×), ST-segment depression (OR 2×) and troponin I elevation (OR 1.6×). ST-segment depression produced a high endpoint increase (31% versus 13%). Troponin I elevation increased the risk in the subgroup without ST-segment depression (20% versus 11%) but did not further modify the risk in the subgroup with ST depression. Nevertheless, the negative ECG and troponin I subgroup showed a non-negligible endpoint rate. Finally, no patient with a negative exercise test presented events compared to 7% of those with a non-negative test (RR 2.5×). They concluded that ED evaluation of chest pain should not focus on a single parameter; on the contrary, the clinical history, ECG, troponin, and early exercise testing must be globally analyzed.

From the Prince Charles Hospital, Australia comes a clinical audit of 630 consecutive patients who presented to the ED in 2001 with chest pain and intermediate-risk features.[126] They applied the Accelerated Chest Pain Assessment Protocol, as advocated by the "Management of unstable angina guidelines—2000" from the National Heart Foundation and the Cardiac Society of Australia and New Zealand. Four hundred nine patients (65%) were reclassified as low risk and discharged at a mean of 14 hours after assessment in the chest pain unit. None had missed MIs, while three (1%) had cardiac events by 6 months (all elective revascularization procedures). Another 110 patients (17%) were reclassified as high risk, and 21 (19%) of these had cardiac events (mainly revascularizations) by 6 months. Patients who were unable to exercise or had nondiagnostic exercise tests (equivocal risk) had an intermediate cardiac event rate (8%).

The Davis group has described their use of immediate exercise testing to evaluate a large, heterogeneous group of low-risk patients presenting with chest pain.[127] Patients presenting to the ED with chest pain compatible with a cardiac origin and clinical evidence of low risk on initial assessment underwent immediate exercise treadmill testing in our chest pain evaluation unit. Indicators of low clinical risk included no evidence of hemodynamic instability, arrhythmias, or ECG signs of ischemia. Serial measurements of cardiac injury markers were not obtained. Exercise testing was performed to a sign- or symptom-limited endpoint in 1000 patients (520 men, 480 women; age range 31 to 82 years) and was positive for ischemia in 13%, negative in 64%, and nondiagnostic in 23% of patients. There were no adverse effects of exercise testing, and all patients with a negative exercise test were discharged directly from the ED. At 30-day follow-up there was no mortality in any of the three groups. Cardiac events in the three groups included: negative group, 1 non-Q-wave MI; positive group, 4 non-Q-wave MIs, and 12 myocardial revascularizations; nondiagnostic group, 7 myocardial revascularizations.

SUMMARY OF THE DIAGNOSTIC UTILIZATION OF EXERCISE TESTING

It is appropriate to compare the newer diagnostic modalities with the standard exercise test, since it is a mature, established technology. The equipment and personnel for performing it are readily available. Exercise testing equipment is relatively inexpensive so that replacement or updating is not a major limitation. The test can be performed in the doctor's office and does not require injections or exposure to radiation. It can be an extension of the medical history and physical exam, providing more than simply diagnostic information. Furthermore, it can determine the degree of disability and impairment to quality of life as well as be the first step in rehabilitation and altering a major risk factor (physical inactivity).

Some of the newer add-ons or substitutes for the exercise test have the advantage of being able to localize ischemia as well as diagnose coronary disease when the baseline ECG negates ST analysis (1mm ST depression, LBBB, Wolff-Parkinson-White syndrome). In addition, nonexercise stress techniques permit diagnostic assessment of patients unable to exercise. Although the newer technologies appear to have better diagnostic characteristics, this is not always the case, particularly when more than the ST segments from the exercise test are used in scores.

Test evaluation has been advanced and so we are now in a better position to evaluate studies of test characteristics. A number of researchers have applied these guidelines along with meta-analysis to come to consensus on the diagnostic characteristics of the available tests for angiographically significant CAD. Table 7-11 presents some of the results from meta-analysis and from multicenter studies. Since sensitivity and specificity are inversely related and altered by the chosen cutpoint for normal/abnormal, the predictive accuracy (percentage of patients correctly classified as normal and abnormal) is a convenient way to compare tests. For instance, while the sensitivity and specificity for ST-segment depression during exercise testing and EBCT are nearly opposite, the predictive accuracies of the tests are similar. This means that altering their cutpoints (i.e., lowering the amount of ST-segment depression or raising the calcium score) would result in similar sensitivities and specificities. Because predictive accuracy can be thought of as the number of individuals correctly classified out of 100 tested, simply subtracting predictive accuracies provides an estimate of how many more patients are classified by substituting one test for another. Predictive accuracy is affected by disease prevalence, so comparisons are only valid in populations with the same disease prevalence.

Although the nonexercise stress tests are very useful, the results shown below are probably better than their actual performance because of patient selection. The results of the CKG multicenter study are included because of its excellent design. To evaluate diagnostic characteristics, patients with a prior MI should be excluded since the diagnosis of coronary disease is not an issue in them.

The ACC/AHA Guidelines for the diagnostic use of the standard exercise test have stated that it is appropriate for testing of adult male or female patients (including those with complete right bundle branch block or with <1mm of resting ST depression) with an *intermediate pretest probability* of CAD based on gender, age, and symptoms. Table 7-13 indicates which patients were in this probability level.

Feinstein[62,63] has promoted criteria for "methodological standards" for diagnostic tests. Their purpose was to improve patient care, reduce healthcare costs, improve the quality of diagnostic test information, and to eliminate useless tests or testing methodologies. The two most important criteria to consider when evaluating such studies are limited challenge and work-up bias. Limited challenge usually results in exaggerated values for sensitivity, specificity, predictive accuracy, and ROC curve area. Work-up bias results in shifting cutpoint performance further along the ROC curve, and when removed shows that the exercise test has a high specificity in office practice. The eponyms SnNout and SpPin help to remember the performance of a test with high values of either sensitivity or specificity. When a test has a very high **sensitiv**ity a **N**egative test rules **out** the diagnosis (SnNout); when a test has a very high **specificity**, a **P**ositive test rules **in** the diagnosis (SpPin). The ACP Journal Club has published an excellent roadmap for systematic reviews of diagnostic test evaluations.[128]

In studies that took into account the number of coronary arteries involved, all found increasing sensitivity of the test as more vessels were involved. The most false negatives have been found among patients with single-vessel disease, particularly if the diseased vessel was not the left anterior descending artery. No matter what techniques are used, there is a reciprocal relationship between sensitivity and specificity. The more specific a test is (i.e., the more able it is to determine who is disease-free), the less sensitive it is, and vice versa. The values for adjusting the criterion can alter sensitivity and specificity for the cutpoint used for abnormal. For instance, when the criterion for an abnormal exercise-induced ST-segment response is altered to 0.2 mV depression, making it more specific for CAD, the sensitivity of the test will be reduced by half.

For patients subgrouped according to beta-blocker administration as initiated by their referring physician, no differences in test performance were found in a consecutive group of males being evaluated for possible CAD. However, *the only way to maintain sensitivity with the standard exercise test in the beta-blocker group who failed to reach target heart rate was to use a treadmill score or 0.5-mm ST depression as the criterion for abnormal.* Thus, in our most recent study of the effects of beta-blockade and heart rate response, we found the sensitivity and predictive accuracy of standard ST criteria for exercise-induced ST depression significantly decreased in male patients taking beta-blockers and do not reach target heart rate. In those who fail to reach target heart rate and are not beta-blocked, sensitivity and predictive accuracy were maintained. Although perhaps optimal, for routine exercise testing it appears unnecessary for physicians to accept the risk of stopping beta-blockers before testing when a patient is exhibiting possible symptoms of ischemia.

The summary from the guidelines are well stated regarding testing women: concern about false-positive ST responses may be addressed by careful assessment of posttest probability and selective use of stress imaging test before proceeding to angiography. Although the optimal strategy for circumventing false-positive test results for the diagnosis of coronary disease in women remains to be defined, there is currently insufficient data to justify routine stress imaging test as the initial test in coronary disease in women.

Studies considering non-ECG data consistently demonstrate that the multivariable equations outperform simple ST-diagnostic criteria. These equations generally provide a predictive accuracy of 80% (ROC area of 0.80). To obtain the best diagnostic characteristics with the exercise test clinical and non-ECG test responses should be considered. Computerized ECG measurements and ECG scores are not superior to visual analysis but can duplicate the results of expert readers. Multivariate scores using computers to make the calculations from logistic regression equations appear to significantly improve on test characteristics. We have validated our simple scores (Figs. 7-16 and 7-17) for both men and women at other institutions and have compared them to physicians. They should be applied during every test along with the DTS score since they are easy to use and significantly improve the prediction of angiographic CAD.

Miranda et al[129] found exercise-induced ST-segment depression in inferior limb leads to be a poor marker for CAD in and of itself. Precordial lead V_5 alone consistently outperformed the inferior lead and the combination of leads V_5 with II, because lead II had such a high false-positive rate. In patients without prior MI and normal resting ECGs, ST depression in precordial lead V_5 along with V_4 and V_6 are reliable markers for CAD, and the monitoring of inferior limb leads adds little additional diagnostic information, but ST elevation in these leads should not be ignored. In patients with a normal resting ECG, exercise-induced ST-segment depression confined to the inferior leads is of little value for the identification of coronary disease.

Once the diagnosis is made, how does this affect outcomes? In Denmark, an observational study evaluated the association among different centers' referral practices for coronary angiography after exercise testing, with 1- and 5-year outcomes.[130] All 10 hospitals and six private consultants in Aarhus and Ringkjoebing counties (900,000 inhabitants) were screened. They found that in 1996, 736 patients with an abnormal bicycle exercise test were considered for referral for coronary intervention. As an immediate consequence of the exercise test, 61% of subjects were referred for cardiac catheterization. Centers were defined as exhibiting low (<33%), intermediate (33%–66%) and high (>66%) referral patterns. A low compared with a high referral fraction was associated with a similar 5-year mortality and MI rate. The same was found for an intermediate, compared with a high fraction, referral center. Estimates were about the same after 1 year of follow-up with no major differences among centers in mortality or MI. Studies like this with a longer follow-up, including costs and quality of life assessment, would be of great import to clinicians.

Obviously the concept of ACS has altered the clinical milieu. The CNR Cardiology Research group in Italy reviewed the literature to see if evidence still supports the use of exercise ECG as first choice of stress testing modality for ACS.[131] They concluded that a large body of evidence supports the use of exercise ECG as a cost-effective tool for prognostic purposes and for quality of life assessment following ACS. This is consistent with the ACC/AHA guidelines.

The guidelines state that patients who are pain-free, have either a normal or nondiagnostic ECG or one that is unchanged from previous tracings, and have a normal set of initial cardiac marker measurements are candidates for further evaluation to screen for nonischemic discomfort versus a low-risk ACS. If the patient is low risk, does not experience any further ischemic discomfort, and a follow-up 12-lead ECG and cardiac marker measurements after 6 to 8 hours of observation are normal, the patient may be considered for an early exercise test to provoke ischemia. This test can be performed before the discharge and should be supervised by an experienced physician. Alternatively, the patient may be discharged and return for the test as an outpatient within 3 days.

The most exciting new area in diagnosis is the use of biomarkers such as BNP. The point of contact analysis techniques available for these assays involves a hand-held battery-powered unit that uses a replaceable cartridge. Finger stick blood samples are adequate for analyses and the results are available immediately. If validated using appropriate study design (similar to QUEXTA), biomarkers could have a big impact on physician and patient confidence in the standard office/clinic exercise test.

REFERENCES

1. Snow V, Barry P, Fihn SD, et al: Evaluation of primary care patients with chronic stable angina: guidelines from the American College of Physicians. Ann Intern Med 2004;141:57-64.
2. Rosanski A, Diamond GA, Berman DS, et al: The declining specificity of exercise radionuclide ventriculography. N Engl J Med 1983;309:518-522.
3. Fagan TJ: Nomogram for Bayes theorem. N Engl J Med 1975;293:257.
4. Wilson RF, Marcus ML, Christensen BV, et al: Accuracy of exercise electrocardiography in detecting physiologically significant coronary arterial lesions. Circulation 1991;83:412-421.
5. Piek JJ, Boersma E, di Mario C, et al: For the DEBATE study group. Angiographical and Doppler flow-derived parameters for assessment of coronary lesion severity and its relation to the result of exercise electrocardiography. Eur Heart J 2000;21:466-474.
6. Pellinen TJ, Virtanen KS, Toivonen L, et al: Coronary collateral circulation. Clin Cardiol 1991;14:111-118.
7. Blackburn H, Katigbak R: What electrocardiographic leads to take after exercise? Am Heart J 1964;67:184-188.
8. Miller TD, Desser KB, Lawson M: How many electrocardiographic leads are required for exercise treadmill tests? J Electrocardiol 1987;20:131-137.
9. Mason RE, Likar I, Biern RO, Ross RS: Multiple-lead exercise electrocardiography. Experience in 107 normal subjects and 67 patients with angina pectoris, and comparison with coronary cinearteriography in 84 patients. Circulation 1967;36:517-525.
10. Sketch MH, Nair CK, Esterbrooks DJ, Mohiuddin SM: Reliability of single-lead and multiple-lead electrocardiography during and after exercise. Chest 1978;74:394-401.
11. Simoons ML, Block P: Toward the optimal lead system and optimal criteria for exercise electrocardiography. Am J Cardiol 1981;47:1366-1374.
12. Miranda CP, Liu J, Kadar A, Janosi A, et al: Usefulness of exercise-induced ST-segment depression in the inferior leads during exercise testing as a marker for coronary artery disease. Am J Cardiol 1992;69:303-308.
13. Viik J, Lehtinen R, Turjanmaa V, et al: Correct utilization of exercise electrocardiographic leads in differentiation of men with coronary artery disease from patients with a low likelihood of coronary artery disease using peak exercise ST-segment depression. Am J Cardiol 1998;81:964-969.
14. Riff DP, Carleton RA: Effect of exercise on the atrial recovery wave. Am Heart J 1971;81:759-763.
15. Weiner DA, McCabe CH, Ryan TJ: Prognostic assessment of patients with coronary artery disease by exercise testing. Am Heart J 1983;105:749-755.
16. Weiner DA, McCabe CH, Ryan TJ: Identification of patients with left main and three vessel coronary disease with clinical and exercise test variables. Am J Cardiol 1980;46:21-27.
17. Mark DB, Hlatky MA, Lee KL, et al: Localizing coronary artery obstructions with the exercise treadmill test. Ann Intern Med 1987;106:53-55.
18. Fortuin NJ, Friesinger GC: Exercise-induced ST segment elevation: Clinical, electrocardiographic and arteriographic studies in twelve patients. Am J Med 1970;49:459-464.
19. Hegge FN, Tuna N, Burchell HB: Coronary arteriographic findings in patients with axis shifts or ST segment elevations on exercise testing. Am Heart J 1973;86:603-615.
20. Chahine RA, Raizner AE, Ishimori T: The clinical significance of exercise-induced ST-segment elevation. Circulation 1976;54:209-213.
21. Longhurst JC, Kraus WL: Exercise-induced ST elevation in patients without myocardial infarction. Circulation 1979;60:616-629.
22. Bruce RA, Fisher LD: Unusual prognostic significance of exercise-induced ST elevation in coronary patients. J Electrocardiol 1987;20(suppl):84-88.
23. De Feyter PJ, Majid PA, Van Eenige MJ, et al: Clinical significance of exercise-induced ST segment elevation. Br Heart J 1981;46:84-92.
24. Kentala E, Luurela O: Response of R wave amplitude to posture changes and to exercise. Ann Clin Res 1975;7:258-263.
25. Bonoris PE, Greenberg PS, Christison GW, et al: Evaluation of R wave amplitude changes versus ST segment depression in stress testing. Circulation 1978;57:904-910.
26. Eenige van MJ, De Feyter PJ, Jong JP, Roos, JP: Diagnostic incapacity of exercise-induced QRS wave amplitude changes to detect coronary artery disease and left ventricular dysfunction. Eur Heart J 1982;3:9-16.
27. Myers J, Ahnve S, Froelicher V, Sullivan M: Spatial R wave amplitude during exercise: Relation with left ventricular ischemia and function. J Am Coll Cardiol 1985;6:603-608.
28. Goldschlager N, Selzer A, Cohn K: Treadmill stress tests as indicators of presence and severity of coronary artery disease. Ann Intern Med 1976;85:277-286.
29. Callaham PR, Thomas L, Ellestad MH: Prolonged ST-segment depression following exercise predicts significant proximal left coronary artery stenosis (abstract). Circulation 1987;76(suppl IV):IV-253.
30. Meyers DG, Bendon KA, Hankins JH, Stratbucker RA: The effect of baseline electrocardiographic abnormalities on the diagnostic accuracy of exercise-induced ST-segment changes. Am Heart J 1990;119:272-276.
31. Tonkon MJ, Lee G, DeMaria AN, et al: Effects of digitalis on the exercise electrocardiogram in normal adult subjects. Chest 1977;72:714-718.
32. Sketch MH, Moss AN, Butler ML, et al: Digoxin-induced positive exercise tests: Their clinical and prognostic significance. Am J Cardiol 1981;48:655-659.
33. Sundqvist K, Atterhog JH, Jogestrand T: Effect of digoxin on the electrocardiogram at rest and during exercise in healthy subjects. Am J Cardiol 1986;57:661-665.
34. LeWinter M, Crawford M, O'Rourke R, Karliner J: The effects of oral propanolol, digoxin and combined therapy on the resting and exercise ECG. Am Heart J 1977;93:202-209.
35. Herbert WG, Dubach P, Lehmann KG, Froelicher VF: Effect of β-blockade on the interpretation of the exercise ECG: ST level versus delta ST/HR index. Am Heart J 1991;122:993-1000.
36. Gauri AJ, Raxwal VK, Roux L: Effects of chronotropic incompetence and beta-blocker use on the exercise treadmill test in men. Am Heart J 2001;142:136-141.
37. Cantwell JD, Murray PM, Thomas RJ: Current management of severe exercise-related cardiac events. Chest 1988;93:1264-1269.
38. Anastasiou-Nana MI, Anderson JL, Stewart JR: Occurrence of exercise-induced and spontaneous wide complex tachycardia during therapy with flecainide for complex ventricular arrhythmias: A probable proarrhythmic effect. Am Heart J 1987;113:1071-1077.
39. Whinnery JE, Froelicher VF, Stuart AJ: The electrocardiographic response to maximal treadmill exercise in asymptomatic men with left bundle branch block. Am Heart J 1997;94:316.

40. Ibrahim NS, Selvester RS, Hagar JM, Ellestad MH: Detecting exercise-induced ischemia in left bundle branch block using the electrocardiogram. Am J Cardiol 1998;82:832-835.
41. Richter WS, Aurisch R, Munz DL: Septal myocardial perfusion in complete left bundle branch block: Case report and review of the literature. Nuklearmedizin 1998;37:146-150.
42. Grady TA, Chiu AC, Snader CE, et al: Prognostic significance of exercise-induced left bundle-branch block. JAMA 1998;279:153-156.
43. Munt B, Huckell VF, Boone J: Exercise-induced left bundle branch block: A case report of false positive MIBI imaging and review of the literature. Can J Cardiol 1997;13:517-521.
44. Whinnery JE, Froelicher VF, Stuart AJ: The electrocardiographic response to maximal treadmill exercise in asymptomatic men with right branch bundle block. Chest 1977;71:335.
45. Blackburn H: Canadian Colloquium on Computer-Assisted Interpretation of Electrocardiograms. VI. Importance of the electrocardiogram in populations outside the hospital. Can Med Assoc J 1973;108:1262-1265.
46. Cullen K, Stenhouse NS, Wearne KL, Compston GN: Electrocardiograms and 13 year cardiovascular mortality in Busselton study. Br Heart J 1982;47:209-212.
47. Aronow WS: Correlation of ischemic ST-segment depression on the resting electrocardiogram with new cardiac event rates in 1,106 patients over 62 years of age. Am J Cardiol 1989;64:232-233.
48. Califf RM, Mark DB, Harrell FE, et al: Importance of clinical measures of ischemia in the prognosis of patients with documented coronary artery disease. J Am Coll Cardiol 1988;11:20-26.
49. Harris PJ, Harrell FE, Lee KL, et al: Survival in medically treated coronary artery disease. Circulation 1979;60:1259-1269.
50. Miranda CP, Lehmann KG, Froelicher VF: Correlation between resting ST segment depression, exercise testing, coronary angiography, and long-term prognosis. Am Heart J 1991;122:1617-1626.
51. Kansal S, Roitman D, Sheffield LT: Stress testing with ST-segment depression at rest. Circulation 1976;54:636-639.
52. Harris FJ, DeMaria AN, Lee G, et al: Value and limitations of exercise testing in detecting coronary disease with normal and abnormal resting electrocardiograms. Adv Cardiol 1978;22:11-15.
53. Roitman D, Jones WB, Sheffield LT: Comparison of submaximal exercise ECG test with coronary cineangiocardiogram. Ann Intern Med 1970;72:641-647.
54. Roger VL, Jacobsen SJ, Pellikka PA, et al: Gender differences in use of stress testing and coronary heart disease mortality: A population-based study in Olmsted County, Minnesota. J Am Coll Cardiol 1998;32:345-352.
55. James FW, Chung EK, (eds). Exercise ECG Test in children. In Exercise electrocardiography: A Practical Approach, 2nd ed. Baltimore, Williams & Wilkins, 1983, p. 132.
56. Lauer MS, Pashkow FJ, Snader CE, et al: Sex and diagnostic evaluation of possible coronary artery disease after exercise treadmill testing at one academic teaching center. Am Heart J 1997;134 (5 Pt 1):807-813.
57. Lee DP, Fearon WF, Froelicher VF: Clinical utility of the exercise ECG in patients with diabetes and chest pain. Chest 2001;119: 1576-1581.
58. Lai S, Kaykha A, Yamazaki T, et al: Treadmill scores in elderly men. J Am Coll Cardiol 2004;43:606-615.
59. Lavoie KL, Fleet RP, Lesperance F, et al: Are exercise stress tests appropriate for assessing myocardial ischemia in patients with major depressive disorder? Am Heart J 2004;148:621-627.
60. Gianrossi R, Detrano R, Mulvihill D, et al: Exercise-induced ST depression in the diagnosis of coronary artery disease: A meta-analysis. Circulation 1989;80:87-98.
61. Morise A, Diamond GA: Comparison of the sensitivity and specificity of exercise electrocardiography in biased and unbiased populations of men and women. Am Heart J 1995;130:741-747.
62. Philbrick JT, Horwitz RI, Feinstein AR: Methodologic problems of exercise testing for coronary artery disease: Groups, analysis and bias. Am J Cardiol 1980;46:807-812.
63. Reid M, Lachs M, Feinstein A: Use of methodological standards in diagnostic test research. JAMA 1995;274:645-651.
64. Guyatt GH: Readers' guide for articles evaluating diagnostic tests: What ACP Journal Club does for you and what you must do yourself. ACP Club 1991;115:A16.
65. Ellestad MH, Savitz S, Bergdall D, Teske J: The false positive stress test. Multivariate analysis of 215 subjects with hemodynamic, angiographic and clinical data. Am J Cardiol 1977;40:681-687.
66. Braitman LE; Davidoff F: Predicting clinical states in individual patients. Ann Intern Med 1996;125:406-412.
67. Yamada H, Do D, Morise A, Froelicher V: Review of studies utilizing multi-variable analysis of clinical and exercise test data to predict angiographic coronary artery disease. Prog Cardiovasc Dis 1997; 39:457-481.
68. Concato J, Feinstein AR, Holford TR: The risk of determining risk with multivariate models. Ann Intern Med 1993;118:201-210.
69. Peterson MC, Holbrock JH, Hales DV, et al: Contributions of the history, physical examination, and laboratory investigation in making medical diagnoses. West J Med 1992;156:163-165.
70. Diamond GA: Future imperfect: The limitations of clinical prediction models and the limits of clinical prediction. J Am Coll Cardiol 1989;14:12A-22A.
71. Harrell FE, Jr, Lee KL, Mark DB: Multivariable prognostic models: Issues in developing models, evaluating assumptions and adequacy, and measuring and reducing errors. Stat Med 1996;15:361-387.
72. Morise A, Diamond G: Estimating probability of coronary artery disease (letter to the editor). 1993;22:340-341.
73. Morise AP, Bobbio M, Diamond G, et al: The effect of disease prevalence adjustments on the accuracy of a logistic prediction model. Med Decis Making 1996;16:133-142.
74. Morise AP, Detrano R, Bobbio M, Diamond GA: Development and validation of a logistic regression - derived algorithm for estimating the incremental probability of coronary artery disease before and after exercise testing. J Am Coll Cardiol 1992;20: 1187-1196.
75. Detrano R, Bobbio M, Olson H, et al: Computer probability estimates of angiographic coronary artery disease: Transportability and comparison with cardiologists's estimates. Comput Biomed Res 1992;25:468-485.
76. Robert AR, Melin JA, Detry JM: Logistic discriminant analysis improves diagnostic accuracy of exercise testing for coronary artery disease in women. Circulation 1991;83:1202-1209.
77. Morise AP, Dalal JN, Duval RD: Value of a simple measure of estrogen status for improving the diagnosis of CAD in women. Am J Med 1993;94:491-496.
78. Harrell FE Jr, Lee KL, Mark DB: Multivariable prognostic models: Issues in developing models, evaluating assumptions and adequacy, and measuring and reducing errors. Stat Med 1996;15:361-387.
79. Froelicher V, Shetler K, Ashley E: Better decisions through science: exercise testing scores. Prog Cardiovasc Dis 2002;44:395-414.
80. Swets JA, Dawes RM, Monahan J: Better decisions through science. Sci Am 2000;283:82-87.
81. Ashley E, Myers J, Froelicher V: Exercise testing scores as an example of better decisions through science. Med Sci Sports Exerc 2002;34:1391-1398.
82. Atwood JE, Do D, Froelicher V, et al: Can computerization of the exercise test replace the cardiologist? Am Heart J 1998;136: 543-552.
83. Morise A: Comparison of the Diamond-Forrester method and a new score to estimate the pretest probability of coronary disease before exercise testing. Am Heart J 1999;138:740-745.
84. Poses RM, Cebul RD, Collins M, Fager SS: The importance of disease prevalence in transporting clinical prediction rules. Ann Intern Med 1986;105:586-591.
85. Do D, West JA, Morise A, Froelicher V: A consensus approach to diagnosing coronary artery disease based on clinical and exercise test data. Chest 1997;111:1742-1749.
86. Raxwal V, Shetler K, Do D, Froelicher V: A simple treadmill score. Chest 2000;113:1933-1940.
87. Morise AP, Lauer MS, Froelicher VF: Development and validation of a simple exercise test score for use in women with symptoms of suspected coronary artery disease. Am Heart J 2002;144:818-825.
88. O'Rourke RA, Brundage BH, Froelicher VF, et al: American College of Cardiology/American Heart Association Expert Consensus Document on electron-beam computed tomography for the diagnosis and prognosis of coronary artery disease. J Am Coll Cardiol 2000;36:326-340.
89. Hlatky M, Bovinick E, Brundage B: Diagnostic accuracy of cardiologists compared with probability calculations using Bayes' rule. Am J Cardiol 1982;49:192-197.
90. Lipinski M, Do D, Froelicher V, et al: Comparison of exercise test scores and physician estimation in determining disease probability. Arch Intern Med 2001;161:2239-2244.

91. Lipinski M, Froelicher V, Atwood E, et al: Comparison of treadmill scores with physician estimates of diagnosis and prognosis in patients with coronary artery disease. Am Heart J 2002;143:650-658.

92. Froelicher VF, Lehmann KG, Thomas R, et al: The electrocardiographic exercise test in a population with reduced workup bias: Diagnostic performance, computerized interpretation, and multivariable prediction. Veterans Affairs Cooperative Study in Health Services #016 (QUEXTA) Study Group. Quantitative Exercise Testing and Angiography. Ann Intern Med 1998;128(12 Pt 1):965-974.

93. Ustin J, Umann T, Froelicher V: Data management: A better approach. Physicians and Computers 1994;12:30-33.

94. Froelicher V, Shiu P. Exercise test interpretation system. Physicians and Computers 1996;14:40-44.

95. Mark D, Hlatky M, Harrell F, et al: Exercise treadmill score for predicting prognosis in coronary artery disease. Ann Intern Med 1987;106:793-800.

96. Reid M, Lachs M, Feinstein A: Use of methodological standards in diagnostic test research. JAMA 1995;274:645-651.

97. Fletcher G, Balady G, Froelicher V, et al: AHA Medical/Scientific Statement. Exercise Standards. Circulation 1995;91:580-615.

98. Detrano R, Leatherman J, Salcedo EE, et al: Bayesian analysis versus discriminant function analysis: Their relative utility in the diagnosis of coronary disease. Circulation 1986;73:970-977.

99. Morise AP, Duval RD: Comparison of three Bayesian methods to estimate posttest probability in patients undergoing exercise stress testing. Am J Cardiol 1989;64:1117-1122.

100. Morise AP, Duval R, Detrano R, et al: Comparison of logistic regression and Bayesian based algorithms to estimate posttest probability in patients with suspected CAD undergoing exercise ECG. Electrocardiol 1992;25:89-99.

101. Shaw LJ, Peterson ED, Shaw LK, et al: Use of a prognostic treadmill score in identifying diagnostic coronary disease subgroups. Circulation 1998;98:1622-1630.

102. Fleischmann KE, Hunink MG, Kuntz KM, Douglas PS: Exercise echocardiography or exercise SPECT imaging? A meta-analysis of diagnostic test performance. JAMA 1998;280(10):913-920.

103. Detrano R, Janosi A, Marcondes G, et al: Factors affecting sensitivity and specificity of a diagnostic test: The exercise thallium scintigram. Am J Med 1988;84:699-710.

104. Weiner DA: Accuracy of cardiokymography during exercise testing: Results of a multicenter study. J Am Coll Cardiol 1985;6:502-509.

105. Gehring J, Koenig W, Donner M, et al: The diagnostic value of signal-averaged stress cardiokymography compared with exercise electrocardiography. J Noninvasive Cardiol 1998;5:32-41.

106. Akdemir I, Aksoy N, Aksoy M, et al: Does exercise-induced severe ischaemia result in elevation of plasma troponin-T level in patients with chronic coronary artery disease? Acta Cardiol 2002;57:13-18.

107. Ashmaig ME, Starkey BJ, Ziada AM, et al: Changes in serum concentrations of markers of myocardial injury following treadmill exercise testing in patients with suspected ischaemic heart disease. Med Sci Monit 2001;7:54-57.

108. Foote RS, Pearlman JD, Siegel AH, Yeo KT: Detection of exercise-induced ischemia by changes in B-type natriuretic peptides. J Am Coll Cardiol 2004;44:1980-1987.

109. Sabatine MS, Morrow DA, de Lemos JA, et al: TIMI Study Group. Acute changes in circulating natriuretic peptide levels in relation to myocardial ischemia. J Am Coll Cardiol 2004;44:1988-1995.

110. Shemesh J, Apter S, Rozenman J, et al: Calcification of coronary arteries: Detection and quantification with double-helix CT. Radiology 1995;197:779-783.

111. Kajinami K, Seki H, Takekoshi N, Mabuchi H. Noninvasive prediction of coronary atherosclerosis by quantification of coronary artery calcification using electron beam computed tomography: Comparison with electrocardiographic and thallium exercise stress test results. J Am Coll Cardiol 1995;26:1209-1221.

112. Detrano R, Hsiai T, Wang S, et al: Prognostic value of coronary calcification and angiographic stenoses in patients undergoing coronary angiography. J Am Coll Cardiol 1996;27:285-290.

113. Budhoff MJ, Georgiou D, Brody A, et al: Ultrafast computed tomography as a diagnostic modality in the detection of coronary artery disease: A multicenter study. Circulation 1996;93:898-904.

114. Gibbons RJ, Abrams J, Chatterjee K, et al: ACC/AHA 2002 guideline update for the management of patients with chronic stable angina: A report of the American College of Cardiology/American Heart Association Task Force on Practice Guidelines (Committee to Update the 1999 Guidelines for the Management of Patients with Chronic Stable Angina). J Am Coll Cardiol 2003;41:159-168.

115. Cannon CP, O'Gara PT: Critical pathways for acute coronary syndromes. In Cannon CP, (ed.): Management of Acute Coronary Syndromes. Totowa, NJ, Humana Press, 1999, pp 611-627.

116. Graff L, Joseph T, Andelman R, et al: American College of Emergency Physicians information paper: Chest pain units in emergency departments: A report from the Short-Term Observation Services Section. Am J Cardiol 1995;76:1036-1039.

117. Brillman J, Mathers-Dunbar L, Graff L, et al: Management of observation units. Ann Emerg Med 1995;25:823-830.

118. Graff LG, Dallara J, Ross MA, et al: Impact on the care of the emergency department chest pain patient from the Chest Pain Evaluation Registry (CHEPER) study. Am J Cardiol 1997;80:563-568.

119. Gomez MA, Anderson JL, Karagounis LA, et al: An emergency department-based protocol for rapidly ruling out myocardial ischemia reduces hospital time and expense: Results of a randomized study (ROMIO). J Am Coll Cardiol 1996;28:25-33.

120. Farkouh ME, Smars PA, Reeder GS, et al: Chest Pain Evaluation in the Emergency Room (CHEER) Investigators. A clinical trial of a chest-pain observation unit for patients with unstable angina. N Engl J Med 1998;339:1882-1888.

121. Newby LK, Mark DB: The chest-pain unit-ready for prime time (editorial)? N Engl J Med 1998;339:1930-1932.

122. Amsterdam EA, Kirk JD, Diercks DB, et al: Early exercise testing in the management of low risk patients in chest pain centers. Prog Cardiovasc Dis 2004;46:438-452.

123. Prina LD, Decker WW, Weaver AL, et al: Outcome of patients with a final diagnosis of chest pain of undetermined origin admitted under the suspicion of acute coronary syndrome: A report from the Rochester Epidemiology Project. Ann Emerg Med 2004;43:59-67.

124. Henrikson CA, Howell EE, Bush DE, et al: Chest pain relief by nitroglycerin does not predict active coronary artery disease. Ann Intern Med 2003;139:979-986.

125. Sanchis J, Bodi V, Llacer A, et al: Predictors of short-term outcome in acute chest pain without ST-segment elevation. Int J Cardiol 2003;92:193-199.

126. Aroney CN, Dunlevie HL, Bett JH: Use of an accelerated chest pain assessment protocol in patients at intermediate risk of adverse cardiac events. Med J Aust 2003;178:370-374.

127. Amsterdam EA, Kirk JD, Diercks DB, et al: Immediate exercise testing to evaluate low-risk patients presenting to the emergency department with chest pain. J Am Coll Cardiol 2002;40:251-256.

128. Pai M, McCulloch M, Enanoria W, Colford JM, Jr: Systematic reviews of diagnostic test evaluations: What's behind the scenes? ACP J Club 2004;141:A11-13.

129. Miranda CP, Liu J, Kadar A, et al: Usefulness of exercise-induced ST-segment depression in the inferior leads during exercise testing as a marker for coronary artery disease. Am J Cardiol 1992;69:303-308.

130. Niemann T, Labouriau R, Sorensen HT, et al: Prognostic impact of different regional referral practices for interventional investigation and coronary treatment after exercise testing: A population-based 5-year follow-up study. J Intern Med 2004;255:478-485.

131. Bigi R, Cortigiani L, Desideri A: Exercise electrocardiography after acute coronary syndromes: still the first testing modality? Clin Cardiol 2003;26:390-395.

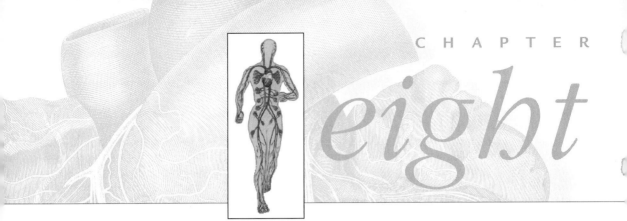

Prognostic Applications of Exercise Testing

RATIONALE

There are two principal reasons for estimating prognosis. The first is to provide accurate answers to patient's questions regarding the probable outcome of their illness. Although discussion of prognosis is inherently delicate, and probability statements can be misunderstood, most patients find this information useful in planning their affairs regarding work, recreational activities, personal estate, and finances. The second reason to determine prognosis is to identify those patients for whom interventions might improve outcome.

Although improved prognosis equates with increased quantity of life, quality of life issues must also be taken into account. In that regard, it is apparent that in certain clinical settings, catheter or surgical interventions provide better therapy than medication. However, these interventions, when misapplied, can have a negative impact on the quality of life (inconvenience, complications, and discomfort), as well as creating a financial burden to the individual and to society.

Part of the Basic Patient Evaluation

Patients with known or suspected coronary disease are usually evaluated initially after a careful cardiac history and physical exam with an exercise test. It can be performed safely and inexpensively and even accomplished in the physician's office.

In addition to diagnostic information, the test gives practical and clinically valuable information regarding exercise capacity and response to therapy. Patients with clinical data and exercise test responses considered abnormal or associated with a high enough probability for cardiac events or for having severe coronary artery disease (CAD) are frequently evaluated further by coronary angiography. A study evaluating the appropriateness of the performance of coronary angiography in clinical practice considered angiography to be inappropriate nearly a quarter of the time due to the failure to obtain an exercise test.[1] However, the indications for angiography have dramatically changed since the eighties. Now, with drug-eluting stents, the risk of reocclusion has been reduced to single digits. The possibility of putting patients at higher risk by performing an intervention has drastically dropped. Fewer patients with (CAD) are experiencing angina pectoris than ever before, thanks to progress in interventional cardiology.

As will be reviewed, numerous investigators have indicated that responses to exercise testing predict the severity of underlying coronary disease and prognosis. However, exercise testing cannot predict angiographic findings or a poor prognosis with absolute certainty. In addition, only certain groups of patients with specific CAD patterns are conferred a survival benefit from coronary artery bypass surgery (CABS).[2] Because of the lack of certainty and the need for a "road map" for coronary intervention, coronary angiography is considered the "gold standard" for evaluating patients for the presence of coronary disease, and for determining which patients might benefit from interventional therapy. Angiography defines static anatomy, because it is performed at rest, but the addition of flow wires into the coronary arteries can quantitate coronary blood flow.[3] Techniques are even being explored to identify subcritical lesions likely to rupture or gather thrombus (i.e., labile plaque). This chapter begins with the pathophysiologic basis of the exercise test responses and then follows with a discussion of the pertinent studies.

Pathophysiology

The basic pathophysiologic features of CAD that determine prognosis include the amount of remaining myocardium (reflected by left ventricular [LV] function), the amount of myocardium in jeopardy, and arrhythmic risk. Arrhythmias usually are the final event, whether primary or secondary to ischemia or LV dysfunction. Arrhythmic risk has become a very active area for research because of the data showing a marked improvement in survival in select patient groups with implantation of defibrillators (ICD). Exercise test-induced ventricular arrhythmias (ETIVA) indicate electrical instability not necessarily related to exercise-induced ischemia (except for the rare ST elevation in a normal ECG that is very arrhythmogenic). Although ETIVA can be due to LV dysfunction, most likely in others it is due to a genetic propensity that has yet to be characterized. Recent studies have highlighted the independent predictive power of exercise test-induced arrhythmias. These findings have been confusing, because they appear to be associated with long rather than short-term events, are relatively weak to other test responses, and a therapy is not readily available. Since primary arrhythmic deaths are relatively rare and ETIVA exert a modest independent risk largely after longer periods of follow-up, ETIVA are dealt with in Chapter 6 of this book.

Myocardium in jeopardy refers to myocardium supplied by a coronary artery that has a critically obstructive lesion or has a plaque that could rupture and/or form a thrombus (labile plaque). The "dirty," subcritical lesion does not cause ischemia during stress; therefore, it cannot be detected by an exercise test. However, interventions other than statins and acetylsalicylic acid (ASA) are not effective in improving outcomes. The obstructive lesion should cause ischemia and be detectable with an exercise test. These lesions can be altered by interventions (for example, percutaneous coronary intervention [PCI] and coronary artery bypass grafting [CABG]) and outcome improved in subsets.

What exercise test responses are due to myocardial ischemia or dysfunction? The exercise responses due to ischemia include angina, ST-segment depression, and ST-segment elevation over ECG areas without Q waves. Predicting the amount of ischemia (i.e., the amount of myocardium in jeopardy) is difficult. It appears to be inversely related to the double product at the onset of signs/symptoms of ischemia.

The only response specifically associated with LV dysfunction is ST elevation over Q waves. This carries an increased risk in patients with Q waves and indicates that they have lower LV function and possibly larger aneurysms as compared to those with Q waves without elevation.[4] If ST elevation decreases with subsequent exercise tests, such patients are thought to have a better prognosis. Those with elevation over Q waves have poorer resting LV function than those without elevation.[5]

The responses resulting from either ischemia or LV dysfunction include chronotropic incompetence or heart rate impairment,[6] systolic blood pressure (SBP) drops,[7] and a poor exercise capacity.[8] Their combined association with ischemia and myocardial damage or dysfunction explains why they are so important in predicting prognosis.

Previous studies have shown that exercise capacity correlates weakly with LV function in patients without signs or symptoms of right-sided failure.[9] Exercise testing is not very helpful in identifying patients with moderate LV dysfunction, which is part of the requirement for improved survival with surgery. This is better recognized by a history of congestive heart failure (CHF), physical exam, resting ECG,[10] echocardiogram, or nuclear imaging.

Who needs to undergo cardiac catheterization among patients with stable CAD? This is easy to decide when symptoms cannot be controlled, but otherwise it is often difficult to decide who should be considered for intervention to prolong life. Modern statistical techniques applied to patient populations followed for cardiac endpoints make it possible to identify low-risk patients, who do not need cardiac catheterization, and those at high risk, who may benefit when it is feasible to attempt intervention.

STATISTICAL METHODS USED FOR SURVIVAL ANALYSIS

To answer these questions regarding patient decisions, follow-up studies must be performed and special statistical methods called survival analysis must be applied. Survival analysis consists of a group of uni- and multivariate mathematical techniques that consider person-time of exposure and use that to calculate hazard or risk. The key difference between survival analysis and other statistical methods is *censoring* or removal from exposure. Censoring is done at time of "lost to follow-up," removal from risk (i.e., CABS, percutaneous transluminal coronary angioplasty), or termination of the study. The two most commonly used techniques are Kaplan-Meier survival curves for univariate analysis and the Cox hazard model for multivariable analysis. Multivariable analysis is necessary because many of the variables interact. Univariately, variables can be associated with death but the association may be through other variables. For instance, the use of digoxin associates with death through CHF and exercise-induced ST elevation associates with death most often through the underlying Q waves.

All variables should be explored by means of Kaplan-Meier survival curves for univariate comparisons and the Cox model for multivariate analysis. A Cox proportional hazards model should be used to determine the effect of a given independent variable on time to death. Many of the variables univariately predictive of death are likely to have overlapping prognostic significance; a multivariate stepwise Cox regression analysis can be employed. The Cox model assumes that the hazard which equals the instantaneous death rate is given by the formula:

$$h_i(t) = h(t)\, C_i,$$

where $C_i = \exp(B_1 X_{1i} + B_2 X_{2i} + \ldots + B_p X_{pi})$

The model assumes that the hazard (h) of death for patient i at time t ($h_i(t)$) equals the hazard of death for an "average patient" at the same time ($h(t)$) multiplied by a factor (C_i) that is a function of the prognostic profile of patient i; this is the proportional hazards assumption that gives the model its name. The proportional hazard coefficient for patient i (C_i) is, in turn, a function of the values for that patient of a set of prognostic factors ($X_{1i}, \ldots, X_{pi}$), multiplied by a corresponding set of regression coefficients ($B_1, \ldots, B_p$) that measure the strength of the association between the prognostic factor and outcomes of large numbers of patients with the same disorder.[11] Cox model also assumes that the effect of a prognostic factor on outcome is linear. Variables of prognostic significance may be discrete or they may be continuous. Many studies analyze the strength of a continuous prognostic factor by setting an arbitrary "cutpoint" and dividing the patients into subgroups with values above and below the cutpoint. Although this technique is helpful in illustrating findings and facilitating drawing of survival curves, it discards valuable prognostic information and may weaken the apparent prognostic significance of a continuous variable.

Endpoints and Censoring

The relative prognostic importance of the ischemic variables can be minimized by not censoring interventions for ischemia (i.e., removal of intervened patients from observation when the intervention occurs in follow-up) because the intervention stops patients from dying. Consideration of all-cause mortality instead of cardiovascular (CV) mortality can have the same effect. This may explain why the ischemic variables included in the Duke score that clearly had diagnostic power[12] do not predict all-cause mortality. While all-cause mortality has advantages over CV mortality as an endpoint,[13] the Duke score was generated using the endpoints of infarction and CV death.[14] Interventions such as CABS or catheter procedures were censored in the Duke study (i.e., subjects were removed from the survival analysis when interventions occurred). Such censoring should increase the association of ischemic variables with outcome, by removing patients whose disease has been alleviated, and thereby would not be as likely to experience the outcome. Often researchers do not censor patients if they had a CV procedure during follow-up because they do not have that information. From a previous study using a similar Veterans Affairs (VA) patient population with an annual all-cause mortality of 3%, our group found that 75% of deaths were CV deaths, and that 6% of patients were censored in follow-up due to CABS.[15] If the proportions are similar in our current population, it would not be unreasonable to expect a bias against the predictive power of these variables. The contradictory results regarding the prognostic power of ischemic variables could also be due to the more effective methods of treatment currently available for ischemic coronary disease compared to LV dysfunction.

The use of coronary interventions as endpoints falsely strengthens the association of ischemic variables with endpoints, because the ischemic responses clinically result in the intervention being performed. Although some investigators have justified their use by requiring a time period to expire after the test before using the intervention/procedure as an endpoint, this still influences the associations. Another problem is that variables predicting infarction can be different than those predicting death, creating a situation where one variable's contrasting effects with respect to two endpoints can cancel each other out.

All-Cause versus Cardiovascular Mortality

Recent studies of prognosis have actually not been superior to the earlier studies that considered CV endpoints and removed patients who had interventions from observation. This is because death data is now relatively easy to obtain, whereas previously investigators had to follow-up the patients and contact them or review their records. Thus, prognostic studies were uncommon because of the expense of follow-up. CV mortality can be determined from death certificates. While death certificates have their limitations, in general, they classify those with accidental, gastrointestinal, pulmonary, and cancer deaths, so that those remaining are most likely to have died of CV causes. This endpoint is more appropriate for a test for CV disease. Whereas all-cause mortality is a more important endpoint for intervention studies, CV mortality is more appropriate for evaluating a CV test (e.g., the exercise test). Identifying those at risk of death due to any cause does not make it possible to identify those who might benefit from CV interventions, one of the two goals of prognostication.

The patient groups that have been studied to determine their prognosis using exercise testing include: (1) patients who have had myocardial infarction (Chapter 9), (2) patients with stable coronary heart disease (discussed in this chapter), (3) patients with CHF (Chapter 10), and (4) asymptomatic individuals (Chapter 11). Patients who have had myocardial infarction, those with CHF, and asymptomatic individuals will be discussed in separate chapters.

PREDICTION OF HIGH RISK AND/OR POOR PROGNOSIS IN PATIENTS WITH STABLE CORONARY HEART DISEASE

This chapter will discuss prognostic studies using exercise testing in patients with stable coronary heart disease predicting the following:

1. Cardiovascular disease endpoints
2. Coronary angiographic findings
3. Improved survival with CABS

In addition, specialized situations for predicting prognosis, including silent ischemia, diabetes, and the elderly, will be targeted separately.

Early Prognostic Studies

In one of the first follow-up studies of treadmill testing, Ellestad and Wan[16] reported the predictive implications of maximal exercise testing in 2700 individuals followed from 6 months to 9 years. ST depression and prior myocardial infarction were both associated with subsequent higher mortality. The first study is from Duke by McNeer et al[17] and the other study is from the Coronary Artery Surgery Study (CASS) data by Weiner et al.[18] Both studies evaluated more than 1000 patients and had at least a 1 year follow-up. Those at high risk in the Duke study had more than 1 mm of ST segment depression at less than 7 METs; the risk was even higher if the maximal heart rate was less than 120 beats per minute. Those at low risk did not have ST-segment depression, were able to exceed 13 METs, or had a maximal heart rate of over 160. CASS patients at high risk either had markers of CHF or ST-segment depression at a low workload. Patients able to exceed 13 METs were at low risk regardless of their other responses.

The study by Podrid et al[19] has placed some doubt on the use of exercise testing to identify high-risk patients. They contend that the prevailing view, "that patients with marked amounts of ST depression have far advanced multivessel disease and that CABS is the only way to improve their outlook" is in error. In their select group of patients with normal ventricular function, who were referred because of profound ST-segment depression, they did not find a bad prognosis. In 142 patients with CAD and severe ST-segment depression with a mean follow-up of 59 months, there was only 1.4% mortality and only 1.3% had CABS per year. This study points out that it is necessary to consider multiple variables when predicting the risk of ischemic heart disease. A relatively low-risk group can be found in any population identified using one-risk predictor, by excluding patients with other risk predictors.

Dagenais et al[20] analyzed the factors influencing the 5-year survival rate in 220 patients with at least 0.2 mV of ST-segment depression during exercise testing. They confirmed previous observations that survival was inversely proportional to the exercise workload: all patients who achieved 10 METs survived and the patient survival rate declined in relation to exercise capacity.

Bruce et al[21] added to their analysis of the Seattle Heart Watch by applying noninvasive criteria in a learning set for exercise-enhanced risk assessment for events resulting from coronary heart disease to a test series in a later population sample. In this series, subsequent follow up in 5308 men enrolled in the learning series of the Seattle Heart Watch from 1971 to 1974 were compared with findings in 3065 men enrolled from 1975 to 1981. Of the 8373 men, 4105, or almost half, were classified before exercise testing as asymptomatic healthy individuals. Another 1374 men had hypertension and 2894 had prior clinical manifestations of coronary heart disease including angina, myocardial infarction (MI), cardiac arrest, or cardiac death. Men in the same age and risk groups for each pretest clinical classification showed similar gradients of risk. Age-standardized event rate showed a reduction longitudinally in healthy men and in patients who underwent CABS. It is important to realize that the majority of events occurred in men with only increased risk rather than high risk. The two exercise predictors of survival were duration of exercise and the ST-segment response.

Follow-up Studies with Clinical, Exercise Test, and Coronary Angiography

Since the pioneering studies from the University of Alabama,[22,23] numerous investigators have utilized clinical, exercise test, and catheterization data to predict prognosis in patients with CAD. Implicit in these studies has been the issue of which variables are predictive, and whether exercise testing and coronary angiography improve prediction sufficiently to merit their performance despite their expense and risk.

Oberman et al[22] found cardiac enlargement on chest x-ray and a history of CHF to be the two most predictive independent clinical variables and that angiography improved prediction of death. They did not consider exercise test results because of incomplete data, but they were the first investigators to demonstrate the poorer prognosis found in those patients unable to perform the exercise test.

From the Seattle Heart Watch, Hammermeister et al[24] assessed 733 medically treated patients by going stepwise, first through clinical markers and then the exercise test. CHF was the most important clinical variable, and maximal double product was the most important treadmill variable.

Maximal SBP, heart rate, and exercise capacity were far less important. Cox's regression analysis showed ejection fraction, age, number of diseased vessels, and resting ventricular arrhythmia, in that order, to be most predictive. From Bad Krozingen, Gohlke et al[25] followed 1034 patients with CAD specifically to answer the question, "Whether exercise testing could provide additional prognostic information when angiographic information was available?". They found exercise workload, angina during the exercise test, and maximal heart rate to independently predict risk of death. Exercise-induced ST depression was the only independently predictive risk factor in the subgroup with three-vessel disease and normal ventricular function.

From the Italian Multicenter Study, Brunelli et al[26] reported their findings in 1083 patients younger than 65 years of age, followed for a mean of 66 months. They found clinical markers to stratify risk and they found that coronary angiography added prognostic information only in patients with moderately severe disease. Q-wave presence and history of infarction were the most important clinical predictors (CHF was not considered). Exercise-induced ST depression was not considered independently but rather was combined with angina and exercise capacity in order to create a marker associated with CV death.

From the CASS, Weiner et al[27] analyzed exercise test, coronary angiographic, and clinical variables in 4083 patients to identify predictors of mortality in medically treated patients with symptomatic CAD. This study was based on analysis of 16% of the registry of patients with no previous CABS who were able to undergo a standard or modified Bruce protocol within 1 month of their catheterization. During the mean follow-up of 4 years, 212 patients, or 5%, died. This represents a very low annual mortality, and approximately 40% of the patients had a prior MI and 36% underwent CABS during a 3-year minimal follow-up. Standard clinical variables, including chest pain, CHF, physical exam, family history, risk factor index, drugs, and cardiac catheterization findings were taken into account. Exercise test variables included limiting symptoms, premature ventricular contractions (PVCs), peak heart rate, peak SBP, ST-segment response, and final exercise stage. Thirty variables were analyzed in 4000 patients. Regression analysis demonstrated that seven variables were independent predictors of survival. A high-risk subgroup (annual mortality about 5%) was identified consisting of patients with either CHF or ST-segment depression and less than 5 METs exercise capacity. When all 30 variables were analyzed jointly, the LV contraction pattern and the number of diseased vessels were the best predictors of survival. In a subgroup of 572 patients with three-vessel disease and good LV function, the probability of survival at 4 years ranged from 53%, for patients only able to achieve stage 1 or 2, to 100%, for patients able to perform 10 METs. Thus, in patients with defined coronary lesions, clinical and exercise variables primarily relating to left ventricle function were helpful in assessing prognosis. The following are some of the univariate risk ratios generated by some of the variables: age above 60 = 2.5x, prior MI = 2.4x, CHF = 5x, cardiac enlargement = 9x, digoxin = 4x, less than stage 1 = 2x, more than 0.1 mV ST-segment depression = 1.4x. The presence of CHF was the most potent clinical predictor of survival when the clinical and exercise test variables were analyzed, and has led us to consider CHF patients separately when doing prognostic evaluation studies.

The Duke Treadmill Score and Nomogram

Mark et al[28] studied 2842 consecutive patients who underwent cardiac catheterization and exercise testing and whose data was entered into the Duke computerized medical information system. The median follow-up for the study population was 5 years and was 98% complete. All patients underwent a Bruce protocol exercise test and had standard ECG measurements recorded. A treadmill angina index was assigned a value of 0 if angina was absent, 1 if typical angina occurred during exercise, and 2 if angina was the reason the patient stopped exercising. Before the test, 54% of the patients had taken propranolol and 11% had taken digoxin. ST measurements considered were sum of the largest net ST depression and elevation, sum of the ST displacements in all 12 leads, the number of leads showing ST displacement of 0.1 mV or more, the product of the number of leads showing ST displacement, and the largest single ST displacement in any lead. To make the score apply to other treadmill protocols, it is necessary to convert minutes in the Bruce protocol to METs with the equation:

$$METs = 1.3 \text{ (minutes)} - 2.2$$

or

$$\text{minutes in the Bruce protocol} = (METs + 2.2) \div 1.3$$

Patients with ST-segment elevation in ECG leads with pathological Q waves were excluded because this ST-segment response has a different meaning.

Six steps were used to derive the prognostic treadmill score. First, the patient population was randomly split into two groups: a training sample of 1422 patients and a validation sample of 1420 patients. Second, the Cox proportional hazards regression model was used in the training sample to assess the strength of association between the primary study endpoint (death of CV cause) and treadmill responses. Treadmill responses were then ranked using the likelihood ratio derived from the Cox model. Third, the most important treadmill response was entered into a Cox regression model, and the remaining responses were then entered in order until the model represented the independent prognostic information available from the exercise test. Fourth, the regression coefficients from this regression model were used to form a linear treadmill score. Fifth, the new score was tested to determine if patients with different levels of scores had a survival pattern similar to that seen in the training sample. Finally, the score was recalculated based on variables derived from the test results in all patients. Kaplan-Meier life table estimates were used to generate cumulative survival curves. Subgroup rates were not calculated beyond the point in follow-up when fewer than 15 patients remained at risk. All patients considered were initially treated nonsurgically. In the 24% of the patients who had CABS, the follow-up was measured to the time of surgery and then they were removed from observation. Seventy percent of the study patients were men and the median age was 49 years. Two thirds had stable angina and one third had progressive anginal symptoms. A history of MI was present in 29%, and 22% had pathological Q waves. At catheterization, the mean ejection fraction was 60%, and 27% had three-vessel or left main CAD.

The largest net ST deviation recorded during exercise in any one of the 12 leads proved to be the single most important variable for predicting prognosis. After adjusting for maximum net ST deviation using the Cox model, only two other variables contained additional prognostic information: the treadmill angina index and exercise time. The results did not change substantially when patients taking beta-blockers or digoxin were excluded. The results also remained unchanged when patients treated surgically were excluded from the study. A score was calculated as follows:

$$\text{exercise time} - (5 \times \text{ST maximum net deviation}) - (4 \times \text{angina index}),$$

where exercise time is measured in minutes and ST deviation is measured in millimeters. Patients at high risk with a score of –11 or lower had a 5-year survival of 72%. Patients at moderate risk with a score of –10 to +4 had a 5-year survival of 91%, and patients with a low risk score of +5 or greater had a 5-year survival risk of 97%. When total cardiac events were considered, the high-risk group had a 5-year survival rate of 65%, the moderate risk group 86%, and the low risk group 93%. The treadmill score contained prognostically important information even after the information provided by clinical and catheterization data was considered. The prognostic stratifying power of the treadmill score was greatest in patients with three-vessel disease and lowest in those with one-vessel disease. Patients at highest risk had the greatest potential to increase their survival duration by having CABS. Patients with three-vessel disease and a treadmill score of –11 or less had a 5-year survival rate of 67%. Patients with three-vessel disease and a risk of this magnitude appear to gain a survival advantage through surgery. Those patients with three-vessel disease and a treadmill score equal to or greater than 7 had an excellent prognosis. This score has been implemented in a nomogram (Fig. 8-1).

Other Prognostic Studies

From the VA randomized trial of CABS, Peduzzi et al[29] reported on the 7-year follow-up of the 245 patients randomized to medical management who had a baseline treadmill test. Univariately and using Cox analysis, ST depression (≥2mm), exercise-induced PVCs, and final heart rate greater than 140 beats per minute were significant predictors. Unfortunately, they did not censor on interventions. These results are in marked contrast to other studies and our findings, in which PVCs did not have an independent predictive power, and high heart rates were found to be protective rather than associated with risk. Peduzzi et al did not find a poor exercise capacity to be predictive as well. These unusual results might be explained by their failure to censor on interventions.

In Buenos Aires, Lerman et al[30] reported 190 patients with exercise test and coronary angiograms who were followed-up for 6 years. Their study began in 1978; patients had a high annual mortality and a low rate of interventions, yet exercise-induced ST depression failed to

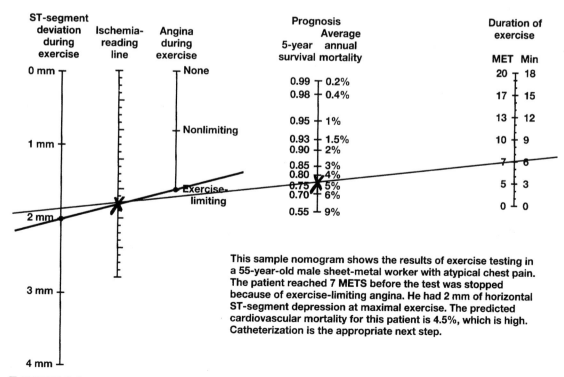

This sample nomogram shows the results of exercise testing in a 55-year-old male sheet-metal worker with atypical chest pain. The patient reached 7 METS before the test was stopped because of exercise-limiting angina. He had 2 mm of horizontal ST-segment depression at maximal exercise. The predicted cardiovascular mortality for this patient is 4.5%, which is high. Catheterization is the appropriate next step.

■ FIGURE 8–1

The Duke treadmill nomogram with a case example.

predict prognosis. Maximal SBP of less than 130 mmHg was the strongest predictor.

Wyns et al[31] evaluated the independent prognostic information provided by exercise testing by calculating the survival rates with the life table method in 372 men referred for coronary angiography. A previous MI was noted in 146 and 248 had typical angina. During a mean follow-up of 29 months, 32 patients died and 27 patients had nonfatal events. Typical angina pectoris and/or an old MI and an abnormal exercise test (angina and/or ST-segment shifts) had significant prognostic value. In patients with an MI and/or angina, the 5-year cumulative survival rate was 76% if the exercise test was abnormal versus 94% if it was normal. Cox regression analysis was performed, and by univariate analysis, the age and the maximal workload were the only noninvasive predictive variables for survival or cardiac events. Exercise capacity provided prognostic information that was not available either from the history or from cardiac catheterization.

A second study from Saint-Luc Hospital in Brussels excluded patients with a prior MI.[32] From 1978 to 1985, 470 consecutive male patients with complaints of chest pain underwent a maximal exercise perfusion test and coronary angiography. During follow-up (1 to 8 years) 32 patients died of CV causes and 30 had a nonfatal MI. The average annual CV death rate was 2%. Of historical variables, only age was chosen as significant multivariately, while angina and pretest likelihood were chosen univariately. A maximal exercise test score based on maximal heart rate, ST_{60} at maximal exercise, angina during the test, maximal workload, and ST slope was chosen in multivariate analysis. This combined score is similar to the ischemic index used in the Italian Study which made a test abnormal if one or more of the following occurred: angina, ST depression, or poor exercise capacity.

In a VA Medical Center, 588 male patients who underwent exercise testing and cardiac catheterization were followed-up to determine whether CV mortality could be predicted by clinical and exercise test data.[33] Over a mean follow-up period of 4 years, there were 39 CV deaths and 45 nonfatal MIs. The Cox proportional hazard model demonstrated the following characteristics to have a significant independent hazards ratio: history of CHF (relative risk = 4×), ST depression on the resting ECG (3×), and a drop of SBP below rest during exercise (5×). Exercise-induced ST depression was not associated with either death or nonfatal MI. From cardiac catheterization, only the ejection fraction added independent information to

the model. A simple score based on one item of clinical information (history of CHF), a resting electrocardiogram finding (ST depression), and an exercise test response (exertional hypotension) stratified our patients for 4 years after testing from 75% with a low risk (annual cardiac mortality of 1%), to 17% with a moderate risk (annual mortality of 7%), and 1% with a high risk (annual cardiac mortality of 12%; hazards ratio of 20, 95% confidence interval 6 to 70×). Three quarters of those usually undergoing cardiac catheterization could be identified by simple noninvasive variables as being at such low risk that invasive intervention is unlikely to improve prognosis.

Also from the Duke database, Califf et al[34] applied clinical measures of ischemia (exercise test results not considered) to predict infarct-free survival in 5896 patients with angina and angiographically significant (>75% lesions) CAD. The Cox regression model chose the following variables in descending order: more than 1 mm of resting ST depression or T-wave inversion, frequency of angina, unstable angina, typical angina, and duration of symptoms. An angina score was derived from the Cox coefficients, and when entered into a model with catheterization data, the following variables were chosen in descending order predicting survival: ejection fraction, number of diseased vessels, left main stenosis, angina score, age, and sex. This score helped predict prognosis even when the catheterization data was considered.

Detre et al[35] developed a multivariate risk function from the 508 patients randomized to medical treatment in the VA randomized study of CABS. The variables, in order of importance, were ST-segment depression on resting ECG, history of MI, history of hypertension, and New York Heart Association functional classification III or IV. Applying the risk function to medical and surgical patients of the 1972–1974 cohort yielded a 5-year probability of dying for each patient. Investigation of treatment effects in approximate terciles, obtained by collapsing the probability distribution into low-, middle-, and high-risk groups, showed that surgery was beneficial for patients in the high-risk tercile even after removal of patients with left main CAD (17% surgical versus 34% medical mortality at 5 years). This finding was accentuated when patients in the 10 hospitals with the lowest operative mortality (3.3%) were compared. Mortality results in the low-risk tercile favored medical treatment (medical versus surgical mortality, 7% versus 17%). The risk function predicted mortality not only for the VA medical group, but also for an independent symptomatic coronary heart disease population from the University of Alabama angiographic registry.

WHY DO PROGNOSTIC STUDIES FAIL TO AGREE?

These nine studies have utilized clinical, exercise test, and catheterization data to predict prognosis in patients with CAD. Implicit in these studies has been the issue of which variables are predictive, and whether exercise testing and coronary angiography

improve prediction sufficiently to merit their performance despite their expense and risk. A careful literature search has yielded the nine studies in Table 8-1 for comparison. All used multivariate survival analysis techniques and the variables chosen are listed in order of predictive power. Some investigators combined variables, and others did not consider key variables or excluded patients with certain clinical features (e.g., CHF, those receiving digoxin). Nevertheless, two of the nine found a history of CHF, two found exercise SBP, and one found resting ST depression to be associated with

TABLE 8-1. Population descriptors including clinical variables and results from exercise testing and coronary angiography in the follow-up studies of multivariate prediction of cardiac events

Descriptors	LB VAMC (No cath)	LB VAMC	VA CABS	CASS	DUKE
Clinical					
Years entered	1984–1990	1984–1990	1970–1974	1974–1979	1969–1981
Population size	2546	588	245	4083	2842
Age	59	59 (mean)	51 (mean)	50	49 (median)
Males (%)	100	100%	100%	80%	70%
Congestive heart failure	5%	8%	9%	8%	4%
Myocardial infarction	23%	45%	54%	40%	29%
Q waves (at least one)	21%	37%	38%	22%	22%
Digoxin	8%	8%	NA	14%	11%
Beta-blockers	22%	35%	14%	40%	54%
Typical angina	21%	52%	100%	50%	47%
Exercise Test					
% with 1 mm ST-segment depression	22%	58%	72%	44%	35%
% angina	4%	35%	66%	80%	50%
Maximal heart rate (beats/min)	137	124	125	138	134
Maximal systolic blood pressure (mmHg)	175	159	156	171	160
METs	8.4	6.6	5.7	NA	7
Premature ventricular contractions	5%	12%	19%	12%	6%
Cardiac Catheterization Findings					
Three-vessel disease (%)	NA	14%	55%	23%	22%
Left main artery disease (%)	NA	7%	13%	7%	5%
No significant lesion (%)	NA	26%	0%	34%	40%
Ejection fraction	NA	60 (mean)		57%	60 (median)
Significant lesion criteria	NA	70%	50%	70%	75%
Follow-up					
Years	5	5	7	5	5
Coronary artery bypass surgery	2%	20%	24%	36%	24%
Annual cardiovascular mortality	1.5%	2.7%	NA	1.0%	1.6%
Annual total mortality	2.8%	3.5%	4.0%	1.6%	1.8%
Independent Predictors of Mortality by Priority					
	CHF/digoxin	CHF	E-I PVCs	CHF	E-I ST depression
	METs	SBP drop	MHR >140	Treadmill stage	Angina index
	Max SBP	Resting ST depression	E-I ST dep >2 mm	E-I ST depression	Treadmill time
	E-I ST depression				

Continued

TABLE 8–1. Population descriptors including clinical variables and results from exercise testing and coronary angiography in the follow-up studies of multivariate prediction of cardiac events—*cont'd*

Italian	Belgian	Belgian (No MI)	German	Seattle	Buenos Aires
1976–1979	1972–1977	1978–1985	1975–1978	1971–1974	1972–1982
1083	372	470	1238	733	180
49 (mean)	48	52	50 (mean)	52 (mean)	51 (mean)
90%	100%	100%	90%	80%	96%
Excluded	1%		Excluded	13%	Excluded
42%	39%	Excluded	>50%	40%	64%
37%	39%	Excluded	50%	45%	
	0%	Excluded	8%	18%	
	0%				
95%	67%	75%	95%	86%	71%
42%	27%	54%	56%		65%
60%	49%	44%	61%		60%
130	148	140	118	145	128
171	NA	186	182	160	151
5.4	9	8	5	6.5	5.2
15%	2%	NA		18%	21%
5%	34%	26%	33%	12%	44%
5%	8%	8%	0%		8
26%	18%	22%	0%	39%	0%
60	NA	65	60	60	
75%	50%	50%	50%	70%	75%
5.5	5	5	5	3.5	6
15%	28%	29%			9%
1.5%	1.8%	2.0%		2.6%	4.6%
2.0%	2.4%		2.4%	3.1%	
Q-wave	Age	Age	Exercise capacity	CHF	Max SBP <130
Prior MI	Exercise capacity	Max exercise score (−2 to +2)	Angina	Max double product	ST elevation
Effort ischemia		(MHR, ST₆₀, AP, watts, ST slope)	MHR	Max SBP	<4 METs
Exercise capacity				Angina Resting ST dep	Inappropriate dyspnea

AP, angina pectoris; CABS, coronary artery bypass surgery; CASS, Coronary Artery Surgery Study; CHF, congestive heart failure; Dep, depression; E-I, exercise-induced; LB, Long Beach; METs, metabolic equivalents; MHR, maximal heart rate; MI, myocardial infarction; PVCs, premature ventricular contractions; SBP, systolic blood pressure; VA, Veterans Affairs; VAMC, Veterans Affairs Medical Center.

death, as we did. However, in contrast to the Long Beach VAMC study three found exercise-induced ST depression and six of the nine found poor exercise capacity to be predictive of death. Unfortunately, for comparison sake, the Duke study did not have maximal SBP collected for consideration. The choice of variables in the Cox hazard models from these studies is tabulated in Table 8-2. Age is not chosen by most of the studies because of the narrow age range for patients submitted to cardiac catheterization. Exertional hypotension has previously been examined in our population and in the other studies reviewed. Note, however, that this is the first time it was chosen by a Cox model rather than just observed univariately.

Because of the differences in the variables chosen to have independent predictive power in the reported studies, we have presented their key characteristics in Table 8-1. Other than the differences detailed previously, the Duke population and the VA CABS study patients appeared to be more "ischemic;" no obvious population, methodological, or test characteristics explain the different results. All studies had to deal with interventions

TABLE 8–2. Meta-analysis of prognosis in stable coronary artery disease studies requiring an exercise test and coronary angiography

Poor exercise capacity	6 of 9 studies
Congestive heart failure	3 of 9 studies
ST-segment depression	
Resting	2 of 9 studies
Exercise	3 of 9 studies
Exercise systolic blood pressure	3 of 9 studies

that alter the natural history but each censored on them as we did, except for the earlier VA CABS study. The first explanation that comes to mind for the failure of ST depression to predict prognosis in six of the nine studies might be that the clinical process was highly effective in selecting high-risk patients with exercise-induced ST depression for interventions. However, all patients were censored at the time of their CABS or PTCA and the same variables were chosen when the patients who received these interventions during follow-up were excluded. Also, in the five comparable studies that did not find ST-segment depression to be predictive, this did not appear to be related to surgical intervention rates.

Ischemic exercise test variables are clearly related to ischemic events during follow-up (i.e., nonfatal MI, CABS, PTCA). This is logical but of little help in clinical decision-making, since the clinician has no trouble in justifying these procedures for patients whose symptoms accelerate after adequate medical management, given the established symptomatic benefit from interventions. The problem lies in justifying intervention to improve survival for patients whose symptoms are satisfactorily managed medically. Our study demonstrates that simple clinical indicators can stratify these patients with stable CAD into high- or low-risk groups. Surprisingly, exercise-induced ischemic variables (ST depression), commonly thought by physicians to identify high risk, did not do so in five of the nine comparable studies.

Spectrum of Cardiac Death

The following discussion of endpoints will attempt to explain why the studies available for making clinical prediction rules do not agree. Cardiac death occurs in a spectrum between patients with myocardial damage who die of CHF (or pump failure) and those with normal ventricles in whom ischemia precipitates death (Fig. 8-2). The clinical and test markers would thus be expected to be quite different for patients who die at the extremes of this spectrum. Whereas markers of myocardial damage (history of CHF, Q waves) track the former, markers of ischemia (angina, ST-segment depression) better track the latter. Arrhythmias, poor exercise capacity, and exertional hypotension are associated with both. Further complicating prediction algorithms, "damage" markers predict short-term deaths, while "ischemic" markers predict deaths occurring 2 or more years later.

Given this etiological milieu, associating clinical and test markers with death as an outcome becomes quite difficult. Other ischemic events (i.e., unstable angina, hospitalization for chest pain) were too "soft" for consideration. In addition, interventions, even if only considered an endpoint if they occur months after testing, are clearly related to the test response (i.e., patients are submitted for interventions because of abnormal tests). Since nonfatal MI most likely is an ischemic event, infarct-free survival is another way of including more ischemic endpoints, but we had similar results when this was considered the endpoint in the Cox model. Differences in populations may have a higher proportion of one or the other type of mortality (pump failure versus ischemia). This may explain why ischemic variables are more predictive in one population and "myocardial damage" variables more predictive in another. One could argue that our population included a majority of patients who died secondary to CHF. However, the same results were obtained after removing patients who either carried that diagnosis or were taking digoxin at time of entry into our study; most of the other studies had a similar proportion of such patients.

Work-Up Bias

All of the above studies selected patients by requiring that they also underwent coronary angiography. To evaluate the effect of this selection process, the Duke group repeated their analysis in an outpatient population that did not undergo cardiac catheterization.[14] The same variables were chosen in their Cox model and the same equation was derived. Similarly, we analyzed 2546 male patients who underwent noninvasive evaluation for CAD, including exercise testing. Over a mean follow-up period of 2.8 years, there were 119 CV deaths and 44 nonfatal MIs. The Cox proportional hazard model demonstrated the following characteristics to have a significant independent hazards ratio: history of CHF and/or taking digoxin, exercise-induced ST depression, exercise capacity in METs, and the response of SBP during exercise. A simple score based on these four factors stratified patients from low risk (annual cardiac mortality of less than 1%) to high risk (annual cardiac mortality of 7%).

The first Duke study used "in-patients," all of whom had a catheterization, while the later report only included outpatients evaluated prior to the decision for cardiac catheterization. Their score, based on treadmill time, exercise-induced ST

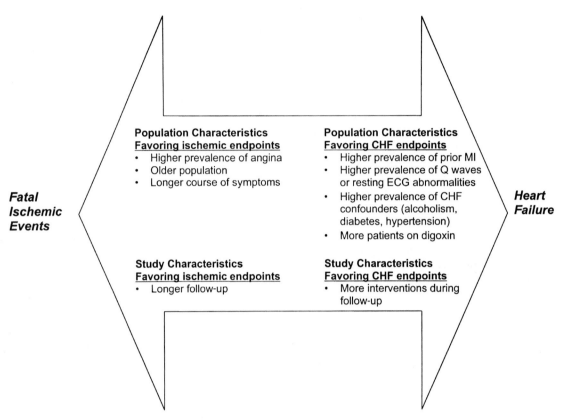

FIGURE 8-2

The spectrum of cardiovascular death. Cardiovascular mortality for individuals and for whole populations occurs in varying degrees as a result of ischemia and left ventricular dysfunction. This range in pathophysiologic characteristics has two consequences: (1) variations in study population and design can produce different results compared with prognostic studies and (2) applying noninvasive variables for prognosis studies, and knowledge of local population characteristics, has the potential for greater precision in prediction.

depression, and angina score during the test, performed as well for prognostication as it did in the first report. Therefore, "work-up" bias did not affect their prognostication model. We have attempted the same type of validation in this study. In contrast to the Duke group, we included exercise SBP and clinical data in our model. Although history of CHF or digoxin was the most powerful variable in both of our VA studies, surprisingly, different exercise test variables were chosen. The model from our first VA study in patients selected for catheterization only chose exertional hypotension, while the model from this second VA study (only noninvasive clinical evaluation) found exercise-induced ST depression, exercise SBP, and exercise capacity to have predictive power.

The "work-up" bias inherent in choosing patients for cardiac catheterization in our first study resulted in a sicker, older, more disabled

group with a higher annual cardiac mortality (2.6% versus 1.5%). This second study included a population with a near normal age-adjusted exercise capacity, while the first study population had an average age-adjusted exercise capacity 75% of normal. Age, as a variable, is not chosen by most of the studies, including ours, because of the narrow age range for patients referred for evaluation of CAD and its relationship to other variables.

LONG-BEACH VA TREADMILL SCORE

Using stepwise selection, the Cox model was allowed to build on each variable group to arrive at the final model that chose history of CHF or digoxin, the change in SBP score, METs, and exercise-induced ST depression.[36] A score was then formed using the coefficients from the Cox model as follows:

$$5 \times (\text{CHF/dig [yes = 1, no = 0]}) + (\text{exercise-induced ST depression in millimeters}) + (\text{change in SBP score}) - (\text{METs})$$

This resulted in a likelihood ratio statistic of 68 with 4 degrees of freedom. Three groups were formed using the score: <–2 (low risk), –2 to +2 (moderate risk), and >2 (high risk). The Kaplan-Meier survival curves are illustrated in Figure 8-3. This score enabled identification of a low-risk group (80% of the population), with an annual mortality of less than 1% over the first 3 years after their exercise test. In addition, a moderate-risk group (14% of the population), with a 4% annual mortality, and a high-risk group (6% of the population), with a 7% annual mortality over the 3 years after their exercise test, were identified.

In addition, the Duke treadmill score (DTS) was calculated for each of our VA patients. The treadmill angina index was modified because we did not have angina coded as the reason for stopping, but was coded as 0 for not present, and 1 as occurring during the test; we used METs instead of minutes of exercise

$$\text{DTMS} = \text{METs} - 5 \times [\text{mm ST depression during exercise}] - 4 \times [\text{treadmill angina index}]$$

Figure 8-4 illustrates the ROC curves for the Duke score and the VA score predicting CV deaths in the total group ($n = 3134$). The area under the VA score curve (0.76) was significantly greater than the area under the Duke score curve (0.68). Similar results were also obtained in the population presented in this study ($n = 2546$). These scores are summarized in Table 8-3. Because of its reproducibility, its applicability in women, and its functionality as a diagnostic score, the DTS is highly recommended.

Unfortunately, one of the only studies to also compare these two scores was carried out on patients who had prior MI and the follow-up was only for 6 months. The GISSI investigators compared the performance of the DTS and the Veteran Affairs Medical Center Score (VAMCS) in predicting 6-month death in GISSI-2 study survivors of acute MI treated with thrombolytic agents to a simple predictive scoring system developed from the same database.[37] Patients of the GISSI-2 study ($n = 6251$) performed a symptom-limited exercise test 1 month after MI. They calculated for each patient the DTS, the VAMCS, and the new GISSI score. All three scores were able to stratify risk into three groups: a low risk of less than 1%, a moderate risk of 2%, and a high risk of 5%. They concluded that exercise test-derived prognostic scores in a population of survivors of acute MI treated with thrombolytic drugs could stratify risk.

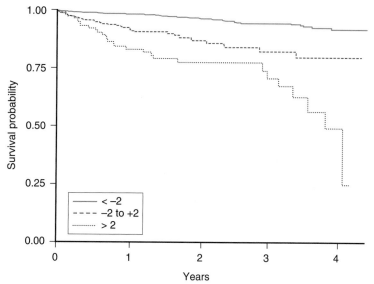

■ **FIGURE 8–3**
The Kaplan-Meier survival curve for the Veterans Affairs (VA) prognostic score.

VA TM score = 5 (CHF [0,1]) + EI ST depression (millimeters) + change SBP score (0–5) – METs

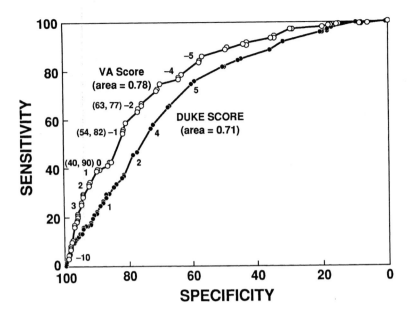

■ FIGURE 8-4
ROC curve for the Veterans Affairs
(VA) score and the Duke score for
predicting cardiovascular death.

However, Morise and Jalisi[38] compared our new simple scores for predicting angiographic CAD to the DTS for predicting all-cause mortality. They utilized 4640 patients without known coronary disease, who underwent exercise testing, to evaluate symptoms of suspected coronary disease between 1995 and 2001. Overall mortality was 3.0% with 3 years of follow-up. All three scores stratified patients into low-, intermediate-, and high-risk groups. No differences were seen when patients were evaluated as subgroups according to gender, diabetes, beta-blockers, or inpatient status. Low-risk patients defined by the DTS had consistently higher mortality and absolute number of deaths compared with low-risk patients using other scores. In addition, the DTS had less incremental stratifying value than the new exercise scores. He concluded that simple pretest and exercise scores risk-stratified patients with suspected coronary disease in accordance with published guidelines and better than the DTS. These results extended to diabetics, inpatients, women, and patients on beta-blockers. It would really be beneficial to see these same analyses performed predicting infarct-free survival with censoring for cardiac interventions.

PROGNOSIS IN "ALL-COMERS" TO THE EXERCISE LAB

Previous prognostic studies focused on specific subsets of patients, so we decided to analyze all patients referred for evaluation at our exercise lab between 1987 and 2000.[39] There were 6213 males (mean age 59 ± 11 years) who had standard exercise ECG treadmill tests over the study period with a mean 6-year follow-up. There were no complications of testing in this clinically referred population, 78% of whom were referred for chest pain, risk factors, or signs or symptoms of ischemic heart disease. Overlapping thirds had typical angina or history of MI. Of the patients, 579 had prior CABS and 522 had a history of CHF. Indications for testing were in accordance with published guidelines. Twenty percent had died over the follow-up, giving rise to an average annual mortality of 2.6%. Cox hazard function chose the following variables in rank order as independently and significantly associated with time to death: METs less than 5, age greater than 65, history of CHF, and history of MI. A score based on simply adding these variables classified patients into low-, medium-, and

---

TABLE 8-3. The two major treadmill prognostic scores

Duke score = METs − 5 × (mm E-I ST depression) − 4 × (TM AP index)
VA score = 5 × (CHF/Dig) + mm E-I ST depression + change in SBP score − METs
Treadmill angina pectoris (TM AP) score: 0 if no angina; 1 if angina occurred during test; 2 if angina was the reason for stopping.
Change in systolic blood pressure (SBP) score: from 0 for rise greater than 40 mmHg to 5 for drop below rest.

high-risk groups. The high-risk group (score of 3 or more) had a hazard ratio of 5 (4.7 to 5.3, 95% CI) and a 5-year mortality of 31% (Fig. 8-5).

When CV mortality was available, we repeated these analyses. Two additional treadmill responses appeared as independently significant: exercise-induced ST depression and arrhythmias (Fig. 8-6).

SPECIFIC PROGNOSTIC ISSUES

Predicting Prognosis in Women

Clinical presentation, performance in diagnostic tests, and prevalence of CAD is different between men and women presenting with chest pain. To demonstrate the value of exercise testing in women, Duke University researchers analyzed data from 976 women referred for evaluation of chest pain and who underwent exercise treadmill test and cardiac catheterization.[40] Women and men differed significantly in DTS, disease prevalence (32% versus 72% significant CAD), and 2-year mortality (1.9% for the study women compared with 4.9% for the men). Mortality increased for high-risk DTS groups in both genders. Two-year mortality for women was 1.0%, 2.2%, and 3.6%, respectively for low-, moderate-, and high-risk groups; For men it was 1.7%, 5.8%, and 16.6%, respectively. Because of the differences in disease prevalence, women had better survival at all values of the DTS. In addition, the DTS actually performed better in women than in men for excluding disease, with fewer low-risk women having mild or severe disease.

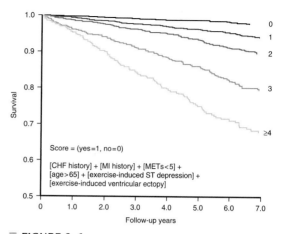

FIGURE 8–6

The "All-comers" treadmill score for predicting cardiovascular mortality.

Within the Women's Ischemia Syndrome Evaluation study, Morise et al[41] evaluated 563 women undergoing coronary angiography for suspected myocardial ischemia. The prevalence of angiographically significant CAD was 26%. Overall, 189 women underwent treadmill testing. Prognostic endpoints included death, MI, stroke, and revascularization. The simple scores and the DTS score stratified women into three probability groups according to the prevalence of coronary disease—pretest: low 20/164 (12%), intermediate 53/245 (22%), and high 75/154 (49%); exercise test: low 11/83 (13%), intermediate 22/74 (30%), and high 17/32 (53%). However, the Duke score did not stratify as well. When pretest and exercise scores were considered together, the best stratification with the exercise test score was in the intermediate pretest group. The Duke score did not stratify this group at all. Pretest and exercise test scores also stratified women according to prognostic endpoints. The exercise test score is most useful in women with an intermediate pretest score, consistent with American College of Cardiology/American Heart Association guidelines.

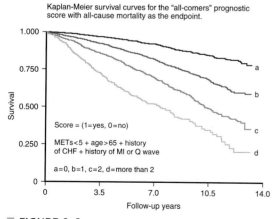

FIGURE 8–5

The "All-comers" treadmill score for predicting all-cause mortality.

Predicting Prognosis in Patients with Resting ST Depression

Kwok et al[42] demonstrated that DTS can effectively risk-stratify patients with ST-T abnormalities on resting the ECG. When patients with ST-T abnormalities were classified into risk groups according to DTS, there were significant overall differences among the risk groups for all outcome endpoints. The 7-year event-free survival was 94%, 88%, and 69% for the low-, intermediate-, and high-risk groups, respectively. More patients with ST-T changes were classified as high-risk (5% versus 2%) and their 7-year survival was lower than that of the control population high-risk patients (76% versus 93%).

Should Heart Rate in Recovery be Included in Prognostic Scores?

Recent studies have highlighted the prognostic value of heart rate recovery (HRR), or the drop in heart rate, after an exercise test. Although earlier physiological studies suggested a rapid HRR response to exercise to be a marker of physical fitness, only recently has its prognostic value been reported. The rate of heart rate return to baseline postexercise is theorized to be due to high vagal tone associated with fitness and good health. While the prognostic value of HRR has recently been highlighted, its relative value compared with other treadmill responses and its diagnostic value remains uncertain. Table 8-4 shows comparisons of the HRR studies across a number of important parameters. In the first study, Cole et al[43] looked at 2428 adults who had been referred for exercise nuclear perfusion scans. Cole et al found that using a drop of 12 beats per minute or less as the definition of an abnormal response exhibited a relative risk of 4.0 for death; the group with a value lower than 12 having a mortality of 19%, and the group with a value higher than 12 having a mortality of 5% over the 6-year period. The study employed the symptom-limited Bruce protocol with a 2-minute cool-down walk, and HRR was measured at 1 minute after peak exercise. Patients on beta-blockers were included in the study, and in these patients no difference was seen in the ability of the test to discriminate between low- and high-risk groups. In this study, the investigators used all-cause mortality and performed survival analysis both with and without censoring of interventions (CABG and PCI), and found no difference in results.

The same investigators then studied a different patient population.[44] Asymptomatic patients enrolled in the Lipid Research Clinics Prevalence Study underwent exercise testing using a Bruce protocol. The tests were stopped when 85% to 90% of peak heart rate was achieved, and there was no cool-down walk. HRR was measured at 2 minutes of recovery. HRR continued to be a strong predictor of all-cause mortality; patients with an abnormal value had a mortality rate of 10% while patients with a normal value had a mortality rate of 4% at 12 years of follow-up.

In order to further elucidate the power of HRR in distinct populations, these same investigators then published another study using patients referred for standard treadmill testing.[45] Using the same methods as the original study, the investigators found similar results, although notably the cut-off value for an abnormal test was different. Patients with abnormal HRR had 8% mortality at 5.2 years, whereas patients with normal HRR had only 2% mortality. Neither this nor the previous study censored for CABG or PCI, and this study had 8% patients with CABG enrolled along with 75% asymptomatic individuals. The investigators also compared the prognostic ability of heart rate recovery to that of the DTS. Whereas the ischemic components of the Duke score did not have prognostic power, METs did, because the DTS produced similar survival curves to HRR. Patients with abnormal DTS and HRR survival were even further compromised.

We attempted to validate the use of HRR for prognosis in a male veteran population.[46] The mortality rate in our study was higher than in previous studies of HRR. Using similar statistical analysis, we found that HRR of less than 22 beats per minute at 2-minute recovery identified a high-risk group of patients. We also found that beta-blockers had no significant impact on the prognostic value of HRR. Through multivariate analysis, we evaluated the power of several other clinical and treadmill variables to see how they compared to HRR in their ability to predict poor outcome. Similar to Cole et al,[43] we found that low MET capacity was the most powerful predictor of mortality.

A distinct advantage over previous studies is that we selected a group who underwent coronary angiography. This made it possible to evaluate the diagnostic ability of HRR. Surprisingly, HRR was not selected among the standard variables to be included in a logistic model and its ROC curve did not indicate any discriminatory value. Therefore, although, HRR has been validated as an important prognostic variable, it did not help in diagnosing coronary disease in this study. Because in general

TABLE 8–4.   Previous published prognostic studies relating to the decrease of heart rate after exercise

Study	Population	Sample size (% women)	Years f/u	Exclusion criteria	Test protocol/ recovery status	Minutes of recovery/ cutpoint	Mortality (all-cause)	Sensitivity/ specificity for death	Other variables studied	Beta-blocker status
Cole* N Engl J Med	Referral for exercise perfusion; 9% with known CAD	2428 (37)	6	CABG, angiography, CHF/digoxin use, LBBB	Bruce, with 2-min cool down symptom-limited	1 min/12 bpm	213 (9%)	(cutpoint = 12 bpm) 56%/77% (cutpoint = 8 bpm) 33%/90%	METs, male sex, age, perfusion defects on scintigraphy, chronotropic incompetence No comparison	Used by 12% of study population No association with abnormal test
Cole Ann Intern Med	Participants in Lipid Research Clinics Prevalence Study, asymptomatic	5234 (39)	12	Beta-blockers, other cardiac medications, h/o cardiovascular disease	Bruce, without cool down 85% age predicted heart-rate	2 min/42 bpm	325 (6.2%), 36% felt to be cardiovascular follow-up 100%	54%/69%		Excluded
Nishime JAMA	Referral for ETT; 8% prior CABG, 75% screening asymptomatic, 9% prior MI	9454 (22)	5.2	CHF, LBBB, digoxin, valvular heart disease	Bruce, with 2-min cool down symptom-limited	1 min/12 bpm	312 (3%)	49%/81%	METs, maximal HR, Duke treadmill score; TM AP score and EI-ST depression not prognostic	Heart rate recovery not predictive of death in beta-blocker group
Watanabe Circulation	Referral for ETT-ECHO	5785 (37)	3	CHF, valve disease, Afib, pacer	N/A no cool down	1 min/18 bpm	190 (3.5%)	33%/87%	Data not available	N/A
Shetler J Am Coll Cardiol	Referral for Standard ETT; 42% with prior MI	2193 (all men)	6.8	CABG, angiography, LBBB, pacer	Ramp without cool down symptom-limited	2 min/22 bpm	413 (19%)	35%/83%	Age, METs, history of typical angina; TM AP score and EI-ST depression not prognostic	Used by 34% of the study population heart rate recovery equally predictive

these studies did not censor on events or consider event-free survival, heart rate recovery may well just be a surrogate for physical fitness or activity level predicting outcome along with medical therapy. Our conclusion is that these studies support the health benefits of a lifestyle of physical activity rather than the addition of HRR to scores designed to help direct patients to appropriate therapies. However, it is still an important addition to every exercise test performed.

The following studies addressed the issues of the ability of HRR to predict CV disease or events rather than all-cause mortality, and its performance in women and diabetics.

Because no prior study considered the association of HRR after exercise with the incidence of coronary heart disease and CV disease, 2967 Framingham study subjects (1400 men, mean age 43 years) free of CV disease were analyzed.[47] During 15 years follow-up, 214 subjects experienced a coronary heart disease event, 312 developed a CV disease event, and 167 died. In multivariable models, continuous HRR indexes were not associated with the incidence of coronary heart disease or CV disease events, or with all-cause mortality. However, in models evaluating quintile-based cutpoints, the top quintile of HRR (greatest decline in heart rate) at 1-minute after exercise was associated with half the coronary heart disease and CV disease as the bottom quintile, but not all-cause mortality.

A total of 2994 asymptomatic women without CV disease, 30 to 80 years of age, performed a near-maximal Bruce-protocol treadmill test as part of the Lipid Research Clinics Prevalence Study (1972–1976).[48] They were followed for 20 years with CV and all-cause mortality as the endpoints. There were 427 (14%) deaths, of which 147 were due to CV causes. Low exercise capacity, low HRR, and not achieving target heart rate were independently associated with increased all-cause and CV mortality. There was no increased CV death risk for exercise-induced ST-segment depression, but there was an age-adjusted 20% increase for every MET decrement and a 36% increase in CV mortality per 10 beats per minute decrement in HRR. After adjusting for multiple other risk factors, women who were below the median for both exercise capacity and HRR had a 3.5-fold increased risk of CV death. Among women with low-risk Framingham scores, those with below median levels of both METs and HRR had significantly increased risk compared with women who had above median levels of these two exercise variables, 45 and four CV deaths per 10,000 person-years, respectively (hazard ratio of 13).

In a cohort study, the Cleveland clinic group examined 2333 male diabetics who underwent a treadmill test at the Cooper Clinic.[49] Hazard ratios for CV and all-cause death were adjusted for age, METs, resting heart rate, fasting blood glucose, body mass index, smoking habit, alcohol consumption, lipids, and history of CV disease. During 15 years follow-up, there were 142 deaths that were considered CV disease related and 287 total deaths. Compared with men in the highest quartile of HRR, the adjusted hazard ratio was 1.5 to 2 for CV death.

Why is Cardiac Catheterization Considered to be Superior for Predicting Prognosis?

Enthusiasm for cardiac catheterization led to an acceptance of invasive measurements as superior to clinical variables for prognostication in patients with CAD. Although clinical variables were mentioned in the early studies, often, key ones were not considered nor were they considered together or defined as accurately as they are today. It was assumed that laboratory methods and images were more accurate and precise than simple clinical data. In addition, the importance of clinical data could have been underestimated because of the nonavailability of modern survival analysis techniques. A further consideration is that the decline in mortality by vessel score recently noted is not actually due to disease treatment but by patient selection (e.g., excluding patients with CHF because of a better recognition of it).

On the basis of clinical and exercise test data, patients with signs and symptoms of coronary heart disease can be classified into low- and high-risk categories. The latter clearly should be considered for cardiac catheterization, while the former should not, unless their symptoms dictate otherwise. The problem lies in justifying intervention to improve survival for patients whose symptoms are satisfactorily managed medically. Simple clinical indicators can stratify these patients with stable CAD into high- or low-risk groups. Cardiac catheterization is not needed to do so in the majority of such patients. Clinical judgment must be applied to decide whether intervention is likely to improve survival in our high-risk patients.

With the number of excellent outcome studies that have been completed but with divergent results to predict outcome, one must conclude that patient population as well as selection has a great impact upon results. The Duke and VA predictive equations appear to be the best and represent the "state of the art" in prognostication.

Does the Addition of Imaging Techniques Improve Prognostication?

Skeptics may say that the standard exercise test must be augmented by either radionuclide imaging or echocardiographic imaging to optimize the ability of the exercise test to predict prognosis. Therefore, a brief review of these technologies is appropriate. Naturally there has been an evolution in the technologies available since their inception, which makes any conclusions regarding their application somewhat of a "moving target." Nuclear techniques were first employed so we will start with them.

Nuclear Ventricular Function Assessment

One of the first techniques added to exercise testing was radionuclear ventriculography (RNV). This involved the intravenous injection of technetium-tagged red blood cells. Using ECG gating of images obtained from a scintillation camera, images of the blood circulating within the LV chamber could be obtained. While regurgitant blood flow from valvular lesions could not be identified, ejection fraction and ventricular volumes could be estimated. The resting values could be compared to those obtained during supine exercise and criteria were established for abnormal. The most common criteria involved a drop in ejection fraction.

Nuclear Perfusion Imaging

Although initially popular, these blood volume techniques have come to be surpassed by perfusion techniques. The first agent used was thallium, an isotopic analog of potassium that is taken up at variable rates by metabolically active tissue. When taken up at rest, images of metabolically active muscle, such as the heart, are possible. With the nuclear camera placed over the heart after intravenous injection of this isotope, images were initially viewed using an x-ray film. The normal complete donut-shaped images gathered in multiple views would be broken by "cold" spots where a scar was present. Defects viewed after exercise could be due to either scar or ischemia. Follow-up imaging confirmed that the "cold" spots were due to ischemia if they filled in later. As computer-imaging techniques were developed, three-dimensional

imaging (SPECT) and subtle differences could be plotted and scored. In recent years, ventriculograms based on the imaged wall, as apposed to the blood in the chambers (as with RNV), could be constructed. Because of the technical limitations of thallium (i.e., source and lifespan), it has largely been replaced by chemical compounds called isonitriles that can be tagged with technetium, which has many practical advantages over thallium as an imaging agent. The isonitriles are trapped in the microcirculation permitting imaging of the heart with a scintillation camera. The differences in technology over the years and the differences in expertise at different facilities can complicate the comparisons of the results and actual application of this technology.

Echocardiography

The impact of the echocardiogram on cardiology has been impressive. This imaging technique comes second only to contrast ventriculography via cardiac catheterization for measuring ventricular volumes, wall motion, and ejection fraction. With Doppler added, regurgitant flows can be estimated as well. Echocardiographers were quick to add this imaging modality to exercise, with most studies showing that supine, post-treadmill assessments were adequate, and the more difficult imaging during exercise was not necessary.

Available Prognostic Studies

The following is a summary of the available literature addressing the added value of these available add-ons to the exercise test.

Radionuclide Ventriculography. Simari et al[50] evaluated the ability of supine exercise ECG and RNV to predict subsequent cardiac events in 265 patients with a normal resting ECG and who were not receiving digoxin, but who had undergone cardiac catheterization. The Cox model chose ST depression, exercise heart rate, and patient gender as equivalent to the RNV data. They concluded that exercise RNV was not justified for use over standard exercise variables. This conclusion was countered by Lee et al[51] in his study of 571 patients in which RNV provided more prognostic information than clinical variables.

Nuclear Perfusion. An elegant review by Brown[53] summarized the available knowledge regarding the prognostic value of nuclear perfusion imaging as of 1991. The two most comparable and comprehensive studies up to that point were those by Kaul et al[53] and Melin et al[54], who concluded that change in heart rate and other exercise test variables were superior to perfusion defects for prognostication.

The group at Cedars-Sinai identified 5183 consecutive patients who underwent stress/rest nuclear perfusion and were followed-up for the occurrence of cardiac death or MI.[55] Over a mean follow-up of 2 years, 119 cardiac deaths and 158 MIs occurred (3.0% cardiac death rate, 2.3% MI rate). Patients with normal scans were at low risk (≤0.5% per year), and rates of both outcomes increased significantly with worsening scan abnormalities. Patients who underwent exercise testing and had mildly abnormal scans had low rates of cardiac death but higher rates of MI (0.7% versus 2.6% per year). After adjustment for prescan information, scan results provided incremental prognostic value toward the prediction of cardiac death. Myocardial nuclear perfusion yielded incremental prognostic information toward the identification of cardiac death. Patients with mildly abnormal scans after exercise stress are at low risk for cardiac death, but intermediate risk for nonfatal MI, and thus may benefit from a noninvasive strategy and may not require invasive management.

A prognostic study was based on 3400 consecutive adults undergoing exercise nuclear perfusion testing at the Cleveland Clinic Foundation between September 1990 and December 1993; none had previous invasive procedures, heart failure, or valve disease.[56] Estimated METs, classified by age and gender, and perfusion defects, expressed as a stress extent score on a 12-segment scale, were analyzed to determine their relative prognostic importance during 2 years of follow-up. Of 3400 patients, 108 (3.2%) died during follow-up; 32 deaths were identified as cardiac related. On univariate analysis, estimated METs was a strong predictor of death, with 62 (57%) deaths occurring in patients achieving less than 6 METs. On multivariable analysis, the strongest independent predictors of all-cause mortality were low METs (relative risk [RR] of 4×) and age. The presence of perfusion defects was a less powerful predictor of death. Cardiac mortality was predicted by decreased METs (RR of 4.4×) and by stress extent score (RR of 1.4×). In this clinically low-risk group, METs was a strong and overwhelmingly important independent predictor of all-cause mortality among patients undergoing exercise perfusion testing. The extent of myocardial perfusion defects was of comparable importance for the prediction of cardiac mortality.

Gibbon's group[57] at Mayo Clinic sought to determine whether their previously validated clinical score could identify patients with a low-risk DTS who had a higher risk of adverse events and, therefore, in whom myocardial perfusion imaging would be valuable for risk stratification. They studied 1461 symptomatic patients with low-risk DTS (≥5) who underwent myocardial perfusion imaging. The score was derived by assigning one point to each of the following variables: typical angina, history of MI, diabetes, insulin use, male gender, and each decade of age over 40 years. A score cut-off equaling or greater than 5 or less than 5 was used to categorize patients as high risk (n = 303 [21%]) or low risk (n = 1158 [79%]). Perfusion scans were categorized as low, intermediate, or high risk on the basis of a score. High-risk scans were more common in patients with a high-risk score. The score and perfusion score were significant independent predictors of cardiac death. However, in patients with a low score, 7-year cardiac survival was excellent, regardless of the nuclear perfusion result (99% for normal and 99% even for severely abnormal scans). In contrast, patients with a high score had a lower 7-year survival rate (92%), which varied with the nuclear perfusion score. They concluded that in symptomatic patients with low-risk DTS and low clinical risk, myocardial perfusion imaging is of limited prognostic value. In patients with low-risk DTS and high clinical risk, annual cardiac mortality (>1%) is not low, and myocardial perfusion imaging has independent prognostic value.

French researchers assessed the long-term prognostic value of the ECG and nuclear perfusion exercise tests in a large population of patients with low to intermediate risk of cardiac events.[58] They followed 1137 patients (857 men, mean age 55 years), referred for typical (62%) or atypical (22%) chest pain, or suspected silent ischemia (16%) for 6 years. Overall mortality was higher after strongly abnormal (ST depression >2 mm, or >1 mm for a workload ≤5 METs) (2.4% per year) or nondiagnostic (1.6% per year) bike test than after normal (0.85% per year) or abnormal (1.4% per year) bike test, and after abnormal nuclear perfusion than after normal perfusion (1.6% per year versus 0.7% per year). The major cardiac event rate (cardiac death or MI) was 0.9%, 1.6%, 2%, and 2% per year after negative, positive, strongly positive, and nondiagnostic exercise test and 0.6%, 1.4%, and 2% per year in patients with 0, 1 to 2, and equal or greater than 3 abnormal segments on nuclear perfusion, respectively. In multivariate analysis, nuclear perfusion had modest incremental prognostic value over clinical and exercise test data for predicting overall mortality and major cardiac events, and the predictive value of nuclear perfusion was maintained over 6 years.

A retrospective study was performed in 388 consecutive patients comparing the prognostic utility of perfusion imaging and exercise ECG in patients with an exercise capacity exceeding 7 METs.[59] Follow-up was performed at 1.5 years for adverse events ($n = 40$), including revascularization, MI, and cardiac death. Of the patients, 19 had revascularization related to the testing or their condition and were not included in further analysis; 17 (12%) with abnormal scan and 4 (2%) with normal scan had adverse cardiac events. In Cox proportional hazards analysis, an abnormal scan had a hazard of eight times, while neither the ECG nor DTS had similar hazards. These contrary results are probably due to a biased selection of patients for scanning and the exclusion of patients due to test results leading to interventions.

The Cleveland Clinic group evaluated nuclear perfusion for prediction of all-cause mortality when considered along with METs and HRR.[60] They followed 7163 consecutive adults referred for symptom-limited exercise nuclear perfusion (mean age 60, 25% women) for 7 years; 855 deaths were found to have occurred. Using information theory, they identified a probable best model relating nuclear findings to outcome in order to calculate a prognostic nuclear score. Intermediate- and high-risk prognostic nuclear scores were noted in 28% and 10% of patients. Compared with those who had low-risk scans, patients with an intermediate-risk score were at increased risk for death (14% versus 9%, hazard ratio 1.7), while those with high-risk scores were at greater risk (24%, hazard ratio 3). Impaired exercise capacity and decreased HRR provided additional prognostic information to the nuclear perfusion score.

To assess the incremental value of exercise nuclear perfusion imaging for the prediction of cardiac events in patients with known or suspected CAD, follow-up was performed in 648 patients.[61] Ten patients underwent early coronary revascularization, and seven lost to follow up were excluded. Endpoints were cardiac death, nonfatal infarction, and late (>60 days) coronary revascularization. An abnormal study was defined as the presence of fixed and/or reversible perfusion defects. A summed stress score (SSS) was derived to estimate the extent and severity of perfusion defects. An abnormal scan was detected in 344 patients (54%). During a mean follow-up period of 4 years, 56 patients (9%) died; 22 of the deaths were caused

by cardiac conditions. Nonfatal MI occurred in 19 patients (3%), and 89 patients (14%) underwent late coronary revascularization. An abnormal scan and SSS were independent predictors of cardiac death (hazard ratio 3.5) and provided incremental information over clinical and exercise test data.

Echocardiography. At the Mayo Clinic the outcome of 1325 patients after normal exercise echocardiography were examined to identify potential predictors of subsequent cardiac events.[62] Endpoints were overall and cardiac event-free survival. Cardiac events were defined as cardiac death, nonfatal MI, and coronary revascularization. Patient characteristics were analyzed in relation of time to first cardiac event in a univariate and multivariate manner to determine which, if any, were associated with an increased hazard of subsequent cardiac events. Overall survival of the study group was significantly better than that of an age- and gender-matched group obtained from life tables. The cardiac event-free survival rates at 1, 2, and 3 years were 99.2%, 97.8%, and 97.4%, respectively. The cardiac event rate per person-year of follow-up was 0.9%. Subgroups with an intermediate or high pretest probability of having CAD also had low cardiac event rates. Multivariate predictors of subsequent cardiac events were angina during exercise testing (RR 4×), low exercise capacity (RR 3×), and echocardiographic LV hypertrophy (RR 2.6×). The outcome after normal exercise echocardiography was good even in those with an intermediate or high pretest probability of having CAD. In a subsequent study, these investigators examined the outcomes of 1874 patients with known or suspected CAD (mean age 64, 64% men) who had good exercise capacity (≥5 METs for women, 7 METs for men) but abnormal exercise echocardiograms and analyzed the association between clinical, exercise, and echocardiographic variables and subsequent cardiac events.[63] Multivariate predictors of time to cardiac death or nonfatal MI were diabetes mellitus (RR 2×), history of MI (RR 2.4×), and an increase or no change in LV end-systolic size in response to exercise (RR 1.6×). Using echocardiographic variables that were of incremental prognostic value, they were only able to further stratify the cardiac risk from 1.6% for patients who had a decrease in LV end-systolic size in response to exercise ($n = 1330$) to 1.2% for patients with normal exercise ECHO ($n = 868$).

Marwick et al[64] collected clinical and exercise testing data on 5375 patients (aged 54 years, 60% men) referred for exercise echocardiography and followed them up for 6 years; 649 patients died.

The Duke score classified 59% of patients as low risk, 39% as intermediate risk, and 2% as high risk. Resting LV dysfunction was present in 27% and the exercise echocardiogram was abnormal in 47%. Those with normal exercise echocardiograms had a mortality of 1% per year. Ischemia was an independent predictor of mortality. In sequential Cox models, the predictive power of clinical data was strengthened by adding the Duke score, resting LV function, and the results of exercise echocardiography. Exercise echocardiography was able to substratify patients with intermediate-risk Duke scores into groups with a yearly mortality of 2% to 7%. They concluded that a normal exercise echocardiogram confers a low risk of death and that the ECHO add-on was particularly useful in patients with intermediate-risk DTS. However, they did not consider CV death or MI as endpoints.

Elhendy et al[65] studied 5679 patients (aged 62; 3231 men) who were followed for a mean of 3 years after treadmill echocardiography. Patients were randomly divided into a modeling and a training group. The modeling group underwent multivariate analysis to define independent predictors of mortality. Three hundred bootstrap resamplings were performed to determine parameter coefficients. Patients were divided into five risk categories according to their composite score. The validation group comprised patients for whom the risk model was applied. Patients were divided into five risk categories based on data obtained from the modeling group. During follow-up, 315 patients died (151 in the modeling group). Independent predictors of mortality were exercise wall motion score index (first), workload (second), male gender (third), and age (fourth). Application of the composite score in the validation group resulted in an effective stratification of patients for mortality and cardiac events. However, it is important to note that exercise capacity and basic demographics provide the majority of the prognostic information.

Summary. What do these findings mean to the clinician? First, it should be noted that all studies have population-specific attributes that may be difficult to define. Nevertheless, if the aim is to predict infarct-free survival, the DTS is preferred because censoring was performed and infarct-free survival was predicted. All of the findings strengthen the importance of exercise capacity—a reflection of the integrity of the cardiopulmonary system and a marker of a physically active lifestyle—as an important predictor of survival along with, or in spite of, modern medical treatment.

COMPARISON OF PREDICTION EQUATIONS WITH CARDIOLOGISTS

To study the accuracy with which long-term prognosis can be predicted in patients with CAD, prognostic predictions from a data-based multivariable statistical model were compared with predictions from senior cardiologists.[66] Test samples of 100 patients each were selected from a large series of medically treated patients with significant coronary disease. Using detailed case summaries, five senior cardiologists each predicted 1- and 3-year survival and infarct-free survival probabilities for 100 patients. Fifty patients appeared in multiple samples for assessing interphysician variability. Cox regression models, developed using patients not in the test samples, predicted corresponding outcome probabilities for each test patient. Overall, model predictions correlated better with actual patient outcomes than did the doctors' predictions. For 3-year survival, rank correlations were 0.61 (model) and 0.49 (doctors). For 3-year infarct-free survival predictions, correlations with outcome were 0.48 (model) and 0.29 (doctors). Comparisons by individual doctor revealed Cox model 3-year survival predictions were better than those of four of five doctors (model predictions added significant [$p < 0.05$] prognostic information to the doctor's predictions, whereas the converse was not true). For infarct-free survival, the Cox model was superior to all five doctors. In cases where multiple doctors made predictions, the interphysician variability was substantial. In CAD, statistical models developed from carefully collected data can provide prognostic predictions that are more accurate than predictions of experienced clinicians, made from detailed case summaries.

A computer algorithm for estimating probabilities of any significant coronary obstruction and triple-vessel/left main obstructions was derived, validated, and compared with the assessments of cardiac clinician angiographers.[67] The algorithm performed at least as well as the clinicians when the latter knew the identity of the patients whose angiograms they had decided to perform. The clinicians were more accurate when they did not know the identity of the subjects but worked from tabulated objective data. Referral and value-induced bias may affect physician judgment in assessing disease probability. Application of computer aids or consultation with cardiologists not directly involved with patient management may assist in more rational assessments and decision-making.

With these two papers as background, we used our database to compare exercise test scores and ST measurements with a physician's estimation of the probability of the presence and severity of angiographically significant CAD and the risk of death.[68,69] A clinical exercise test was performed and an angiographic database was used to print patient summaries and treadmill reports. The clinical and treadmill test reports were sent to expert cardiologists and to two other groups, including randomly selected cardiologists and internists. They classified the patients summarized in the reports as having a high-, low-, or intermediate probability for the presence of any and also severe angiographically significant disease using a numerical probability from 0% to 100%. The Social Security Death Index was used to determine survival status of the patients. Of the patients, 26% had severe angiographically significant disease, and the annual mortality rate for the population was 2%. Forty-five expert cardiologists returned estimates on 473 patients, 37 randomly chosen practicing cardiologists returned estimates on 202 patients, 29 randomly chosen practicing internists returned estimates on 162 patients, 13 academic cardiologists returned estimates on 145 patients, and 27 academic internists returned estimates on 272 patients. When probability estimates for presence and severity of angiographically significant disease were compared, in general, the treadmill scores were superior to physicians' and ST analysis at predicting severe angiographic disease. When prognosis was estimated, treadmill prognostic scores did as well as expert cardiologists and better than most other physician groups.

PREDICTING SEVERE ANGIOGRAPHICALLY SIGNIFICANT CAD

Using Clinical Variables

Pryor et al[70] examined clinical characteristics predictive of severe disease in 6435 consecutive symptomatic patients referred for suspected CAD between 1969 and 1983. Eleven of 23 characteristics were important for estimating the likelihood of severe angiographically significant disease. These included chest pain type, previous MI, age, sex, duration of chest pain symptoms, risk factors, carotid bruit, and chest pain frequency. A model using these characteristics accurately estimated the likelihood of severe disease in an independent sample of 2342 patients referred to Duke since 1983. The model also accurately estimated the prevalence of severe CAD in a large series of patients reported in the literature. Hubbard et al[71] performed a similar study from the Mayo Clinic. Five variables were found to be predictive of severe disease: age, gender, diabetes, typical angina, and history of prior MI. An international cross-validation study was performed by Detrano et al[72] concluding that use of their algorithm could avert at least 10 angiograms on patients with less severe disease for every missed case of severe disease. These studies demonstrate that the clinician's initial evaluation even without a treadmill test can identify patients at high or low risk of anatomically severe CAD. These important studies emphasize that cost-conscious quality care can be accomplished by consideration of simple clinical variables to identify patients at higher risk for severe CAD who are most likely to benefit from further evaluation.

Using Exercise Test Responses

Studies have tried to predict left main disease using exercise testing.[17,73-74] Different criteria have been used with varying results. Predictive value here refers to the percentage of those with the abnormal criteria that actually had left main disease. Naturally, most of the "false positives" actually had CAD but in a less severe form. Sensitivity here refers to the percentage of those with left main disease only that are detected. These criteria have been refined over time and the last study by Weiner et al[18] using the CASS data deserves further mention. Weiner et al[18] defined a markedly positive exercise test in a study of 436 consecutive patients referred for suspected or known CAD who were able to undergo both exercise testing and coronary angiography. All patients underwent treadmill testing using the Bruce protocol, and 12-lead ECG were obtained during exercise. A lesion of the left main coronary artery was considered significant if it had greater than 50% diameter narrowing and this criterion was 70% in other vessels. Fifty-five patients were excluded because of LV hypertrophy, digoxin therapy, left bundle branch block, and for the attainment of less than 85% maximal predictive heart rate. Of these 55, two had left main CAD, and four had three-vessel disease, therefore the predictive value of being excluded was about 10%. Four patient groups were defined by angiographic findings: (1) 35 with left main disease, (2) 89 with three-vessel disease without left main disease, (3) 188 patients with either one-or two-vessel disease, and (4) 124 patients with no significant coronary disease. Of the 35 patients with left main disease, most had disease of other coronary arteries and nearly half had three-vessel disease. Exercise test responses that were considered included the amount of ST-segment depression, configuration, onset, and duration, and the number of leads in which it occurred. Hemodynamic responses included treadmill time, SBP, and maximal heart rate. Other measurements included angina, PVCs, and abnormal R-wave response in lead V_5.

Nearly all patients with left main disease had at least 0.1 mV of ST depression and 91% had 0.2 mV or more of ST-segment depression. Patients with left main disease as a group were distinguished from patients with three-vessel disease by an early onset and longer persistence of ST-segment depression, as well as by a greater number of leads in which the depression occurred. A fall in SBP occurred in 23% of the patients with left main disease versus 17% of those with triple-vessel disease and 6% of those with single- or double-vessel disease. As an indicator of either left main or three-vessel disease, a fall in SBP had a predictive value of 66% and a sensitivity of 19%. The criterion of 0.3 mV or more of ST-segment depression occurred in 44% of such patients and had only a slightly lower predictive value (64%). Combined analysis of test variables (i.e., a markedly abnormal response, Table 8-5) disclosed that the development of 0.2 mV or more of downsloping ST-segment depression beginning at 4 METs, persisting for at least 6 minutes into recovery, and involving at least five ECG leads had the greatest sensitivity (74%) and predictive value (32%) for left main coronary disease. This abnormal pattern identified either left main or three-vessel disease with a sensitivity of 49%, a specificity of 92%, and a predictive value of 74%.

It appears that individual clinical or exercise test variables are unable to detect left main coronary disease because of their low sensitivity or predictive value. However, a combination of the amount, pattern, and duration of ST-segment response was

highly predictive and reasonably sensitive for left main or three-vessel coronary disease. The question still remains of how to identify those with abnormal resting ejection fractions, those that will benefit the most with prolonged survival after CABS. Perhaps those with a normal resting ECG will not need surgery for increased longevity because of the associated high probability of normal ventricular function.

Blumenthal et al[75] validated the ability of a strongly positive exercise test to predict left main coronary disease even in patients with minimal or no angina. The criteria for a markedly positive test included: (1) early ST-segment depression, (2) 0.2 mV or more of depression, (3) downsloping ST depression, (4) exercise-induced hypotension, (5) prolonged ST changes after the test, and (6) multiple areas of ST depression.

While Lee et al[76] included many clinical and exercise test variables, only three variables were found to help predict left main disease: angina type, age, and the amount of exercise-induced ST-segment depression. Using a Bayesian approach, the pretest likelihood of left main disease was best determined by the type of angina and age. In spite of the many clinical markers considered, such as unstable angina, history of MI, and others, only age and the angina type were found best to predict pretest probability of disease. The only exercise test variable that was found to then improve the post-test probability was the amount of ST-segment depression. There is a low pretest probability of left main disease in 40-year-old men with atypical angina and a high pretest probability of left main disease in older men with typical angina. Given a pretest probability of 50%, for example, the post-test probability could range from 20% to 75% according to the degree of ST-segment depression.

The problem with using the amount of depression as the sole predictor is that in many exercise labs, an exercise test is stopped at 2 mm of ST depression for safety reasons or because of severe angina. In addition, some physicians stop the test at an age-predicted maximal heart rate. Surprisingly, exercise-induced hypotension and exercise duration did not impact on post-test probability in their analysis.

TABLE 8–5. The markedly positive responses identified by Weiner

>0.2 mV downsloping ST-segment depression
Involving five or more leads
Occurring at less than 5 METs
Prolonged late into recovery

Meta-Analysis of Studies Predicting Angiographic Severity

To evaluate the variability in the reported accuracy of the exercise ECG for predicting severe coronary disease, Detrano et al[77] applied meta-analysis to 60 consecutively published reports comparing exercise-induced ST depression with coronary angiographic findings. The 60 reports included 62 distinct study groups comprising 12,030 patients who underwent both tests. Both technical and methodologic factors were analyzed. Wide variability in sensitivity and specificity was found (*mean sensitivity 86%* [range 40% to 100%]; mean *specificity 53%* [range 17% to 100%]) for left main or triple-vessel disease. All three variables found to be significantly and independently related to test performance were methodological. Exclusion of patients with right bundle branch block or who were receiving digoxin improved the prediction of triple vessel or left main CAD and comparison with a "better" exercise test decreased test performance.

Hartz et al[78] compiled results from the literature on the use of the exercise test to identify patients with severe CAD. Pooled estimates of sensitivity and specificity were derived for the ability of the exercise test to identify three-vessel or left main CAD. *One millimeter criteria averaged a sensitivity of 75% and a specificity of 66%* while *two millimeters* criteria averaged a *sensitivity of 52% and a specificity of 86%*. There was great variability among the studies examined in the estimated sensitivity and specificity for severe CAD that could not be explained by their analysis.

Multivariable Equations and Scores to Predict Severe Angiographically Significant CAD

The most common statistical methods employed include Bayesian statistics, logistic regression, and discriminant function analysis. The Bayesian approach, which considers pretest clinical variables, is a logical method in clinical practice and helps one decide which tests are appropriate. However, it appears that logistic regression or discriminant function analysis permits a more robust prediction of disease.

Multivariable analysis is a statistical technique that seeks to separate subjects into different groups on the basis of measured variables.[79] Clinical investigators have commonly used two types of analysis: discriminate function and logistic regression analysis. Logistic regression has been preferred since it models the relationship to a sigmoid curve (which often is the mathematical relationship between a risk variable and an outcome) and its output is between 0 and 1 (i.e., from 0% to 100% probability of the predicted outcome). Thus, the output of a discriminate function is a unitless

numerical score, while a logistic regression provides an actual probability; this, however, may vary from one population to another.

Logistic regression results in an equation that takes the form:

$$\text{Probability} = 1 / (1 + e^{-(a + bx + cy \dots)})$$

where a is the intercept; b and c are coefficients; x and y are variable values such as 0 or 1 for gender, diabetes, or chest pain; and there is a continuous value for age or heart rate.

Studies Using Multivariate Techniques to Predict Severe Angiographically Significant CAD

Since 1979, 13 studies reported combining the patient's medical history, symptoms of chest pain, hemodynamic data, exercise capacity, and exercise test responses to calculate the probability of severe angiographic CAD.[72,80-89] The results are summarized in Table 8-6. Of the 13 studies, 9 excluded patients with previous CABS or prior PCI and in the remaining 4 studies, exclusions were unclear. The definition of significant percentage stenosis for angiographically significant disease ranged from 50% to 70%. The percentage of patients with one-, two-, and three-vessel disease was described in 10 of the 13 studies. The definition of severe disease

TABLE 8-6. A summary of the results from the 13 studies (14 equations) predicting disease severity

Clinical variables	Significant predictors	
Gender	7/9	78%
Chest pain symptoms	8/11	73%
Diabetes mellitus	6/10	60%
Age	8/14	57%
Abnormal resting ECG	4/8	50%
Elevated cholesterol	4/10	40%
Family history of CAD	1/4	25%
Smoking history	2/8	25%
Hypertension	1/6	17%
Exercise test variables		
ST-segment depression	11/14	79%
ST-segment slope	6/8	75%
Double product	4/7	57%
Delta systolic BP	5/11	45%
Exercise capacity	4/13	31%
Exercise induced angina	4/13	31%
Maximal HR	1/10	10%
Maximal systolic BP	0/4	0%

or disease extent (multivessel versus three-vessel or left main artery disease) also differed. In 5 of the 13 studies disease extent was defined as multivessel disease (i.e., more than one vessel involved). In the remaining 8 studies, it was defined as three-vessel or left main disease and in one of them as only left main artery disease and in another the impact of disease in the right CAD on left main disease was considered. The prevalence of severe disease ranged from 16% to 48% in the studies defining disease extent as multivessel disease and from 10% to 28% in the studies using the more strict criterion of three-vessel or left main disease.

Not all of the publications of the reviewed studies included the equations derived from the multivariable analyses they performed. These equations are critical to the validation of their findings.[90] The actual equations developed in the studies were available for only 4 of the 13 studies predicting disease extent or severity.

Some notable results were obtained in 1 of the 13 studies that did not produce a score because discriminate function analysis was utilized. Ribisl et al[91] studied 607 male patients to determine whether patterns and severity of CAD could be predicted using standard clinical and exercise test data. Left main disease produced responses significantly different from three-vessel disease only when accompanied by a 70% or greater narrowing of the right coronary artery. The maximum amount of horizontal or downsloping ST depression in exercise and/or recovery was the most powerful predictor of disease severity, with 2-mm ST depression yielding a sensitivity of 55% and specificity of 80% for prediction of severe CAD (three-vessel plus left main disease). Patients with increasingly severe disease also demonstrated a greater frequency of abnormal hemodynamic responses to exercise. It appears that the exercise test will best distinguish left main or left main equivalent disease only when there is significant disease in the right coronary artery (i.e., similar to three-vessel disease). Otherwise, the exercise responses are similar to patients with two-vessel disease. The exercise test did not function worse in patients selected for beta-blocker administration and that standard ST analysis outperforms the ST/HR index in either situation.[92]

Chosen Predictors. Surprisingly, some of the variables chosen for predicting severe disease are different than those for predicting disease presence for diagnosis. While gender and chest pain were chosen to be significant in more than half of the severity studies, age was less important and

resting ECG abnormalities and diabetes were the only other variables chosen in more than half the studies. In contrast, the most consistent clinical variables chosen for diagnosis were: age, gender, chest pain type, and hypercholesterolemia. ST depression and slope were frequently chosen for severity, but METs and heart rate were less consistently chosen than for diagnosis. Double product and delta SBP were chosen as independent predictors in more than half of the studies predicting severity.

History of Myocardial Infarction as a Clinical Predictor. Although it makes little sense to consider a history of MI or Q-wave evidence for MI in studies dealing with diagnosis, there is some justification for considering them in studies dealing with disease severity. This variable has been defined in numerous ways, including patient history (or chart review) or by review of resting ECG for Q waves. One coding scheme called for a 1 if by history only, 2 if diagnostic Q waves were present, and 3 if both history and Q waves were present. The amount of LV damage (considered to be the result of severe coronary disease) has been estimated in some studies by a Q-wave score or by summing the number of diagnostic Q waves. This variable was a significant predictor in 2 of the 8 studies that considered it. Due to the inaccuracy of historical data alone, emphasis should also be given to objective measures such as diagnostic criteria for Q waves for a prior infarction.

Consensus or Agreement to Improve Prediction

Only two of the studies (Detrano et al[72] and Morise et al[85]) have published equations that have been validated in large patient samples. Although validated, the equations from these studies must be calibrated before they can be applied clinically. For example, a score can be discriminating but provide an estimated probability that is higher or lower than the actual probability. The scores can be calibrated by adjusting them according to disease prevalence; most clinical sites, however, do not know their disease prevalence and even if known, it could change from month to month.

At the National Aeronautics and Space Administration (NASA), trajectories of spacecraft are often determined by agreement between three or more equations calculating the vehicle path. With this in mind, we developed an agreement method to classify patients into high, no agreement, or low-risk groups for probability of severe disease by requiring agreement in all three equations (Detrano, Morise and ours [Long Beach and Palo Alto]).[93] This approach adjusts the calibration and makes the equations applicable in clinical populations with varying prevalence of CAD.

We demonstrated that using simple clinical and exercise test variables could improve the standard application of ECG criteria for predicting severe CAD. By setting probability thresholds for severe disease at less than 20% and greater than 40% for the three prediction equations, the agreement approach divided the test set into populations with low risk, no agreement, and high risk for severe CAD. Since the patients in the no-agreement group would be sent for further testing and would eventually be correctly classified, *the sensitivity of the agreement approach was 89% and the specificity was 96%*. The agreement approach appeared to be unaffected by disease prevalence, missing data, variable definitions, or even by angiographic criterion. Cost analysis of the competing strategies revealed that the agreement approach compares favorably with other tests of equivalent predictive value, such as nuclear perfusion imaging, reducing costs by 28%, or $504, per patient in the test set.

Requiring diagnosis of severe coronary disease to be dependent on agreement between these three equations has made them likely to function in all clinical populations. Excellent predictive characteristics can be obtained using simple clinical data entered into a computer. Cost analysis suggests that the agreement approach is an efficient method for the evaluation of populations with varying prevalence of CAD, limiting the use of more expensive noninvasive and invasive testing to patients with a higher probability of left main or three-vessel CAD. This approach provides a strategy for assisting the practitioner in deciding when further evaluation is appropriate or interventions indicated.

PREDICTING IMPROVED SURVIVAL WITH CORONARY ARTERY BYPASS SURGERY

Which exercise test variables indicate those patients who would have an improved prognosis if they underwent CABS? *The limitation of the available studies is that the patients were not randomized to surgery according to their exercise test results and the analysis is retrospective.*

Bruce et al[94] demonstrated noninvasive screening criteria for patients who had improved 4-year survival after CABS. Their data came from 2000 men with coronary heart disease enrolled in the Seattle Heart Watch who had a symptom-limited maximal treadmill test; these subjects received usual community care, which resulted in 16% of them having CABS in nonrandomized fashion. The diagnosis of coronary heart disease was based on a history of angina, MI, or cardiac arrest. Cardiomegaly was determined by physical and chest x-ray examinations. The patients were divided into three groups. One group had only myocardial ischemia manifested by exercise test-induced normal ST-segment elevation or depression and/or angina. The second group could have myocardial ischemia, but had to have "LV dysfunction" manifested by at least two of the following: cardiomegaly, less than 4 METs exercise capacity, and less than 130 mmHg maximal SBP. A third group had none of the above. Comparisons were then made within each group between the operated and unoperated patients and surprisingly little difference was found. However, life table analysis showed a significantly higher survival rate of 94% at 4 years among the operated patients, as compared with the 68% survival of the unoperated patients in the group with LV dysfunction. If the 4.6% death rate due to surgery in those with "ischemia" only was reduced, perhaps the patients who were operated on in that group would have had a significantly improved survival as well. Thus, patients with cardiomegaly, less than 5 MET exercise capacity and/or a maximal SBP of less than 130 mmHg would have a better outcome if treated with surgery. Two or more of the above parameters present the highest risk and the greater differential for improved survival with bypass. In this group, 4-year survival would be 94% for those who had surgery versus 67% for those who received medical management (in those who had two or more of the above factors). In the European surgery trial,[95] patients who had an exercise test response of 1.5 mm of ST-segment depression had improved survival with surgery. This also extended to those with baseline ST segment depression and those with claudication.

From the CASS study group,[96] in more than 5000 nonrandomized patients, although there were definite differences between the surgical and nonsurgical groups, this could be accounted for by stratification in subsets. The surgical benefit regarding mortality was greatest in the 789 patients with 1-mm ST-segment depression at less than 5 METs. Among the 398 patients with triple-vessel disease with this exercise test response, the 7-year survival was 50% in those medically managed versus 81% in those who underwent CABS.

There was no difference in mortality in patients able to exceed 10 METs exercise capacity. From the VA CABS randomized trial, Hultgren et al[97] reported a 79% survival rate with CABS versus 42% for medical management in patients with two or more of the following: 2 mm or more of ST depression, heart rate of 140 or greater at 6 METs, and/or exercise-induced PVCs. The results from those four studies are summarized in Table 8-7.

SPECIALIZED SITUATIONS FOR PREDICTING POOR PROGNOSIS AND/OR SEVERE CAD

- In the elderly
- In diabetic patients and those with silent ischemia

The Elderly

The decline in function that accompanies aging is a consequence of age-related decrements in CV, pulmonary, and musculoskeletal structure. Ultimately, these result in impaired physical function in the elderly.[98] Whereas the DTS was validated in patients in the age range when CAD first

appears, in the elderly, data is limited. To determine the prognostic value of the treadmill test in the elderly, researchers from the Mayo Clinic and the Olmsted Medical Group compared the prognostic value of the test in patients less than 65 and older than 65 years of age.[99] Elderly ($n = 514$) and younger ($n = 2593$) patients who underwent treadmill testing between 1987 and 1989 were identified retrospectively and followed-up for 6 years. Compared to younger patients, elderly patients had more comorbid conditions, a higher prevalence of abnormal ST depression (28% versus 9%) and achieved lower workloads (6 versus 11 METs). A poor exercise capacity and angina during the exercise test were associated with future cardiac events. Exercise-induced ST depression did not carry significant value in the elderly and was associated with future cardiac events only in younger patients. An increase of 1 MET in the workload was associated with a 14% decrease in risk for a cardiac event in younger patients and with an 18% risk reduction among the elderly. After adjustment for clinical factors, there was a strong inverse association between exercise capacity and outcome. METs was the only treadmill exercise-testing variable that provided prognostic information for mortality and cardiac events. In the elderly, exercise capacity was also inversely associated with the likelihood of nursing home placement. Spin et al[100] also demonstrated the strong association between METs estimated from exercise testing and all-cause mortality in the elderly.

Kwok et al[101] found that the DTS could not predict death, MI, and cardiac interventions in patients 75 years or older. Lai et al[102] considered both death and angiographic endpoints and found age-specific scores to be necessary in the elderly. Given this last study, we entered the DTS and age into the Cox analysis and found them to have similar coefficients but opposite sign so that a new score equation was expressed as DTS minus age. Thus, age was as strong a prognostic predictor as the DTS in our population. A score of DTS minus age provided a significant improvement in area under the curve compared to DTS alone in the whole population and the subset of younger subjects, but there was no improvement in the elderly.

Why do the exercise test variables other than METs not provide prognostic information in those over 75 years of age? Possibly it is due to the many competing causes of mortality in the elderly compared to younger subjects, who are more likely to die of one cause. It is also possible that the elderly are survivors who, for instance, have coronary disease but have extensive collaterals that protect

TABLE 8-7. Studies evaluating exercise test responses indicate improved survival with coronary artery bypass surgery

Study	Markers of improved survival with coronary artery bypass surgery
Seattle heart watch	• Cardiomegaly • Less than 5 METs exercise capacity • Maximal systolic blood pressure less than 130
European surgery trial	• ST-segment depression at rest • 1.5 mm of ST-segment depression with exercise • Claudication
Coronary artery surgery study (CASS)	• 1 mm of ST-segment depression at less than 5 METs • No difference if 10 METs exceeded
Veterans affairs coronary artery bypass surgery study	Two or more of the following: • 2 mm of ST-segment depression • Heart rate less than 140 at 6 METs • Exercise-induced premature ventricular contractions

them from death, but not ischemia. Reduced exercise capacity in the elderly is partially explained by the high prevalence of coexisting medical problems, such as deconditioning, muscle weakness, orthopedic problems, neurological problems, and peripheral vascular disease. Elderly patients are also more likely to have a nondiagnostic exercise ECG because of the greater prevalence of resting ECG abnormalities. These factors could confound the association between exercise test responses and outcomes.

To further study this issue, we classified our patients into subsets based on age. METs were chosen by the Cox hazard model most consistently in the age groups using either endpoint. Even when age was added to the DTS, prediction of death did not improve in those over 70 years of age because of the nonlinear relationship between age, the exercise test variables, and time to death. The most important age cutpoints for clinically important differences in exercise test predictors appeared to be 70 and 75 years of age. In the patients 70 to 75 years of age, METs was the only variable predictive of all-cause mortality and exercise-induced ST depression was the only predictor of CV death; in the patients older than 75 years of age, none of the exercise test responses were predictive of either death outcome (Table 8-8). None of the treadmill variables were selected as a predictor of outcome in those 45 years old or younger. This is probably due to the small number of deaths and our lack of data regarding cardiac interventions during follow-up. Exercise-induced ST depression was significantly more prevalent in those who died, but it

was independently associated with CV mortality only in those 45 to 55 years of age. The failure of DTS to have prognostic value in our population remains a mystery since in the very same population it is one of the important predictors for the presence of angiographic disease.[103] Results of this study are provided in Table 8-8.

Our study considered a large number of patients who underwent treadmill testing for clinical indications in a general hospital or clinic setting. Patients with prior MI and/or coronary artery revascularization were excluded from the study, leaving 3745 male veterans. Exercise testing variables were analyzed within the age groups to evaluate the effect of age and the choice of outcome, CV, or all-cause death. Our results show the importance of age and the endpoint used in the Cox hazard analyses to develop prognostic scores. We also showed that age has a nonlinear relationship to the variables, and outcomes such as adding age to scores does not improve prediction in the elderly. This is most likely because other clinical predictors (comorbidities, psychosocial factors, and subclinical conditions) overpower the treadmill responses in the elderly even in a population such as ours, in which patients with recognized heart disease were removed. Both age and the outcome selected as an endpoint affect the exercise test responses chosen for scores to predict prognosis. Differences in age of the subjects tested and/or the outcome selected as the endpoint can explain the differences in the studies using exercise testing to predict prognosis.

TABLE 8-8. Results of cox-hazard model with cardiovascular mortality as the endpoint for age groupings illustrating how the predictive power of the treadmill responses change with age

Age	<45	45-55	55-65	65-75	>75	
N	619	987	1081	717	174	
CV death	8	35	72	77	22	
METs	−0.22	−0.18	−0.13	−0.13	NS	Regression coefficient/
	0.81	0.83	0.87	0.87		Hazard ratio
	0.67–0.97	0.75–0.93	0.81–0.94	0.80–0.95		95% CI hazard
Exercise-induced ST depression	NS	0.61	NS	NS	NS	
		1.85				
		1.39–2.46				
Duke Angina score	NS	NS	NS	NS	NS	
Max SBP	NS	0.014	NS	NS	NS	Regression coefficient
		1.01				Hazard ratio
		1.00–1.03				95% CI hazard
Max HR	NS	NS	NS	NS	NS	1st in Cox
						2nd in Cox
						3rd in Cox
Resting ST depression	NS	NS	NS	0.81	NS	
				2.27		
				1.26–4.07		

Modified from Yamazaki T, Myers J, Froelicher VF. Effect of age and end point on the prognostic value of the exercise test. Chest 2004;125:1920-1928.

Exercise myocardial perfusion was evaluated in elderly patients with interpretable exercise ECG tests by considering clinical, ECG, scan, and follow-up data for 626 outpatients aged 65 years or older with interpretable ECGs between 1992 and 1996.[104] Follow-up was for 4 years. After exclusion of the 27 patients who underwent revascularization within 90 days, there were 361 men and 217 women with a mean age of 70. By univariate analysis, numerous variables (including male gender, age, rest ECG, poor exercise capacity, peak heart rate, and exercise ST-segment depression) predicted death or MI. By multivariable modeling, only increasing patient age, male sex, poor exercise capacity, and the number of ischemic scan segments were predictive of subsequent death or MI.

In Diabetics and Those with Silent Ischemia

These two situations are discussed together because of the widespread belief that silent ischemia is more common in diabetics. An open mind should be taken in this regard, however, since the basis of evidence for this belief is weak.

Silent Ischemia during Exercise Testing

The interest in silent ischemia (i.e., ST depression without anginal symptoms) has come about because of five clinical observations: (1) the increased risk of coronary events when screening asymptomatic men, (2) the frequency of painless ST-segment depression during exercise testing in patients with coronary heart disease, (3) episodes of painless ST-segment depression noted during Holter ambulatory monitoring, (4) the clinical impression that silent ischemia is more common in diabetics, and (5) the apparent high risk of painless ST-segment depression in patients with unstable ischemic syndromes. Potential dangers of silent ischemia include asymptomatic progression to sudden death and myocardial fibrosis (leading to CHF) due to lack of a warning mechanism.

As for many other clinical syndromes, dividing silent ischemia into subsets can be very helpful. The types of silent ischemia described by Cohn are particularly useful:

- Type I—occurring in asymptomatic, apparently healthy individuals
- Type II—occurring in patients after an MI
- Type III—occurring in patients with known CAD

Preliminary studies led to the hypothesis that "silent" myocardial ischemia had a worse prognosis than angina pectoris because patients with it do not have an intact "warning system." However, in studies of patients referred for diagnostic purposes or with stable coronary syndromes, silent myocardial ischemia detected by exercise testing has been associated with either a lesser or similar prognosis compared to patients with angina pectoris. Because exercise testing has advantages over ambulatory monitoring with regard to the leads monitored, chest pain description, and fidelity of the recording apparatus, confirmation of these findings would help resolve the controversy over the relative prognostic impact of silent myocardial ischemia. Exercise testing studies give us one means of evaluating the risk of silent ischemia. Unfortunately these exercise test studies do not evaluate patients with true silent ischemia. The patients are being tested because of some symptoms, usually angina, although they may not have angina at the time of their test. However, patients with true silent ischemia are rare. Therefore, the following data from exercise test studies gives us a good idea of how the usual patients seen in clinical practice with silent ischemia, at least in some occasions, are likely to perform.

Ellestad and Wan[16] reported the predictive implications of maximal exercise testing in 2700 individuals followed for 6 months to 9 years. ST depression and prior MI were both associated with subsequent higher mortality. From the CASS registry of patients who underwent coronary angiography and exercise testing and were followed up for 7 years, the significance of ischemic ST segment depression without associated chest pain during exercise testing was studied.[105] Of the 2982 patients, those with proven CAD were grouped according to whether they had at least 1 mm of ST-segment depression or anginal chest pain during exercise testing: 424 had ischemic ST depression without angina, 232 had angina but no ischemic ST depression, 456 had both ischemic ST depression and angina, and 471 had neither ischemic ST depression nor angina. The 7-year survival rates were similar for patients in all groups (77%), except for patients without ST depression or angina, who did better (88%). Among silent ischemia patients, survival was related to severity of CAD. The 7-year survival rate was significantly worse than that in a separate group of 282 patients with ischemic ST depression but without angina during exercise testing who had no CAD (95% survival). This study demonstrated that in patients with silent myocardial ischemia during exercise testing the extent of CAD and the 7-year survival rate were similar to those of patients with angina during exercise testing. Prognosis was determined primarily by the severity of CAD.

At Duke, Marks et al[106] evaluated the clinical correlates and long-term prognostic significance of silent ischemia during exercise. They analyzed 1698 consecutive symptomatic patients with CAD who had both treadmill testing and cardiac catheterization. These patients were classified into three groups; group 1 included patients with no exercise ST deviation ($n = 856$), group 2 included patients with painless exercise ST deviation ($n = 242$), and group 3 included patients with both angina and ST-segment deviation during exercise ($n = 600$). Patients with exercise angina had a history of a longer and more aggressive anginal course (with a greater frequency of angina, with nocturnal episodes and/or progressive symptom pattern) and more severe CAD (almost two thirds had three-vessel disease). The 5-year survival rate among the patients with painless ST deviation was similar to that of patients with ST deviation (86% and 88%, respectively) and was significantly better than that of patients with both symptoms and ST deviation (5-year survival rate 73% in patients with exercise-limiting angina). Similar trends were obtained in subgroups defined by the amount of CAD present. In the total study group of 1698 patients, silent ischemia on the treadmill was not a benign finding (average annual mortality rate 2.8%) but, compared with symptomatic ischemia, did indicate a subgroup of patients with CAD who had a less aggressive anginal course, less CAD, and a better prognosis. Other smaller angiographic studies agree with this finding,[107,108] which may reflect the bluntness of the tool which is exercise-induced ST depression. It is possible that those patients with no pain had less severe disease despite similar levels of ST depression.

To evaluate whether patients with angiographic evidence of CAD with silent myocardial ischemia during exercise testing are at increased risk for developing a subsequent acute MI or sudden death, another analysis from the CASS registry was performed.[109] The study involved 424 patients with silent ischemia who were compared with another 456 patients with CAD who had both ischemic ST depression and angina pectoris during exercise testing, and with 1019 control patients without CAD. The probability of remaining free of a subsequent acute MI or sudden death at 7 years was 80% and 91%, respectively, for patients with silent ischemia; 82% and 93%, respectively, for patients with ST depression and angina

pectoris (difference not significant), and 98% and 99%, respectively, for the control patients. Among patients with silent ischemia the probability of remaining free of MI and sudden death at 7 years was related to the severity of CAD and presence of LV dysfunction, and ranged from 90% for patients with one-vessel CAD and preserved LV function to 38% for patients with three-vessel CAD and abnormal LV function. Thus, patients with either silent or symptomatic ischemia during exercise testing have a similar risk of developing an acute MI or sudden death, except in the three-vessel CAD subgroup, where the risk is greater in silent ischemia.

Callaham et al[110] performed a study to determine the effect of silent ischemia on prognosis in patients undergoing exercise testing. In addition, we took the opportunity to demonstrate if differences in the prevalence of silent ischemia and its impact on the prognosis of patients with silent ischemia could be explained by age or by their MI and diabetes mellitus status. The design was retrospective with a 2-year mean follow-up. The patient population was inpatient and outpatient referrals for exercise testing at a 1000-bed VA hospital. Exercise test responses were analyzed separately for the four subgroups: angina plus ST depression, silent ischemia, angina only, and no ischemia. Mean maximal heart rate, maximal SBP, and maximal MET level attained were significantly higher for patients with silent ischemia than patients with angina plus ST depression. Mean maximal ST segment depression was significantly greater among patients with angina plus ST depression than patients with silent ischemia. The prevalence of silent ischemia increased with age, while the prevalence of angina plus ST depression did not. There was a 7% prevalence of silent ischemia among patients less than 50 years of age, 17% prevalence in patients aged 50 to 59 years, 20% prevalence in patients aged 60 to 69 years, and 36% prevalence for patients aged 70 or greater. Among 326 patients undergoing cardiac catheterization, the mean number of vessels diseased (two) and LV ejection fraction (58%) were not significantly different according to ischemia status. During 2-year follow-up, 71 patients died, 68 patients underwent CABS, 51 patients underwent PCI as their sole revascularization procedure, and 13 patients underwent both CABS and PCI. Patients in the angina plus ST depression and silent ischemia groups had significantly higher overall 2-year mortality than patients without ST-segment depression. Overall mortality in patients with angina and ST depression and patients with silent ischemia was not significantly different. We recently repeated these analyses in a larger data set of veterans, including those from Palo Alto VA, with a longer follow-up (Fig. 8-7).

Prior MI and Silent Ischemia. We investigated whether prior MI influenced silent ischemia and prognosis. Patients who had recently suffered an MI (within 2 weeks), and patients who had suffered an MI in the past (>2 weeks) were grouped separately. No significant difference was seen in the prevalence of silent ischemia angina plus ST depression among the three groups. Prognosis was significantly worse among patients with a recent MI, particularly when ischemic ST segment depression was present.

Diabetes and Silent Ischemia. Ninety-three insulin-dependent and 87 non-insulin-dependent patients with diabetes mellitus were tested. Of those with ischemic ST-segment depression, 64% of insulin-dependent and 61% of non-insulin-dependent diabetic patients had silent myocardial ischemia. The prevalence of silent ischemia among the nondiabetic patients (60%) and diabetic patients (62%) was not significantly different. Mortality was significantly greater among patients with abnormal ST-segment depression compared with those without ST segment depression. The presence or absence of angina pectoris during exercise testing was not significantly related to death. The prevalence of silent ischemia is not statistically different during exercise testing in patients with recent MI, remote MI, or no history of MI, or those with insulin–dependent or non-insulin-dependent diabetes mellitus. Thus, silent ischemia is associated with a similar prognosis as ST depression associated with angina pectoris. These findings demonstrate that silent ischemia occurring with treadmill testing does not confer an increased risk for death relative to patients experiencing angina. Thus, therapy should not be guided by the false hypothesis that patients with silent ischemia are at higher risk for death than those with angina and ST depression. Recently we repeated these analyses in diabetics in a larger veteran population, with a longer follow-up (Figure 8-8).

Dagenais et al[20] reported 6-year cumulative survival in 298 moderately treated patients with exercise-induced ST-segment depression equal or greater than 2 mm. In those with silent myocardial ischemia, survival was 85%, while it was significantly lower (80%) in those with angina pectoris. Patients with silent myocardial ischemia reached a greater heart rate and higher MET level than those with painful ischemia. Cumulative survival was very much related to the MET level achieved. Those who reached 10 METs had very few deaths, while those with less than 5 METs had approximately a 50% survival. In a small study of less than 100 diabetics from the CASS registry, contrary results were reported.[111] These data suggested that, among patients with diabetes and CAD, silent myocardial ischemia during exercise testing adversely affects survival, and that CABS improves the survival of diabetic patients with silent myocardial ischemia and three-vessel CAD.

The Cedars group studied 1271 consecutively registered patients with diabetes and 5862 patients without diabetes with known or suspected

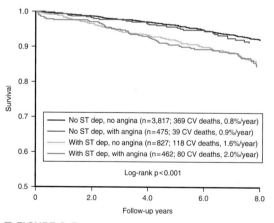

■ FIGURE 8-7

Silent ischemia Kaplan-Meier curves for the general population.

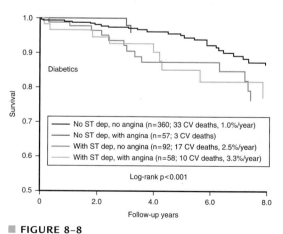

■ FIGURE 8-8

Silent ischemia Kaplan-Meier curves in diabetic patients.

CAD undergoing nuclear perfusion myocardial perfusion imaging with exercise or adenosine pharmacologic testing.[112] Patients were followed-up for at least 1 year except for the 6% lost to follow-up. Over the follow-up period, patients with diabetes had significantly higher rates of "hard" events (cardiac death or nonfatal MI) (4.3% versus 2.3% per year) and higher total event rates (hard events and late revascularization) (9.0% versus 5.3% per year) compared with rates among patients without diabetes. Cox proportional hazards analysis revealed that nuclear testing added incremental value over clinical and historical variables among patients with diabetes. The event rates rose significantly as a function of summed stress score and summed difference score among both patients with diabetes and patients without diabetes. The patients with diabetes with normal scans had relatively low hard event rates (1% to 2% per year), those with mildly abnormal scans had intermediate hard event rates (3% to 4% per year), and those with moderately to severely abnormal scans had relatively high hard event rates (>7% per year).

Giri et al[113] followed-up patients with symptoms of CAD, who were undergoing nuclear perfusion imaging from five centers for 2.5 years, for the subsequent occurrence of cardiac death, MI, and revascularization. Perfusion scan results were categorized as normal or abnormal (fixed or ischemic defects). Of 4755 patients, 929 (20%) were diabetic. Patients with diabetes, despite an increased revascularization rate, had twice as many cardiac events (8.6%; 39 deaths and 41 MIs) compared to the nondiabetics (5%; 69 deaths and 103 MIs). Abnormal perfusion was an independent predictor of cardiac death and MI in both populations. Diabetics with ischemic defects had an increased number of cardiac events, with the highest MI rates (17%) observed with three-vessel ischemia. Similarly, a multivessel fixed defect was associated with the highest rate of cardiac death (14%) among diabetics. In multivariable Cox analysis, both ischemic and fixed defects independently predicted cardiac death alone or cardiac death/MI.

Angiographic Studies of Silent Ischemia

Visser et al[108] from the Netherlands studied 280 patients with anginal complaints, without prior MI and with an abnormal exercise test. They were divided into two groups: one with ($n = 67$) with exercise-induced silent ischemia ($n = 67$) and the other with exercise-induced angina pectoris ($n = 213$). Both underwent coronary angiography and were compared with each other with respect to various exercise and angiographic parameters. Patients with exercise-induced silent ischemia exercised longer, reached a higher peak exercise heart rate, and a higher peak exercise rate pressure product than patients with exercise-induced angina pectoris. In the latter group, more patients showed exercise-induced ST-segment depression greater than 2 mm. The group of patients with silent ischemia encompassed more individuals with normal coronary arteries. More patients with exercise- induced angina pectoris had three-vessel disease. The exclusion of patients with normal coronary arteries (23% in those with silent ischemia group and 6% in those with exercise-induced angina) had no influence on the level of significance for peak heart rate, mean exercise duration, and exercise duration greater than 10 minutes. As in most other studies, exercise-induced silent myocardial ischemia was associated with better exercise performance and less extensive coronary disease than in exercise-induced angina pectoris.

Miranda et al[114] performed a retrospective analysis of 416 male veterans referred for exercise testing and selected for cardiac catheterization. We found that exercise-induced ST depression was a better marker for CAD than exercise test-induced angina and that symptomatic ischemia (ST depression plus angina) was a better indicator of severe angiographically significant CAD than silent ischemia. As part of the Program on the Surgical Control of the Hyperlipidemias (POSCH), subjects with hyperlipidemia who had one healed MI were studied and followed-up for 9 years.[115] Of the 417 control subjects, 279 had a treadmill test result that was definitely positive or negative. There was no difference in survival between subjects with a positive or negative test result with or without angina and as regards to blood lipids, type of MI (Q or non-Q wave), and LV function.

The angiographic studies of silent ischemia reviewed by Miranda et al[114] are summarized in Table 8-9. In this review encompassing almost 6000 patients, a consistent finding was that patients with symptomatic ischemia had a higher prevalence of severe angiographically significant CAD than did patients with silent ischemia.

Comparison of Treadmill Testing to Ambulatory Monitoring

In one of only a few studies comparing the prognostic value of the treadmill test and ambulatory

TABLE 8–9. Studies of silent ischemia during exercise testing with angiographic correlation

Investigator	No. patients	Exclusions	NOISCH MVD (%)	NOISCH 3V/LM (%)	APO MVD (%)	APO 3V/LM (%)	SI MVD (%)	SI 3V/LM (%)	STAP MVD (%)	STAP 3V/LM (%)
Amsterdam	92	No CAD, coronary stenoses <70%, normal ET	—	—	62	—	77	—	82	—
Deligonul	390	No CAD, coronary stenoses <50%, digoxin, LBBB, LM, LVH, failed PTCA	49	10	50	5	64	18	71	23
Erikssen	103	Coronary stenoses <50%, previously known CAD, "other" heart disease, HTN, DM, malignancy, musculoskeletal disorders, any other advanced disease	50	—	45	—	45	—	75	—
Falcone	473	No CAD, coronary stenoses <50%, digoxin, LBBB, CHF, valvular disease, variant angina, no exercise ST depression	—	—	—	—	85	56/5	84	55/7
Mark	1698	No CAD, coronary stenoses <75%, LBBB, exercise ST elevation, USA, valvular disease, congenital heart disease, cardiac surgery	—	27	—	37	79	48/12	88	60/12
Miranda	200	Digoxin, coronary stenoses <75%, LVH, LBBB, CABG/PCI, women, prior MI, resting ST depression	16	6	13	9	50	20	51	30

Study	N	Description								
Ouyang	60	Coronary stenoses <70%, no exercise ST depression	—	—	—	—	74	29/11	81	54/6
Stern	480	No CAD, coronary stenoses <70%, no exercise ST depression, digoxin, "baseline ECG changes," valvular disease, cardiomyopathy	—	—	—	—	66	33	72	36
Visser	280	No CAD, coronary stenosis <50%, no exercise ST depression, LVH, LBBB, CHF, valvular disease, cardiomyopathy, prior MI, congenital heart disease	—	—	—	—	38	13	74	38
Weiner	1583	No CAD, coronary stenoses <70%	42	13	55	23	63	29	74	38
Weiner	302	Coronary stenoses <70%, digoxin, LBBB, LVH, valvular disease, patients without exercise angina or ST depression that did not achieve 85% of submaximal heart rate	21	—	67	—	51	—	94	—
Total:	5877	Means:	36	13	46	17	63	31	76	41

APO, Angina pectoris only during exercise test; CABG, coronary artery bypass graft; CAD, coronary artery disease; DM, diabetes mellitus; ET, exercise test; HTN, hypertension; LBBB, left bundle branch block; LM, left main coronary artery disease is >50% narrowing; LVH, left ventricular hypertrophy; MI, myocardial infarction; MVD, multivessel disease (two-, three-vessel, or LM CAD); NOISCH, normal exercise test; PTCA, percutaneous transluminal coronary angioplasty; SI, ST-segment depression only during exercise test; STAP, ST-segment depression and angina pectoris during exercise test; 3V/LM, three-vessel/left main coronary artery disease; USA, unstable angina pectoris.

monitoring, Tzivoni et al[116] followed 224 low-risk patients with prior MI for a mean of 28 months (range 12 to 58 months). Seventy-four patients developed ischemic changes during daily activity, of which 44 (60%) were silent, 14 (19%) were symptomatic, and 16 (21%) were both. All 74 patients had ischemic responses to treadmill testing, but in addition, of the 150 patients with ischemic changes on Holter, 44 did show ischemia with the treadmill test. The incidence of cardiac events (i.e., cardiac death, nonfatal MI, development of unstable angina, CABG, or angioplasty), was significantly greater in patients with positive Holter and treadmill tests (38/74 = 51%) compared to abnormal exercise tests but negative Holter (9/44 = 20%). As might be expected, the group with the least cardiac events had a normal Holter and exercise test (9/106). Interestingly, of the 74 patients with ischemic events on the Holter, there was no correlation between symptoms (silent or symptomatic) and prognosis.

Two representative studies comparing exercise testing to ambulatory monitoring that make an interesting comparison are those of Mody et al[117] and Mulcahy et al.[118] Mody et al studied 97 patients who were not on antianginal medications. Sixty-three patients had no ischemia (poor sensitivity), 22 patients had 1 to 60 minutes of ischemia during 24 hours, and 12 patients exceeded 60 minutes for 24 hours. There was no correlation with exercise duration or time to ST-segment depression. However, prolonged ischemia on Holter correlated with the angiographically severe CAD. Conversely, Mulcahy et al[118] found that in patients whose exercise test was negative, or who do not develop ST-segment depression before 5 METs, rarely had silent myocardial ischemia during ambulatory monitoring. They found that ST-segment depression occurs at a lower heart rate with ambulatory monitoring than with exercise testing, but the results were highly correlated. Stern et al[119] found that in 544 patients (299 with abnormal angiograms and 241 had prior MI, all of whom had abnormal treadmill tests) 47% had silent myocardial ischemia while 53% had chest pain. The age, prior MI, medications, number of diseased vessels, heart rate, blood pressure, and maximal ST depression were similar in both groups. At 1 mm of ST-segment depression, patients with silent ischemia had a higher heart rate and exercise level, reached a higher double product, and had a faster recovery postexercise. However, if the ST-segment depression exceeded 2 mm, there were no differences between the two groups. Flugelman et al[120] studied painless persistent ST-segment depression after exercise testing. There were 31 patients with angina and ST-segment depression. The angina pectoris disappeared at 3 minutes while the ST-segment depression disappeared at 6 minutes in recovery. There was no change in this with nitroglycerin and the persistence was longer in more elderly people. They found that silent myocardial ischemia persists after disappearance of exercise-induced angina pectoris.

The most important study is that of Hedblad et al[121] performed in "men born in 1914 in Malmo." It essentially shows that pretest probability (i.e., chest pain symptoms) affects ambulatory monitoring for screening as it does for exercise testing.

Silent Ischemia More Prevalent in Diabetics?

Not all studies have shown a difference in the prevalence of silent myocardial ischemia between diabetics and the general population. In a landmark Danish study,[122] the prevalence of ischemia was compared in a random sample of 120 users of insulin and 120 users of oral hypoglycemic agents aged 40 to 75 years. The observed prevalence of silent ischemia on treadmill or Holter testing in diabetics was 13.5% and was no different in matched controls. No association was found between silent ischemia and gender or diabetes type. Although hypertension was highly predictive of silent ischemia in the diabetic subjects, other variables did not have a predictive value. This finding is hard to explain. Scandinavian populations have previously been noted to have increased CV disease prevalence[123] and it is possible that a high level of baseline disease in the nondiabetic population masks the population differences seen in other studies.

Data from the Asymptomatic Cardiac Ischemia Pilot[124] revealed that asymptomatic ST-segment depression during Holter monitoring was 94% in diabetics and 88% in nondiabetics. In addition, the time to onset of 1-mm ST-segment depression and time to onset of angina were similar in both groups. Unlike the previous study, however, entry into the Asymptomatic Cardiac Ischemia Pilot required a cardiac event, so the disease was not consistently silent.

Making sense of these seemingly contradictory findings is not straightforward. Silent myocardial ischemia has been found to be associated with the same, lower, and higher risk as nonsilent ischemia. It has also been found to occur with the same or higher frequency in diabetics. What is clear, however, is that, whether silent or not, ischemia during treadmill testing in the general population predicts increased risk for death. However, in general, these study patients presented for testing *with chest pain symptoms*. That is, their ischemia was 'silent' only with respect to the exercise test itself. This inconsistent appearance of pain could represent a different process in the general population (e.g., a different severity of disease) than in the diabetic population, where autonomic dysfunction is known to be present. This idea is supported by Weiner's studies, in which patients with silent ischemia and either three-vessel disease or diabetes had a poorer outcome.

Screening Studies in Diabetics

The inherent uncertainty of assessing the prevalence and risk of silent CAD retrospectively has led some investigators to assess the impact of truly silent disease by carrying out prospective screening studies. We found only four studies which took a truly asymptomatic diabetic population and screened for CV disease. Koistinen[125] found that 29% of diabetics and 5% of control patients had ischemic results in one or more noninvasive tests whilst Gerson et al[126] found a quarter of 110 asymptomatic, insulin-requiring, diabetic patients had abnormal ST depression or an inadequate heart rate response. Janand-Delenne et al[127] found 16% of noninvasive tests to be positive in 203 patients screened for 1 year with exercise ECG and perfusion scans followed-up with coronary angiography. Angiographically significant (>50% stenosis) disease was found in 9.3%. Finally, May et al[122] found the prevalence of silent ischemia to be 13.5% in a randomly chosen diabetic population.

It seems likely then that the prevalence of silent CV disease in diabetic populations is high, and probably of the order 10% to 30%, compared with a control rate of around 5%. However, the diagnostic tools available to assess coronary disease in the general population need to be re-evaluated for the diabetic population, in light of the significantly higher preprobability of disease, and the potential confounding factor of silent ischemia.

The Mayo clinic group examined nuclear perfusion exercise imaging in asymptomatic diabetic patients. The results of stress nuclear perfusion in patients without prior MI or coronary revascularization were compared in asymptomatic diabetics ($n = 1738$) versus symptomatic diabetic patients ($n = 2998$), asymptomatic nondiabetic patients ($n = 6215$), and symptomatic nondiabetic patients ($n = 16,214$).[128] Abnormal scans were present in 59% of asymptomatic diabetic patients, approximately

equal to the percentage in symptomatic diabetic and higher than in asymptomatic nondiabetic (46%) and symptomatic nondiabetic (44%) patients. The breakdown of high-risk scans followed a similar pattern in the four patient subsets, roughly about 20%. Patients with diabetes had more ECG and scan evidence for silent MI versus those without diabetes. The finding that approximately one in five of these individuals has a high-risk scan suggests a potentially more widespread application of screening stress nuclear perfusion in asymptomatic diabetic patients to identify those with severe CAD.

THE ACC/AHA GUIDELINES FOR THE PROGNOSTIC USE OF THE STANDARD EXERCISE TEST

The task force to establish guidelines for the use of exercise testing has met and produced guidelines in 1986, 1997, and 2002. The following is a synopsis of these evidence-based guidelines.

Indications for exercise testing to assess risk and prognosis in patients with symptoms or a prior history of CAD:

Class I (Definitely Appropriate). Conditions for which there is evidence and/or general agreement that the standard exercise test is useful and helpful to assess risk and prognosis in patients with symptoms or a prior history of CAD.

- Patients undergoing initial evaluation with suspected or known CAD. Specific exceptions are noted below in Class IIb.
- Patients with suspected or known CAD previously evaluated with significant change in clinical status.

Class IIb (Maybe Appropriate). Conditions for which there is conflicting evidence and/or a divergence of opinion that the standard exercise test is useful and helpful to assess risk and prognosis in patients with symptoms or a prior history of CAD but the usefulness/efficacy is less well established.

- Patients who demonstrate the following ECG abnormalities:
- Pre-excitation (Wolff-Parkinson-White) syndrome
- Electronically paced ventricular rhythm
- More than 1 mm of resting ST depression
- Complete left bundle branch block

- Patients with a stable clinical course who undergo periodic monitoring to guide management

Class III (Not Appropriate). Conditions for which there is evidence and/or general agreement that the standard exercise test is not useful and helpful to assess risk and prognosis in patients with symptoms or a prior history of CAD and in some cases may be harmful.

- Patients with severe comorbidity likely to limit life expectancy and/or candidacy for revascularization

The evidence supporting these guidelines has been presented in this chapter.

SUMMARY

The two principal reasons for estimating prognosis are to provide accurate answers to patient's questions regarding the probable outcome of their illness and to identify those patients in whom interventions might improve outcome. There is a lack of consistency in the available studies because patients die along a pathophysiologic spectrum ranging from those that die due to CHF with little myocardium remaining to those that die from an ischemic-related event with ample myocardium remaining. Clinical and exercise test variables most likely associated with CHF deaths (CHF markers) include a history or symptoms of CHF, prior MI, Q waves, and other indicators of LV dysfunction. Variables most likely associated with ischemic deaths (ischemic markers) are angina, ST depression at rest, and exercise ST depression. Some variables can be associated with either extremes of the type of CV death; these include exercise capacity, maximal heart rate, and maximal SBP that may explain why they are reported most consistently in the available studies. A problem exists that ischemic deaths occur later in follow-up and are more likely to occur in those lost to follow-up, whereas CHF deaths are more likely to occur early (within 2 years) and are more likely to be classified. Work-up bias probably explains why exercise-induced ST depression fails to be a predictor in most of the angiographic studies. Ischemic markers are associated with a later and lesser risk, whereas CHF or LV dysfunction markers are associated with a sooner and greater risk of death (these concepts are illustrated in Fig. 8-2).

Recent studies of prognosis have actually not been superior to the earlier studies that considered CV endpoints and removed patients from observation who had interventions. This is because death data is now relatively easy to obtain, whereas previously investigators had to follow the patients and contact them or review their records. CV mortality can be determined from death certificates. While death certificates have their limitations, in general, they classify those with accidental, gastrointestinal, pulmonary, and cancer deaths so that those remaining are most likely to have died of CV causes. This endpoint is more appropriate for a test for CV disease. Whereas all-cause mortality is a more important endpoint for intervention studies, CV mortality is more appropriate for evaluating a CV test (i.e., the exercise test). Identifying those at risk of death due to any cause does not make it possible to identify those who might benefit from CV interventions, one of the two goals of prognostication.

Rather than the differences perhaps it is better to stress the consistencies. Considering simple clinical variables can assess risk. A good exercise capacity, no evidence or history of CHF or ventricular damage (Q waves, history of CHF), no ST depression, or having only one of these clinical findings are associated with a very low risk. These patients are low risk in exercise programs and need not be considered for interventions to prolong their life. High-risk patients can be identified by groupings of two or more clinical markers. Exertional hypotension is particularly ominous. Identification of high risk implies that in exercise training programs such patients should have lower goals and should be monitored. Such patients should also be considered for coronary interventions to improve their longevity. Furthermore, with each drop in METs there is a 10% to 20% increase in mortality, so simple exercise capacity has consistent importance in all patient groups.

The mathematical models for determining prognosis are usually more complex than those used for identifying angiographically severe disease. Diagnostic testing can utilize multivariate discriminant function analysis to determine the probability of the presence or absence of angiographically severe disease. Prognostic testing must utilize survival analysis, which includes censoring for patients with uneven follow-up due to "lost to follow-up" or other cardiac events (e.g., CABS, PCI) and must account for time-person units of exposure. Survival curves must be developed and the Cox proportional hazards model is often preferred. We have proposed the rules in Table 8-10 to assess prognostic studies. The newest kid on the block: heart rate recovery has yet to be validated with the

TABLE 8-10. Proposed criteria for studies assessing prognostic value of clinical and exercise test variables

1. *Study population:* inclusion criteria such as catheterization should be specified. Prevalences of congestive heart failure, congestive heart failure-associated conditions (prior myocardial infarction, Q waves on resting ECG), and angina should be stated.
2. *Avoidance of "work-up bias":* limited study populations, such as patients referred for catheterization, should be avoided, or validation studies in different populations or bootstrapping techniques should be used.
3. *Exercise testing procedures:* protocols used and criteria for abnormal values should be well described.
4. *Clinical and exercise test variables:* variables must be clearly defined and entered into the statistical analysis separately.
5. *Study endpoints:* cardiovascular death and nonfatal myocardial infarction should be used.
6. *Avoidance of "overfitting the data":* the ratio of events to the number of variables studied should be at least 10 to ensure enough "hard" outcomes per given variable studied.
7. *Follow-up:* length and completeness should be documented.
8. *Treatment of interventions:* coronary artery bypass surgery and percutaneous transluminal coronary angioplasty should not be used as endpoints.
9. *Censoring:* patients should be censored on interventions (coronary artery bypass surgery or percutaneous transluminal coronary angioplasty) and on "lost to follow-up."
10. *Relationship between censored events and studied variables:* it should be determined whether censoring is random or correlated with specific clinical and exercise test markers.
11. *Multivariate survival analysis techniques:* Cox proportional hazard model or discriminate analysis should be used.
12. *Concordance with the hierarchical nature of clinical data acquisition:* variables should be entered into multivariate analysis in an order similar to clinical practice (i.e., clinical parameters followed by exercise test variables and then invasive test variables).
13. *Interactions between variables:* associations between variables (i.e., digoxin use and congestive heart failure or ST elevation over Q waves) should be noted and treated appropriately.
14. *Avoidance of test-review bias:* investigators should be blinded to patient characteristics and results of other diagnostic and prognostic tests.

more appropriate endpoint of CV mortality. In fact, it appears to predict non-CV death better than CV death.

From this perspective, it is obvious that there is much information supporting the use of exercise testing as the first noninvasive step after the history, physical exam, and resting ECG in the prognostic evaluation of CAD patients. It accomplishes both of the purposes of prognostic testing: to provide information regarding the patient's status and to help make recommendations for optimal management. The exercise test results help us make reasonable decisions for selection of patients who should undergo coronary angiography. Since the exercise test can be performed in the doctor's office and provides valuable information for clinical management in regard to activity levels, response to therapy, and disability, the exercise test is the reasonable first choice for prognostic assessment. This assessment should always include calculation of the estimated annual mortality using the DTS though its ischemic elements have less power in the elderly.

REFERENCES

1. Chassin MR, Kosecoff J, Solomon DH, Brook RH: How coronary angiography is used. Clinical determinants of appropriateness. JAMA 1987;258:2543-2547.

2. Yusuf S, Zucker D, Peduzzi P, et al: Effect of coronary artery bypass graft surgery on survival: Overview of 10-year results from randomised trials by the Coronary Artery Bypass Graft Surgery Trialists Collaboration. Lancet 1994;344:563-570.
3. Marcus ML, Wilson FR, White CW: Methods of measurement of myocardial blood flow in patients: A critical review. Circulation 1987;76:245-251.
4. Stone PH, Turi ZG, Muller JE, et al: Prognostic significance of the treadmill exercise test performance 6 months after myocardial infarction. J Am Coll Cardiol 1986;8:1007-1017.
5. Haines DE, Beller GA, Watson DD, et al: Exercise-induced ST segment evaluation 2 weeks after uncomplicated myocardial infarction: Contributing factors and prognostic significance. J Am Coll Cardiol 1987;9:996-1003.
6. Hammond HK, Kelly TL, Froelicher VF: Radionuclide imaging correlatives of heart rate impairment during maximal exercise testing. J Am Coll Cardiol 1983;2:826-833.
7. Dubach P, Froelicher VF, Klein J, et al: Exercise-induced hypotension in a veteran population — criteria, causes, and prognosis. Circulation 1988;78:1380-1387.
8. Morris CK, Ueshima K, Kawaguchi T, et al: The prognostic value of exercise capacity: A review of the literature. Am Heart J 1991;122:1423-1430.
9. McKirnan MD, Sullivan M, Jensen D, Froelicher VF: Treadmill performance and cardiac function in selected patients with coronary heart disease. J Am Coll Cardiol 1984;3:253-261.
10. Bounous EP, Califf RM, Harrell FE, et al: Prognostic value of the simplified Selvester QRS score in patients with coronary artery disease. J Am Coll Cardiol 1988;11:35-41.
11. Hlatky MA, Califf RM, Harrell FE, et al: Clinical judgment and therapeutic decision making. J Am Coll Cardiol 1990;15:1-14.
12. Shaw LJ, Peterson ED, Shaw LK, et al: Use of a prognostic treadmill score in identifying diagnostic coronary disease subgroups. Circulation 1998;98:1622-1630.
13. Lauer MS, Blackstone E, Young J, Topol E: Cause of death in clinical research: Time for a reassessment? J Am Coll Cardiol 1999;34:618-620.
14. Mark DB, Shaw L, Harrell FE, Jr, et al: Prognostic value of a treadmill exercise score in outpatients with suspected coronary artery disease. N Engl J Med 1991;325:849-853.

15. Froelicher VF, Morrow K, Brown M, et al: Prediction of artherosclerotic cardiovascular death in men using a prognostic score. Am J Cardiol 1994;73:133-138.
16. Ellestad M, Wan M: Prediction implications of stress testing. Circulation 1975;51:363-369.
17. McNeer JF, Margolis JR, Lee KL, et al: The role of the exercise test in the evaluation of patients for ischemic heart disease. Circulation 1978;57:64-70.
18. Weiner DA, McCabe CH, Ryan TJ: Identification of patients with left main and three vessel coronary disease with clinical and exercise test variables. Am J Cardiol 1980;46:21-27.
19. Podrid PJ, Graboys T, Lown B: Prognosis of medically treated patients with coronary artery disease with profound ST segment depression during exercise testing. N Engl J Med 1981;305:1111-1116.
20. Dagenais GR, Rouleau JR, Christen A, Fabia J: Survival of patients with a strongly positive exercise electrocardiogram. Circulation 1982;65:452-456.
21. Bruce RA, Fisher LD, Hossack KF: Validation of exercise-enhanced risk assessment of coronary heart disease events: Longitudinal changes in incidence in Seattle community practice. J Am Coll Cardiol 1985;5:875-881.
22. Oberman A, Jones WB, Riley CP, et al: Natural history of coronary artery disease. Bull NY Acad Med 1972;48:1109-1125.
23. Reeves TJ, Oberman A, Jones WB, Sheffield LT: Natural history of angina pectoris. Am J Cardiol 1974;33:423-430.
24. Hammermeister KE, DeRouen TA, Dodge HT: Variables predictive of survival in patients with coronary disease. Selection by univariate and multivariate analyses from the clinical, electrocardiographic, exercise, arteriographic, and quantitative angiographic evaluation. Circulation 1979;59:421-430.
25. Gohlke H, Samek L, Betz P, Roskamm H: Exercise testing provides additional prognostic information in angiographically defined subgroups of patients with coronary artery disease. Circulation 1983;68:979-985.
26. Brunelli C, Cristofani R, L'Abbate A, for the ODI Study Group: Long-term survival in medically treated patients with ischemic heart disease and prognostic importance of clinical and electrocardiographic data. (The Italian CNR Multicenter Prospective Study ODI). Eur Heart J 1989;10:292-303.
27. Weiner DA, Ryan T, McCabe CH: Prognostic importance of a clinical profile and exercise test in medically treated patients with coronary artery disease. J Am Coll Cardiol 1984;3:772-779.
28. Mark DB, Hlatky MA, Harrell FE, et al: Exercise treadmill score for predicting prognosis in coronary artery disease. Ann Intern Med 1987;106:793-800.
29. Peduzzi P, Hultgren H, Thomsen J, Angell W: Prognostic value of baseline exercise tests. Prog Cardiovasc Dis 1986;28:285-292.
30. Lerman J, Svetlize H, Capris T, Perosio A: Follow-up of patients after exercise test and catheterization. Medicina (Buenos Aires) 1986;46:201-211.
31. Wyns W, Musschaert-Beauthier E, Van Domburg R, et al: Progostic value of symptom limited exercise testing in men with a high prevalence of coronary artery disease. Eur Heart J 1985;6:939-945.
32. Detry JM, Luwaert J, Melin J, et al: Non-invasive data provide independent prognostic information in patients with chest pain without previous myocardial infarction: findings in male patients who have had cardiac catheterization. Eur Heart J 1988;9:418-426.
33. Morris CK, Morrow K, Froelicher VF, et al: Prediction of cardiovascular death by means of clinical and exercise test variables in patients selected for cardiac catheterization. Am Heart J 1993;125:1717-1726.
34. Califf RM, Mark DB, Harrell FE, et al: Importance of clinical measures of ischemia in the prognosis of patients with documented coronary artery disease. J Am Coll Cardiol 1988;11:20-26.
35. Detre K, Peduzzi P, Murphy M, et al: Effect of bypass surgery on survival in patients in low- and high-risk subgroups delineated by the use of simple clinical variables. Circulation 1981;63:1329-1338.
36. Morrow K, Morris CK, Froelicher VF, Hideg A: Prediction of cardiovascular death in men undergoing noninvasive evaluation for CAD. Ann Intern Med 1993;118:689-695.
37. Villella M, Villella A, Santoro L, et al: Ergometric score systems after myocardial infarction: Prognostic performance of the Duke Treadmill Score, the Veterans Administration Medical Center Score, and of a novel score system, GISSI-2 Index, in a cohort of survivors of acute myocardial infarction. Am Heart J 2003;145:475-483.

38. Morise AP, Jalisi F: Evaluation of pretest and exercise test scores to assess all-cause mortality in unselected patients presenting for exercise testing with symptoms of suspected coronary artery disease. J Am Coll Cardiol 2003;42:842-850.
39. Prakash M, Froelicher V, Myers J, et al: Clinical and exercise test predictors of all-cause mortality: Results from over 6,000 consecutive referred male patients. Chest 2001(in press).
40. Alexander K, Shaw L, Delong E, et al: Value of exercise treadmill testing in women. J Am Coll Cardiol 1998;32:1657-1664.
41. Morise AP, Olson MB, Merz CN, et al: Validation of the accuracy of pretest and exercise test scores in women with a low prevalence of coronary disease: The NHLBI-sponsored Women's Ischemia Syndrome Evaluation (WISE) study. Am Heart J 2004;147: 1085-1092.
42. Kwok JM, Miller TD, Christian TF, et al: Prognostic value of a treadmill exercise score in symptomatic patients with nonspecific ST-T abnormalities on resting ECG. JAMA 1999;282:1047-1053.
43. Cole CR, Blackstone EH, Pashkow FJ, et al: Heart-rate recovery immediately after exercise as a predictor of mortality. N Engl J Med: 1999;341:1351-1357.
44. Cole CR, Foody JM, Blackstone EH, Lauer MS: Heart rate recovery after submaximal exercise testing as a predictor of mortality in a cardiovascularly healthy cohort. Ann Intern Med 2000;132: 552-555.
45. Nishime EO, Cole CR, Blackstone EH, et al: Heart rate recovery and treadmill exercise score as predictors of mortality in patients referred for exercise ECG. JAMA 2000;284:1392-1398.
46. Shetler K, Marcus R, Froelicher VF, et al: Heart rate recovery: Validation and methodologic issues. J Am Coll Cardiol 2001;38:1980-1987.
47. Morshedi-Meibodi A, Larson MG, Levy D, et al: Heart rate recovery after treadmill exercise testing and risk of cardiovascular disease events (The Framingham Heart Study). Am J Cardiol 2002;90:848-852.
48. Mora S, Redberg RF, Cui Y, et al: Ability of exercise testing to predict cardiovascular and all-cause death in asymptomatic women: A 20-year follow-up of the lipid research clinics prevalence study. JAMA 2003;290:1600-1607.
49. Cheng YJ, Lauer MS, Earnest CP, et al: Heart rate recovery following maximal exercise testing as a predictor of cardiovascular disease and all-cause mortality in men with diabetes. Diabetes Care 2003;26:2052-2057.
50. Simari RD, Miller TD, Zinsmeister AR, Gibbons RJ: Capabilities of supine exercise electrocardiography versus exercise radionuclide angiography in predicting coronary events. Am J Cardiol 1991; 67:573-577.
51. Lee KL, Pryor DB, Pieper KS, et al: Prognostic value of radionuclide angiography in medically treated patients with coronary artery disease. A comparison with clinical and catheterization variables. Circulation 1990;82:1705-1717.
52. Brown KA: Prognostic value of thallium-201 myocardial perfusion imaging. A diagnostic tool comes of age. Circulation 1991;83:363-381.
53. Kaul S, Lilly DR, Gasho JA, et al: Prognostic utility of the exercise thallium-201 test in ambulatory patients with chest pain. Circulation 1988;77:745-748.
54. Melin JA, Robert A, Luwaert R, et al: Additional prognostic value of exercise testing and thallium-201 scintigraphy in catheterized patients without previous myocardial infarction. Int J Cardiol 1990;27:235-243.
55. Hachamovitch R, Berman DS, Shaw LJ, et al: Incremental prognostic value of myocardial perfusion single photon emission computed tomography for the prediction of cardiac death: Differential stratification for risk of cardiac death and myocardial infarction. Circulation 1998;97:535-543.
56. Snader CE, Marwick TH, Pashkow FJ, et al: Importance of estimated functional capacity as a predictor of all-cause mortality among patients referred for exercise thallium single-photon emission computed tomography: Report of 3,400 patients from a single center. J Am Coll Cardiol 1997;30:641-648.
57. Poornima IG, Miller TD, Christian TF, et al: Utility of myocardial perfusion imaging in patients with low-risk treadmill scores. J Am Coll Cardiol 2004;43:194-199.
58. Vanzetto G, Ormezzano O, Fagret D, et al: Long-term additive prognostic value of thallium-201 myocardial perfusion imaging over clinical and exercise stress test in low to intermediate risk patients: Study in 1137 patients with 6-year follow-up. Circulation 1999;100: 1521-1527.

59. Chatziioannou SN, Moore WH, Ford PV, et al: Prognostic value of myocardial perfusion imaging in patients with high exercise tolerance. Circulation 1999;99:867-872.
60. Diaz LA, Brunken RC, Blackstone EH, et al: Independent contribution of myocardial perfusion defects to exercise capacity and heart rate recovery for prediction of all-cause mortality in patients with known or suspected coronary heart disease. J Am Coll Cardiol 2001;37:1558-1564.
61. Schinkel AF, Elhendy A, van Domburg RT, et al: Incremental value of exercise technetium-99m tetrofosmin myocardial perfusion single-photon emission computed tomography for the prediction of cardiac events. Am J Cardiol 2003;91:408-411.
62. McCully RB, Roger VL, Mahoney DW, et al: Outcome after normal exercise echocardiography and predictors of subsequent cardiac events: Follow-up of 1,325 patients. J Am Coll Cardiol 1998;31:144-149.
63. McCully RB, Roger VL, Mahoney DW, et al: Outcome after abnormal exercise echocardiography for patients with good exercise capacity: Prognostic importance of the extent and severity of exercise-related left ventricular dysfunction. J Am Coll Cardiol 2002;39:1345-1352.
64. Marwick TH, Case C, Vasey C, et al: Prediction of mortality by exercise echocardiography: A strategy for combination with the Duke treadmill score. Circulation 2001;103:2566-2571.
65. Elhendy A, Mahoney DW, McCully RB, et al: Use of a scoring model combining clinical, exercise test, and echocardiographic data to predict mortality in patients with known or suspected coronary artery disease. Am J Cardiol 2004;93:1223-1228.
66. Lee KL, Pryor DB, Harrell FE, Jr, et al: Predicting outcome in coronary disease. Statistical models versus expert clinicians. Am J Med 1986;80:553-560.
67. Detrano R, Bobbio M, Olson H, et al: Computer probability estimates of angiographic coronary artery disease: Transportability and comparison with cardiologists' estimates. Comput Biomed Res 1992;25:468-485.
68. Lipinski M, Do D, Froelicher V, et al: Comparison of exercise test scores and physician estimation in determining disease probability. Arch Intern Med 2001;161:2239-2244.
69. Lipinski M, Froelicher V, Atwood E, et al: Comparison of treadmill scores with physician estimates of diagnosis and prognosis in patients with coronary artery disease. Am Heart J 2002;143:650-658.
70. Pryor DB, Shaw L, Harrell FE, et al: Estimating the likelihood of severe coronary artery disease. Am J Med 1991;90:553-562.
71. Hubbard BL, Gibbons RJ, Lapeyre AC, 3rd, et al: Identification of severe coronary artery disease using simple clinical parameters. Arch Intern Med 1992;152:309-312.
72. Detrano R, Janosi A, Steinbrunn W, et al: Algorithm to predict triple-vessel/left main coronary disease in patients without myocardial infarction. An international cross validation. Circulation 1991;83(suppl):III89-96.
73. Cheitlin MD, Davia JE, de Castro CM, et al: Correlation of "critical" left coronary artery lesions with positive submaximal exercise tests in patients with chest pain. Am Heart J 1975;89:305-310.
74. Goldschlager N, Selzer A, Cohn K: Treadmill stress tests as indicators of presence and severity of coronary artery disease. Ann Intern Med 1976;85:277-286.
75. Blumenthal DS, Weiss JL, Mellits ED, Gerstenblith G: The predictive value of a strongly positive stress test in patients with minimal symptoms. Am J Med 1981;70:1005-1010.
76. Lee TH, EF Cook, Goldman L: Prospective evaluation of a clinical and exercise-test model for the prediction of left main coronary artery disease. Med Decis Making 1986;6:136-144.
77. Detrano R, Gianrossi R, Mulvihill D, et al: Exercise-induced ST segment depression in the diagnosis of multivessel coronary disease: A meta analysis. J Am Coll Cardiol 1989;14:1501-1508.
78. Hartz A, Gammaitoni C, Young M: Quantitative analysis of the exercise tolerance test for determining the severity of coronary artery disease. Int J Cardiol 1989;24:63-71.
79. Concato J, Feinstein AR, Holford TR: The risk of determining risk with multivariate models. Ann Intern Med 1993;118:201-210.
80. Cohn K, Kamm D, Feteih N, et al: Use of treadmill score to quantify ischemic response and predict extent of coronary artery disease. Circulation 1979;59:286-296.
81. Fisher L, Kennedy J, Chaitman B, et al: Diagnostic quantification of CASS (Coronary Artery Surgery Study) clinical and exercise test results in determining presence and extent of coronary artery disease. Circulation 1981;63:987-1000.
82. McCarthy D, Sciacca R, Blood D, Cannon P: Discriminant function analysis using thallium 201 scintiscans and exercise stress test variables to predict the presence and extent of coronary artery disease. Am J Cardiol 1982;49:1917-1926.
83. Hung J, Chaitman BR, Lam J, et al: A logistic regression analysis of multiple noninvasive tests for the prediction of the presence and extent of coronary artery disease in men. Am Heart J 1985;110:460-469.
84. Christian T, Miller T, Bailey K, Gibbons R: Exercise tomographic thallium-201 imaging in patients with severe coronary artery disease and normal electrocardiograms. Ann Intern Med 1994;121:825-832.
85. Morise A, Bobbio M, Detrano R, Duval R: Incremental evaluation of exercise capacity as an independent predictor of coronary artery disease presence and extent. Am Heart J 1994;127:32-38.
86. Morise A, Diamond G, Detrano R, Bobbio M: Incremental value of exercise electrocardiography and thallium-201 testing in men and women for the presence and extent of coronary artery disease. Am Heart J 1995;130:267-276.
87. Moussa I, Rodriguez M, Froning J, Froelicher VF: Prediction of severe coronary artery disease using computerized ECG measurements and discriminant function analysis. J Electrocardiol 1992;25: 49-58.
88. Christian TF, Miller TD, Bailley KR, Gibbons RJ: Noninvasive identification of severe coronary artery disease using exercise tomographic thallium-201 imaging. Am J Cardiol 1992;70:14-20.
89. Hung J, Chaitman BR, Lam J, et al: Noninvasive diagnostic test choices for the evaluation of coronary artery disease in women: A multivariate comparison of cardiac fluoroscopy, exercise electrocardiography and exercise thallium myocardial perfusion scintigraphy. J Am Coll Cardiol 1984;4:8-16.
90. Diamond GA: Future imperfect: The limitations of clinical prediction models and the limits of clinical prediction. J Am Coll Cardiol 1989;14:12A-22A.
91. Ribisl PM, Morris CK, Kawaguchi T, et al: Angiographic patterns and severe coronary artery disease. Arch Intern Med 1992;152:1618-1624.
92. Herbert WG, Lehmann KG, Dubach P, et al: Effect of beta blockade on the exercise ECG: ST level versus delta ST/HR index. Am Heart J 1991;122:993-1000.
93. Do D, West JA, Morise A, Froelicher VF: Agreement predicting severe angiographic coronary artery disease using clinical and exercise test data. Am Heart J 1997;134:672-679.
94. Bruce RA, Hossack KF, DeRouen TA, Hofer V: Enhanced risk assessment for primary coronary heart disease events by maximal exercise testing: 10 years' experience of Seattle Heart Watch. J Am Coll Cardiol 1983;2:565-573.
95. European Cooperative Group: Long-term results of prospective randomized study of coronary artery bypass surgery in stable angina pectoris. Lancet 1982;2:1173-1180.
96. Weiner DA, Ryan TJ, McCabe CH, et al: The role of exercise testing in identifying patients with improved survival after coronary artery bypass surgery. J Am Coll Cardiol 1986;8:741-748.
97. Hultgren HN, Peduzzi P, Detre K, Takaro T: The 5 year effect of bypass surgery on relief of angina and exercise performance. Circulation 1985;72:V79-V83.
98. Brechue W, Pollock M: Exercise training for coronary artery disease in the elderly. Clin Geriatr Med 1996;12:207-229.
99. Goraya T, Jacobsen S, Pellikka P, et al: Prognostic value of treadmill exercise testing in elderly persons. Ann Intern Med 2000;132:862-870.
100. Spin JM, Prakash M, Froelicher VF, et al: The prognostic value of exercise testing in elderly men. Am J Med 2002;112:453-459.
101. Kwok JM, Miller TD, Hodge DO, et al: Prognostic value of the Duke treadmill score in the elderly. J Am Coll Cardiol 2002;39:1475-1481.
102. Lai S, Kaykha A, Yamazaki T, et al: Treadmill scores in elderly men. J Am Coll Cardiol 2004;43:606-615.
103. Raxwal V, Shetler K, Morise A, et al: Simple treadmill score to diagnose coronary disease. Chest 2001;119:1933-1940.

104. Steingart RM, Hodnett P, Musso J, Feuerman M: Exercise myocardial perfusion imaging in elderly patients. J Nucl Cardiol 2002;9:573-580.

105. Weiner DA, Ryan TJ, McCabe CH, et al: Significance of silent myocardial ischemia during exercise testing in patients with coronary artery disease. Am J Cardiol 1987;59:725-729.

106. Mark DB, Hlatky MA, Califf RM, et al: Painless exercise ST deviation on the treadmill: Long-term prognosis. J Am Coll Cardiol 1989;14:885-892.

107. Falcone C, de Servi S, Poma E, et al: Clinical significance of exercise-induced silent myocardial ischemia in patients with coronary artery disease. J Am Coll Cardiol 1987;9:295-299.

108. Visser FC, van Leeuwen FT, Cernohorsky B, et al: Silent versus symptomatic myocardial ischemia during exercise testing: A comparison with coronary angiographic findings. Int J Cardiol 1990;27:71-78.

109. Weiner DA, Ryan TJ, McCabe CH, et al: Risk of developing an acute myocardial infarction or sudden coronary death in patients with exercise-induced silent myocardial ischemia. A report from the Coronary Artery Surgery Study (CASS) Registry. Am J Cardiol 1988;62:1155-1158.

110. Callaham P, Froelicher VF, Klein J, et al: Exercise-induced silent ischemia. J Am Coll Cardiol 1989;14:1175-1180.

111. Weiner DA, Ryan TJ, Parsons L, et al: Significance of silent myocardial ischemia during exercise testing in patients with diabetes mellitus: A report from the Coronary Artery Surgery Study (CASS) Registry. Am J Cardiol 1991;68:729-734.

112. Kang X, Berman DS, Lewin HC, et al: Incremental prognostic value of myocardial perfusion single photon emission computed tomography in patients with diabetes mellitus. Am Heart J 1999;138(6 Pt 1):1025-1032.

113. Giri S, Shaw LJ, Murthy DR, et al: Impact of diabetes on the risk stratification using stress single-photon emission computed tomography myocardial perfusion imaging in patients with symptoms suggestive of coronary artery disease. Circulation 2002;105:32-40.

114. Miranda C, Lehmann K, Lachterman B, et al: Comparison of silent and symptomatic ischemia during exercise testing in men. Ann Intern Med 1991;114:649-656.

115. Karnegis JN, Matts JP, Tuna N, et al: Positive and negative exercise test results with and without exercise-induced angina in patients with one healed myocardial infarction: Analysis of baseline variables and long-term prognosis. Am Heart J 1991;122:701-708.

116. Tzivoni D, Gavish A, Zin D, et al: Prognostic significance of ischemic episodes in patients with previous myocardial infarction. Am J Cardiol 1988;62:661-664.

117. Mody FV, Nademanee K, Intarachot V, et al: Severity of silent myocardial ischemia on ambulatory electrocardiographic monitoring in patients with stable angina pectoris: Relation to prognostic determinants during exercise stress testing and coronary angiography. J Am Coll Cardiol 1988;12:1169-1176.

118. Mulcahy D, Keegan J, Crean P, et al: Silent myocardial ischemia in chronic stable angina: A study of its frequency and characteristics in 150 patients. Br Heart J 1988;60:417-423.

119. Stern S, Weisz G, Gavish A, et al: Comparison between silent and symptomatic ischemia during exercise testing in patients with coronary artery disease. J Cardiopulm Rehabil 1988;12:507-512.

120. Flugelman MY, Halon DA, Shefer A, et al: Persistent painless ST-segment depression after exercise testing and the effect of age. Clin Cardiol 1988;11:365-369.

121. Hedblad B, Juul-Moller S, Svensson K, et al: Increased mortality in men with ST segment depression during 24 h ambulatory long-term ECG recording. Results from prospective population study "Men born in 1914", from Malmo, Sweden. Eur Heart J 1989;10:149-158.

122. May O, Arildsen H, Damsgaard EM, Mickley H: Prevalence and prediction of silent ischaemia in diabetes mellitus: A population-based study. Cardiovasc Res 1997;34:241-247.

123. Keys A: Coronary heart disease in seven countries. Circulation 1970;41-42: I1-I211.

124. Caracciolo EA, Chaitman BR, Forman SA, et al: Diabetics with coronary disease have a prevalence of asymptomatic ischemia during exercise treadmill testing and ambulatory ischemia monitoring similar to that of nondiabetic patients. An ACIP database study. ACIP Investigators. Asymptomatic Cardiac Ischemia Pilot Investigators. Circulation 1996;93:2097-2105.

125. Koistinen MJ: Prevalence of asymptomatic myocardial ischaemia in diabetic subjects. BMJ 1990;301:92-95.

126. Gerson MC, Khoury JC, Hertzberg VS, et al: Prediction of coronary artery disease in a population of insulin-requiring diabetic patients: Results of an 8-year follow-up study. Am Heart J 1988;116:820-826.

127. Janand-Delenne B, Savin B, Habib G, et al: Silent myocardial ischemia in patients with diabetes: Who to screen. Diabetes Care 1999;22:1396-1400.

128. Miller TD, Rajagopalan N, Hodge DO, et al: Yield of stress single-photon emission computed tomography in asymptomatic patients with diabetes. Am Heart J 2004;147:890-896.

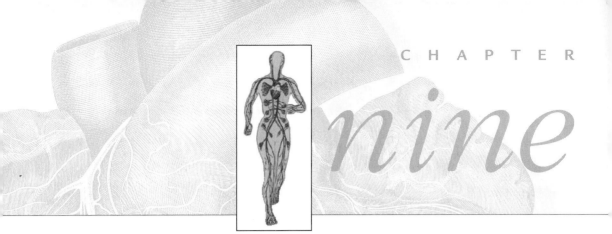

Exercise Testing of Patients Recovering from Myocardial Infarction

INTRODUCTION

Although the death rate for coronary heart disease (CHD) has been decreasing steadily since the mid 1960s, it still remains the leading cause of death in the United States.[1] Four of every 10 deaths are due to cardiac disorders and 90% of these can be attributed to CHD. The four distinct clinical manifestations of CHD are primary cardiac arrest, stable angina pectoris, acute coronary syndromes (ACS),[2] and acute myocardial infarction (MI). The resting electrocardiogram (ECG) is critical to guiding therapy, with ST elevation indicating the prompt application of thrombolysis or percutaneous coronary intervention (PCI) and ST depression requiring antiplatelet drugs (Fig. 9-1).

Each year 900,000 people in the United States experience acute MI. Of these, roughly 225,000 die, including 125,000 who die before obtaining medical care. The case fatality rate in MI patients is temporally related to onset. The risk of death is highest within the first 24 hours of onset of signs and/or symptoms and declines throughout the following year. Following the onset of a first MI in middle-aged males, 30% to 50% die within 30 days and 85% of these deaths occur within the first 24 hours. Those patients with a first MI who actually reach a hospital alive have a 10% to 18% risk of dying before discharge. The mortality thereafter falls from an annualized rate of 9% for

months 2 through 6, to 4% for months 7 through 30, and to 3% for the next 3 years. Other studies have suggested a mortality rate of 11% in the first 3 months after hospital discharge, with lower rates thereafter. In comparison with standard medical therapy, thrombolytic therapy exerts a highly significant one-fifth reduction in 35-day mortality among patients with acute MI and ST elevation, corresponding to an overall reduction of 21 deaths per 1000 patients treated. All of these statistics are probably less meaningful because of two changes in healthcare: (1) the use of troponin to define MI[3] and, (2) data supporting emergency PCIs over thrombolysis.[4] Temporal comparison studies have suggested a contemporary reduction in mortality as a result of modern therapies and prevention.[5,6] The impact of the 30% reduction in mortality with implantable defibrillators in patients with history of MI with left ventricular (LV) dysfunction has not even been factored in yet.

The pathophysiologic determinates of prognosis are (1) the amount of viable myocardium and (2) the amount of myocardium in jeopardy. Inferences can be made regarding these two determinates clinically if a patient has had congestive heart failure (CHF) or cardiogenic shock and continued chest pain or ischemia. Using cardiac catheterization, they can be assessed by ejection fraction (EF) and the number of vessels occluded. The clinical findings manifested by abnormalities of these two

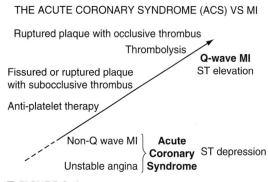

THE ACUTE CORONARY SYNDROME (ACS) VS MI

FIGURE 9–1

ACS and MI extend on a continuum and treatment is directed by the ECG.

determinates are the basis for several indices that have been used to predict risk. Clinical data have also been very useful in triaging patients in regard to the necessary length of stay in the hospital. The criteria for a complicated MI are listed in Table 9-1. Patients without these criteria, that is, those with uncomplicated MIs, can be discharged within 3 to 5 days, whereas those with these criteria require longer hospitalization and closer observation.

Healthcare professionals must be able to advise patients with history of MI as to what they should or should not do to improve their prognosis. One strategy has been to identify high-risk patients by using various clinical markers and test results.[7] Clinical markers that have indicated high risk include history of MI, CHF, cardiogenic shock, tachycardia, continued chest pain, older age, stroke or transient ischemic attack, and complicating illnesses. Procedures used to determine risk with some success have included the chest x-ray scan, routine ECG, ambulatory monitoring, radionuclide cardiac tests, and exercise testing. The assumption has been that patients at high risk should be considered for intervention; the interventions are coronary artery bypass surgery (CABS) and PCI. Because of easy access to these procedures nearly

TABLE 9–1. Characteristics that classify an myocardial infarction as being complicated

Congestive heart failure
Cardiogenic shock
Large myocardial infarction—as determined by creatine phosphokinase, troponin, and/or electrocardiogram
Pericarditis
Dangerous arrhythmias, including conduction problems
Concurrent illnesses
Pulmonary embolus
Continued ischemia
Stroke or transient ischemic attack

all patients with history of MI undergo cardiac catheterization before discharge, particularly because PCI is superseding thrombolysis.[8] Exercise testing is now rarely used to decide who needs cardiac catheterization because it is the clinical norm. Furthermore, success of PCI is being promoted as superior to exercise testing and clinical risk status for providing criteria for early discharge after acute MI.[9]

AHA/ACC EXERCISE TESTING GUIDELINES: RECOMMENDATIONS FOR EXERCISE TESTING AFTER MYOCARDIAL INFARCTION

This chapter begins with a synopsis of the American College of Cardiology (ACC)/American Heart Association (AHA) Guidelines for the Use of the Standard Exercise Test after MI.[10] Specifically with regard to testing post MI, the issue of the effects of new therapies, particularly thrombolysis and PCI, were addressed.[11]

Class I (Definitely Appropriate). Conditions for which there is evidence and/or general agreement that the standard exercise test is useful and helpful in patients recovering from an MI.

1. Before discharge for prognostic assessment, activity prescription, evaluation of medical therapy (submaximal at about 4 to 6 [rather than 7] days)
2. Early after discharge for prognostic assessment, activity prescription, evaluation of medical therapy, and cardiac rehabilitation, if the predischarge exercise test was not done (symptom-limited at about 14 to 21 days)
3. Late after discharge for prognostic assessment, activity prescription, evaluation of medical therapy, and cardiac rehabilitation, if the early exercise test was submaximal

Exceptions are noted below under Class IIb and III.

Class IIa (Probably Appropriate). Conditions for which there is conflicting evidence and/or a divergence of opinion that the standard exercise test is useful and helpful in patients recovering from an MI but the weight of evidence for usefulness or efficacy is in favor of the exercise test.

1. After discharge for activity counseling and/or exercise training as part of cardiac rehabilitation

in patients who have undergone a coronary revascularization procedure

Class IIb (Maybe Appropriate). Conditions for which there is conflicting evidence and/or a divergence of opinion that the standard exercise test is useful and helpful in patients recovering from an MI and/or the usefulness or efficacy is less well established.

1. Before discharge in patients who have undergone cardiac catheterization to identify ischemia in the distribution of a coronary lesion of borderline severity
2. In patients with an abnormal resting ECG as a result of left bundle branch block, interventricular conduction delay, electronically paced, LV hypertrophy, digoxin therapy, or those demonstrating major ST-segment depression (>1 mm) in several leads
3. Periodic follow-up exercise testing in patients who continue to participate in exercise training or as part of supervised or unsupervised cardiac rehabilitation

Class III (Not Appropriate). Conditions for which there is evidence and/or general agreement that the standard exercise test is not useful and helpful in patients recovering from an MI, and in some cases may be harmful.

1. Severe comorbidity likely to limit life expectancy and/or candidacy for revascularization.
2. At any time to evaluate patients with acute MI who have uncompensated CHF, arrhythmia, or cardiac conditions that severely limit their ability to exercise (level of evidence C).
3. Before discharge to evaluate patients who have already been selected for, or undergone, cardiac catheterization. Although a stress test may be useful before or after catheterization to evaluate or identify ischemia in the distribution of a coronary lesion of borderline severity, stress imaging tests are recommended (level of evidence C).

The following sections provide the literature support for these guidelines as well as a summary of early studies and methodological studies that have provided useful information regarding the use of exercise testing post MI. The studies that have compared exercise test results with coronary angiography are also presented. The main part is devoted to a critique of the follow-up studies. It is good to keep in mind, though, that although our approach is evidence-based, mainly empirical

clinical experience has demonstrated the benefits of the treadmill test following an MI in the following two areas:

1. Demonstration of exercise capacity for activity prescription after hospital discharge—this includes domestic and occupational work evaluation and exercise training as part of comprehensive cardiac risk reduction and rehabilitation
2. Evaluation of the adequacy of medical therapy and the need to employ other diagnostic or treatment options

METHODOLOGICAL STUDIES

Safety of Exercise Testing Early Post MI

The risk of death and major arrhythmias by performing an exercise test early after MI is very small. However, the major experience is based on clinically selected MI patients; those without major complications such as heart failure, severe arrhythmia or ischemia, LV dysfunction, or other severe diseases. Risk is highest in those rejected for testing for these clinical reasons. The incidence of fatal cardiac events, including fatal MI and cardiac rupture, is 0.03%, the incidence of nonfatal MI and unsuccessfully resuscitated cardiac arrest is 0.09%, and complex arrhythmias, including ventricular tachycardia, is 1.4%. Symptom-limited protocols have an event rate that is twice that of submaximal tests, although the overall fatal event rate is quite low.[12–14] Exercise testing after MI is safe. Submaximal testing can be performed at 4 to 6 days, and a symptom-limited test can be performed 3 to 6 weeks later. Alternatively, symptom-limited tests can be conducted early after discharge at about 14 to 21 days.

Submaximal Testing

The exercise test can determine the possible risk the patient may incur with exercise. It is certainly safer that adverse reactions be observed in controlled circumstances. Arbitrarily, a heart rate limit of 140 beats per min and a MET level of 7 is used for patients younger than 40 years of age, and 130 beats per min and a MET level of 5 for patients more than 40 years of age. Particularly for patients on beta-blockers, a Borg perceived exertion level in the range of 15 is used to end the test. In addition, conservative clinical indications for stopping the test should be applied. The physician providing medical care for the patient can gain valuable information about the patient by being there during the test and interacting with the patient.

Studies have evaluated symptom-limited protocols at 5 to 7 days after an MI and have included patients treated with thrombolytic agents. These studies demonstrate that such testing yields ischemic responses nearly twice as often as submaximal tests and are a better estimate of actual maximal exercise capacity.[15] Thus, early symptom-limited tests have potential to be more useful in activity prescription before discharge.

Historical Methodological Studies

Torkelson[16] reported results in 10 patients following an uncomplicated MI. During the sixth week of an in-hospital rehabilitation program, a low-level treadmill test was performed using 1.7 mph at a 10% grade. He concluded that the treadmill test was valuable for discerning the exercise responses of MI patients. Ibsen et al[17] reported the results of a maximal bicycle test in the third week after an MI in 209 patients. Niederberger[18] presented the values and limitations of exercise testing after MI in a monograph published in Vienna in 1977. Markiewicz et al[19] studied 46 men younger than 70 years of age with treadmill tests at 3, 5, 7, 9, and 11 weeks after their MI. The test at 3 to 5 weeks, and the test at 7 to 11 weeks, appeared to provide most of the information obtained in all five tests performed. The Washington University group evaluated 41 patients with a history of MI.[20] They assessed symptoms, signs, and hemodynamic and ECG responses during and after three activities: sitting upright, walking to an adjacent toilet, and walking on a treadmill. These activities were studied at 3, 6, and 10 days, respectively, after infarction. They concluded that successful performance of these three activities provided useful criteria for discharge of a patient with an MI.

Effect on Patient and Spouse Confidence

Taylor et al[21] evaluated the effects of the involvement of the wife in her husband's performance of a treadmill test 3 weeks after an uncomplicated acute MI.[21] They compared wives who did not observe the test, those who observed the test, and those who observed and performed the test themselves. In a counseling session after the treadmill test, wives were fully informed about the patient's capacity to perform activities. Perceived confidence in their husbands' physical and cardiac capabilities were significantly greater among those wives who also performed the test than in the other two groups. In a similar study, Ewart et al[22] demonstrated that the patients' confidence was enhanced by the test also.

Protocol Comparison

Handler and Sowton[23] compared the Naughton and modified Bruce treadmill protocols in 20 patients 6 weeks after a MI. Estimated exercise capacity and ischemic responses were similar using both protocols. Starling et al[24] evaluated 29 patients with uncomplicated MIs with heart rate-limited and symptom-limited modified Naughton treadmill test and 31 similar patients with a symptom-limited modified Naughton and standard Bruce test at 6 weeks following an MI. Predischarge, the symptom-limited Naughton test identified a greater number of patients with ST-segment depression or angina than did the heart rate-limited test. At 6 weeks following MI, the standard Bruce test identified significantly more ischemic abnormalities than did the symptom-limited modified Naughton test. During the Bruce test, a higher double product was reached in a shorter time.

Reproducibility

Starling et al[25] evaluated the comparative predictive value of ST-segment depression or angina in 93 patients with history of MI tested predischarge and 36 tested again at 6 weeks. They concluded that angina alone, irrespective of the presence of ST-segment depression, was a better predictor of multivessel disease than ST-segment depression alone. Handler and Sowton[26] evaluated the diurnal variation and reproducibility of abnormalities occurring during predischarge treadmill testing in 41 patients. Each patient was exercised using a symptom-limited Naughton protocol in the morning and the afternoon on 2 consecutive days. Ischemic abnormalities were poorly reproducible in any patient but no significant diurnal variation occurred. The reproducibility of an ischemic result in all four tests was 66%. Starling et al[27] evaluated 89 patients with predischarge and 6 weeks' treadmill tests to determine the importance of doing repeat tests to identify abnormalities of known prognostic value. Nineteen patients completed only a predischarge exercise test, nine of whom experienced an early cardiac event precluding repeat testing. ST-segment depression was highly reproducible. Angina, inadequate BP response, and ventricular arrhythmia have limited reproducibility and substantial individual variability.

Spontaneously Improved Exercise Capacity Post MI

Wohl et al[28] studied 50 patients after an acute MI. They found that in stable patients, there was an improvement at 3 weeks of the relationship between myocardial oxygen supply and demand as detected by ST-segment changes. There was a delayed improvement between 3 and 6 months in exercise capacity associated with increased stroke volume and cardiac output. Haskell et al[29] reported the cardiovascular responses to repeated treadmill testing at 3, 7, and 11 weeks after acute MI. Two symptom-limited tests were performed on 24 males several days apart. All test variables measured at maximum effort increased significantly between 3 and 11 weeks. Other studies have documented that exercise capacity increases spontaneously after an MI, even in patients not in a formal exercise program.

Effect of Q-Wave Location on ST-Segment Shifts

Castellanet et al[30] studied 97 patients with a prior transmural MI who underwent coronary angiography and treadmill testing. In patients with a previous inferior wall infarction, the ST-segment response had a high degree of sensitivity and specificity (approximately 90%) in detecting additional coronary disease. However, in patients with a previous anteroseptal MI, the ST response had much less sensitivity. In this group, a positive test suggested the presence of ischemia in the lateral or inferior posterior region. It was thought that the aneurysm generated an ischemic vector canceling ST-segment changes and producing a false-negative treadmill test. If the anterior infarction extended beyond V_4, the sensitivity rate of treadmill testing dropped even further. Ahnve et al[31] used thallium scintigraphy and computerized ST-vector shifts to evaluate the effect of Q-wave location on the relationship of ST shifts to ischemia. Anterolateral MIs had large ST-segment spatial shifts that did not indicate ischemia, whereas when shifts occurred in patients with inferior or subendocardial MIs, ischemia was detected by thallium defects.

It appeared that large anterior MIs behave as if left bundle branch block was present and the ST shifts have a very low specificity for ischemia. However, a subsequent study by Miranda et al[32] demonstrated that severe angiographic disease could be recognized in spite of Q waves using ST depression.

THE RESULTS OF EXERCISE TESTING AND CORONARY ANGIOGRAPHY

Exercise testing after MI has been used to decide who needs PCI or CABS to improve their outcome. The angiographic studies are summarized in Table 9-2 and summarized below.

Weiner[33] reported 154 patients with a single MI who had exercise testing and coronary angiography. Patients averaged being 1 year post-MI. Eighty-three patients developed ST depression only, 22 had elevation with depression in other leads, 19 had elevation only, and 30 had no changes. ST depression (with or without ST elevation) predicted multi-vessel disease, ST elevation alone, or no ST shift suggested single vessel involvement and elevation predicted LV aneurysm. Paine et al[34] studied 100 consecutive patients with exercise testing and cardiac catheterization at a median of 4 months after MI. Of 31 patients with 0.1 mV of ST depression, 87% had two- or three-vessel disease, whereas of 21 patients with no depression, 38% had two- or three-vessel disease. Fourteen patients had ST elevation, and they had more LV damage. Dillahunt and Miller[35] exercise tested 28 patients from 10 to 18 days after MI and catheterized the same patients 4 to 20 weeks later. Among 11 patients with no symptoms, ST-segment changes, or arrhythmia during the treadmill test, eight had single-vessel disease (73%) and three had two-vessel disease. In contrast, among the 17 patients with any abnormality, 14 (82%) had three- or four-vessel disease.

Sammel et al[36] reported the results of exercise testing and coronary angiography in 77 men younger than 60 years of age studied one month after MI. The 22 patients with exercise-induced angina had a greater proportion of myocardium supplied by significant lesions compared with the 55 patients free of angina. The combination of ST segment changes and angina was 91% predictive of triple vessel disease. All four patients with significant left main disease had both angina and ST segment changes. Fuller et al[37] performed submaximal exercise tests on 40 MI patients before discharge and performed catheterization 5 to 12 weeks after MI. Among the 15 patients with an

TABLE 9-2. Studies in which results of exercise testing were used to predict results of coronary angiography after acute myocardial infarction exercise test characteristics

Investigator	Year published	Patients tested	Endpoints for testing	ECG leads	Protocol	Time after MI	Angiography time after MI
Weiner	1978	154	SS, SBPd, >4 mm, RVA	12LD	Bruce	2–36 mo	2–36 mo
Paine	1978	100	90% MHR, SS, IVCD, 1 mm	V_{4-6}	Bruce	4 mo	4 mo
Dillahunt	1979	28	SS, 1 mm, >3 PVC/min, 5 min	CM_5, V_2	Naughton	10–18 days	4–20 wk
Samuel	1980	77	SS, 6 METs	12LD	Green Lane	1 mo	1 mo
Fuller	1981	40	HR 120, SS, 1 mm, >5 PVCs	12LD	Low Bruce	9–18 days	5–12 wk
Starling	1981	57	SS, VT, SBPd, HBP	12LD	Naughton	9–21 days	3–12 wk
Boschat	1981	65	85% MHR, 1 mm	12LD	Bruce	2–12 mo	2–12 mo
Schwartz	1981	48	SS, SBPd VT, 2 mm, 75% MHR	12LD	Low Bruce	18–22 days	3 wk
De Feyter	1982	179	SS, VT	12LD	Bruce	6–8 wk	6–8 wk
Akhras	1984	119	SS	12LD	Bruce	2 wk	6 wk
Morris	1984	110	SS	12LD	UPR Bike	>6 wk	<3 mo
van der Wall	1985	176	SS	12LD	Bruce/TH	6–8 wk	6–8 wk

Exercise test characteristic columns: CM_5, a bipolar lead; *HBP*, high blood pressure; *HR*, heart rate; *IVCD*, intraventricular conduction defect; *MET*, a maximal exercise level allowed to be reached as estimated from work load; *MHR*, heart rate at maximal effort; *mm*, amount in millimeters of ST shift taken as an endpoint; *(percent heart rate)*, percentage of age-predicted maximal heart rate chosen as a limit; *SPBd*, systolic blood pressure drop; *SS*, signs or symptoms, or both; *12LD*, the full set of 12 leads; V_5, fifth precordial lead; *VT*, ventricular tachycardia.

Protocol, type of exercise study done: *Bruce*, Bruce protocol stopped at 85% of the age-predicted maximal heart rate; *low Bruce*, Bruce protocol with 0 and $1/2$ stages, which are 0% and 5% grade at 1.7 mph before stage 1 (10% grade at 1.7 mph); *Bruce/TH*, Bruce protocol with thallium imaging; *Green Lane*, Green Lane Hospital treadmill protocol; *Naughton*, Naughton treadmill test; *UPR*, upright bicycle combined with radionuclide testing. *Time after MI*, mean time after myocardial infarction that the exercise test or angiography was done.

abnormal response (angina and/or ST segment depression), 13 (87%) had multivessel disease versus 7 of 25 patients (28%) with a negative test. In a subgroup of 30 patients with a first MI, 89% with an abnormal test had multivessel disease compared with 19% of those with a negative test. Among the 15 patients with an abnormal test, 73% later had angina compared with 16% among the 25 patients with a negative test.

Boschat et al[38] from France have reported their results in 65 patients who sustained their first transmural MI and within four months had undergone coronary angiography and treadmill testing. These 65 who had a treadmill test were from a group of 80 patients (81%) who had coronary angiography. Approximately 33% had post-MI angina. Only half of the vessels supplying the infarcted areas remained occluded, meaning that half had undergone spontaneous recanalization. Only 28 (43%) had an abnormal test by ST-segment depression criteria and abnormal tests were more common in the inferior MIs (54%). The clinical severity of the angina was directly related to abnormal tests, whereas exercise aerobic impairment closely correlated with the number of diseased vessels.

ST-segment elevation was noted in patients with wall motion abnormalities in the leads facing the areas of infarction and was associated with a lower EF but was a poor indicator of multivessel disease. ST-segment depression was only about 60% sensitive for multivessel disease. The occurrence of ST-segment elevation in the leads facing the infarcted zone along with significant depression in the opposed leads always indicated that another major vessel was involved, but this occurred in only 25% of the cases presented. Patients who had both angina and ST-segment depression usually had multivessel disease.

Schwartz et al[39] reported 48 patients studied with an exercise test and coronary angiography 3 weeks after their MI. Among the 21 patients with abnormal responses, 90% had multivessel disease versus 55% among the 27 patients with a normal test. Exercise-induced ST-segment elevation in 24 patients was associated with lower EF and more abnormally contracting segments. Starling et al[40] evaluated 57 uncomplicated patients with a symptom-limited Naughton treadmill test 9 to 21 days after MI and with coronary angiography within 12 weeks. They found that ST-segment depression and/or angina during the exercise test had a superior sensitivity (88%) for detecting multivessel disease compared with ST-segment depression alone (54%). Patients with inadequate BP response had multivessel disease (12 of 13) and they had mean reduced EF (EF 39%) compared with patients with a normal systolic blood pressure (SBP) response (EF 58%).

De Feyter et al[41] found the prevalence of multivessel disease was 63% in inferior and 42% in anterior MIs. Left ventricle impairment was more severe in anterior and prior MIs more prevalent than in inferior or nontransmural MIs. When they considered an abnormal exercise response to be ST-segment depression and/or angina, the sensitivity and specificity for multivessel disease was low for anterior and inferior transmural MIs. However, 80% sensitivity and 91% specificity was obtained in 21 patients with non-Q-wave MIs. With the definition of an abnormal test as depression and/or angina and elevation, they analyzed the diagnostic value for combined multivessel disease and wall motion abnormalities and a sensitivity of 41% and a specificity of 87% was obtained.

Summary of the Angiographic Studies

These studies involve populations that are much selected, often containing a higher prevalence of patients with angina than the usual population with history of MI, because they were more likely to undergo angiography. Review of the studies demonstrates a limited sensitivity and specificity for multivessel disease.

PROGNOSTIC STUDIES

This portion is based on the analysis of reports published between 1972 and 1987 of longitudinal studies using exercise testing in the early period after an MI with a follow-up for cardiac events. The most commonly cited studies and those of particular instructive value were chosen. These studies have been carefully analyzed for their: (1) methodology, (2) sample selection, (3) detailed description of sample, and, (4) description of statistical methods to permit identification of differences that might be due to their lack of agreement or commonality. The cardiac event endpoints chosen are reinfarction and death. Some studies combine these two endpoints to predict outcome. Some investigators combine reinfarction and death with soft endpoints such as angina, worsening of

symptoms, or CABS. The latter is especially worrisome, because the results of the test can influence who will have CABS, and CABS may affect mortality. These studies are summarized in Table 9-3. The studies are grouped and combined for meta-analysis by the institution at which they were performed. Each column is explained in the legend.

Ericsson et al[42] reported their results of treadmill testing 3 weeks after an acute MI in 100 of 228 MI patients. Ventricular dysrhythmias were classified as occurring during monitoring, during rest before the test, and during and after the treadmill test. They considered premature ventricular contractions (PVCs) if equal to or greater than five per minute and specifically as to patterns, ventricular tachycardia, and ventricular fibrillation. During rest before the treadmill test, two patients had unifocal and multifocal PVCs. During and after the treadmill test, six had unifocal, eight had multifocal, seven had two or three in a row, and one had four or more PVCs in a row.

Kentala[43] have reported their findings in consecutive male patients discharged after acute MI in 1969 from the University of Helsinki Hospital. During this period, 298 males younger than 65 years old were treated. Forty-five died in-hospital and the patients were selected for follow-up because of their availability and willingness to participate in a randomized trial of cardiac rehabilitation. The prognostic power of clinical and ECG variables recorded soon after MI, and in connection with the exercise test, were analyzed by stepwise multiple discriminant analysis. Patients dying within 2 years had a low exercise SBP. With longer follow-up, the exercise blood pressure had a weaker impact. At the 4- and 6-year points, an abnormal resting terminal P wave was the best predictor of poor prognosis, probably identifying a group with CHF. Patients with a high level of physical activity before infarction were less prone to die suddenly. Exercise-induced ST-segment depression did not identify a high-risk group at any point during follow-up. Abnormal apical impulses, T-wave inversion after exercise, prior resuscitation, sedentary life style, and PVCs during exercise were predictive of sudden death.

Granath et al[44] performed exercise tests at 3 and 9 weeks after an acute MI in 205 patients and followed them for up to 5 years. The investigators chose not to evaluate the ST segments because of the accepted difficulties of evaluating ST shifts after MI and because of medications. The appearance of tachycardia at low workloads, major ventricular dysrhythmias, or anginal complaints during these early exercise tests was associated with a significantly increased mortality during the

TABLE 9–3. Summary of 24 prospective studies evaluating the ability of exercise test after acute myocardial infarction to predict morbidity and mortality

Investigator	Year	MI pop. size	Exercise tested n	Exercise tested %	End points	ECG leads	Protocol	Weeks after MI	Age/% of women	Exclusions	MI % PR	MI % SE	Transmural A	Transmural IP	Meds (Dig or BB)
1 Ericsson	73	184	100	54	HR 140, SS	PC	TM	3	59/7	>65	25	?	51	43	35%D, 1%BB
2 Kentala	75	298	158	53	Max	CH$_{1-6}$	Bike	6-8	53/0	>65, Rehab	28	13	42	58	66%D, 10%BB
3 Granath	77	430	205	48	HR 140,SS	12LD	Tm/Bike	3&9	59/11	>65	18	?	48	33	?
4 Smith	79	109	62	57	60%HR	12LD	GXT	3	60/?	?	?	5	?	?	?
5 Hunt	79	633	56	9	70%HR, SS	7LD	Bike	6	57/11	No complic	?	0	47	53	?
Srinivasan	81		154			7LD					?	?	?	?	
6 Sami	79	461	200		SS	12LD	Naughton	3-52	57/10	CHF, USAP	8	9	29	62	8%D
Davidson	80		195	42	HR/SS	12LD	Stanford	3	53/0	>70, drgs, CHF	8	10	29	61	None
DeBusk	83	702	338	48	SS	12LD	Naughton	3	54/0	>70, CHF, USAP	?	?	?	?	3%D
7 Theroux	79	326	210	64	5 METs, 70%HR	CM5	Naughton	1.6	52/0	>70, CHF, USAP	34	18	31	50	40%BB, 1%D
Waters	85	330	225	68					53/16		25	21	43	55	6%D, 32%BB
8 Koppes	80	410	108	26	Submax Max	12LD	Bruce	3&8	52/13	CHF, drgs, ANG	?	24	28	48	None
9 Starling	80	190	130	68	HR130/SS	V$_{1,5,6}$	Naughton	2	53/14	USAP, CHF	24	29	34	37	26%D, 16%BB
10 Weld	81	325	236	73	4 METs, SS	V5	Low Bruce	2	54/12	>70	21	?	?	?	12%BB, 41%D
11 Saunamaki	81	404	317	78	SS	PC	Bike	3	57/20	Age, CHF, ANG	10	?	32	?	20%D, 2%BB
12 Velasco	81	958	200	21	30 w, SS	PC	SupBike	2.5	60/22	>66, se, w	3	0	46	55	11%D, 9%BB
13 De Feyter	82	222	179	81	SS	12LD	Bruce	6-8	52/0	>65, referrals ANG, CHF	8	12	35	45	Stopped
14 Jelinek	82	188	188		Symptoms	V$_{4-6}$	Bike	1.5	52/10		18	28	29	42	?
15 Madsen	83	886	456	52	SS	9LD	Bike	2.6	51/?	>75, CHF, USAP	31	6	35	?	12%D, 2%BB
16 Gibson	83	229	140	61	HR 120, SS	3LD	Naughton	1.6	63/13	>65, CHF	19	26	35	53	2%D, 61%BB
17 Norris	84	395	315	80	SS	?	2.5 mph	4	51/13	>60	0	27	29	42	30%BB
18 Williams	84	226	205	91	6 METs	3LD	Bruce	1.7	50/0	>70	23	23	33	46	16%D, 90%BB
19 Jennings	84	503	103	20	5 METs, SS	V$_5$	2 mph	1.7	56/18		?	?	51	49	4%D, 10%BB

Exercise test characteristics | Population characteristics | MI %

20 Fioretti	84	293	214	72	Symptoms	XYZ	Bike	2	54/13	>66, CHF, ANG		?			40%BB
	85	405	300	74					54/16	CHF, ANG	27		36	?	18%D, 52%BB
21 Krone	85	1417	667	47	5 METs	3LD	Low Bruce	2	?/20	>70	22	22	31	42	28%D, 31%BB
Dwyer	85								60%	<60					
22 Handler	85	296	222	75	5 METs, 70%HR	3LD	Naughton	1.4	54/16	>65, CABS, BBB	?	21	42	37	1%D, 17%BB
23 SCOR	85	1469	295	20	75%HR, SS	12LD	Mixed TM	1.7	58/18	MD judgment	21	18	38	44	26%D, 53%BB
24 Jespersen	85		126		Max, SS	II, $V_{4,6}$	Bike	3.4	57/14	>71, CHF, USAP	0	36	31	33	13%D, 20%BB
25 Paolila	85	362	263	73	Max	12	Bike	7	50/0	>65, CHF, USAP, w	3	11	32	57	2%D, 2%BB
26 Murray	86	350	300	86	Sub		TM	2	53/17	>66, CHF	?	?	?	?	20%BB
27 Cleempoel	86	202	198	98	Sub	4	TM	1.6	58/0	>70, w, CHF	?	?	?	?	10%D, 50%BB
28 Stone	86	719	473	66	Max	12	TM	24	54/21	>75, USAP, CHF, PVCs	22	28	?	?	26%D, 39%BB
			—												
TOTAL			7029												

	Follow-up period			Exercise test risk markers							
Investigator	Mean or median	Range	%CABS	Mortality if ET performed yes/no	Repeat MI if ET performed yes/no	SBP	PVC	ExCap	Angina	ST	Statistical method
Ericsson	3 mo	3 mo-?	?	5%/		NR	4×	?	?	NR	Descriptive
Kentala	6 yr	?	0%	32%/	?	+	+	NR	NR	+*	UV; some DF
Granath	2-5 yr	2-5 yr	?	25%/		NR	2×*	2×	2×	NR	UV
Smith	1.5 yr	?	?	10%/17%	?	NR	—	NR	NR	6×*	UV
Hunt	1 yr	?	?	14%/18%	?	NR	1	NR	4×*	3×*	Descriptive, UV
Srinivasan	1.25 yr	1-2 yr	?	8%	?	NR	?	NR	3×*	7×*	Not cited (UV)
Sami	19 mo	2-51 mo	10%	2%/	5%/	NR	—	1	NR	3×*	UV
Davidson	26 mo	1-60 mo	10%	1.5%/	6%/	?	?	+*	1	+*	MV-LR, LT, K-M, est
DeBusk	34 mo	?	6%	2.1%/5.5%	2%/	NR	NR	NR	NR	8×*	UV; Cox to select some variables
Theroux	1 yr	1 yr	5.7%	9.5%	6%/	NR	2×	NR	—	13×*	UV
Waters	2 yr	5-7 yr	16%	11%-3%		+*	+	+	NR	8×*	UV (Cox), MV-Cox
Koppes	2 yr	?		2%/		?	?	?	?	?	UV
Starling	11 mo	6-20 mo	?	8%/	9%/	5×	2×	NR	4×	4×	UV
Weld	1 yr	?	?	9%/		5×*	2×*	19×*	2×	2×	MV-LR; UV est
Saunamaki	5.7 yr	5-6 yr	?	35.6%/	?	3×*	2×*	NR	NR	1	LT w/in clinical subsets

Continued

TABLE 9–3. Summary of 24 prospective studies evaluating the ability of exercise test after acute myocardial infarction to predict morbidity and mortality—cont'd

| Investigator | Follow-up period | | %CABS | Exercise test risk markers | | | | | | | Statistical method |
	Mean or median	Range		Mortality if ET performed yes/no	RE MI if ET performed yes/no	SBP	PVC	ExCap	Angina	ST	
Velasco	3 yr	3 mo-6 yr	?	11%/	3%/	3x	2x	NR	3x*	4x*	UV
De Feyter	28 mo	13-40 mo	13%	6%/	7%/	NR	3x	+	2x	1	UV
Jelinek	2.3 yr	10 days-62 mo	?	7%/	19%/	—	NR	+	2x*	1	UV
Madsen	1 yr	mo	0%	6.6%/28%	4%/12%	+*	+*	+*	?	1	MV-DF, Cox; algoritham
Gibson	1.3 yr	1-3 hr	14%	5%/	6%/	NR	NR	NR	+	+	UV
Norris	3.5 yr	1-6 yr	24%	13%/33%	12%/	NR	NR	?	?	1	UV-LT; Cox cited
Williams	1 yr	1 yr	12%	6%/31%	6.8%	2x	—	2x*	2x	1	MV-DF; UV est
Jennings	1 yr	?	5%	9%/21%	3%/	8x*	1	8x*	?	2x	UV
Fioretti	1.2 yr	?	8%	9%/23%		+*	2x	+	1	1	UV
	1 yr	1 yr	8%	7%/28%	4%/	+*	+	+*	1	1	MV-DF, algorithm
Krone	1 yr	1 yr	8%	5%/14%		8x*	2x	3x*	3x*	?	UV;MV-LR
Dwyer	1 yr		12%		5%/10%	NR	?	?	?	1	UV;MV-LR
Handler	1.2 yr	6-36 mo	9%	7%/	4%/	5x*	1	8x*	1	2x	UV
SCOR	1 yr	?	?	7%/15%		1%	2x	9x*	2x	3x	UV, MV-DF
Jespersen	1 yr	1 yr	>1%	7%	2%	1	1	1	1	3x*	UV, K-M
Paolila	2.6 yr	3-57 mo	6%	4.1%/	8.3%/	1	1	1	1	4x	UV
Murray	13 mo	6 mo-?	?	18%/	13%/	NR	NR	NR	+	+	UV
Cleempoel	0.16 yr	2 mo	?	5%/	?	NR	NR	+	NR	1	UV, MV-DF

Stone	1 yr	?	2	3/16 SPB RR	5%/ PVC RR	5× ExCap RR	6× Ang RR	6× ST RR	1	1	UV, MV, LT
			*Number of studies demonstrating significant risk predictor	9	5	9	5	9			
			Number with positive risk	13	14	14	12	15			
			Number with reported effect	18	23	18	20	24			

Investigator, the first author; SCOR, Specialized Center of Organized Research; year; year of publication; MI Pop. size, number of patients admitted to the hospital with myocardial infarction over the period of the study; Exercise tested: n, number, and %, percentage, of patients out of this MI population who underwent exercise testing.

Exercise test characteristics: SS, signs or symptoms, or both; HR with a heart rate value—a heart rate limit; max, maximal effort; (percent heart rate), percentage of age-predicted maximal heart rate chosen as a limit; MET, a maximal exercise level allowed to be reached as estimated from work load; Symptoms, symptoms alone were the endpoint; PC, precordial leads; 12LD, the full set of 12 leads; CM_5, a bipolar lead; V_5, fifth precordial lead (among others); XYZ, Frank vector leads; Protocol, Type of exercise study done; TM, treadmill; GXT, Bruce protocol stopped at 85% of the age-predicted maximal heart rate; Stanford, Stanford version of the Naughton test; low Bruce, Bruce protocol with 0 and ½ stages, which are 0% and 5% grade at 1.7 mph before stage 1 (10% grade at 1.7 mph). The Norris study at Green Lane used a 2.5-mph tradmill protocol with increasing grade; Weeks after MI, mean time after MI that the exercise test or tests were done.

Population characteristics including age, sex, exclusions, MI mix, and medications: Age/% of women, mean age of patients and the percentage of women included in the study; Exclusions, > (greater-than symbol) excludes patients above a certain age; other exclusion factors were CHF, congestive heart failure; USAP, unstable angina pectoris; drgs, cardiac drugs; ANG, angiography; se, subendocardial MI; w, women; complic, complications; Rehab, not in a rehabilitation program; PVCs, abnormal premature venticular contractions; MI%, percentage of the types of infarctions included in the study; PR, prior MI; SE, subendocardial or non-Q-wave MIs; A, transmural (Q wave) anterior wall MI; IP, transmural inferior and/or posterior MI; Meds, percentage of patients on digoxin (Dig, D) or a beta-blocker (BB) at the time of treadmill testing and often through the follow-up period. CABS, coronary artery bypass surgery; Mortality, in those patients included in the study who underwent exercise testing (ET) (yes) and in those who were excluded from exercise testing for clinical reasons (no); RE MI, recurrent MI, the percentage who had a repeat MI if exercise tested (yes, left of/) or if not exercise tested (no right of/).

Exercise test risk markers: SBP, abnormal systolic blood pressure response; PVC, abnormal premature venticular contractions seen; Excap, abnormally low exercise capacity tolerance; Angina (Ang), angina induced by test; ST, abnormal ST-segment response (usually only depression). These are the responses to exercise testing that have been most commonly reported as having prognostic value. RR, Risk ratio—univariate (UV) or multivariate (MV) analysis risk ratio. If significant statistically, the risk ratio has an asterisk.*Nonsignificant risk ratios permit trends across studies to be detected. The risk ratio means that if the cutpoint value for this abnormality was reached, those with that abnormality have a certain times (×) risk of death (high risk) as opposed to those without the abnormality. Only the hard endpoints of death (and in some studies, reinfarction) are considered. NR < Results of prediction with the exercise test marker were not reported; LT, clinical life table, usually stratified; LR, logistic regression; K-M, Kaplan-Meier; est, estimates; w/in, within; DF, discriminant function analysis; ?, insufficient data to test significance; I, null effect; +, a positive nonsignificant association of usual high-risk with death; -, a negative nonsignificant association of usual high risk level with death; Cox, proportion hazard regression model for survival analysis; algorithm, detailed specific algorithm displayed for clinical use.

observation period. Exercise-induced PVCs proved to be of greater prognostic significance than those recorded at rest. During exercise testing, 9 weeks after infarct, PVCs were seen in 23% of the patients. During follow-up, 16 of them died compared with 25 of 134 without arrhythmia. Tachycardia during a submaximal workload (greater than 130 beats per minute) identified a high-risk group at both periods.

Smith et al[45] from Arizona did treadmill tests on 62 patients 18 days after admission for acute MI. Death and MI were similarly high, both in the group with elevation and in the group with depression. Of the patients who developed ST-segment depression, 30% (6 of 20) either died or had another MI after discharge from the hospital versus only 2 (5%) of 42 patients who did not have ST-segment depression during exercise.

Australia

Hunt et al[46] reported findings from the Royal Melbourne Hospital in 75 patients younger than 70 years of age. They selected their patients on the basis of having survived an MI complicated by arrhythmia and/or mechanical abnormalities. Of 11 patients with ST depression of 1 mm or more, 36% died whereas 4 of 45 (11%) without depression died. A second study of exercise testing was performed in patients with electrical and/or mechanical complications during their acute MI.[47]

Jelinek et al,[48] also from Melbourne, presented their findings in 188 patients with an uncomplicated MI. All underwent bicycle testing on the day of discharge (about day 10) and returned to work at a median of 6 weeks post MI. They considered the total duration of exercise, maximal heart rate, maximal blood pressure, and ST-segment shifts. Secondary risk factors for recurrence of heart attack were found to be angina before the MI, angina on the exercise test, and CHF. There was no difference between the two groups for maximal workload, maximal heart rate, maximal SBP, or maximal double product. The risk factors for total events were angina before MI, angina during exercise testing, and x-ray findings of CHF. No other variables were predictive, including ST depression, but only chi-square analysis was performed.

Stanford Studies

Sami et al[49] studied the prognostic value of treadmill testing in 200 males who were tested serially approximately five times each from 3 to 52 weeks

after an MI. At 3 weeks, 100% of those who subsequently had an episode of cardiopulmonary resuscitation and 60% of those who required CABS had 0.2 mV of ST-segment depression during treadmill testing. Only 35% of those without an event had a similar amount of ST-segment depression. At 5 weeks and beyond, recurrent PVCs during serial treadmill testing occurred in 90% of those who had a recurrent MI and in only 47% of those without an event. Exercise-induced PVCs or ischemic ST-segment depression 11 weeks after infarction identified patients with an increased risk of subsequent coronary events, whereas the absence of either identified a group of patients who were free of problems.

Davidson and DeBusk[50] reported results of treadmill testing in 195 men tested 3 weeks after acute MI. Stepwise logistic analysis on a subset of 92 with at least 2-year follow-up showed ST-segment depression equal or greater than 0.2 mV, angina, and a work capacity of less than 4 METS to be risk markers. These results were confirmed in the 195 men using stratified life table analysis with log rank tests. The patients were followed for 1 year and had a 19% event rate; however, more than half of these endpoint events were CABS. PVCs on a single treadmill test 3 weeks after MI had no independent prognostic value.

DeBusk and Dennis[51] applied a stepwise risk stratification procedure sequentially combining historical, then clinical characteristics and finally treadmill test results in a study population of 702 consecutive men less than 70 years of age and alive 21 days after an acute MI. Prior MI or angina, or recurrence of pain in the cardiac care unit (CCU) identified 10% of the patients with the highest rate of reinfarction and death within 6 months (18%). Clinical contraindications to exercise testing identified another 40% with an intermediate risk (6%). Exercise test results included ST-segment shifts, the MET level, angina pectoris, peak heart rate, peak SBP, exertional hypotension, and PVCs. In the patients who underwent treadmill testing, an abnormal test identified a high-risk group (10%), whereas those with a negative test had a 4% incidence of hard medical events. No other treadmill responses were predictive.

Montreal Heart Institute Studies

Theroux et al[52] studied the prognostic value of a limited treadmill test performed 1 day before hospital discharge after an MI in 210 consecutive patients. These patients were followed for cardiovascular endpoints for 1 year. Exercise capacity and the BP response were not considered. Sixty-five percent (28 of 43) who had angina during treadmill testing reported the onset of angina subsequently, according to the authors. In those with a normal ECG response to exercise testing, there was 2% mortality and a 0.7% sudden death rate; in those with ST-segment depression, there was a 27% mortality (17 of 64) and a sudden death rate of 16%.

Waters et al[53] reported an expansion of the initial study from the same institution. During 1976 to 1977, 12% of all patients admitted died in the hospital, 28% were excluded from the study and 60% were included and underwent exercise testing. Over the 5- to 7-year follow-up of the 225 patients tested, 16% had CABS. ST elevation and ST depression were similar risk predictors, and so they were combined. Target heart rate was considered to be 70% of predicted maximal heart rate and the maximal workload was 5 METs. In the first year, overall mortality was 11% and it was 3% per year afterward. Exercise-induced ST-segment depression was present in 31% and generated a risk ratio of 8× for 1 year mortality; 12% had ST elevation and the risk ratio was slightly less than with ST-segment depression; 28% had PVCs and 9% had a flat BP response. Predictors by the Cox regression model differed from the first year to the second year of follow-up. During the first year, ST-segment shift in either direction or a flat BP response were predictors. During the second year, a history of MI, the QRS score, or PVCs were independent risk predictors.

Wilford Hall USAF Medical Center

Koppes et al[54] have presented their results in a highly selected group of 108 patients with MI of a group of 410 admitted to Wilford Hall Air Force Medical Center from 1975 to 1978. Starling et al[55] have reported results using treadmill testing in 130 patients after an uncomplicated MI.

Denmark

Saunamaki and Andersen[56] in Copenhagen reported the prognostic value of the exercise test 3 weeks post MI. They considered the general prognostic importance of ventricular arrhythmia associated with the exercise test, LV function, and ST-segment changes. ST-segment deviation was not associated with endpoints. The change of

rate-pressure product (HR × SBP) from rest to maximal exercise adjusted for age was empirically found to be discriminating. Mortality increased among patients with major PVCs. Those with a small increase in rate pressure product and/or arrhythmia had a 5-year survival of 55% versus 80% in the others. In their 1982 study, they considered clinical parameters as well. Clinical subgroups were defined as (1) patients with clinical heart failure during hospitalization and/or previous MI, (2) patients with anterior MI versus inferior or indefinite MI. Within each clinical group, exercise tests still determined a high-risk and low-risk group. Follow-up was complete at 6 years.

Madsen and Gilpin[58] reported findings from symptom-limited bike testing at Grostrup Hospital in Denmark. The study population included 886 patients discharged between 1977 and 1980 after an MI. During the 1-year follow-up, few patients were on beta-blockers and no one underwent CABS. Madsen considered angina, ST-segment depression, PVCs, duration of exercise, maximal heart rate, and maximal rate pressure product as possible risk markers. The most important exercise test variables were duration of exercise and PVCs. Prediction of death was not different with clinical or exercise test variables or their combination. For reinfarction, the predictive value was significantly higher for the exercise test variables than the combined set.

Jespersen et al[59] from two Danish Hospitals have reported a series of 126 consecutive patients selected because they could exercise and had no evidence of prior MI, unstable angina pectoris, or severe heart failure and were younger than 71 years of age. The nine patients with ST-segment depression and subsequent cardiac events did not differ in any of their clinical or exercise test features from the patients without ST-segment depression. One patient who had ST-segment depression underwent CABS because of angina refractory to medical management. During the year of follow up, there were nine major cardiac events, six being fatal, in the 46 patients who developed ST-segment depression. Only three cardiac events (all deaths) occurred in 80 patients without exercise-induced ST-segment depression. The subgroup with exercise-induced ST-segment depression had annual death rates and reinfarction of 13% and 17%, respectively, and the annual rate of cardiac death was 4% in the subgroup without ST-segment depression. The estimates of cardiac event-free probability showed a significantly worse prognosis for patients with ST-segment depression. Exercise-induced angina pectoris was not predictive for further cardiac events. There was no significant difference for rate pressure product, estimated VO_2 or arrhythmia in those with cardiac events.

Spain

Velasco et al[60] reported their findings using exercise testing after an uncomplicated transmural MI. From 1973 to 1978, 958 patients with a preliminary diagnosis of MI were admitted to their CCU. Men younger than 66 years old with a transmural MI, who survived, were considered for the studies. This study is flawed by the large dropout rate (over 50% of those tested chose not to be followed) and by the use of only univariate analysis.

Houston

Weld[61] reported the results of low-level exercise testing on 236 of 250 patients who had diagnosed acute MIs. Angina was not found to be useful in predicting outcome. The exercise test variables ranked in the following order: (1) exercise duration, (2) PVCs, and (3) ST-segment depression. Patients unable to reach an exercise capacity of 4 METS had a relative risk of 15×. Exertional hypotension (a maximal SBP of less than 130) generated an odds ratio of 5 but a drop in SBP was not predictive. Standardized regression coefficients showed that all three exercise variables had a stronger association with 1-year cardiac mortality than any of the clinical variables. However, by this multivariate analysis, ST-segment depression was not statistically associated with 1-year mortality.

The Netherlands

De Feyter et al[41] from the Free University Hospital in Amsterdam have reported the prognostic value of exercise testing and cardiac catheterization 6 to 8 weeks after MI. Their study provides data on a consecutive series of 179 survivors of acute MI who had a symptom-limited Bruce test. They considered the number of vessels, EF, LV end-diastolic pressure, wall motion abnormalities, and left anterior descending coronary artery (LAD) involvement. Fifty-eight patients with at least 10 METs had a very low risk for cardiac death or reinfarction. Patients having no treadmill markers resulted in a higher risk group, whereas three-vessel disease or a LV EF of 30% or less did predict high risk. The mortality rate was 22% in patients with an EF less than 30% or

with triple-vessel disease; 1% in patients with an EF greater than 30% or with one- or two-vessel disease.

Fioretti et al[62] from the Thorax center in Rotterdam have evaluated the relative merits of resting EF by radionuclide ventriculography and the predischarge exercise test for predicting prognosis in hospital survivors of MI. The Frank leads were computer processed; 43% had abnormal ST-segment depression and approximately 40% were on beta-blockers. The hospital mortality was 13% and 19 additional patients of 214 died in the subsequent follow-up (9%). Mortality was 33% for patients with an EF less that 20%, 19% for patients with EF between the 20 and 39, and 3% for patients with an EF greater than 40%. Mortality was high (23%) in 47 patients excluded from performing exercise tests because of heart failure or other limitations. The patients could be stratified further into intermediate, low-risk groups according to an increase in SBP during exercise. Maximal workload, angina, ST-segment changes, and PVCs were less predictive. After discharge, 14% of the patients had clinical signs or symptoms of heart failure and 38% had angina; 17 were treated with bypass surgery or angioplasty. This study was later expanded to 405 patients and similar results were obtained. Discriminant function analysis demonstrated that the combination of clinical and exercise variables gave better predictive accuracy than either used alone.

New Zealand

Norris et al[63] from Greenlane Hospital reported the determinants of reinfarction and sudden death in male survivors of a first MI who were younger than 60 years of age. All underwent exercise testing and coronary angiography 4 weeks after their MI. Between January 1977 and June 1982, 425 suitable men were admitted to the hospital. Of these, 7% died in the hospital, leaving 395 survivors. Of these 395, 315 (80%) underwent exercise testing and 325 (82%) underwent coronary angiography. Exercise testing was performed at 2.5 mph starting at 0% grade and gradually increasing to 15%. Total cardiac mortality was best predicted by EF and by a coronary prognostic index dependent on age, history of infarct, and chest x-ray scan. Neither the severity of coronary artery lesions nor the results of exercise testing predicted mortality. Reinfarction could not be predicted by any clinical or angiographic variable.

United Kingdom

Jennings et al[64] at Newcastle on Tyne considered 1253 patients admitted over 1 year to their CCU; 503 sustained an MI but only 289 were younger than 66 years of age. Of these 289, 18% died in the hospital and 36% were excluded from study because of left bundle branch block, ischemic pain, or other complications; 49 could not be tested before discharge for logistic reasons. Using univariate analysis, exertional hypotension generated a risk ratio of 8×, inability to complete the protocol a risk ratio of 8×, and an excessive HR response a risk ratio of 4×. No survival analysis techniques were employed; only chi-square and t-tests were used.

Handler[65] from Guy's Hospital in London reported using submaximal predischarge exercise testing on 339 consecutive patients' age 66 years or younger. Although abnormal ST-segment depression generated a risk ratio of 6, which was not significant, ST elevation and combined elevation and depression had risk ratios greater than 10 that were statistically significant. An abnormal BP response and ST-segment elevation also predicted heart failure.

Multicenter Post-MI Research Group

Krone et al[66] reported the experience of the Multicenter Post-MI Research Group using low level exercise testing after MI. Fourteen hundred and seventeen patients met their criteria and 866 consented. Of those who consented to be in the study, 77% performed the treadmill test. Of those who exceeded a SBP of 110 during testing, there was 3% mortality versus 18% for those unable to do so. In those that had an absence of couplets, there was 4% mortality, whereas it was 13% in those with couplets. In patients with a normal exercise blood pressure and no pulmonary congestion on the chest x-ray scan, there was a 1% mortality versus 13% in those with either abnormality. Most of the results are presented in univariate form with Fisher's exact test evaluation. Further analysis of selected clinical and demographic variables using stepwise logistic regression demonstrated that exercise results significantly improved the prediction model for cardiac death. In this same study population, Dwyer et al[67] reported the experience with nonfatal events in the year following an acute MI. Radionuclide ventriculography and Holter monitoring were performed on all subjects and treadmill tests were performed in 76%.

Thirty-two percent were readmitted (7% for CABS) with a death rate of 14%. The relative risk of death in the first year after readmission was 2.6× greater than for patients who did not have a readmission. Only an EF less than 40% and angina following an MI were predictive of readmission. Reinfarction was best predicted by predischarge angina that carried a risk ratio of 2.5×. Failure to perform the exercise test was significantly associated as well with reinfarction, but none of the treadmill variables were discriminating.

Canada

Williams et al[68] from Ottawa Civic Hospital compared clinical and treadmill variables for the prediction of outcome after MI. They considered the relative prognostic merits of 15 clinical and 10 predischarge exercise test variables in 226 patients. A submaximal treadmill test was performed on 205 patients (88%) to a mean workload of 6 METs after an average of 12 days after MI. During the first year of observation, 3.4% of the patients developed unstable angina, 6.8% had a recurrent infarction, and 6% died. Twelve percent underwent coronary bypass surgery. Among those who did not have a treadmill test, there was a 31% death rate. The predictors of death were found to be resting ST-segment depression, a high creatine phosphokinase, a poor exercise tolerance, and a history of prior MI.

University of California San Diego (UCSD) Specialized Center for Organized Research (SCOR)

Madsen and Gilpin[69] attempted to answer two important questions: Can an "ischemic" exercise test response and the exercise capacity be predicted from historical and clinical data available during hospitalization? Can the patients at low or high risk of death or new MI be identified by the exercise test? To answer these questions, they analyzed data from 1469 patients discharged after an acute MI from four hospitals. Of these patients, 466 or 32% underwent a treadmill test at discharge. The exercise test was an optional part of the SCOR multicenter study protocol. The main reasons for not performing an exercise test were advanced age, poor general condition, severe cardiac dysfunction, or complicating diseases. The 466 patients, who underwent exercise testing, had a lower frequency of clinical risk factors than patients that did not undergo exercise testing. Various treadmill protocols were used but MET levels were calculated. Limiting conditions of exercise tests were angina in 16%, marked ST-segment changes in 7%, fatigue in 44%, shortness of breath in 17%, claudication in 4%, and severe arrhythmia in 2%. If no symptoms developed the patients continued exercise until they approached 75% of maximal age-adjusted heart rate. In the 9% of patients without limiting symptoms, where the exercise test was stopped at a low heart rate, the test was considered indeterminate. Patients taking beta-blockers were included if a heart rate greater than 100 beats per minute were achieved above 6 METS. Medications taken during the testing time included digoxin in 26% and beta-blockers in 53%. Ninety-two patients with indeterminate test results were excluded, leaving 374 patients.

Four historical variables from hospitalization were chosen as predicting an ischemic exercise test response by discriminate analysis. These included previous angina, ST-segment depression at rest, beta-blocking agents on discharge, and age; however, prediction was poor. In the 295 patients followed 1 year with satisfactory exercise tests, among exercise test variables tested univariately, only exercise capacity in METS and the occurrence of exercise-induced ST-segment depression were important for predicting death and/or new MI within 1 year. A discriminate analysis using all exercise test variables selected only the exercise capacity in METS. Total correct classification was 75%. In the low-risk group of patients (72% of patients with an exercise capacity greater than 4 METS), fewer than 2% died or had a new MI within 1 year. In the high-risk group of patients (29% of patients with an exercise capacity less than or equal to 4 METS), 18% had a cardiac endpoint. They concluded that an ischemic exercise test response could not be reliably predicted from historical or clinical variables from the hospitalization. Using age and ST-segment changes at rest would identify patients likely to have good exercise capacity. Good exercise capacity is the most important exercise test variable for identifying those with a very low risk of death and new MI within a year. A group of patients at relatively high risk can be identified by a poor exercise capacity.

Summary of Prognostic Indicators from Exercise Tests

The inconsistencies found in these studies make it difficult to develop an algorithm for intervention in patients with history of MI. One of the best means of selecting a high-risk group is to exclude an individual for clinical reasons from undergoing exercise testing. Possible biases as a result of this clinical selection process, as well as the characteristics associated with being admitted to the academic centers from which these reports come, must be considered. Specific summaries grouped by each of the exercise test risk markers follow. Only studies reporting statistically significant results are explicitly cited. From the previous summaries of each study, where the definitions for an abnormal responses were given, it is apparent that often several different responses under each heading are being considered together by summarizing across studies (i.e., the thresholds for abnormal PVCs, exercise capacity, or SBP response differ). In addition, the various investigators considered not all of the exercise predictors; such studies are indicated in Table 9-3 with an NR for "not reported" in the appropriate test response column.

The five exercise test variables suggested to have prognostic importance are ST-segment depression (and sometimes elevation), exercise test-induced angina, poor exercise capacity, or excessive heart rate response to a low workload, a blunted SBP response (or exertional hypotension), and PVCs. Because they involve the same populations and institutions and usually obtained the same results, the following studies are grouped together: Theroux and Waters (Montreal Heart Institute); Sami, Davidson, and DeBusk (Stanford); Hunt and Srinivasan (Royal Melbourne Hospital), Krone and Dwyer (Multicenter Post-MI Group), and Fioretti (1984 and 1985, Thoraxcenter). Thus, the results from a total of 24 centers are considered.

Exercise-Induced ST-Segment Shifts

ST Depression. Of the 28 centers, 9 found ST-segment depression to be significantly predictive of subsequent death; additional 6 centers reported a positive, but insignificant, association; and 9 centers reported a null effect with 4 of the 28 failing to report data on ST-segment depression.

ST Elevation. Sullivan et al[70] evaluated the prognostic importance of exercise-induced ST-segment elevation in 64 patients who underwent submaximal exercise testing a mean of 11 days after an acute infarct. Follow-up was for 1 year. The presence of exercise-induced ST-segment elevation was the only exercise test variable that predicted cardiac death. De Feyter et al[41] found that ST-segment depression indicated multivessel disease, whereas ST-segment elevation indicated advanced LV wall motion abnormalities and a low EF. Both shifts indicated that both multivessel disease and advanced LV wall motion abnormalities existed. In Water's study, ST-segment elevation generated the same univariate risk as did depression and so they were considered together. However, location of the ST shift was not specified. Saunamaki and Andersen considered ST-segment depression and elevation separately, but did not specify its location. In their study, the ST responses were found to have little prognostic value. Handler[65] found ST-segment elevation and combined depression and elevation to generate significant risk ratios. Elevation was more common in anterior MIs. ST-segment elevation also predicted heart failure. These results are too inconsistent to make a conclusion.

Exercise-Induced Arrhythmia

Only 5 of 28 centers reported exercise test-induced PVCs to indicate a significant increase in risk. Four centers did not include results regarding PVCs; nine centers reported null or negative associations of PVCs with mortality.

Exercise Capacity

Nine centers of 28 reported that a low exercise capacity and/or an excessive heart rate (HR) response to exercise indicated a high-risk group. Five additional centers reported nonsignificant positive associations, Stanford reported a positive association in only one of three studies, whereas 10 of the 28 centers failed to report sufficient data on this variable to assess its effect.

Exercise-Induced Angina

Only 5 of 28 centers reported exercise test-induced angina to indicate a significantly increased risk group. Eight centers failed to report angina data. Seven of the remaining 11 reported nonsignificant positive associations.

Systolic Blood Pressure Response to Exercise

Nine of 28 centers found that inadequate or abnormal SBP response to exercise significantly identified a high-risk group; 11 of the centers failed to report data, and four of the remaining six reported a nonsignificant positive association.

Comparison of Exercise Data to Clinical Data

An important question to be resolved is does the exercise test give more predictive information than the standard clinical risk predictors do?

Attempts to establish risk have included scores based on clinical features of the MI and historical information such as the Norris and Peel indices. There are reasons other than prognostication for performing exercise testing, but given the need to cost-account, all possible justification for performing a procedure is needed.

Kentala et al assessed clinical parameters, including a careful history of prior activity level. The prognostic power of clinical and ECG variables recorded soon after MI, and in connection with the exercise test, were analyzed by stepwise multiple discriminant analysis. They found that both clinical and exercise variables were important. Patients dying within 2 years had a low exercise systolic BP. With longer follow-up, the exercise BP had a weaker impact. At the 4- and 6-year points, an abnormal resting terminal P wave was the best predictor of poor prognosis. This probably identified a group with mild heart failure. For patients who suddenly died after 2 years, the T-wave changes after exercise, which possibly indicated subendocardial injury, were common. Patients with a high level of physical activity before their MI were less prone to die suddenly. Of the many factors considered, an abnormal apical impulse, T-wave inversion after exercise, prior CPR, sedentary lifestyle before infarction, and occurrence of PVCs during exercise were of discriminatory value in relation to sudden death.

Granath et al[44] found that analysis of clinical data in the CCU failed to produce any differences between survivors and those who died, although there were more deaths among those patients who had a previous MI. Saunamaki and Andersen[57] demonstrated that exercise testing variables, including PVCs, and a poor SBP HR change in response to exercise still were able to predict risk within the strata of CHF, prior MI, and anterior MI. The exercise variables outperformed these important clinical parameters. Weld[61] found the exercise test variables of duration, PVCs, and ST-segment depression to be ranked in that order ahead of the clinical variables of x-ray vascular congestion, prior MI, and x-ray cardiomegaly in predictive value.

De Feyter et al[41] were unable to identify a higher risk group from treadmill markers, whereas three-vessel disease or a LV EF of 30% or less did. Madsen and Gilpin[58] found that in those who underwent testing, clinical variables were better able to predict outcome than in the nontested group. The most important exercise test variables were exercise duration and PVCs; however, they improved prediction of reinfarction but not death. Although exercise test variables were selected by discriminant analysis, the correct total classification of deaths and survivors was not improved. The total correct prediction was 71% for clinical data alone, 67% for exercise data alone, and 71% for both combined.

DeBusk et al[51] found that prior MI or angina, or recurrence of pain in the CCU identified the 10% of patients with the highest rate of reinfarction and death within 6 months (18%). Clinical contradictions to exercise testing identified another 40% with an intermediate risk (6.4%). In those who underwent treadmill testing, ST-segment depression and low peak workload were selected before any clinical variables or ambulatory ECG data in the logistic regression analysis.

Norris et al[63] found that total cardiac mortality was best predicted by EF and by an index dependent of age, history of MI, and chest x-ray scan. Neither the severity of coronary lesions nor the results of exercise testing predicted mortality. Any clinical exercise test or angiographic variable could not predict reinfarction. Williams et al[68] considered the relative prognostic merits of 15 clinical and 10 predischarge exercise test variables in 226 patients. The predictors of death were found to be resting ST depression, a high creatine phosphokinase, a poor exercise tolerance, and a history of MI.

Jennings et al[64] found that the Norris index score (age, prior MI, x-ray scan abnormalities) of less than 3 was associated with a 12% mortality and a score of more than 12 with a mortality of 85%. Fioretti et al[62] evaluated the relative merits of resting EF by radionuclide ventriculography and the predischarge exercise test. Mortality was 33% for patients with an EF less than 20%, 19% for patients with EF between 20% and 39%, and 3% for patients with an EF greater than 40%. Mortality was high (23%) in 47 patients excluded from performing exercise tests because of heart failure or other limitations.

Krone et al[66] found that among those not able to take a treadmill test, there was a 14% mortality compared with 5% in those who were able to take it. In patients with a normal exercise blood pressure and no pulmonary congestion on the chest x-ray scan, there was a 1% mortality versus 13% in those with either abnormality. In this same population, Dwyer et al[67] reported the experience with nonfatal events in the year following an MI. Thirty-two percent were readmitted (7% for CABS) with a death rate of 14% and a risk ratio of 2.6. Only an EF less than 40% and post-infarction angina were predictive of readmission. Reinfarction was best predicted by predischarge angina. Failure to perform the exercise test was significantly associated with

these events, but none of the treadmill variables was discriminating.

Waters et al[53] found that predictors by the Cox regression model were different in the first and the second year of follow-up. During the first year, ST-segment shift in either direction, a flat BP response or angina within the 48 hours after admission were predictors ("markers of ischemia"). During the second year, a history of MI, the QRS score, or PVCs was independent risk predictors ("markers of LV dysfunction").

In summary, the results are mixed regarding whether the exercise test gives information that can predict death and reinfarction better than the clinical features. Remember that clinical judgment to exclude patients from testing identifies the highest risk group and that the threshold for doing so must be quite variable between locations.

Clinical Design Features

The column headings used in Table 9-3, and separately listed in Table 9-4, are the important features of the study design that could affect the findings. Following is a discussion of these features.

TABLE 9–4. Characteristics that could differ as to methodology among studies

Patients excluded
Entrance criteria
Age range; gender
Infarct mix (i.e., non-Q wave, inferior/anterior/lateral Q wave)
Patients with prior MI and those with complications included or not
Prior coronary artery bypass surgery or PCI
History of congestive heart failure and angina
MI size
Follow-up thoroughness and length
Percentage of patients undergoing CABS or PCI during follow-up and whether they are censored
Cardiac events (problems with using CABS as an endpoint)
Mortality during follow-up (are they a high- or low-risk group?)
Reinfarction rate
Exercise protocol
Time post-MI test performed
Endpoints of test
Leads monitored
Medications taken after discharge from hospital and at time of exercise test
Test responses considered (PVCs, ST segment, blood pressure, exercise capacity, angina)
Statistical methods

CABS, coronary artery bypass surgery; MI, myocardial infarction; *PCI*, percutaneous coronary intervention; PVCs, premature ventricular contractions.

Exercise Protocol. Bike protocols, especially a supine protocol, can give different responses than a treadmill. Most protocols were continuous but some were not progressive in workload increments. The standard Bruce protocol starts at a relatively high workload (4–5 METS). The protocol as well as beta-blockade, fitness, and anxiety can affect heart rate responses at submaximal levels.

Endpoints of Exercise Test. If stopped at a certain amount of ST-segment shift, MET level, or heart rate, then this response could not be considered as a continuous variable nor could a higher value, which might be more discriminating, be reached.

ECG Leads Monitored. Use of different electrode placements can make comparisons between studies difficult, but probably does not have a great impact.

Time Post MI When Exercise Test was Performed. "Stunned" myocardium and deconditioning affect predischarge testing more than they affect hemodynamic responses later. ST-segment responses appear more labile earlypost MI. The responses differ at various times post MI as well, with a spontaneous improvement in hemodynamics occurring by 2 months. The spontaneous improvement in both EF and exercise capacity, but their failure to correlate with each other, makes them difficult to interpret. The studies that included exercise testing at multiple times found the same responses to have a different predictive value at the specific times the tests were performed. There is a spontaneous improvement during the first year post MI in the blunted BP response to exercise that occurs particularly in large anterior MIs.

MI Mix (i.e., Q-Wave Location). Each have a different prognosis and different "normal" response to exercise. Exercise predictors may be different in each type.

Inclusion of Non-Q-Wave MIs. After much controversy regarding the risk of having a "subendocardial" MI, a study from Mayo clinic appears to clarify the situation.[70] From 1960 to 1979, 1221 residents of Rochester, Minnesota had an MI as the first manifestation of CHD; 784 had a transmural (Q wave) and 353 had a non-Q-wave MI. The 30-day fatality rate was 18% among transmural and 9% in subendocardial MIs. No significant difference was found in the rates of reinfarction, CABS, or mortality over the next 5 years. CHF was more common among patients with transmural MIs, and angina

was more common among patients with non-Q-wave MIs. This review and other data support the concept that ST depression with exercise effectively stratify patients following a non-Q-wave MI. This group is now considered in the ACS category with unstable angina.

The failure of exercise-induced ST-segment depression to consistently be associated with increased risk in patients after MI was hard to explain. This failure could be a result of population differences and the resting ECG. To test this we studied 198 males who survived an MI, underwent a submaximal predischarge treadmill test, and were followed-up for cardiac events for 2 years.[71] Abnormal ST-segment depression was associated with twice the risk for death and the risk increased to 11 times in patients without diagnostic Q waves, similar to the results by Krone et al[72] in patients with an initial non-Q-wave MI. These results suggest that the difference in the prognostic value of the post-MI exercise ECG between studies is due to variations in the prevalence of the patterns of the rest ECG among study populations. Angiographic studies, however, have demonstrated that exercise-induced ST depression is associated with severe coronary artery disease whether Q waves are present. The conflicting results from follow-up and angiographic studies most probably relate to the fact that early mortality is strongly associated with LV damage, whereas later mortality is associated with ischemia and severe coronary artery disease.

Thoroughness and Length of Follow-Up. Those lost to follow-up most likely have a higher percentage of deaths. In addition, follow-up affects analysis if censored data cannot be handled adequately with the statistical program. Mortality changes over time and predictors change.

Percentage of Patient Undergoing CABS (or PCI) During Follow-Up. CABS could alter mortality and affect outcome prediction. In addition, patients with ischemic predictors would be selected to have this procedure more frequently. These patients should be censored at the time of intervention but such censoring is not random.

Cardiac Events Considered as Endpoints. The only hard endpoints that should be considered, from an epidemiological point of view, are death and reinfarction. Separation or distinction of sudden death makes little sense and may confuse the analysis, particularly if those with sudden death are compared with all others (including nonsudden cardiac death). Noncardiac deaths are often difficult to distinguish and lead to biased results but may play a confusing role, particularly in older populations. CABS is not a valid endpoint and should be considered as a censored outcome. It is clearly related to certain exercise test results that physicians feel motivated to "fix" with that procedure. "Instability" or progression of symptoms (CHF or angina) is a soft endpoint that should not be used for epidemiological purposes.

Mortality During Follow Up. If there is a low mortality rate, more patients are needed to find a statistical difference between those with or without certain variables. Some studies have compensated for this by using soft endpoints and combining endpoints.

Prior MI Patients Included or Not. Prior MI is an important predictive variable that depends on the severity of the prior MI or MIs. Patients with prior large MIs are biased toward being admitted with non-Q-wave MIs, because another transmural MI increases their likelihood of dying before hospitalization. Few studies have tried to account for the number or severity of prior MIs.

Exclusion Criteria. Clearly, clinical judgment applied to the population who had a prior MI, to exclude patients from exercise testing, identifies the highest risk group. Though this process considers complicating illnesses and age, cardiac dysfunction and ischemia are considered as well. Because of this, alternative testing methods that have been compared favorably with exercise testing have included right atrial pacing and electrophysiologic stimulation studies.

Age Range and Gender. Women are thought to have a higher MI mortality and certainly are known to respond differently than men to exercise testing. Because of this, they should be considered separately, but the studies do not contain a sufficient number for valid analysis. Death rates are directly related to age.

Medications Taken After Discharge from Hospital and at the Time of the Test. Digoxin causes ST depression, but it is usually taken for CHF, thus implicating an ischemic etiology for a potential death because of dysfunction. Digoxin administration post-MI may actually be an independent risk predictor and act by predisposing to ventricular dysrhythmias. Beta-blockers affect BP and heart rate response and improve survival but do not seem to impact the value of the exercise test.[73-75]

Although beta-adrenergic blockade attenuates the ischemic response, two long term follow-up studies have demonstrated that these agents do not interfere with poor exercise capacity as a marker of adverse prognosis.[76,77] Patients taking beta-blockers after an MI should continue to do so at the time of exercise testing. Because patients will take these medications for an indefinite period after infarction, the exercise test response while on beta-blockers will provide information regarding the adequacy of medical therapy in preventing ischemia and arrhythmias as well as controlling the heart rate and BP response during exercise. Moreover, discontinuation of beta-blockers solely for the purpose of exercise testing may expose the patient to the unnecessary risks of recurrent ischemia, arrhythmia, and exaggerated hemodynamic responses during exercise.

Statistical Critique of the Prognostic Studies

There are several general problems that are apparent across many of the studies. The purpose of a specific study is not always clear; there is confusion evident between the desire to develop a prediction algorithm that will be of practical clinical use in patient treatment and the desire to demonstrate an association of exercise testing responses to subsequent cardiac events in any form. Development of a prediction algorithm requires an approach to validation that is quite different from the testing of the statistical significance of an effect, as is done in many of the studies. Although effect size estimation is probably the most clinically relevant procedure, most of the studies report only significance test results, perhaps with some means or frequency differences cited. None of the studies reported effect size estimates with confidence intervals, even though this is the well-established method of reporting estimation results.

Finally, many of the studies reviewed failed to provide enough details about the data to allow independent evaluation of the investigators' conclusions. Such details are especially necessary to compare results across different studies. Recompilation of effects may be required to compare studies that have reported results in different formats. The number of "?" appearing in the exercise test risk markers column of Table 9-3 illustrates how often data reported were insufficient to compute even the direction of the associations in the study (whether the association is "significant").

Common areas of difficulty include selection biases, a relatively rare outcome of interest, use of multiple endpoints, and unequal follow-up times.

Many of the studies fail to be specific enough about the target population of interest. Selection biases in the patients studied may be too severe for the results to be considered representative of the general population. However, the limited target population is carefully designing further research, even if the results are not generally applicable. Evaluation of possible biases requires information on patients who were eligible for the study but declined to participate, or who dropped out of the study after their initial entry. A few of the investigators have reported on such nonparticipants or follow-up losses, but many do not report more than the number of individuals involved.

The most desirable endpoint for analyses in these studies is cardiovascular death because the aim of the test is to identify those benefiting from cardiac interventions. One approach to attempt to deal with small numbers of deaths is the use of multiple endpoints, often combined. However, this practice may obscure underlying relationships for several reasons. Endpoints other than death, such as angina, cannot be well enough defined to avoid extensive misclassification errors. A potentially more serious issue when endpoints are combined is independent of the precision of the endpoint measurement. Different endpoints may be related to different mechanisms and thus may have different associations with the test markers. Such differences confound any attempt to measure associations using combined endpoints. Perhaps the worst pitfall is the use of an endpoint to assess associations that may be influenced by the exercise test result; studies that have included CABS or PCI as an endpoint have fallen prey to this trap.

Finally, the problem of unequal follow-up periods of patients cannot be ignored. This problem can be circumvented in the design of a study by using a limited period for entry into the study, with follow-up that allows the study to be completed with sufficient events. This approach requires that the follow-up time be limited enough to minimize loss-to-follow-up problems. Adjustments for unequal follow-up time can also be made in the analysis phase of the study, but these were not used in most of the studies.

Only one fourth of the research centers reported any use of multivariate techniques. Computer programs for such analyses were certainly widely available after 1980; only 5 of the 28 centers have reports limited to before 1981, when access to such analysis tools may have been more difficult. None of the studies reported multivariate estimates of effect, even though the effect estimate is at least as sensitive to error from exclusive univariate analysis as

significance tests. It is true that multivariate techniques often have stricter assumptions than some of the univariate techniques available and should not be used without initial screening with univariate analysis. Even if univariate estimates are given for comparison to other studies, the multivariate results should be reported so that the extent of adjustment necessary for inter-relationships can be assessed.

The other major analysis issue is the problem of unequal follow-up. Unequal follow-up that is not controlled in the design of a study must be handled in the analysis of the data. Unequal follow-up of patients can be treated as censored data. A typical approach in biomedical research for analysis of censored time-to-response data is to use survival analysis techniques. This approach was used in several of the more recent studies. However, a fundamental assumption of most survival techniques is that the censoring is random with respect to the outcome of interest. This assumption cannot be evaluated without reporting on those patients who were lost to follow-up either because of dropping out of the study or because of lack of complete follow-up due to late entry into the study. Information on those who have dropped out could be gathered by death certificate searches or other techniques; reports on such persons are often missing from the studies reviewed. Including patients who are censored observations because of short follow-up time must be considered carefully, because the risk of subsequent cardiac events is known to change with time. Multivariate approaches to survival analysis are available using proportional hazard regression models or other hazard functions. However, these models may be relatively insensitive to modeling of interactions among the variables. In addition, the results may not be readily interpretable in terms useful to clinicians.

Other approaches to the problem of censored data are possible. One solution often used in epidemiological research is computations in the form of events/person-time or person-time incidence. Another approach that avoids the inclusion of short-term follow-up patients is to stop entry into the study early enough so that all patients available can be followed for a fixed time. A limited, fixed time of follow-up can also help reduce the number of dropouts, because the likelihood of losing a patient from the study increases with time. One approach to be avoided that was used in several of the studies is to merely count events in various subgroups without regard to differences in follow-up time. Data that is reported in such a way is essentially meaningless.

Survival analysis is appropriate when outcome measurements represent the time to occurrence of some event (i.e., death or reinfarction). If differences in important covariates or prognostic variables exist at entry between the groups to be compared, the investigator must be concerned with the analysis of the survival experience as influenced by that difference. To adjust for these differences in prognostic variables, stratified analysis or a covariance type of survival analysis could be done. If there are many covariates the number of strata can quickly become large, with few subjects in each. Moreover, if a covariate is continuous, it must be divided into intervals and each interval assigned to a score or rank before it can be used in a stratified analysis. Cox proposed a regression model that allows analysis of censored survival data adjusting for continuous and discrete covariates, thus, avoiding these two problems. This model, also called the proportional hazard model, assumes that the hazard rate or "force of mortality" can be expressed as a product of two terms. Available statistical packages allow incomplete data; that is, there are cases for which the response is not observed but the data (time in study) are included in the analysis. This could occur in the study of survival where an individual may remain alive at the close of the observation period or may drop out before the end. The Cox survival analysis allows covariates that can be selected in a stepwise fashion. The covariates or prognostic factors usually represent either inherent differences among the study subjects or constitute a set of one or more indicator variables representing different groups. The covariates may also describe changes in a patient's prognostic status as a function of time. The Cox proportional hazards regression model presumes death rates may be modeled as log-linear functions of the covariates. A regression coefficient is estimated, which relates the effect of each covariate to the survival function.

The Cox model is currently favored; however, few investigators have compared the various techniques in one data set. Madsen et al[78] compared two software versions of the Cox multivariate analysis, stepwise discriminant analysis, and recursive partitioning. They concluded that all four techniques gave equally precise prognostic evaluations but that recursive partitioning was easier to use and the Cox models were more accurate. The UCSD SCOR group evaluated several multivariate statistical methods in two different hospital populations to predict 30-day mortality and survival following MI.[79] The methods evaluated were linear discriminant analysis, logistic regression, recursive partitioning, and nearest neighbor. Variables used were identified as predictive univariately from the base hospital and were obtained during the first 24 hours. Linear discriminant analysis assumes normality among the predictor variables, whereas logistic regression is based on the assumption that the log of the classification function is a linear function of the fitted coefficients. Recursive partitioning makes no assumption regarding normality and can detect interactions among variables and handles missing data. The nearest neighbor procedure is based on the concept that in the multidimensional space defined by the variables, a patient would likely have the same outcome as another patient in that space. It cannot detect interaction or assign importance. Linear discriminant analysis, logistic regression, and recursive partitioning performed similarly within a given population, although each used the information contained in the prognostic variables differently. Application between different populations of prediction schemes based on linear discriminant analysis and logistic regression was shown to be feasible but prior validation is essential.

Temporal changes in risk. It is well documented that changes in the risk of subsequent cardiac events occur within the first year post MI. Such underlying changes in the hazard function suggest that there may be temporal changes in the effects of any related risk markers. Evaluation of this effect requires time-dependent modeling or conditional analysis with respect to time. Waters et al[53] are the only investigators to have addressed this problem. One expected effect of not considering the temporal changes in risk is that estimates of effect size may be biased toward the null over intervals that span several risk periods.

Meta-Analysis Considerations

Meta-analysis is a statistical approach to develop a consensus from an existing body of research. It is a quantitative approach to reviewing research using a variety of statistical techniques for sorting, classifying, and summarizing information from the findings of many studies. It is also the application of research methodology to the characteristics and findings of studies. This includes problem selection, hypothesis formulation, the definition and measurement of constructs and variables, sampling, and data analysis.

The application of meta-analysis to a body of research involves three stages. First, a complete literature search is conducted which is analogous to the collection of data in an experimental study.

28 reports met the criteria providing information on 15,613 tested patients. For myocardial perfusion imaging, eight studies reported on 1247 patients. Ventricular function-imaging reports included nine radionuclide angiography studies (1357 patients) and two echocardiographic imaging studies (107 patients). A total of eight pharmacologic stress-imaging reports reported on 1550 patients; 301 for perfusion and 1338 for echocardiography. The mean ages of patients were similar (54 to 57 years); 80% of the patients were male. Only 18 reports included patients receiving thrombolytic therapy, and a quarter of all patients had a prior MI.

Outcomes (see Table 9-6). The pooled 1-year cardiac death rate was 3.3% for the 28 exercise ECG reports; the combined cardiac death and MI rate was 8.1%. Pooled cardiac death and combined death and repeat MI rates from the eight exercise myocardial perfusion reports at 1 year were higher at 4.8% and 13.9%, respectively. The cardiac death rate was higher yet for exercise radionuclide angiography (9.3%); the combined "hard" event rate of death and MI was 13.2%. For the two exercise echocardiography reports, the rates of cardiac death and combined events at 1 year were 5.6% and 15.9%, respectively. The cardiac death rate among the eight pharmacologic stress reports was 2.5% for echocardiography and 6.6% for perfusion imaging, whereas cardiac death and MI rates were 5.0% and 15.0%, respectively.

Table 9-7 synthesizes all the predictive values of risk markers from the 54 noninvasive reports stratified by the total number of cardiac deaths. When the number of cardiac deaths was small, predictive values for cardiac death were often much larger than for cohorts with more frequent events.

Risk Indices. Table 9-8 provides a breakdown of various risk indices for high-risk markers obtained during exercise or pharmacologic examination.

The pooled values for individual markers were quite low. The sensitivity of risk markers derived from exercise treadmill or bicycle tests ranged from 23% to 56% for cardiac death. Sensitivity values obtained from myocardial perfusion and radionuclide angiographic imaging reports were higher (56% to 100%), but this most likely is spurious because of their smaller numbers. The positive predictive values for cardiac death (percentage of those with an abnormal test that have the outcome) were low for most risk markers, with values of less than 10% for exercise-induced ST depression, chest pain, any reversible or multiple myocardial perfusion defects, and the presence of new stress-induced wall motion abnormality. Higher positive predictive values were noted for the combined endpoint of cardiac death or MI but remained less than 20%. The positive predictive values of a peak exercise EF less than 40% (cardiac death 27%, cardiac death or MI 31%) were higher than those of other noninvasive predictors. In 33 patients with a new or worsening wall motion abnormality after exercise, the positive predictive value for cardiac death or MI was 48%. In contrast to the low positive predictive values for most markers, negative predictive values (percentage of those with a negative test result that do not experience the outcome during follow-up) exceeded 90% in most cases.

Summary Odds Ratio (OR) for Cardiac Death and Death or Reinfarction

Exercise ECG. Figures 9-2 through 9-4 provide pooled cardiac event rates and summary OR of cardiac death and cardiac death or nonfatal MI for the 54 reports. The summary OR for cardiac death was significantly higher for patients with 1-mm ST depression (OR 1.7, 95% confidence interval [CI] 1.2 to 2.5), impaired SBP (OR 4.0, 95% CI 2.5 to 6.3), or limited exercise capacity (OR 4.0, 95% CI 1.9 to 8.4). A similar pattern was noted for the

TABLE 9-7. Predictive value of noninvasive testing for cardiac death based upon total number of observed cardiac deaths

Total no. deaths	Average no. deaths per study	Average sample size	Sensitivity	Specificity	Summary or (95% ci)
0–5 (21 studies)	2	89	0.63	0.77	4.92 (1.15, 21.12)
6–10 (9 studies)	7	145	0.46	0.62	1.92 (0.85, 4.35)
11–19 (9 studies)	16	328	0.55	0.58	1.63 (0.84, 3.15)
≥20 (15 studies)	39	1840	0.43	0.73	1.52 (1.05, 3.51)

Note: A positive test was identified from the most predictive risk marker from each testing technique.
Modified from Shaw LJ, Peterson ED, Kesler K, et al: Am J Cardiol 1996;78:1327-1337.

TABLE 9–8. Predischarge risk stratification with noninvasive testing

	Sensitivity		Specificity		(+) Predictive Value		(–) Predictive value	
	Cardiac death	Cardiac death/MI	Cardiac death	Cardiac death/MI	Cardiac death	Cardiac death/MI	Cardiac death	Cardiac death/MI
Exercise Electrocardiography								
ST depression	0.42	0.44	0.75	0.70	0.04	0.16	0.98	0.91
Impaired systolic BP	0.44	0.23	0.79	0.87	0.11	0.21	0.96	0.88
Limited exercise duration	0.56	0.53	0.62	0.65	0.10	0.18	0.95	0.91
Exercise chest pain	0.23	0.29	0.83	0.82	0.08	0.19	0.94	0.89
Exercise Myocardial Perfusion Imaging								
Reversible perfusion defect	0.89	0.80	0.38	0.48	0.07	0.16	0.98	0.95
Multiple perfusion defects	0.64	0.75	0.71	0.76	0.07	0.17	0.98	0.97
Pharmacologic Stress Imaging								
Reversible perfusion defect	0.56	0.71	0.46	0.49	0.10	0.19	0.90	0.91
Multiple perfusion defects	—	0.50	—	0.64	—	0.17	—	0.90
Exercise Radionuclide Angiography								
Peak EF ≤40%	0.63	0.60	0.77	0.75	0.27	0.31	0.94	0.91
Change in EF ≤5%	0.80	0.55	0.67	0.74	0.15	0.18	0.98	0.94
New dyssynergy	—	0.78	—	0.50	—	0.17	—	0.94
Exercise Echocardiography								
Change in EF ≤5%	—	0.56	—	0.60	—	0.14	—	0.92
New dyssynergy	1.00	0.62	0.62	0.79	0.18	0.48	1.00	0.86
Pharmacologic Stress Imaging (ECHO)								
New dyssynergy	0.67	0.55	0.56	0.54	0.05	0.08	0.98	0.94

BP, blood pressure; EF, ejection fraction; MI, myocardial infarction.
Modified from Shaw LJ, Peterson ED, Kesler K, et al: Am J Cardiol 1996;78:1327-1337.

combined endpoint. Although not as predictive of cardiac death, exercise-induced chest pain was better in predicting death or reinfarction (OR 2.1, 95% CI 1.4 to 3.2).

Exercise and Pharmacologic Stress Myocardial Perfusion Imaging. Among the 1247 patients who underwent exercise myocardial perfusion imaging, the occurrence of a reversible defect (either within or remote from the infarction site) was associated with a 1-year cardiac death rate of 7.1% and a death or nonfatal MI rate of 15.8% (Fig. 9-3). Similar rates were reported for multiple perfusion defects. For a reversible perfusion defect, the summary odds of cardiac death was 3.1 (95% CI 1.6 to 4.6) and for death or reinfarction was 3.6 (95% CI 1.2 to 12.6).

For pharmacologic stress perfusion imaging, the summary OR for cardiac death with a reversible perfusion defect was only 1.2 times (95% CI 0.4 to 3.7) higher. Patients who had a dipyridamole-induced reversible perfusion defect had a 1.8 times (95% CI 0.8 to 4.1) higher risk of 1-year cardiac death or MI.

Exercise and Pharmacologic Ventricular Function Imaging. Rates of cardiac death (27%) and combined events (31%) were highest for patients who

Cardiac event rates by test result

	Pos	Neg	Cardiac death rate	Pos	Neg	Cardiac death or MI rate	For cardiac death	For cardiac death or MI
Exercise electrocardiography			3.3%			7.8%		
ST depression	4.6% (2,735)	2.1% (9,943)		15.7% (1,083)	9.9% (2,358)			
Impaired systolic BP	4.9% (1,796)	1.9% (7,093)		21.4% (182)	12.3% (1,061)			
Limited exercise duration	3.4% (3,019)	1.5% (4,557)		17.5% (634)	9.1% (1,074)			
Exercise chest pain	4.6% (864)	2.8% (3,889)		18.9% (360)	10.9% (1,502)			

Summary odds ratio (x-fold) — 0.1 1 10 100

FIGURE 9–2

Summary odds of cardiac death and combined death or reinfarction for exercise electrocardiographic risk predictors. Cardiac death or reinfarction rates are in boldface in the table at left; abnormal test rates by test result are given, as well as the number of patients with a normal or abnormal test (in parentheses). Chi-square tests for homogeneity results were non-significant except for blood pressure predicting cardiac death or myocardial infarction.

Cardiac event rates by test result

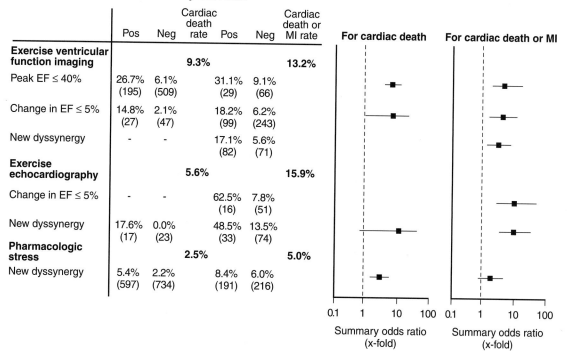

	Pos	Neg	Cardiac death rate	Pos	Neg	Cardiac death or MI rate
Exercise ventricular function imaging			9.3%			13.2%
Peak EF ≤ 40%	26.7% (195)	6.1% (509)		31.1% (29)	9.1% (66)	
Change in EF ≤ 5%	14.8% (27)	2.1% (47)		18.2% (99)	6.2% (243)	
New dyssynergy	-	-		17.1% (82)	5.6% (71)	
Exercise echocardiography			5.6%			15.9%
Change in EF ≤ 5%	-	-		62.5% (16)	7.8% (51)	
New dyssynergy	17.6% (17)	0.0% (23)		48.5% (33)	13.5% (74)	
Pharmacologic stress			2.5%			5.0%
New dyssynergy	5.4% (597)	2.2% (734)		8.4% (191)	6.0% (216)	

For cardiac death — Summary odds ratio (x-fold) — 0.1 1 10 100

For cardiac death or MI — Summary odds ratio (x-fold) — 0.1 1 10 100

FIGURE 9–3

Summary odds of cardiac death and combined death or reinfarction for stress myocardial perfusion scintigraphy risk predictors. Chi-square tests for homogeneity results were non-significant.

had a peak exercise EF less than 40% (Fig. 9-4). Summary odds of cardiac death were 3.2, 4.2, and 1.2 times for EF less than 40%, EF change less than 5%, and new echocardiographic wall motion abnormality, respectively. For the same markers, summary odds of cardiac death or MI were 4.4, 3.6, and 1.7 times higher.

Rates of cardiac events were lower (5.4% to 8.4%) for patients with a pharmacologically induced new or worsening wall motion abnormality. The odds of cardiac death with pharmacologic stress-induced new wall motion abnormality were 2.7 times higher (95% CI 1.4 to 5.2). For cardiac death or MI, the 95% CI included 1.0 for the summary pharmacologic echocardiography data.

Comparative Predictive Value in the Thrombolytic Era

The average cardiac death rates were lower in studies including thrombolytic-treated patients than in those that did not (4% versus 7%). In Figure 9-5, the positive predictive values for cardiac death and cardiac death or MI are illustrated for patients who had ST-segment depression, a reversible perfusion defect, or a peak exercise EF less than 40%. Positive predictive values were usually decreased in patients receiving thrombolytic therapy. For example, the positive predictive value

for cardiac death or MI in patients who had a reversible perfusion defect was 24% in the non-thrombolytic-treated versus 6% in thrombolytic-treated patients.

Noninvasive measurements taken during (or at peak) stress can be divided into those estimating the degree of residual ischemia and LV reserve, however many reflect both. The degree and extent of residual ischemia correlate with the extent of jeopardized myocardium. Such ischemic markers include exercise-induced ST-segment depression, angina, and reversible perfusion defects. In the meta-analysis, exercise test-induced chest pain was not associated with an increased risk of death. The odds of cardiac death in patients with ST-segment depression of 1 mm were half that reported for patients with hemodynamic and exercise limitations. Approximately 20% of patients undergoing exercise ECG testing had an abnormal test based upon exercise-induced ST depression or chest pain.

Single versus Multiple Reperfusion Defects. The presence of a single redistribution abnormality, which relates to poststenotic flow and infarct artery patency, may be insufficient to stratify patients. The decrease in specificity may relate to a lower threshold for "abnormality"; more than half of the patients who underwent myocardial perfusion imaging were considered to have had an

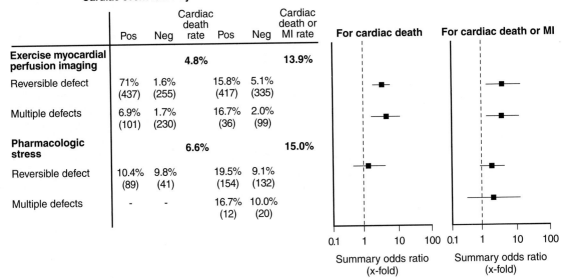

Cardiac event rates by test result

	Pos	Neg	Cardiac death rate	Pos	Neg	Cardiac death or MI rate
Exercise myocardial perfusion imaging			4.8%			13.9%
Reversible defect	71% (437)	1.6% (255)		15.8% (417)	5.1% (335)	
Multiple defects	6.9% (101)	1.7% (230)		16.7% (36)	2.0% (99)	
Pharmacologic stress			6.6%			15.0%
Reversible defect	10.4% (89)	9.8% (41)		19.5% (154)	9.1% (132)	
Multiple defects	-	-		16.7% (12)	10.0% (20)	

For cardiac death — Summary odds ratio (x-fold)

For cardiac death or MI — Summary odds ratio (x-fold)

■ **FIGURE 9–4**

Summary odds of cardiac death and combined death or reinfarction for stress radionuclide angiographic (RNA) and echocardiographic risk predictors. *EF,* ejection fraction; see Figure 9-2 for other definitions. Chi-square tests for homogeneity results were non-significant.

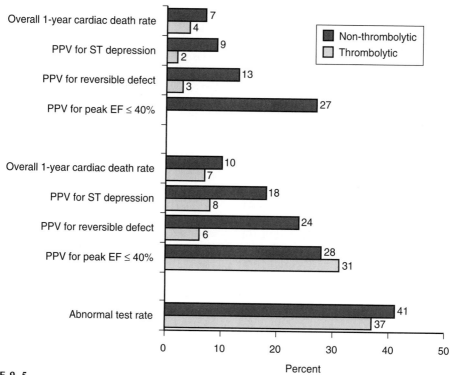

FIGURE 9-5

Positive predictive values (PPV) of noninvasive tests in non-thrombolytic and thrombolytic-treated patients. The PPVs for cardiac death or MI are illustrated for patients who had ST-segment depression, a reversible perfusion defect, or a peak exercise ejection fraction ≤40%. PPVs were usually decreased in patients receiving thrombolytic therapy. For example, the PPV for cardiac death or MI in patients who had a reversible perfusion defect was 24% in the non–thrombolytic-treated versus 6% in thrombolytic-treated patients. *EF*, ejection fraction; *MI*, myocardial infarction.

abnormal scan. Risk stratification with pharmacologic stress perfusion imaging resulted in equally high event rates in patients with normal and abnormal test results. The size and extent of the perfusion defect and the number of abnormal ECG leads may be better predictors of 1-year outcome, but this information was not available.

Risk increases with LV dysfunction and is largely determined by the degree of myocardial damage/dysfunction secondary to the MI. The increase in risk of death was greater than 4 times higher in patients with exertional LV dysfunction (approximately 30% of patients) and for patients with a peak EF less than 40%, the positive predictive value for cardiac death was 27%.

For patients who underwent treadmill or bicycle exercise with no additional imaging agents, evidence of an impaired SBP or exercise response was more prognostic of death than ischemic markers of risk (ST depression and angina), even in thrombolytic trials. The risk of cardiac death was four times higher in patients who had exertional

hypotension or who could not complete the exercise test. This is not surprising given that these markers are due to both LV dysfunction and ischemia.

Effect of Low Prevalence (e.g., "The Reperfusion Era"). The positive predictive values of noninvasive risk markers for cardiac death and combined cardiac death or nonfatal MI are low in studies with low mortality rates. The therapy clinicians apply, as a result of an abnormal predischarge test, should subsequently lower a patient's post-test likelihood for events. A significant proportion of acute MI survivors have single-vessel disease and, even with an abnormal test for ischemia, have a good prognosis making prediction difficult. This can be seen in cohorts where sensitivity is high but specificity is low. An example of lower positive predictive values in lower-risk groups was observed in reports of patients treated with thrombolytics. Predischarge testing after reperfusion therapy may have a limited predictive value for several reasons.

Successful reperfusion results in less myocardial damage and may leave patients with nonsignificant angiographic lesions and a negative stress test who still have an increased likelihood of reinfarction. Additionally, patients who receive thrombolytic agents have a generally lower risk than other patients with history of MI because they are younger and less likely to have complicating illnesses.

Choice of Predischarge Stress Test

Although sensitivity and specificity values are not affected by disease prevalence, the predictive value of the test is. Adjusting the risk by the threefold higher baseline risk for patients included in the exercise radionuclide angiography studies lessens the predictive accuracy of ventricular function abnormalities. Thus, if underlying risk was equal, all abnormal noninvasive risk markers would be equally ineffective at predicting adverse outcome, although the predictive estimates would not decrease linearly with the underlying risk in the population. Although adjusted values allow comparisons among the various modalities, these differences in baseline risk and subsequent post-test predictive estimates may be used to guide appropriate referral to predischarge testing. Lower-risk patients should be referred to exercise ECG whereas higher-risk patients should be considered for a radionuclide angiogram. Using this rule, low-risk patients with an uncomplicated MI who exercise beyond 5 METs without ECG or hemodynamic abnormalities are at low risk of a recurrent cardiac event during the ensuing year. This reassurance to the patient and family as well as the minimal cost of this test may be the overriding reasons for performing this test during the predischarge phase. However, the role of myocardial perfusion imaging is unclear because of its poor specificity, similar predictive values to those of exercise ECG, and fivefold higher cost. Perfusion imaging may have a role in patients subsets for whom the ECG or exercise capacity may not be accurately interpreted as well as for those whose risk of recurrent MI may be high (i.e., non-Q-wave MI).

When assessing the literature on the prognostic value of noninvasive tests, several methodological considerations of note were encountered. Marx and Feinstein[85] published an extensive review of the literature on prognosis following an MI. Their results show that prognostic studies in this setting frequently have methodological limitations and explain the variation in predictive ability. Among the 54 reports, few were prospective series; more often, they were highly select and had various lengths of follow-up with small samples. Thus, the variation in predictive accuracy of noninvasive measures could, in part, reflect the primarily observational nature of these reports. Further, many of the studies contained few outcome events. Early in the development of new imaging agents or techniques, small patient series may be more likely to be published because of excitement about the possible impact of this new modality. Substantial concern exists when negative trials remain unpublished.[86] This problem of publication bias has been shown to lead to significant overestimation of treatment effect.

There are certain patient subsets for whom the sensitivity and specificity of noninvasive measures may be affected (e.g., those receiving beta-blockers or those with pulmonary disease, resting ST–T-wave changes, obesity, inability to exercise, or submaximal stress). There is a potential for an increased accuracy of exercise-induced ST depression in patients with non-Q-wave MI that must be confirmed.[87] For the predischarge noninvasive test to improve upon initial pretest risk estimates, the statistical and clinical incremental value of noninvasive measures must be established. The positive predictive value of clinical history and ECG measures in predicting preserved LV function has been reported as 94%,[88] which could obviate the need for echocardiography or radionuclide imaging to estimate systolic function in otherwise low-risk patients.

The DUKE researchers observed little improvement in the quality of the data compared to our similar meta-analysis published 10 years earlier.[89] The impact of methodological limitations on subsequent predictive accuracy is difficult to quantify but should prompt more rigorous, well-controlled studies in the future to elucidate the relative impact of these tests on patient outcome. Although quality-assessment tools have been devised for use with randomized trial data, these are not applicable to retrospective data.[90] Given all of the limitations, this scholarly meta-analysis provides the best synopsis of the knowledge regarding noninvasive stress testing for risk stratification post MI.

THE REPERFUSION ERA

Contemporary management of the patient with acute MI includes one or more of the following: medical therapy, thrombolytic agents, and coronary revascularization. The first striking improvement in survival in all subsets is with beta-blockers

(25% reduction in the first year post MI). The next dramatic change in treatment of patients with acute MI was the broad use of thrombolytic therapy beginning in 1988. Equally important has been the widespread use of aspirin, beta-adrenergic-blocking agents, vasodilator therapy, common use of angiotensin converting enzyme inhibitors, and a far more aggressive use of revascularization therapy in patients who have clinical markers of a poor prognosis. It is this constellation of new therapy, and not solely the administration of thrombolytic therapy, that marks what is generally called *reperfusion era*. This period has witnessed an impressive reduction in early and 1-year mortality rates for patients with acute MI, which is particularly striking in patients who have received thrombolytic therapy and revascularization during hospitalization. The '90s brought the widespread application of cardiac catheterization negating the use of the exercise test to select patients for this procedure, as had been the situation earlier. Currently, the evidence supports the use of angiography when possible instead of thrombolysis and even "facilitated" PCI, where thrombolysis is only used to hold the patient until angiography is possible. In any circumstance, once the coronary arteries are visualized it is hard for the angiographer not to open closed arteries with drug-eluting stents. CABS only remains for patients with difficult lesions. Most patients recover from their MI with minimal loss of myocardium and reperfused myocardium as well. Thus, the exercise test plays a different role than it did in the past.

Shorter hospital stays, widespread use of thrombolytic agents, greater uses of revascularization strategies, implantable cardiac defibrillators, and increased use of beta-adrenergic-blocking agents and angiotensin converting enzyme inhibitors or angiogenesis receptor blockers continue to change the clinical presentation of the patient with history of MI. Not all patients have received each of these various therapies; hence, survivors of MI are quite heterogeneous. The CAMI study reported that among 3178 consecutive patients with acute MI, 45% received thrombolytic agents, 20% underwent PCI, and 8% had CABS.[91] Medications at the time of hospital discharge included beta-blockers in 61%, angiotensin converting enzyme inhibitors in 24%, and aspirin in 86%.

Although exercise testing was helpful in the management of patients with a history of MI in the prethrombolytic era, the impact over the past decade of thrombolytic therapies could have decreased the value of exercise testing.[92] The GISSI-2 database has enabled reevaluation of the prognostic role of exercise testing in patients who have received thrombolysis.[93] Exercise tests were performed on 6296 patients at an average of 28 days after randomization for thrombolysis post MI. The test was not performed on 3923 patients (40%) because of contraindications. The test was positive for ischemia in 26% of the patients, negative in 38%, and nondiagnostic in 36%. Among the patients with an ischemic test result, 33% had symptoms, whereas 67% had silent myocardial ischemia. The mortality rate was 7.1% among patients who did not have an exercise test and 1.7% for those with an ischemic test, 0.9% for those who had a normal test, and 1.3% for those with nondiagnostic tests. In an adjusted analysis, symptomatic-induced ischemia, ischemia at a submaximal work load, low work capacity, and abnormal SBP were independent predictors of 6-month mortality (relative risks of 2× for each). However, when these variables were considered simultaneously, only symptomatic-induced ischemia and low work capacity were confirmed as independent predictors of mortality (Cox hazard ratio of 2 and 1.8, respectively). The GISSI investigators concluded that patients with a normal exercise response have an excellent medium-term prognosis and do not need further investigation as shown by others.[94] However, evaluation must be directed to the patients who cannot undergo exercise testing because the mortality was five to seven times greater in that group. The GISSI-2 researchers[95] calculated the Duke treadmill score (DTS) and the Veterans Affairs Medical Center Score (VAMCS) for each patient and used coefficients of a multivariate analysis to develop a simple predictive scoring system. Six-month mortality rates in the subgroups of each scoring system were as follows: DTS: low risk 0.6%, moderate risk 1.8%, high risk 3.4%; VAMCS: low risk 0.6%, moderate risk 2%, high risk 5%; GISSI-2 Index: low risk 0.5%, moderate risk 2%, high risk 6%. The results of multivariate analysis were as follows: DTS: moderate risk 2.5×, high risk 5×; VAMCS: moderate risk 3×, high risk 6×; GISSI-2 Index: moderate risk 3×, high risk 9×.

The prognosis among survivors of MI continues to improve as newer treatment strategies are applied. The 1-year postdischarge mortality in the CAMI study was 8.4% and was distinctly lower in the 45% of patients who received thrombolytic therapy (4% mortality) and in the 28% who underwent coronary angioplasty (3% mortality) or CABS (3.7% mortality).[96] Data from the GUSTO trial[97] demonstrate that 57% of the 41,021 patients who received thrombolytic therapy were uncomplicated (no recurrent ischemia, reinfarction, heart failure, stroke, or invasive procedures) at 4 days after MI. The mortality rate at 1 month was 1% and at 1 year was 3.6%. Recurrent ischemia occurred in 7% of this group. These and other data from large thrombolytic trials[98,99] demonstrate that those patients unable to perform an exercise test have the highest adverse cardiac event rate, whereas uncomplicated stable patients have a low cardiac event rate even before undergoing further risk assessment by exercise testing.

The two meta-analyses summarized earlier of 30 studies, including more than 20,000 patients, found that exercise incapacity and abnormal SBP response were more predictive of adverse cardiac events after MI than measures of exercise-induced ischemia. Although most of the studies included were performed before the reperfusion era, similar results were found in the GISSI report that considered 6000 patients who received thrombolysis.

ACTIVITY COUNSELING

Exercise testing after MI is useful in counseling patients and their families regarding domestic, recreational, and occupational activities that can be safely performed after hospital discharge. Exercise capacity in METs derived from the exercise test can be applied to estimate an individual's tolerance for specific activities. Published charts that estimate energy requirements of various activities are available[100] but should be used only as a guide, realizing that the intensity at which activities performed directly influence the amount of energy required. Most domestic chores and activities require less than 5 METs, hence a submaximal test at the time of hospital discharge can be useful in counseling with regard to the first several weeks after an MI.

The follow-up symptom-limited testing performed at 3 to 6 weeks after MI can assist in further activity prescription and issues regarding return to work. Most occupational activities require less than 5 METs. In the 15% of individuals in the work force whose work involves heavy manual labor,[101] the exercise test data should not be used as the sole criterion for recommendations regarding return to work. Energy demands of lifting heavy objects, temperature, environmental, and psychological stresses are not assessed by routine exercise tests and must be taken into consideration. In patients with low exercise capacity, LV dysfunction, exercise-induced ischemia, and in those who are otherwise apprehensive about returning to a physically

demanding occupation, simulated work tests can be performed.[102,103]

Exercise testing in cardiac rehabilitation is essential in the development of the exercise prescription to establish a safe and effective training intensity, in risk stratification of patients to determine the level of supervision and monitoring required during exercise training sessions, and in evaluation of training program outcome.[104] For these reasons, symptom-limited exercise testing before program initiation is needed for all patients in whom cardiac rehabilitation is recommended (recent MI, recent CABS, recent coronary angioplasty, chronic stable angina, and controlled heart failure).[105] Although there are no available studies to assess its value, it is the consensus of this committee based on practical experience that exercise testing in the stable cardiac patient who continues an exercise training program be performed after the initial 8 to 12 weeks of exercise training and at least yearly thereafter, or sooner as needed depending on changes in symptoms or medications that may affect the exercise prescription. Such testing may be useful to rewrite the exercise prescription, evaluate improvement in exercise capacity, and provide feedback to the patient.

SUMMARY

The benefits of performing an exercise test in patients with history of MI are listed in Table 9-9. Submitting patients to exercise testing can expedite and optimize their discharge from the hospital.

TABLE 9–9. Benefits of exercise testing post myocardial infarction

PREDISCHARGE SUBMAXIMAL TEST
Setting safe exercise levels (exercise prescription)
Optimizing discharge
Altering medical therapy
Triaging for intensity of follow-up
First step in rehabilitation—assurance, encouragement
Reassuring spouse
Recognizing exercise-induced ischemia and dysrhythmias

MAXIMAL TEST FOR RETURN TO NORMAL ACTIVITIES
Determining limitations
Prognostication
Reassuring employers
Determining level of disability
Triaging for invasive studies
Deciding upon medications
Exercise prescription
Continued rehabilitation

The patients response to exercise, their work capacity, and limiting factors at the time of discharge can be assessed by the exercise test. An exercise test before discharge is important for giving patient guidelines for exercise at home, reassuring them of their physical status, and determining the risk of complications. It provides a safe basis for advising the patient to resume or increase his or her activity level and return to work. The test can demonstrate to the patient, relatives, or employer the effect of the MI on the capacity for physical performance. Psychologically, it can cause an improvement in the patient's self-confidence by making the patient less anxious about daily physical activities. The test has been helpful in reassuring spouses of patients who had an MI of their physical capabilities. The psychological impact of performing well on the exercise test is impressive. Many patients increase their activity and actually rehabilitate themselves after being encouraged and reassured by their response to this test.

Exercise testing is useful in activity counseling after hospital discharge. It is also an important tool in exercise training as part of comprehensive cardiac rehabilitation, where it can be used to develop and modify the exercise prescription, assist in providing activity counseling, and assess the patient's response into, and progress in, the exercise training program.

One consistent finding in the review of the exercise test studies following an MI that included a follow-up for cardiac endpoints is that patients who met whatever criteria set forth for exercise testing were at lower risk than patients not tested. This finding supports the clinical judgment of the skilled clinician. In the complete data set from the review, only an abnormal SBP response or a low exercise capacity was significantly associated with a poor outcome. These responses are so powerful because they can be associated with either ischemic events or CHF events (see Chapter 8, Prognostic Applications of Exercise Testing).

The DUKE meta-analysis compared the available noninvasive tests results to outcomes in patients recovering from acute-MI. Studies published from 1980 to 1995 had to fulfill these criteria: only MI patients, most patients enrolled after 1980, tested within 6 weeks of MI, follow-up rates greater than 80%, and having outcome prevalence rates for test results, and only the latest results if there were multiple reports from the same institution. Sensitivity, specificity, and predictive values were calculated for test results for 1-year outcomes (cardiac death, cardiac death, or reinfarction). Univariable and summary OR were calculated for

test results. The qualifying reports ($n = 54$) included 19,874 patients and three quarters were retrospective (76%) and a third were small samples with less than five deaths. One-year mortality in the studies ranged from 2.5% for pharmacologic stress echocardiography to 9.3% for exercise radionuclide angiography studies, consistent with population differences. Positive predictive values (the percentage of those with an abnormal test that have the outcome during follow-up) for most noninvasive risk markers were less than 10% for cardiac death and less than 20% for death or reinfarction. ECG, symptomatic, and scintigraphic markers of ischemia (ST-segment depression, angina, and a reversible defect) were less sensitive (average about 44%) for identifying morbid and fatal outcomes than markers of both LV dysfunction and ischemia (exercise duration, exertional hypotension, and peak LVEF). The positive predictive value of predischarge noninvasive testing is low. Markers of LV dysfunction or both dysfunction and ischemia were better predictors than markers of myocardial ischemia alone.

The two meta-analyses summarized of 30 studies, including more than 20,000 patients, found that exercise incapacity and abnormal SBP response were more predictive of adverse cardiac events after MI than measures of exercise-induced ischemia. Although most of the studies included were performed before the reperfusion era, similar results were found in the GISSI report that considered 6000 patients who received thrombolysis.

The evaluation of the patient with an MI has dramatically changed with the issue of who needs cardiac catheterization being resolved: cardiac catheterization is the preferred treatment before and possibly after thrombolysis (facilitated PCI). Patients with LV dysfunction post MI can expect a 30% reduction in mortality with an implantable defibrillator. The clinical value of exercise testing post MI most likely will be resolved by studies like the ROSETTA[106] and PERISCOP[107] study which have evaluated the value of functional testing after interventions. However, the exercise test remains helpful to estimate prognosis in the post-MI patient.

REFERENCES

1. Hunink MG, Goldman L, Tosteson AN, et al: The recent decline in mortality from coronary heart disease, 1980-1990. The effect of secular trends in risk factors and treatment. JAMA 1997;277: 535-542.
2. Braunwald E, Antman EM, Beasley JW, et al: Committee on the Management of Patients With Unstable Angina. ACC/AHA 2002

guideline update for the management of patients with unstable angina and non-ST-segment elevation myocardial infarction—summary article: A report of the American College of Cardiology/American Heart Association task force on practice guidelines (Committee on the Management of Patients With Unstable Angina). J Am Coll Cardiol 2002;40:1366-1374.

3. Dargie H. Myocardial infarction: Redefined or reinvented? Heart 2002;88:1-3.

4. Dalby M, Bouzamondo A, Lechat P, Montalescot G: Transfer for primary angioplasty versus immediate thrombolysis in acute myocardial infarction: A meta-analysis. Circulation 2003;108:1809-1814. Epub 2003 Oct 6.

5. Arciero TJ, Jacobsen SJ, Reeder GS, et al: Temporal trends in the incidence of coronary disease. Am J Med 2004;117:228-233.

6. Goldman L, Phillips KA, Coxson P, et al: The effect of risk factor reductions between 1981 and 1990 on coronary heart disease incidence, prevalence, mortality and cost. J Am Coll Cardiol 2001;38:1012-1017.

7. Guidelines for risk stratification after myocardial infarction. American College of Physicians. Ann Intern Med 1997;126:556-560.

8. Cucherat M, Bonnefoy E, Tremeau G: Primary angioplasty versus intravenous thrombolysis for acute myocardial infarction. Cochrane Database Syst Rev 2003(3):CD001560.

9. Heggunje PS, Harjai KJ, Stone GW, et al: Procedural success versus clinical risk status in determining discharge of patients after primary angioplasty for acute myocardial infarction. J Am Coll Cardiol 2004;44:1400-1407.

10. Gibbons RJ, Balady GJ, Beasley JW, et al: ACC/AHA Guidelines for Exercise Testing. A report of the American College of Cardiology/American Heart Association Task Force on Practice Guidelines (Committee on Exercise Testing). J Am Coll Cardiol 1997;30:260-311.

11. Antman EM, Anbe DT, Armstrong PW, et al: ACC/AHA guidelines for the management of patients with ST-elevation myocardial infarction—executive summary. A report of the American College of Cardiology/American Heart Association Task Force on Practice Guidelines (Writing Committee to revise the 1999 guidelines for the management of patients with acute myocardial infarction). J Am Coll Cardiol 2004;44:671-719.

12. Juneau M, Colle SP, Theroux P, et al: Symptom-limited versus low level exercise testing before hospital discharge after myocardial infarction. J Am Coll Cardiol 1992;20:927-933.

13. Hamm LF, Crow RS, Stull A, Hannan P: Safety and characteristics of exercise testing early after myocardial infarction. Am J Cardiol 1989;63:1193-1197.

14. Jain A, Myers GH, Sapin PM, O'Rourke RA: Comparison of symptom-limited and low level exercise tolerance tests early after myocardial infarction. J Am Coll Cardiol 1993;22:1816-1820.

15. Jespersen CM, Hagerup L, Hollander N, et al: Exercise-provoked ST segment depression and prognosis in patients recovering from acute myocardial infarction. Significance and pitfalls. J Intern Med 1993;233:27-32.

16. Torkelson LO: Rehabilitation of the patient with acute myocardial infarction. J Chronic Dis 1964;17:685-704.

17. Ibsen H, Kjoller E, Styperek J, Pedersen A: Routine exercise ECG three weeks after acute myocardial infarction. Acta Med Scand 1975;198:463-469.

18. Niederberger M: Values and limitations of exercise testing after myocardial infarction (monograph). Wien, Verlag Bruder Hollinek, 1977; pp 3-45.

19. Markiewicz W, Houston N, DeBusk RF: Exercise testing soon after myocardial infarction. Circulation 1977;56:26-31.

20. Sivarajan ES, Bruce RA, Lindskog BD, et al: Treadmill test responses to an early exercise program after myocardial infarction: A randomized study. Circulation 1982;65:1420-1428.

21. Taylor CB, Bandura A, Ewart CK, et al: Exercise testing to enhance wives' confidence in their husbands' cardiac capability soon after clinically uncomplicated acute myocardial infarction. Am J Cardiol 1985;55:635-638.

22. Ewart CK, Taylor CB, Reese LB, DeBusk RF: Effects of early post-myocardial infarction exercise testing on self-perception and subsequent physical activity. Am J Cardiol 1983;51:1076-1080.

23. Handler CE, Sowton E: A comparison of the Naughton and modified Bruce treadmill exercise protocols in their ability to detect ischaemic abnormalities six weeks after myocardial infarction. Eur Heart J 1984;5:752-755.

24. Starling MR, Crawford MH, O'Rourke RA: Superiority of selected treadmill exercise protocols predischarge and six weeks postinfarction for detecting ischemic abnormalities. Am Heart J 1982;104:1054-1059.

25. Starling MR, Crawford MH, Kennedy GT, O'Rourke RA: Exercise testing early after myocardial infarction: Predictive value of subsequent unstable angina and death. Am J Cardiol 1980;46:909-914.

26. Handler CE, Sowton E: Diurnal variation in symptom-limited exercise test responses six weeks after myocardial infarction. Eur Heart J 1985;6:444-450.

27. Starling MR, Crawford MH, Kennedy GT, O'Rourke RA: Treadmill exercise tests predischarge and six weeks post-myocardial infarction to detect abnormalities of known prognostic value. Ann Intern Med 1981;94:721-727.

28. Wohl AJ, Lewis HR, Campbell W, et al: Cardiovascular function during early recovery from acute myocardial infarction. Circulation 1977;56:931-937.

29. Haskell WL, Savin W, Oldridge N, DeBusk R: Factors influencing estimated oxygen uptake during exercise testing soon after myocardial infarction. Am J Cardiol 1982;50:299-304.

30. Castellanet MJ, Greenberg PS, Ellestad MH: Comparison of S-T segment changes on exercise testing with angiographic findings in patients with prior myocardial infarction. Am J Cardiol 1978;42:29-35.

31. Ahnve S, Savvides M, Abouantoun S, et al: Can ischemia be recognized when Q waves are present on the resting electrocardiogram? Am Heart J 1986;110:1016-1020.

32. Miranda C, Herbert W, Dubach P, et al: Post MI exercise testing: Non Q wave vs Q wave. Circulation 1991;84:2357-2365.

33. Weiner DA: Prognostic value of exercise testing early after myocardial infarction. J Cardiac Rehabil 1983;3:114-122.

34. Paine TD, Dye LE, Roitman DI, et al: Relation of graded exercise test findings after myocardial infarction to extent of coronary artery disease and left ventricular dysfunction. Am J Cardiol 1978;42:716-723.

35. Dillahunt PH, Miller AB: Early treadmill testing after myocardial infarction. Chest 1979;76:150-155.

36. Sammel NL, Wilson RL, Norris RM, et al: Angiocardiography and exercise testing at one month after a first myocardial infarction. Aust NZ J Med 1980;10:182-187.

37. Fuller CM, Raizner AE, Verani MS, et al: Early post-myocardial infarction treadmill stress testing. An accurate predictor of multivessel coronary disease and subsequent cardiac events. Ann Intern Med 1981;94:734-739.

38. Boschat J, Rigaud M, Bardet J, et al: Treadmill exercise testing and coronary cineangiography following first myocardial infarction. J Cardiac Rehab 1981;1:206-211.

39. Schwartz KM, Turner JD, Sheffield LT, et al: Limited exercise testing soon after myocardial infarction. Correlation with early coronary and left ventricular angiography. Ann Intern Med 1981;94:727-734.

40. Starling MR, Crawford MH, Richards KL, O'Rourke RA: Predictive value of early postmyocardial infarction modified treadmill exercise testing in multivessel coronary artery disease detection. Am Heart J 1981;102:169-175.

41. De Feyter PJ, van den Brand M, Serruys PW, Wijns W: Early angiography after myocardial infarction: What have we learned? Am Heart J 1985;109:194-199.

42. Ericsson M, Granath A, Ohlsen P, et al: Arrhythmias and symptoms during treadmill testing three weeks after myocardial infarction in 100 patients. Br Heart J 1973;35:787-790.

43. Kentala E: Physical fitness and feasibility of physical rehabilitation after myocardial infarction in men of working age. Ann Clin Res 1972;4(suppl9):1-84.

44. Granath A, Sodermark T, Winge T, et al: Early work load tests for evaluation of long-term prognosis of acute myocardial infarction. Br Heart J 1977;39:758-763.

45. Smith JW, Dennis CA, Gassmann A, et al: Exercise testing three weeks after myocardial infarction. Chest 1979;75:12-16.

46. Hunt D, Hamer A, Duffield A, et al: Predictors of reinfarction and sudden death in a high-risk group of acute myocardial infarction survivors. Lancet 1979;1:233-236.

47. Srinivasan M, Young A, Baker G, et al: The value of postcardiac infarction exercise stress testing. Identification of a group at high risk. Med J Aust 1981;2:466-467.

48. Jelinek VM, Ziffer RW, McDonald IG, et al: Early exercise testing and mobilization after myocardial infarction. Med J Aust 1977;2:589-593.

49. Sami M, Kraemer H, DeBusk RF: The prognostic significance of serial exercise testing after myocardial infarction. Circulation 1979;60:1238-1246.

50. Davidson DM, DeBusk RF: Prognostic value of a single exercise test 3 weeks after uncomplicated myocardial infarction. Circulation 1980;61:236-241.

51. DeBusk RF, Dennis CA: "Submaximal" predischarge exercise testing after acute myocardial infarction: Who needs it? Am J Cardiol 1985;55:499-500.

52. Theroux P, Marpole DGF, Bourassa MG: Exercise stress testing in the post-myocardial infarction patient. Am J Cardiol 1983;52: 664-667.

53. Waters DA, Bosch X, Bouchard A, et al: Comparison of clinical variables and variables derived from a limited predischarge exercise test as predictors of early and late mortality after myocardial infarction. J Am Coll Cardiol 1985;5:1-8.

54. Koppes GM, Kruyer W, Beckmann CH, Jones FG: Response to exercise early after uncomplicated acute myocardial infarction in patients receiving no medication: Long-term follow-up. Am J Cardiol 1980;46:764-769.

55. Starling MR, Kennedy GT, Crawford MH, O'Rourke RA: Comparative predictive value of ST-segment depression or angina during early and repeat postinfarction exercise tests. Chest 1984;86:845-849.

56. Saunamaki KI, Andersen JD: Early exercise test in the assessment of long-term prognosis after acute myocardial infarction. Acta Med Scand 1981;209:185-191.

57. Saunamaki KI, Andersen JD: Early exercise test vs clinical variables in the long-term prognostic management after myocardial infarction. Acta Med Scand 1982;212:47-52.

58. Madsen EB, Gilpin E: Prognostic value of exercise test variables after myocardial infarction. J Cardiac Rehabil 1983;3:481-488.

59. Jespersen CM, Kassis E, Edeling CJ, Madsen JK: The prognostic value of maximal exercise testing soon after first MI. Eur Heart J 1985;6:769-772.

60. Velasco J, Tormo V, Ferrer LM, et al: Early exercise test for evaluation of long-term prognosis after uncomplicated myocardial infarction. Eur Heart J 1981;2:401-407.

61. Weld FM: Exercise testing after myocardial infarction. J Cardiac Rehabil 1985;5:20-27.

62. Fioretti P, Deckers JW, Brower RW, et al: Predischarge stress test after myocardial infarction in the old age: Results and prognostic value. Eur Heart J 1984;5:101-104.

63. Norris RM, Barnaby PF, Brandt PWT, et al: Prognosis after recovery from first acute myocardial infarction: Determinants of reinfarction and sudden death. Am J Cardiol 1984;53:408-413.

64. Jennings K, Reid DS, Hawkins T, Julian DJ: Role of exercise testing early after myocardial infarction in identifying candidates for coronary surgery. Br Med J 1984;288:185-187.

65. Handler CE: Exercise testing to identify high risk patients after myocardial infarction. J R Coll Physicians Lond 1984;18: 124-127.

66. Krone RJ, Gillespie JA, Weld FM, et al: Low-level exercise testing after myocardial infarction: Usefulness in enhancing clinical risk stratification. Circulation 1985;71:80-89.

67. Dwyer EM, McMaster P, Greenberg H: Nonfatal cardiac events and recurrent infarction in the year after acute myocardial infarction. J Am Coll Cardiol 1984;4:695-702.

68. Williams WL, Nair RC, Higginson LA, et al: Comparison of clinical and treadmill variables for the prediction of outcome after myocardial infarction. J Am Coll Cardiol 1984;4:477-486.

69. Madsen EB, Gilpin E. How much prognostic information do exercise test data add to clinical data after acute myocardial infarction. Int J Cardiol 1983;4:15-27.

70. Sullivan ID, Davies DW, Sowton E: Submaximal exercise testing early after myocardial infarction: Difficulty of predicting coronary anatomy and left ventricular performance. Br Heart J 1985;53: 180-185.

71. Connolly DC, Elveback LR: Coronary heart disease in residents of Rochester, Minnesota. VI. Hospital and posthospital course of patients with transmural and subendocardial myocardial infarction. Mayo Clin Proc 1985;60:375-381.

72. Klein J, Froelicher V, Detrano R, et al: Does the resting electrocardiogram after myocardial infarction determine the predictive value of exercise-induced ST depression? A two year follow-up in a veteran population. J Am Coll Cardiol, 1989;14:305-311.

73. Krone R, Dwyer E, Greenberg H, et al: Risk stratification in patients with first non-Q wave infarction: Limited value of the early low level exercise test after uncomplicated infarcts. J Am Coll Cardiol 1989;14;31-37.

74. Ades PA, Thomas JD, Hanson JS, et al: Effect of metoprolol on the submaximal stress test performed early after acute myocardial infarction. Am J Cardiol 1987;60:963-966.

75. Curtis Jl, Houghton JL, Patterson JH, et al: Propranolol therapy alters estimation of potential cardiovascular risk derived from submaximal postinfarction exercise testing. Am Heart J 1991;121: 1655-1664.

76. Krone RJ, Miller JP, Gillespie JA, et al: Usefulness of low level exercise testing early after acute myocardial infarction in patients taking beta blocking agents. Am J Cardiol 1987;60:23-27.

77. Ronnevik PK, VonderLippe G: Prognostic importance of predischarge exercise capacity for long term mortality and nonfatal myocardial infarction in patients admitted for suspected acute myocardial infarction and treated with Metoprolol. Eur Heart J 1992;13: 1468-1472.

78. Murray DP, Tan LB, Salih M, et al: Does beta adrenergic blockade influence the prognostic implications of post-myocardial infarction exercise testing? Br Heart J 1988;60:474-479.

79. Madsen EB, Gilpin E, Henning H: Short-term prognosis in acute myocardial infarction: Evaluation of different prediction methods. Am Heart J 1984;107:1241-1251.

80. Gilpin E, Olshen R, Henning H, Ross J: Risk prediction after myocardial infarction. Comparison of three multivariate methodologies. Cardiology 1983;70:73-84.

81. Dominguez H, Torp-Pedersen C, Koeber L, Rask-Madsen C: Prognostic value of exercise testing in a cohort of patients followed for 15 years after acute myocardial infarction. Eur Heart J. 2001;22: 300-306.

82. Awad-Elkarim AA, Bagger JP, Albers CJ, et al: A prospective study of long term prognosis in young myocardial infarction survivors: The prognostic value of angiography and exercise testing. Heart 2003;89:843-847.

83. Shaw LJ, Peterson ED, Kesler K, et al: A meta-analysis of predischarge risk stratification after acute myocardial infarction with stress electrocardiographic, myocardial perfusion, and ventricular function imaging. Am J Cardiol 1996;78:1327-1337.

84. Baker DW, Jones R, Hodges J, et al: Management of heart failure. III. The role of revascularization in the treatment of patients with moderate or severe left ventricular systolic dysfunction. JAMA 1994;272:1528-1534.

85. Eddy DM, Hasselblad C, Shachter R: An introduction to a Bayesian method for meta-analysis: The confidence profile method. Med Decis Making 1990;10:15-23.

86. Marx BE, Feinstein AR: Methodologic sources of inconsistent prognoses for post-acute myocardial infarction. Am J Med 1995;98:537-550.

87. Simes RJ: Confronting publication bias: a cohort design for meta-analysis. Stat Med 1987;6:11-29.

88. Silver MT, Rose GA, Paul SD, et al: A clinical rule to predict preserved left ventricular ejection fraction in patients after myocardial infarction. Ann Intern Med 1994;121:750-756.

89. Froelicher VF, Perdue S, Pewen W, Risch M: Application of meta-analysis using an electronic spreadsheet to exercise testing in patients with myocardial infarction. Am J Med 1987;83:1045-1054.

90. Chalmers TC: Problems induced by meta-analyses. Stat Med 1991; 10:971-979.

91. Rouleau JL, Talajic M, Sussex B, et al: Myocardial infarction patients in the 1990's - Their risk factors, stratification and survival in Canada: The Canadian Assessment of Myocardial Infarction (CAMI) study. J Am Coll Cardiol 1996;27:1119-1127.

92. Stevenson R, Muachandran V, Ranjadayalan K, et al: Reassessment of treadmill stress testing for risk stratification in patients with acute myocardial infarction treated by thrombolysis. Br Heart J 1993;70:415-420.

93. Villella A, Maggioni AP, Villella M, et al: Prognostic significance of maximal exercise testing after myocardial infarction treated with thrombolytic agents: The GISSI-2 data-base. Lancet 1995 Aug 26;346(8974):523-529.

94. Piccalo G, Pirelli S, Massa D, et al: Value of negative predischarge exercise testing in identifying patients at low risk after acute myocardial infarction treated by systemic thrombolysis. Am J Cardiol 1992;70:31-33.

95. Villella M, Villella A, Santoro L, et al: Ergometric score systems after myocardial infarction: Prognostic performance of the DUKE Treadmill Score, Veterans Administration Medical Center Score, and of a novel score system, GISSI-2 Index, in a cohort of survivors of acute myocardial infarction. Am Heart J. 2003 Mar; 145:475-483.

96. Newby LK, Califf RM, Guerci A, et al: Early discharge in the thrombolytic era: an analysis of criteria for uncomplicated infarctions from the GUSTO trial. J Am Coll Cardiol 1996;27:625-632.

97. Chaitman BR, McMahon RP, Tarrin M, et al: Impact of treatment strategy on predischarge exercise tests in the Thrombolysis in Myocardial Infarction (TIMI) II trial. Am J Cardiol 1993;71:131-138.

98. Volpi A, DeVita C, Franzosi MG, et al: Predictors of nonfatal reinfarction in survivals of myocardial infarction after thrombolysis. Results of the GISSI-2 database. J Am Coll Cardiol 1994;24:608-615.

99. Fletcher GF, Balady GJ, Froelicher VF, et al: American Heart Association Exercise Standards. Circulation 1995;91:580-615.

100. U.S. Department of Health and Human Services. Clinical practice guideline #17: Cardiac rehabilitation. AHCPR Publication No. 96-0672. 1995.

101. Wilke NA, Sheldahl LM, Dougherty SM, et al: Baltimore Therapeutic Equipment work simulator: Energy expenditure of work activities in cardiac patients. Arch Phys Med Rehabil 1993;74:419-424.

102. Sheldahl LM, Wilke NA, Tristani FE: Exercise prescription for return to work. J Cardiopulm Rehabil 1985;5:567-575.

103. Balady GJ, Fletcher BJ, Froelicher ES, et al: American Heart Association Scientific Statement Cardiac Rehabilitation Programs. Circulation 1994;90:1602-1610.

104. American College of Sports Medicine. Guidelines for exercise testing and prescription. Philadelphia, Williams & Wilkins, 1995.

105. Mak KH, Eisenberg MJ, Tsang J, et al: Clinical impact of functional testing strategy among stented and non-stented patients: Insights from the ROSETTA Registry. Int J Cardiol 2004;95: 321-327.

106. Sellier P, Chatellier G, D'Agrosa-Boiteux MC, et al: Use of non-invasive cardiac investigations to predict clinical endpoints after coronary bypass graft surgery in coronary artery disease patients: Results from the prognosis and evaluation of risk in the coronary operated patient (PERISCOP) study. Eur Heart J 2003;24:916-926.

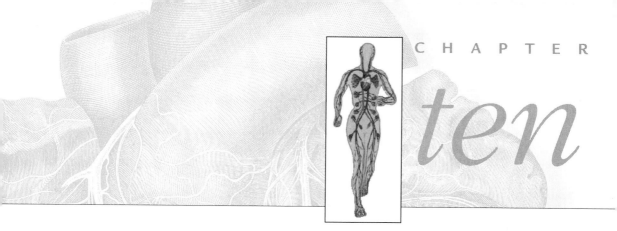

Exercise Testing in Patients with Heart Failure and Left Ventricular Dysfunction

PATHOPHYSIOLOGY

Myocardial damage or dysfunction is the pathophysiologic basis of heart muscle disease. Myocardial damage or dysfunction can be divided into systolic and diastolic dysfunction. Systolic function relates to the emptying characteristics of the left ventricle, and diastolic function relates to its filling properties. Systolic dysfunction due to myocardial damage is most common in clinical practice and usually leads to left ventricular dilation. The ventricle dilates as a compensatory mechanism to take advantage of the Frank-Starling relationship (i.e., increased contractility with stretching of the sarcomeres), which can eventually worsen ventricular performance over time. Anything that causes ventricular damage or scarring (e.g., muscle loss) usually leads to systolic dysfunction.

Approximately 70% of patients with the syndrome of chronic heart failure (HF) have systolic dysfunction, while the remainder has diastolic dysfunction. In patients with the latter, systolic function and ejection fraction (EF) can be normal, but filling pressure is usually elevated due to a stiff, noncompliant ventricle.[1] Usually, diastolic dysfunction is secondary to hypertension, pathological hypertrophy, infiltrative diseases of the myocardium and, at times, ischemia. All patients with systolic dysfunction have some degree of diastolic dysfunction, and when systolic dysfunction is compensated, diastolic dysfunction often remains. Currently, the treatment for acute congestive HF

in both conditions is the same. This is fortunate since they can be difficult to distinguish clinically without echocardiography. However, it appears that treatment and prognosis with diastolic dysfunction is more related to the conditions underlying it and the treatment of these conditions,[2] while the treatment of systolic dysfunction has been clarified by numerous randomized trials. An issue requiring further clarification is whether ischemic systolic dysfunction can be improved by revascularization. Several randomized trials are in progress comparing percutaneous coronary intervention and coronary artery bypass grafting versus medical management in such patients.

Definition of Heart Failure

Congestive heart failure can be defined as a syndrome consisting of:

- Signs and symptoms of intravascular and interstitial volume overload (hypervolemia), including shortness of breath, rales, hepatomegaly and edema
- Manifestations of inadequate tissue perfusion, such as fatigue and poor exercise tolerance

Chronic heart failure can be defined as the same syndrome that is either well compensated or appropriately treated so that the manifestations of acute hypervolemia are minimized.

Key Points

- HF is the major manifestation of left ventricular damage caused by systolic dysfunction and a dilated cardiomyopathy. Patients with systolic dysfunction usually have diastolic dysfunction and the latter often remains after the systolic component is compensated.
- Left-sided failure can lead to right-sided failure.
- Diastolic dysfunction can exist independently and is frequently associated with a stiff, hypertrophied (but normal-sized) ventricle caused by chronic high blood pressure and/or congenital abnormalities.
- Abnormalities in the periphery (anemia, beriberi heart disease, A-V fistulas, thyrotoxicosis) can cause high-output HF.

PREVALENCE AND PROGNOSIS IN HEART FAILURE

HF (when due to dilated cardiomyopathy) has a 15% to 25% annual cardiac mortality. Analysis of 34 years of follow-up of Framingham Study data provides clinically relevant insights into the prevalence, incidence, secular trends, prognosis, and modifiable risk factors for the occurrence of HF in a general population sample.[3] HF was found in about 1% of persons in their fifties and 10% of persons in their eighties. The annual incidence also increased with age, from about 0.2% in persons 45 to 54 years to 4.0% in men aged 85 to 94 years, with the incidence approximately doubling with each decade of age. Women had a lower incidence at all ages. Male predominance was due to coronary heart disease, which conferred a fourfold increased risk of HF. Once HF was present, one third of men and women died within 2 years of diagnosis. The 6-year mortality rate was 82% for men and 67% for women, which corresponded to a death rate four- to eightfold greater than that of the general population of the same age. Sudden death was common, accounting for 28% and 14% of the cardiovascular deaths in men and women, respectively, with HF. Hypertension and coronary disease were the predominant causes of HF and accounted for more than 80% of all clinical events. Factors reflecting deteriorating cardiac function were associated with a substantial increase in risk of overt HF. These include low vital capacity, sinus tachycardia, and left ventricular hypertrophy by ECG. In 2003, more than 550,000 cases of HF were diagnosed in the U.S., but only 2000 heart transplants were performed.[4] For the remainder, quality of life decreases and

less than 40% are living 4 years after diagnosis. We will address the issue of whether exercise testing can improve risk stratification beyond clinical variables.[5,6]

Clinical Risk Markers

Despite important advances in therapy for patients with chronic HF, the mortality rate for this condition remains high and continues to be one of the important challenges facing the clinician who manages these patients. Cardiac transplantation has evolved into an important treatment option for patients with severe HF, but this option remains limited to a relatively small number of patients with end-stage disease because there continues to be a severe shortage of donor hearts. The high mortality rate and widening gap between patients listed for transplantation and available donor hearts have magnified the need for reliable prognostic markers in HF. In addition, revascularization techniques for ischemic cardiomyopathies carry a risk that must be balanced against the benefits.

To direct the limited number of donor hearts to patients who need them the most, a great deal of effort has been directed toward stratifying risk among patients with severe HF through the use of clinical, hemodynamic, and exercise test data. Consensus statements from the American Heart Association and American College of Cardiology[7] and a Bethesda Conference position statement[8] have helped establish guidelines for selection criteria among patients considered for transplantation. The major risk markers in HF include New York Heart Association functional class, reduced EF, reduced cardiac index, renal insufficiency (creatinine clearance <60 mL/min), persistent signs of congestion (orthopnea, jugular venous distension, edema, weight gain, or increased need for diuretics), persistent elevated filling pressure, and reduced exercise capacity. Interestingly, in many studies performed over the last decade, exercise capacity has been demonstrated to be the most important component of the risk profile among patients with HF. Since the early 1990s, more than 100 studies have demonstrated that peak VO_2 is a significant univariate or multivariate predictor of outcomes in patients with HF. Some of the larger studies are outlined in Table 10-1.

Increased reliance on the role of exercise testing for decision-making in HF has occurred for several reasons. The recognition that exercise capacity, expressed simply as workload achieved (i.e., METs) or exercise time, was a significant prognostic marker in patients with cardiovascular disease

TABLE 10–1. Summary of major studies using ventilatory gas exchange to predict outcomes in chronic heart failure

Investigator	Year	No. of subjects	Mean age (years)	Mean follow-up (months)	Annual mortality (%)	Findings
Szlachcic	1985	27	56	12	40	Peak $VO_2 \leq 10$ mL/kg/min had 77% mortality; peak $VO_2 > 10$ mL/kg/min had 21% mortality
Likoff	1987	201	62 ± 10	28	23	Peak $VO_2 > 13$ mL/kg/min was independent predictor of increased mortality
Willens	1987	30	58	6	24.6	Peak VO_2 was best independent predictor of survival by multivariate analysis
Stevenson	1990	42	48 ± 9	14 ± 6	—	Patients who survived more than 6 months on sustained medical therapy achieved peak VO_2 comparable to that of patients surviving after cardiac transplantation
Stevenson	1990	107	53 ± 11	6 ± 5	3	Ability to increase peak VO_2 by ≥ 2 mL/kg/min to a level ≥ 12 mL/kg/min) was an indication to defer transplantation in favor of more compromised candidates
Mancini	1991	122	50 ± 11	11 ± 9	—	Peak $VO_2 > 14$ mL/kg/min had 6% 1-year mortality versus 53% in patients with peak $VO_2 \leq 14$ mL/kg/min
Parmeshwar	1992	127	55.1 ± 9.3	14.6	18	By both univariate and multivariate analysis, peak VO_2 (13.7 mL/kg/min) was one of several independent predictors of outcome
Saxon	1993	528	50 ± 12	12 ± 14	24	By both univariate and multivariate analysis, peak $VO_2 < 11$ mL/kg/min was independent predictor of heart failure death but not of sudden death
Cohn	1993	V-HEFT I = 642, V-HEFT II = 804	59.5 ± 8	60	8	Peak VO_2 was highly significant univariate and multivariate predictor of survival
Roul	1994	75	58 ± 10	12	12	Peak VO_2 (threshold value 14 mL/kg/min) was independent prognostic factor and best predictor of risk of death
Stevenson	1995	265	52 ± 13	12	32	Peak $VO_2 \leq 10$ mL/kg/min was one of several predictors of death or urgent transplantation in patients with Class IV symptoms
DiSalvo	1995	67	51 ± 10	14	24	Percent VO_2 rather than peak VO_2 predicted survival. RVEF was more potent predictor than peak VO_2 or percent VO_2
Aaronson	1995	272	52 ± 12	24 ± 18	33 ± 3	Peak $VO_2 \geq 14$ mL/kg/min predicted survival. Peak VO_2 was better predictor than percentage-predicted VO_2
Wilson	1995	64	49 ± 10	—	—	Low peak exercise VO_2 (< 14 mL/kg/min) could not be used to accurately identify patients with heart failure who had severe hemodynamic dysfunction during exercise
Rickenbacher	1996	116	46.6 ± 10	25 ± 15	2	Peak VO_2 predicted subsequent heart transplantation, but not cardiac death
Chomsky	1996	185	51.4 ± 10	10 ± 6	17	Peak VO_2 (dichotomized at 10 mL/kg/min) was independent predictor of survival both by univariate analysis and multivariate analysis

Continued

TABLE 10–1. Summary of major studies using ventilatory gas exchange to predict outcomes in chronic heart failure—*contd*

Investigator	Year	No. of subjects	Mean age (years)	Mean follow-up (months)	Annual mortality (%)*	Findings
Levine	1996	60	50 ± 9	27 ± 11	17	Peak VO$_2$ (≥16 mL/kg/min) was used as criteria for delisting patients from the waiting list for transplantation Consequent improvement was observed in exercise performance and hemodynamic parameters in these patients after the 27 ± 11 month follow-up period
Haywood	1996	141	—	12	—	All deaths among patients on a transplant waiting list occurred in those with cardiac index <2 L/min/m2 or peak VO$_2$ < 12 mL/kg/min
Aaronson	1997	Derivation sample = 268; validation sample = 199	51 ± 10	36	20	Noninvasive multivariate model outperformed invasive model in predicting risk
Kao	1997	76	51 ± 10	12 ± 3	11.8	In patients at extremes of exercise performance spectrum (VO$_2$ max < 12 or >17 mL/kg/min), VO$_2$ max related to mortality. In patients with moderate to severe exercise intolerance (VO$_2$ max 12–17 mL/kg/min), prognostic value of VO$_2$ max was limited
Richards	1997	76	51 ± 1	12 ± 3	Women 10.5; men 14.5	Percent of predicted peak VO$_2$ achieved described degree of functional impairment in women more accurately than peak VO$_2$
Ponikowski	1997	102	58 ± 10	20 ± 14	12	Peak VO$_2$ < 14 mL//kg/min was one of several independent predictors of death
Cohen Solal	1997	178	52	32	12	Both peak VO$_2$ > 17 mL//kg/min and age-predicted peak VO$_2$ (>63%) were predictors of survival by univariate analysis, but only age-predicted peak VO$_2$ was independent predictor of survival in multivariate analysis
Osada	1998	500	50 ± 10	25 ± 17	15	Peak VO$_2$ ≤ 14 mL//kg/min was univariate and multivariate predictor of mortality. Peak exercise SBP < 120 mmHg and percent predicted peak VO$_2$ ≤ 50% predicted mortality in patients with peak VO$_2$ ≤ 14 mL/kg/min
Opasich	1998	653	52 ± 9	17 ± 13	24	Peak VO$_2$ stratified by <10, 10–18, and >18 mL/kg/min identified high, medium, and low risk
Myers	1998	644	48 ± 11	47 ± 28	5.3	Peak VO$_2$ was better predictor of survival than clinical, hemodynamic, or other exercise variables
Metra	1999	219	55 ± 10	19 ± 25	14.5	Peak exercise stroke work index was most powerful marker of 1-year survival, peak VO$_2$ was most powerful marker of 2-year survival
Myers	2000	644	48 ± 11	47 ± 28	5.3	Peak VO$_2$ was strongest predictor of survival among clinical and exercise test variables. Different cutoffs for peak VO$_2$ (between 10 and 17 mL/kg/min) all had roughly 20% differences in survival

TABLE 10–1. Summary of major studies using ventilatory gas exchange to predict outcomes in chronic heart failure—*cont'd*

Investigator	Year	No. of subjects	Mean age (years)	Mean follow-up (months)	Annual mortality (%)*	Findings
Cohen-Solal	2002	175	53 ± 10	25 ± 10		Peak circulatory power (the product of systolic blood pressure and VO_2) was the only multivariate predictor of prognosis
Mezzani	2003	570	60 ± 10	20 ± 14		Patients who achieve peak RER >1.15 have markedly better survival even when peak VO_2 is ≤10 mL/kg/min
deGroote	2004	407	57 ± 11	26	≈8	B-natriuretic peptide, in combination with % age-predicted peak VO_2 achieved, were strong predictors of survival

CHF, congestive heart failure; RER, respiratory exchange ratio; RVEF, right ventricular ejection fraction.

was made in the early 1970s. Expired gas analysis techniques are now much more widespread, in part because of computerization and increased automation, but also due to an appreciation for their applications to various cardiovascular and pulmonary disorders. Justification for their use in patients with HF has been strengthened by studies describing clinical applications of ventilatory and gas-exchange abnormalities in HF.[9] Cardiopulmonary exercise testing is now part of the standard workup of the patient with HF, and the guidelines on transplantation consider this procedure an integral component of the decision-making process regarding transplantation. The widespread use of cardiopulmonary exercise testing in patients with HF over the past 15 years has provided many groups the opportunity to evaluate the role of peak VO_2 in prognosis.

Although previous studies assessing risk using exercise testing have varied widely in terms of severity of HF, the use of different outcomes for assessing risk, application of different cutpoints for peak VO_2, and inclusion or exclusion of other clinical, exercise, and hemodynamic variables, peak VO_2 is clearly one of the more robust markers of risk in HF. Directly measured peak VO_2 has been shown to outperform clinical, hemodynamic, and other exercise test data in predicting 1- to 2-year mortality. Several investigators have reported that patients who achieve a peak VO_2 greater than 14 mL/kg/min appear to have a prognosis similar to that among patients who receive transplantation (approximately 90% survival at 1 year). This finding implies that transplantation can be safely deferred among these patients. This cutpoint has emerged as a clinically practical prognostic marker in HF; a value less than 14 mL/kg/min is a

relative indication for transplantation in the guidelines. However, as discussed later in this chapter, there are a number of caveats that must be considered when applying specific cutpoints to assess risk.

Questions That Remain to Be Clarified

The questions that remain to be clarified include the following:

- What is the place of cardiopulmonary exercise testing relative to clinical, hemodynamic, and other data in the risk paradigm in patients with HF?
- What is the optimal cutpoint for peak VO_2 when selecting patients for transplantation listing?
- Should peak VO_2 be expressed as an absolute value or corrected for age or body weight?
- How well do other ventilatory gas exchange responses (e.g., the VE versus VCO_2 slope, ventilatory threshold, rate of recovery of VO_2) predict risk?

Each of these issues is discussed in this chapter relative to risk stratification and decision-making in patients with HF.

Exercise Tolerance and Selection of Transplant Recipients

Because there are only approximately 5000 donor hearts available each year in the U.S., recipients must be carefully selected. In this regard, factors associated with 1 to 2-year survival among potential candidates are critical. Historically, the major factors associated with poor short-term outcome without transplantation have included an EF less than 15%, complex ventricular ectopy, sympathetic nervous system activation, and impaired exercise capacity, although there are many other clinical markers that have been associated with risk in HF (Table 10-2). With advances in the treatment for HF, many patients once thought to have end-stage HF can be stabilized by aggressive medical therapy. Although predicting the clinical course in individual patients is imprecise, transplantation has been safely deferred in many patients by combinations of angiotensin-converting enzyme (ACE) inhibition or ACE-II blockade, diuretics, beta-blockade, and careful monitoring of patient status, including weight, electrolytes, and renal function. Other patients will deteriorate despite intensive medical management. Multidisciplinary HF management programs have been set up to manage and monitor patients, and these programs appear to improve survival.[10] For this reason, many heart transplant centers have evolved into "heart failure management" clinics.

Increasing numbers of patients have undergone cardiac transplantation for end-stage HF, and today approximately three quarters of these patients remain alive after 5 years. Because the transplant patient's heart is denervated, some intriguing hemodynamic responses to exercise are observed. The heart is not responsive to the normal actions of the parasympathetic and sympathetic systems. The absence of vagal tone explains the high resting heart rates in these patients (100 to 110 beats per minute) and the relatively slow adaptation of the heart to a given amount of submaximal work. As a result, the delivery of oxygen to the working tissue is slower, contributing to earlier than normal metabolic acidosis and hyperventilation during exercise. Maximal heart rate is lower in transplant patients than in normal subjects, which contributes to a reduction in cardiac output and exercise capacity.

Cardiopulmonary Exercise Testing and Prognosis in HF

Early Studies

Several small studies were published in the early to mid-1980s that addressed factors associated with the risk of death in HF, in which the inclusion of directly measured VO_2 was seemingly incidental. Among the earliest studies was that of Szlachcic et al[11] who performed resting and exercise hemodynamic measurements, ventilatory gas exchange, and radionuclide ventriculography in 27 patients with HF and observed them for 1 year. Patients were dichotomized by those achieving a peak VO_2 less than or equal to 10 versus those achieving a peak VO_2 greater than 10 mL/kg/min. The group of patients achieving less than or equal to 10 mL/kg/min were found to have worse hemodynamic responses, including higher pulmonary capillary wedge pressures, lower left ventricular and right ventricular EFs, and lower exercise heart rates and cardiac indexes, and the mortality rate over the subsequent year was higher among those with limited peak levels of VO_2 (77% vs. 21%, $P < 0.001$).

Likoff et al[12] evaluated 201 patients with HF and prospectively observed them for 28 months. Fifteen clinical, hemodynamic, and exercise variables were entered into a Cox proportional hazards model. Three characteristics at study entry predicted an increased mortality risk: the presence of a third heart sound, low peak VO_2, and diagnosis of ischemic cardiomyopathy. For patients with a third heart sound, ischemic cardiomyopathy, and peak VO_2 less than the sample mean of 13 mL/kg/min, the 1-year mortality rate was 36%, whereas among patients without any of these risk markers the 1-year mortality rate was only 10% ($P < 0.001$).

Willens et al[13] studied 30 patients whose baseline evaluation included radionuclide angiography, echocardiography, 24-hour Holter monitoring,

---

TABLE 10-2. Variables associated with risk in chronic heart failure

Reduced ejection fraction
Poor exercise capacity:
- NYHA Functional Class III or IV
- Dyspnea on exertion
- Peak $VO_2 < 14$ mL/kg/min
Heightened neurohormonal markers (BNP, ANP, endothelins, norepinephine)
Complex ventricular ectopy
Reduced cardiac index (<2.0 L/min/m²)
Renal insufficiency (creatinine clearance <60 mL/min)
Persistent signs of congestion (orthopnea, jugular venous distension, edema, weight gain, increased need for diuretics)
Left ventricular end-diastolic dimension >80 mm
Duration of heart failure
Hyponatremia (serum sodium <134 mEq/L)
High pulmonary capillary wedge pressure

ANP, atrial natriuretic peptide; BNP, brain natriuretic peptide; NYHA, New York Heart Association.

and exercise testing and observed them for a mean of 15 months. Univariate predictors of survival included peak VO_2, age, estimated VO_2 (from exercise time), presence of left bundle branch block, left ventricular end-diastolic dimensions, and frequency of ventricular arrhythmias. Importantly, the best multivariate predictor of survival was peak VO_2.

These early studies were the first to suggest that peak VO_2 may have an important place in risk stratification among patients with HF, and they provided an important springboard for the routine use of gas exchange techniques in the evaluation of transplant candidates today. The study of Szlachcic et al[11] was the first to suggest that a single cutpoint, 10 mL/kg/min, can have considerable importance in risk-stratifying patients with severe HF. However, the 12 deaths in that study, like the eight deaths in the study carried out by Willens et al[13] made them too small to perform valid multivariate analyses.

Multivariate Studies in the 1990s

In a landmark 1991 study that provided an impetus for many others, Mancini et al[14] observed three groups of patients referred for transplantation over 2 years. One group comprised patients accepted for transplant on the basis of achieving a peak VO_2 less than 14 mL/kg/min; a second group comprised patients considered too well for transplant (peak VO_2 >14 mL/kg/min); and a third group comprised patients with a peak VO_2 less than 14 mL/kg/min but rejected from transplantation for noncardiac reasons. Patients with preserved exercise capacity (>14 mL/kg/min) had 1- and 2-year survival rates of 94% and 84%, respectively, roughly equivalent to those observed after transplantation. This was in contrast to patients with poor exercise capacity (peak VO_2 <14 mL/kg/min) who were rejected for transplantation, among whom 1- and 2-year survival rates were only 47% and 32%, respectively. By both univariate and multivariate analysis, peak VO_2 was the best predictor of survival. This study fostered the concept that a single cutpoint, 14 mL/kg/min, provides a clinically applicable cutpoint between patients who require transplantation for survival benefit and those who do not.

Stevenson et al[15] studied 500 patients who were discharged on tailored medical therapy after evaluation for transplantation, and the risk of death or need for urgent transplantation was studied over the subsequent 2 years. Low cardiac index and high filling pressures did not confer a higher risk, but serum sodium levels less than 133 mEq/L and left ventricular diastolic dimensions greater than 80 mm were associated with 34% and 23%

2-year survival rates, respectively. Patients with an initial peak VO_2 greater than 10 mL/kg/min had a 2-year event (death or transplant) rate of 28%, whereas among patients with a peak VO_2 less than 10 mL/kg/min, the event rate was 52%.

Opasich et al[16] evaluated predictors of survival 6 months, 1 year, and 2 years after consideration for transplantation among 653 patients. The presence of a contraindication to exercise testing identified very high-risk patients, which confirmed observations made by Stevenson et al[15] and many studies in patients with coronary disease. Peak VO_2 stratified into three levels (≤10, 10 to 18, and >18 mL/kg/min) identified groups at high, medium, and low risk, respectively. However, in patients in New York Heart Association Class III or IV, peak VO_2 did not have prognostic power.

Haywood et al[17] studied patients accepted for heart transplantation listing between 1986 and 1994 at Stanford University. Of 141 consecutive patients accepted for cardiac transplant, all deaths and 88% of patients who deteriorated to status one while on the waiting list had either a cardiac index less than 2.0 L/min/m^2 or a peak VO_2 less than 12 mL/kg/min. In those with a cardiac index less than 2.0 L/min/m^2 *and* a peak VO_2 less than 12 mL/kg/min, 38% died or deteriorated to status one during the first year on the waiting list. Conversely, all patients with a cardiac index equal or greater than to 2.0 L/min/m^2 *and* peak VO_2 equal or greater than 12 mL/kg/min survived throughout the follow-up. These investigators later studied patients referred for heart transplantation but selected for medical management. One hundred sixteen patients were observed for a mean of 25 ± 15 months. In this comparatively healthy group (mean peak VO_2 17.4 ± 4.3 mL/kg/min, mean pulmonary capillary wedge pressure 16 ± 9 mmHg), there were only eight cardiac deaths, and no clinical, exercise, or hemodynamic variable significantly predicted death by logistic regression. By multivariate regression, only pulmonary artery systolic pressure and duration of HF predicted the need for later transplantation.

Saxon et al[18] studied 528 consecutive patients hospitalized for advanced HF. Predictors of death or hemodynamic deterioration requiring transplantation were evaluated over the subsequent year; a total of 129 patients (24%) experienced one of these outcomes. A serum sodium level equal to 134 mEq/L, pulmonary arterial diastolic pressure greater than 19 mmHg, left ventricular diastolic dimension greater than 44 mm/m^2, peak VO_2 less than 11 mL/kg/min, and the presence of a permanent pacemaker were independent predictors of hemodynamic deterioration or death. In the absence of any of these risk factors, the risk of a negative outcome was only 2%. The presence of hyponatremia and any two additional risk factors raised the risk to greater than 50%.

Cohn et al[19] studied 1446 patients prior to randomization in a vasodilator multicenter trial. Patients were followed up to 5 years. EF, peak VO_2, cardiothoracic ratio, and plasma norepinephrine were independent predictors of mortality. An interesting interaction between EF and peak VO_2 was observed; EF was more influential as a prognostic factor among patients whose peak VO_2 was above the median (14.5 mL/kg/min). Likewise, peak VO_2 was a significant additional prognostic marker only among patients whose EF was above the median (28%). The increase in risk for patients with EFs below the median more than doubled when peak VO_2 was above the median (risk ratio 2.43) compared to when peak VO_2 was below the median (risk ratio 1.43). Similarly, the increase in risk for patients with peak VO_2 values below the median more than doubled when EF was above the median (risk ratio 2.17) compared to when EF was below the median (risk ratio 1.27).

A comprehensive evaluation of clinical, hemodynamic, and exercise variables was performed during a 10-year period among 644 patients referred for evaluation of HF at Stanford.[20] The longer follow-up period (mean, 4 years), large number of deaths (187), and the inclusion of both measured and predicted VO_2 made it unique among the multivariate studies, and one of the more robust data sets to evaluate prognosis. Univariately, the most powerful predictors of death were from the exercise test; peak VO_2, VO_2 at the ventilatory threshold, VO_2 expressed as a percentage of the predicted value, peak systolic blood pressure lower than 130 mmHg, and watts achieved were significant predictors of death. Age was the only predictor of death among clinical variables, and hemodynamic variables, including EF, pulmonary capillary wedge pressure, and left ventricular dimensions were not important predictors of outcome. By multivariate analysis, peak VO_2 was the only significant predictor of death. This study provided the strongest evidence to date that directly measured peak VO_2 not only outperforms clinical and hemodynamic data but also was a better predictor of death than exercise duration or watts achieved.

Osada et al[21] reported results from 500 patients observed for a mean of 25 months. Patients who achieved a peak VO_2 greater than 14 mL/kg/min had a 3-year survival rate of 93%, compared with 68% among patients whose peak VO_2 was between

10 and 14 mL/kg/min.[37] Patients whose peak VO_2 was less than 14 mL/kg/min but greater than 50% of their age and gender-predicted value had a 3-year survival rate similar to patients who achieved a peak VO_2 greater than 14 mL/kg/min (93% versus 91%). Patients with limited exercise capacity had a particularly poor survival if they were unable to raise peak exercise systolic blood pressure to at least 120 mmHg; the 3-year survival rate among these patients was 55%, compared to an 83% survival rate among patients with a measurement less than 14 mL/kg/min whose peak exercise blood pressure was greater than 120 mmHg.

Roul et al[22] prospectively studied 75 patients with clinical, radionuclide, and right heart catheterization data and observed them for 1 year.[5] The cohort was divided into two groups based on peak VO_2 greater or less than 14 mL/kg/min. Patients with preserved exercise capacity had lower left ventricular filling pressures, lower total peripheral resistance, lower creatinine and blood urea nitrogen levels, and higher exercise duration. During the 1-year follow-up, nine patients died in the group with peak VO_2 levels less than 14 mL/kg/min, whereas there were no deaths in the group with levels more than 14 mL/kg/min. Seven major events requiring hospitalization occurred in the limited exercise capacity group versus only three in the preserved group.

Kao et al[23] studied survival rates among 178 patients who underwent exercise testing at a baseline evaluation. Patients whose peak VO_2 levels were less than 12 mL/kg/min had a higher mortality rate when compared to patients with peak VO_2 levels greater than 17 mL/kg/min. However when patients were compared by tertiles of peak VO_2 within the intermediate range (12 to 17 mL/kg/min), no differences in survival were observed between the tertiles. These investigators suggested that although peak VO_2 differentiates patients who do and do not survive at the extremes of the exercise performance spectrum, the prognostic value of peak VO_2 in the intermediate range (in which most patients fall) is limited.

Cardiopulmonary Markers of Risk Other than Peak VO$_2$

Although peak VO_2 defines the limits of the cardiopulmonary system, there are other cardiopulmonary responses which are important in defining the severity of HF and prognosis. These responses are to one extent or another related to the ventilatory response to exercise, the capacity of the cardiopulmonary system to adapt to the demands of a given work rate, or the ability of the cardiopulmonary system to recover from a bout of exercise. Responses such as the anaerobic threshold (AT), the VE/VCO$_2$ slope, oxygen uptake kinetics, rate of recovery of VO$_2$, and the oxygen uptake efficiency slope (OUES) have been used with greater frequency to classify functional limitations and stratify risk in patients with heart disease. Examples of these are illustrated in Figure 10-1. Some of these responses have been demonstrated to have greater prognostic value than peak VO$_2$, and these studies are summarized in Table 10-3.

Ventilatory Threshold

The ventilatory threshold, one important submaximal marker of cardiopulmonary function with a long history, has been employed in surprisingly few multivariate models to predict risk in HF.

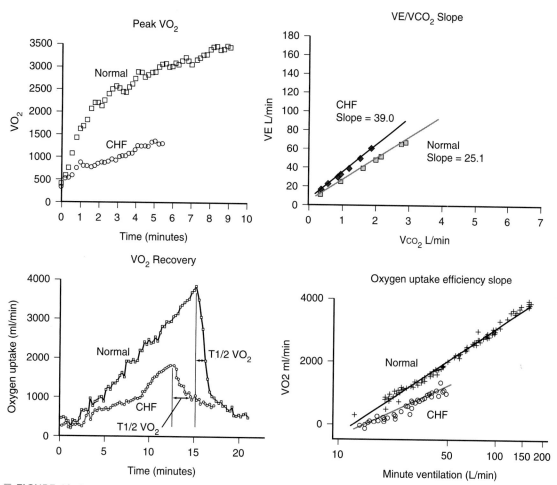

■ FIGURE 10–1

Examples of four different cardiopulmonary exercise test methods that have been used to estimate prognosis in patients with cardiovascular disease. The peak VO$_2$ responses *(upper left)* are taken from a normal subject and a typical patient with chronic heart failure the same age. The VE/VCO$_2$ slope *(upper right)* is derived from the slope of the regression line between VE and VCO$_2$, excluding data points beyond the ventilatory threshold. VO$_2$ in recovery *(lower left)* shows a more graded recovery response in the CHF patient (i.e., longer recovery time), despite the lower exercise capacity. T1/2 represents the time required for a 50% fall from the peak VO$_2$ value. The OUES *(lower right)* is derived by plotting VO$_2$ against the log of VE; a steeper slope reflects a lower VE for any given VO$_2$, that is, more efficient ventilation. From Myers J: Applications of cardiopulmonary exercise testing in the management of cardiovascular and pulmonary disease. Int J Sports Med 2005;26:S49-S55.

TABLE 10-3. Prognostic studies on ventilatory gas exchange responses other than peak Vo_2

Study (Ref) VE/VCO$_2$ slope	Year	Subjects, (N)	Mean follow-up Mean age, Y	Period, Mo	Findings
Chua	1997	CHF (173)	59±12	–	VE/VCO$_2$ slope (>34) provided stronger prognostic information than peak VO$_2$
Francis	2000	CHF (303)	59 ± 11	47	Peak VO$_2$ and VE/VCO$_2$ slope similar in prognostic power
Robbins	1999	CHF (470)	52 ± 11	18	VE/VCO$_2$ slope and low chronotropic index most powerful multivariate predictors of death
Gitt	2002	CHF (223)	63 ± 11	21	VO$_2$ at the anaerobic threshold <11 mL/kg/min and VE/VCO$_2$ slope best predictors of risk
Kleber	2000	CHF (142)	52 ± 10	16*	VE/VCO$_2$ slope outperformed peak VO$_2$ as predictor of death, Tx, or LVAD
Arena	2003	CHF (213)	57±13	32	VE/VCO$_2$ slope stronger predictor of cardiac mortality than peak VO$_2$
Corra	2002	CHF (600)	57 ± 9	26	VE/VCO$_2$ slope was strongest predictor of death or Tx. Peak VO$_2$ ≤10mL/kg/min and VE/VCO$_2$ slope ≥35 had similar mortality rate
Bol	2000	CHF (72)	63 ± 12	–	VE/VO$_2$ slope was more powerful predictor of mortality than clinical variables or peak VO$_2$ in recovery
de Groote (15)	1996	DCM (153)	50 ± 12	15*	VO$_2$ recovery significantly delayed in DCM versus normals; ratio of exercise and recovery VO$_2$ independently predicted survival
VO$_2$ Kinetics					
Rickli	2003	CHF (202)	52 ± 11	29	Mean response time >50 sec was strongest predictor of death or Tx, followed by predicted VO$_2$ <50%
Schalcher	2003	CHF (146)	52 ± 10	25	Mean response time was strongest predictor of survival or freedom from Tx or hospitalization, followed by VE/VCO$_2$ slope
Brunner-LaRocca	1999	CHF (48)	55 ±10	22	Mean response time >60 sec was significant predictor of mortality, and was more powerful than peak VO$_2$
Oxygen Uptake Efficiency Slope					
Pardaens	2000	CHF (284)	52 ± 11	16*	Peak VO$_2$ was stronger predictor of death or cardiovascular events than OUES or VE/VCO$_2$ slope

*Median
DCM, dilated cardiomyopathy; LVAD, left ventricular assist device implantation; OUES, oxygen uptake efficiency slope; Tx, transplantation.

Studies that have included the ventilatory threshold have demonstrated that VO$_2$ at this point significantly predicts outcome. This point has the potential to be a particularly useful marker of outcome, since for many patients with HF, "maximal" exercise is not achieved for various reasons or is difficult to define. In the Stanford study, VO$_2$ at the ventilatory threshold was a significant univariate predictor of death in patients evaluated for HF, but in a multivariate analysis, peak VO$_2$ was a stronger predictor of death.[20] Gitt et al[24] recently tested 223 consecutive patients with HF in Germany. They compared the prognostic power of peak VO$_2$, VO$_2$ at the ventilatory threshold, and the VE/VCO$_2$ slope in predicting all-cause death. Cutpoints for VO$_2$ less than or equal to 14 mL/kg/min, VO$_2$ at the ventilatory threshold (VO$_2$AT) less than 11 mL/kg/min, and a VE/VCO$_2$ slope more than 34 were used as threshold values for high risk of death. Patients with a peak VO$_2$ less than or equal to 14 mL/kg/min had a greater than three-fold increased risk while a VO_2AT less than 11 mL/kg/min or a VE/VCO_2 slope greater than 34 had fivefold increased risks for early death. In patients with both VO_2AT less than 11 mL/kg/min and VE/VCO_2 slope greater than than 34, the risk of early death was 10-fold higher. After correction for age, gender, EF, and New York Heart Association class in a multivariate analysis, the combination of VO_2AT less than 11 mL/kg/min and VE/VCO_2 slope greater than 34 was the best predictor of 6-month mortality (relative risk = 5.1).

VE/VCO₂ Slope

There is an impressive body of recent data demonstrating the role of the VE/VCO_2 slope in predicting prognosis in HF. These studies have shown that the VE/VCO_2 slope predicts mortality at least as well as, and independent from, peak VO_2. This response is usually expressed as the slope of the best-fit linear regression line relating VE and VCO_2 below the ventilatory compensation point for exercise lactic acidosis (see Figure 3-1). While the slope of this relationship is normally between 20 and 30, values in the thirties are common in patients with mild-to-moderate HF, and values in the forties are often observed in patients with more severe HF.[6,25-27] An elevated VE/VCO_2 slope is a reflection of the pathophysiology of the abnormal ventilatory response to exercise in HF.[6,26-28] Thus, the VE/VCO_2 slope is elevated in the presence of early lactate accumulation, ventilation/perfusion mismatching in the lungs (e.g., poor cardiac output response to exercise), or the deconditioning that is commonly observed in HF.

Corra et al[27] performed cardiopulmonary exercise testing in 600 patients with HF and followed them for major cardiac events (death or urgent transplantation) over a 2-year period. The VE/VCO_2 slope was the strongest independent predictor of a cardiac event (outperforming peak VO_2, EF, and other clinical and exercise test variables). The best cutpoint for predicting risk was 35 (relative risk = 3.2 for a VE/VCO_2 slope >35). The total mortality rate in patients with a VE/VCO_2 slope greater than or equal to 35 was 30% versus 10% in patients with a VE/VCO_2 slope less than 35. Patients with a VE/VCO_2 slope greater than or equal to 35 had a similar mortality rate as those with a peak VO_2 less than or equal to 10 mL/kg/min.

Arena et al[25] from our laboratory compared the prognostic power of peak VO_2 and the VE/VCO_2 slope in 213 patients with HF. Peak VO_2 and the VE/VCO_2 slope were demonstrated with univariate

Cox regression analysis both to be significant predictors of cardiac-related mortality and hospitalization ($P < 0.01$). Multivariate analysis revealed that peak VO_2 added additional value to the VE/VCO_2 slope in predicting cardiac-related hospitalization, but not cardiac mortality. Patients who exhibited a VE/VCO_2 slope greater than or equal to 34 had a particularly high probability of hospitalization (> 50% 1-year following evaluation, Figure 10-2). The VE/VCO_2 slope was demonstrated with receiver operating characteristic curve analysis to be significantly better than peak VO_2 in predicting cardiac-related mortality ($P < 0.05$). Although area under the receiver operating characteristic curve for the VE/VCO_2 slope was greater than peak VO_2 in predicting cardiac-related hospitalization (0.77 versus 0.73), the difference was not statistically significant ($P = 0.14$).

Kleber et al[29] evaluated the cardiopulmonary response to exercise in 142 patients with HF and followed then for a mean of 16 months. Forty-four events (37 deaths and seven instances of heart transplantation, cardiomyoplasty, or left ventricular assist device implantation) occurred. Among peak VO_2, NYHA class, EF, total lung capacity, and age, the most powerful predictor of event-free survival was the VE/VCO_2 slope; patients with a VE/VCO_2 slope greater than or equal to 130% of age-and gender-adjusted normal values had a significantly better 1-year event-free survival (88.3%) than patients with a slope greater than 130% (54.7%; $P < 0.001$).

Robbins et al[30] studied 470 consecutive patients with HF who were not taking beta-blockers and

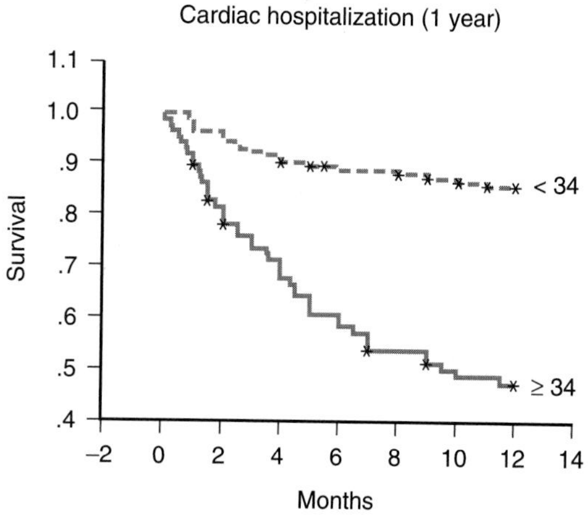

■ FIGURE 10–2

Kaplan-Meier survival curves for 1-year cardiac-related hospitalization using a VE/VCO_2 slope threshold <34 versus ≥34 ($P < 0.0001$). From Arena R, Myers J, Aslam S, et al: Peak VO_2 and VE/VCO_2 slope in patients with heart failure: A prognostic comparison. Am Heart J 2004;147:354-360.

followed them a mean of 1.5 years. Chronotropic index and peak VO_2 were considered abnormal if in the lowest 25th percentile of the patient cohort, whereas VE/VCO_2 was considered abnormal if in the highest 25th percentile. There were 71 deaths during the follow-up period. In univariate analyses, predictors of death included high VE/VCO_2, low chronotropic index, low VO_2, low resting systolic blood pressure, and older age. Nonparametric Kaplan-Meier plots demonstrated that by dividing the population according to peak VE/VCO_2 and peak VO_2, it was possible to identify low, intermediate, and very high risk groups. In multivariate analyses, the only independent predictors of death were high VE/VCO_2 (adjusted relative risk 3.20) and low chronotropic index (adjusted relative risk 1.94).

These and other studies[31-34] suggest that the VE/VCO_2 slope appears to have greater prognostic power than peak VO_2. It is likely that an abnormal VE/VCO_2 slope reflects many of the physiologic processes that lead to hyperventilation during exercise and thus are associated with disease severity (e.g., early lactate accumulation and ventilation/perfusion mismatching in the lungs caused by a poor cardiac output response to exercise). Importantly, the most useful risk stratification paradigm includes the VE/VCO_2 slope in addition to peak VO_2 and other clinical or exercise test variables in a multivariate model.[24,25,27,30] Consideration should be given to revising the clinical guidelines to reflect the prognostic importance of the VE/VCO_2 slope.

VO$_2$ Kinetics

The rate in which oxygen uptake responds to a given level of work, often expressed as oxygen uptake kinetics, has also been shown to have prognostic value. Indices of oxygen kinetics are easy to determine with current automated gas exchange technology, and offer promise as supplemental indices to more precisely stratify risk in patients with HF. Since these measures can be derived when exercise is submaximal, they may be particularly useful in HF patients unable to exercise maximally.

Rickli et al[35] studied the mean response time (MRT), defined as the time required to reach 63% of the steady state VO_2, in patients with HF. They observed that the MRT was the strongest univariate and multivariate predictor of cardiac mortality, and for patients who exhibited an abnormal MRT, a peak VO_2 less than 50% of the age-predicted value, and resting systolic blood pressure less than 105 mmHg, the 1-year event rate was 59%. Schalcher et al[36] studied 146 patients with HF and reported

that, over a mean follow-up period of 25 months, the MRT more powerfully predicted death, need for urgent cardiac transplantation, or hospitalization than peak VO_2 as well as other exercise test and clinical variables.

In an additional study from this group, VO_2 kinetics at exercise onset, expressed as a mean response time greater 60 seconds to a standardized protocol, was a stronger predictor of survival than peak VO_2, the VE/VCO_2 slope, and a variety of clinical and laboratory markers known to be related to HF mortality.[37] While the measurement of VO_2 kinetics has been expressed in many different ways, all of them reflect the capacity of the cardiopulmonary system to adapt to the demands of a given work rate. This measurement appears to have important prognostic value, and has an advantage in that it does not require judgment about the patient's maximal effort.

Oxygen Uptake Efficiency Slope

Another proposed index of ventilatory efficiency, the OUES, has been suggested as a useful measure to stratify the functional reserve of patients undergoing exercise testing, and this index has also been shown to have prognostic value. The OUES is determined by regressing oxygen uptake against the logarithm of total ventilation; thus, it reflects the ventilatory requirement for work performed (VO_2) throughout exercise. Baba et al[38] reported that the OUES was as effective as peak VO_2 for discriminating between HF functional classifications, and that it was strongly correlated to peak VO_2. The purported value of the OUES is that it does not require maximal effort, it has been shown to be reproducible, and it has been suggested to reflect the combination of cardiovascular, musculoskeletal, and pulmonary influences that result in inefficient breathing, which are characteristic of HF and pulmonary disease.[38-40]

However, other studies have suggested that the OUES has limited clinical utility. Mourot et al[41] studied the effects of endurance training on the OUES among 15 healthy women, and observed that while training increased peak VO_2 and VO_2 at the ventilatory threshold, the OUES response was highly variable, and was not a sensitive maker of the response to training. Similarly, Pichon et al[42] studied the OUES in 50 healthy males and reported that the wide variability in the OUES response relative to peak VO_2 limited its usefulness. Pardaens et al[43] studied 284 cardiac transplant candidates who underwent cardiopulmonary exercise testing and followed them for a median of 16 months.

Both peak VO_2 and the OUES were significant predictors of death or other cardiovascular events. However, whereas the prognostic power of peak VO_2 was independent of the OUES, the prognostic significance of the OUES was lost after controlling for peak VO_2.

Oxygen Uptake in Recovery

The time required for oxygen uptake to return to the resting state in recovery from exercise (oxygen uptake recovery kinetics) has also been shown to be an important functional and prognostic marker.[44-46] A delay in the rate of recovery of VO_2 has been explained by a delay in the recovery of energy stores in the muscle, with skeletal muscle metabolic abnormalities, microcirculatory changes, and a prolongation of elevated cardiac output being contributing factors.[47] Importantly, the recovery response does not appear to be affected by the exercise level achieved.[47,48] Hayashida et al[45] reported that the delay in recovery of VO_2 among patients with HF was related to exercise intolerance and the degree of hyperventilation during exercise. de Groote et al[44] observed that recovery oxygen uptake was delayed in patients with dilated cardiomyopathy relative to healthy controls, and that the ratio of total VO_2 during exercise and recovery was an independent predictor of survival.[44] Similarly, Scrutinio et al followed 196 patients with HF for a mean of 18 months, and found that the half-time for VO_2 in recovery was a significant independent predictor of death.

Cutpoints for Peak VO_2

The application of a single cutpoint for peak VO_2, which can provide clinically meaningful separation between patients with high and low likelihood of survival, is inherently attractive to clinicians because it greatly simplifies many of the complexities involved in predicting risk in HF. In the mortality studies, it has been common to dichotomize patients above and below the median peak VO_2 value for a given sample. A peak VO_2 lower than 14 mL/kg/min has been commonly applied for selecting patients for transplantation, and is a relative indication for transplantation in the guidelines. However, many other cutpoints for peak VO_2 have been advocated for stratifying risk in patients with HF; differences between studies likely reflect differences in the severity of HF.

In order to determine whether an "optimal" peak VO_2 criteria for stratifying risk could be determined, we studied 644 patients who were evaluated for HF over a 10-year period.[50] After pharmacologic stabilization at entrance into the study, all participants underwent cardiopulmonary exercise testing. Survival analysis was performed with death as the endpoint. Transplantation was considered a censored event. Four-year survival was determined for patients who achieved peak oxygen uptake values greater than or less than values ranging between 10 and 17 mL/kg/min. Follow-up information was complete for 98.3% of the cohort. During a mean follow-up period of 4 years, 187 patients (29%) died and 101 underwent transplantation. Actuarial 1- and 5-year survival rates were 90.5% and 73.4%, respectively. Peak VO_2 was an independent predictor of survival and was a stronger predictor than work rate achieved and other exercise and clinical variables. A difference in survival of approximately 20% was achieved by dichotomizing patients above versus below each peak VO_2 value ranging between 10 and 17 mL/kg/min. These results are illustrated in Figure 10-3. Survival rate was significantly higher among patients achieving a peak VO_2 above than among those achieving a peak VO_2 below each of these values ($P < 0.01$), but each cutpoint was similar in its ability to separate survivors from nonsurvivors. Although 14 mL/kg/min has been widely applied to stratify risk in patients with HF, these results suggest that an optimal cutpoint may not exist, and it may be better to apply peak VO_2 as a continuous variable in multivariate models to predict prognosis.

Interaction Between Peak VO_2 and Hemodynamic Variables in Stratifying Risk

Survival is most accurately predicted when exercise variables are combined with other clinical and hemodynamic data.[15,17,19,20,30,51,52] Reduced left ventricular performance has been a common reason for referring a patient to a HF management clinic, and many studies have identified EF as a predictor of survival. However, EF by itself is an inadequate reflection of left ventricular performance and a patient's degree of hemodynamic compromise. While EF has been reported to lose its prognostic value in the very low range (i.e., <25%, the most clinically relevant range in patients considered for transplantation),[53] others[19] have shown that EF is associated with a marked increase in mortality once it is below 20%. Adding further confusion to this issue is the fact that EF and peak VO_2 are poorly related.[54] Wilson et al observed that more than 50% of potential heart transplant candidates

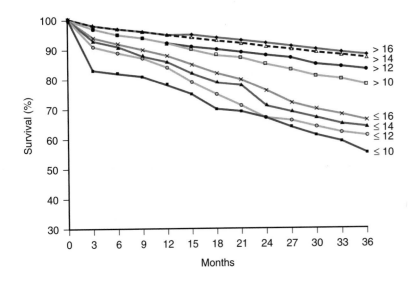

FIGURE 10-3

Survival curves for patients achieving values above 10, 12, 14, and 16 mL/kg/min as compared to below each cutpoint for peak oxygen uptake. There was an approximate 20% difference in survival comparing below vs. above each cutpoint. From Myers J, Gullestad L, Vagelos R, et al: Cardiopulmonary exercise testing and prognosis in severe heart failure: 14 mL/kg/min revisited. Am Heart J 2000;139:78-84.

with reduced peak VO_2 (mean 13.3 ± 2.7 mL/kg/min) had only mild or moderate hemodynamic dysfunction during exercise, as evidenced by relatively normal increases in cardiac output and pulmonary wedge pressure.[55] In the V-Heft studies, EF and peak VO_2 had an intriguing interaction; EF was more influential prognostically when peak VO_2 was comparatively high (approximately twice as predictive when peak VO_2 was >14.5 mL/kg/min).[19] Bol et al[34] reported that the VE/VCO_2 slope was a particularly powerful prognostic marker when EF was comparatively high in patients with HF.

Right heart catheterization has been performed in HF patients to more directly assess cardiovascular performance and stratify risk. Variables such as low resting cardiac output and high intrapulmonary pressures have been associated with higher risk. However, some patients remain markedly symptomatic despite normalization of cardiac output and left ventricular filling pressures. The level of exercise intolerance perceived by patients with HF has a questionable relation to objective measures of circulatory, ventilatory, or metabolic dysfunction during exercise. In addition, these hemodynamic variables have not consistently been shown to be useful in prognosis.[14,15,20]

Peak VO_2 has functioned synergistically with hemodynamic responses in some studies. Haywood et al[17] observed that the combination of resting cardiac index and peak VO_2 was 100% specific for identifying patients who could survive or avoid deterioration to "status one" (highest priority for transplantation) during the year after listing for heart transplantation. These investigators constructed tables based on a Cox proportional hazards model to predict the statistical chance of

survival for any given cardiac index and peak VO_2. Osada et al[21] and the Stanford group[20] observed that the combination of peak VO_2 and systolic blood pressure achieved during exercise increased the accuracy for predicting risk in patients evaluated for HF. The inability to increase systolic blood pressure above 120 to 130 mmHg appears to be associated with a higher risk.

Chomsky et al[56] measured the cardiac output response to exercise along with gas exchange responses in 185 patients referred for evaluation for transplantation. The cardiac output response to exercise was considered normal in 83 patients and reduced in 102. By univariate analysis, patients with normal cardiac output responses had a better 1-year survival rate (95%) than did those with reduced cardiac output responses (72%). Survival in patients with a peak VO_2 greater than 14 mL/kg/min (88%) was not different from that of patients with a peak VO_2 less than or equal to 14 mL/kg/min (79%). However, survival was worse in patients with a peak VO_2 less than or equal to 10 mL/kg/min (52%) versus those with peak VO_2 greater than 10 mL/kg/min (89%). By Cox regression analysis, the cardiac output response to exercise was the strongest independent predictor of survival (risk ratio 4.3), with peak VO_2 dichotomized at 10 mL/kg/min (risk ratio 3.3) as the only other independent predictor. Patients with reduced cardiac output responses and peak VO_2 less than or equal to 10 mL/kg/min had an extremely poor 1-year survival rate (38%).

Metra et al[57] performed cardiopulmonary exercise testing and direct hemodynamic monitoring in 219 consecutive patients with HF, and followed them for mean of 19 months. During the follow-up period, 32 patients died and six underwent urgent transplantation, resulting in a 71% cumulative major event-free 2-year survival. Peak exercise stroke work index was the most powerful prognostic variable selected by Cox multivariate analysis, followed by serum sodium and left ventricular EF for 1-year survival. However, peak VO_2 and serum sodium were the strongest determinants of 2-year survival. Two-year survival was 54% in the patients with peak exercise stroke work index less than or equal to 30 gm/m^2 versus 91% in those with a stroke work index greater than 30 g/m^2 ($P < 0.0001$). A significant percentage of patients (41%) had a normal cardiac output response to exercise with an excellent two-year survival (87% versus 58% in the others) despite a relatively low peak VO_2 (15.1 ± 4.7 mL/kg/min). In a comparatively small 3-year follow-up, Bol et al[34] observed that patients with HF and a relatively high-EF (28%) but normal VE/VCO$_2$ slope had the greatest survival rate (78%), whereas those in the high EF group with an abnormal VE/VCO$_2$ slope had the lowest survival rate (33%).

Although obtaining direct hemodynamic information during exercise is invasive, carries some added risk, and is time consuming, studies that have included these measurements in addition to cardiopulmonary exercise responses have shown that they add independent prognostic information. However, in general the data sets have not been large enough or consistent enough to widely recommend invasive hemodynamic exercise testing to optimize risk assessment in all patients with HF.

Peak VO$_2$ Combined with Plasma Biomarkers in Predicting Risk

The degree of neurohumoral activation assessed by plasma levels of norepinephrine, natriuretic peptides, and endothelins has been recognized as a marker of increased risk in HF. Some investigators have suggested the application of neurohormones in combination with cardiopulmonary exercise testing to optimize predicting risk in patients with HF. The potential advantages of including these markers in multivariate risk models include the fact that they are more objective than peak VO_2 (e.g., peak VO_2 can be difficult to define in some patients), and as discussed above, many patients have a peak VO_2 that falls within the "grey zone" of intermediate risk.

Isnardet al[59] studied 264 consecutive patients with HF referred to two hospitals in France.

Plasma atrial natriuretic peptide (ANP), norepinephrine, and endothelin-1 were measured at rest in all patients, who also underwent symptom-limited maximal exercise. After a median follow-up of 789 days, 52 deaths and 31 heart transplantations occurred, of which four were urgent. In univariate analysis, New York Heart Association functional class, systolic blood pressure at rest, left ventricular end-diastolic diameter, left ventricular EF, peak VO_2, percent of predicted peak VO_2, plasma ANP, plasma norepinephrine, and plasma endothelin-1 were associated with survival without urgent heart transplantation. In a multivariate stepwise regression analysis, only plasma ANP, left ventricular EF, and plasma norepinephrine, but neither peak VO_2 nor percentage of predicted peak VO_2, were independent predictors of death or urgent heart transplantation.

de Groote et al[59] evaluated 407 consecutive patients referred to their department for evaluation of HF. Clinical and cardiopulmonary exercise variables, along with B-type natriuretic peptide (BNP) were assessed in a multivariate model to predict death or transplantation. After a median follow-up period of 787 days, there were 75 cardiac-related deaths and three urgent transplantations. Independent predictors of cardiac survival were percent of maximal predicted VO_2 (%VO_2, relative risk = 2.84), BNP (relative risk = 3.17), left atrial diameter (LAD) (relative risk = 2.04), age (relative risk = 1.93), and aldosterone (relative risk = 1.84). In patients with intramedian levels of BNP (<109 pg/mL), age was the only independent predictor of cardiac survival. However, in patients with supramedian levels of BNP, independent predictors of cardiac survival were %VO_2 achieved (relative risk = 3.76) and LAD (relative risk = 1.90).

Summary of Cardiopulmonary Exercise Testing and Risk Stratification in HF

Directly measured VO_2 has an established place in predicting outcomes in patients with HF. Peak VO_2 has been demonstrated in more than 100 studies to be an independent marker for risk of death or other endpoints. Increased automation of gas exchange systems has made these data easier to obtain, and this objective information is replacing the former dependence on subjective measures of clinical and functional status. Peak VO_2 is now a recognized criterion for selecting patients who could potentially benefit from heart transplantation. It is often a more powerful predictor of death when combined with other clinical, hemodynamic, and exercise data.

The commonly used cutpoint for peak VO_2 of 14 mL/kg/min to separate survivors from nonsurvivors, and thus help select patients for transplantation listing, is too simplistic. The combination of cardiopulmonary exercise data and other clinical and hemodynamic responses in multivariate scores has been shown to more powerfully stratify risk. It is also important to note that peak VO_2 is influenced by age, gender, body weight, and mode of exercise, and some studies have demonstrated that peak VO_2 expressed as a percentage of the predicted value (taking these variables into account) is a more powerful predictor of outcome than absolute peak VO_2.[21,60] However, previous studies are split in regard to whether VO_2 adjusted to percentage of normal outperforms absolute peak VO_2. Several studies have suggested that the estimate of survival using percentage of age-predicted VO_2 is enhanced in women,[61,62] but this observation requires further study. Another study reported that these two expressions did not differ in their prognostic power.[63] This approach is further complicated by the fact that there are many age- and gender-predicted "standards" for peak VO_2.[64]

An increasing number of studies has shown that cardiopulmonary variables other than peak VO_2 have important prognostic value in HF. The focus of these studies has centered on the VE/VO_2 slope, although other expressions of ventilatory efficiency, including the maximal ventilatory equivalent for CO_2, the OUES, various measures of oxygen kinetics, and oxygen uptake in recovery have all been shown to be strong prognostic markers. Among studies that have included both peak VO_2 and the VE/VCO_2 slope, all but one has reported that the VE/VCO_2 slope more powerfully predicts risk than peak VO_2. Although one must be cautious when two related variables are entered into a multivariate model, these studies give the impression that the VE/VCO_2 slope better predicts risk than peak VO_2. Summary reports from metabolic systems should be configured to provide both the VE/VCO_2 slope and peak VO_2, and consideration should be given to including the VE/VCO_2 slope in the HF and transplantation guidelines.

Relative to peak VO_2 or other cardiopulmonary exercise variables, hemodynamic variables are inconsistent in their ability to predict risk of death or clinical deterioration. The dissociation between hemodynamic observations and exercise responses underscores the complex nature of HF. Exertional symptoms and hemodynamic variables should be treated as separate entities; the former is influenced by musculoskeletal metabolism and strength, body composition, and motivation, in addition to cardiac function, whereas the latter is influenced largely by the degree of pump dysfunction. Nevertheless, more powerful estimates of risk have been demonstrated when peak VO_2 is combined with one or more hemodynamic variables.

Comparing or summarizing studies that have used different outcomes is also problematic. Many studies have used, in addition to death, softer endpoints such as hospitalizations, transplantation, change in listing status for transplantation, and others. Although this is often done to increase the number of study endpoints, such a study can no longer be considered one of "survival," and the subjectivity of many of these endpoints introduces the potential for significant bias and other errors that reduce the confidence in the study results. Although endpoints other than death are important outcomes clinically, they generally should not be used in survival analysis, and transplantation should be a censored event because this procedure completely changes the natural course of treatment for the disease. Future studies should also make every effort to classify causes of death by sudden verses progressive HF or noncardiac. The latter has rarely been done in previous studies, yet it is an important distinction clinically if the cardiologist is to know whether an intervention to prevent a lethal arrhythmia or to improve pump function is the more reasonable therapeutic approach to a given patient.

Although it seems clear that peak VO_2 has a vital role in predicting risk in HF populations, it has also been demonstrated that peak METs estimated from work rate also predicts risk in HF. Because maximal exercise time and peak VO_2 are correlated during exercise, some have suggested that these two variables could be used interchangeably when assessing exercise tolerance, and this raises the issue as to whether directly measured VO_2 offers any additional prognostic power over exercise time or workload achieved. This question is not a trivial one, because if exercise time has equivalent prognostic power, it would obviate the need for specialized laboratory equipment, time, expense, and patient discomfort associated with gas exchange analysis. However, compared with exercise time or workload achieved, the direct cardiopulmonary response is not only more precise but also offers a great deal of additional insight into the pathophysiology of exercise intolerance. Again, previous studies have generally not been large enough nor have data been gathered prospectively in a manner that would permit the comparison between measured and estimated VO_2 in prognosis; only one study has performed such a comparison. In that study, both peak VO_2 and watts achieved on a cycle ergometer were significant univariate predictors of death, although measured peak VO_2 was clearly a more important variable; by multivariate analysis, it was the only predictor of death.[20] Similar findings were implied in the study of Willens et al[13], and the V-Heft data,[19] but the former study involved only eight deaths (out of 30 patients over 15 months), and in the latter study the predictive power of exercise time was not presented, although it was stated that peak VO_2 was a better predictor of survival.

EVALUATION OF THERAPIES FOR HF

There are a number of medications indicated for treatment of systolic dysfunction that influence exercise responses, including vasoactive, antiarrhythmic, inotropic, and beta-blocking agents. In addition, cardiac resynchronization therapy (CRT) using pacemakers has evolved as an important therapy in selected HF patients, and the exercise test has been used to document the efficacy of CRT.

Angiotensin-Converting Enzyme Evaluation by Exercise Testing

Despite well-documented benefits of ACE inhibitors on prognosis in patients with HF, there is a lack of consistency in the results of trials investigating the effects of ACE inhibitors on exercise capacity. The inconsistencies cannot be readily explained by variations in effects on known neurohumoral or conventional hemodynamic factors. One potential reason for the observed inconsistencies is that the often-used parallel-group study design (which is ideal for mortality studies) may not be suitable for investigating drug effects on exercise capacity because dropouts from such studies tend to introduce selection biases, thereby confounding treatment effects. Kiowski et al[65] performed a meta-analysis of six placebo-controlled, randomized 3-month trials and reported a modest improvement in exercise test results associated with ACE inhibitor therapy. However, results from larger studies have not been supportive of an exercise benefit. The TRAndolapril Cardiac Evaluation (TRACE) study was a randomized controlled trial designed

to evaluate the effect of trandolapril on mortality in 1749 consecutive Danish patients with systolic dysfunction after a myocardial infarction.[66] In a prospective substudy, 254 patients underwent exercise tests at 1, 3, and 12 months. There was no improvement in exercise capacity or functional class associated with the drug. They felt that the results emphasize the importance of explaining to patients that ACE inhibitors provide protection against death and hospitalization but may not have any significant effect on symptoms.

Russell et al[67] contend that historically studies that used exercise testing as an endpoint to evaluate the efficacy of pharmacologic interventions in HF have been confounded by methodologic differences involving protocols, exercise endpoints, absence or misuse of gas-exchange data, and study design. A meta-analysis by Narang et al[68] would appear to confirm the suggestion that results of studies on the effects of ACE inhibitors on exercise capacity are influenced by differences in methodology. Thirty-five published, double-blind, randomized placebo-controlled trials, involving a total of 3411 patients, which compared the effects of ACE inhibitors versus placebo on exercise capacity in patients with symptomatic HF were identified. Studies were examined in relation to whether they used cross-over or parallel-group study designs, study size, use of treadmill versus bicycle exercise tests, year of publication, patient entry criteria, duration of follow-up, and the particular ACE inhibitor used. Exercise duration improved in 23 of the studies, while symptoms improved in 25 of the 33 studies which evaluated symptoms. In the majority of the trials (27 of 33), there was concordance between the effect of ACE inhibitors on symptoms and exercise capacity. There were six trials which showed discrepant results. Study size, duration of follow-up, and method of exercise testing used were found to be major factors affecting the outcome. Trials using treadmill exercise tests were more likely to be positive than those using bicycle ergometry. All nine trials with a study size more than 50, follow-up of 3 to 6 months, and using treadmill exercise tests showed improved exercise capacity as well as symptoms. These findings suggest that ACE inhibitors are more likely to show a favorable effect on exercise tolerance when more robust methodology is used; for example, those that are larger and involve a longer treatment period.

A small cross-over study suggested another explanation for the failure to find improvement in exercise tolerance with ACE therapy. Twelve patients with HF completed a randomized double-blind crossover trial of lisinopril 5 mg and 20 mg for 24 weeks, crossing over the doses at 12 weeks.[69] The primary endpoint was aerobic exercise capacity and cardiac performance at peak exercise. Peak VO_2 was significantly higher during the 5 mg per day dosage compared to the 20 mg dosage. Contrary to expectation, peak VO_2 was found to be greater with the lower dose of lisinopril, suggesting that therapy with ACE inhibitors for HF may require tailoring the doses to the individual to optimize functional benefits in relation to the assumed prognostic benefits.

Beta-Blocker Evaluation by Exercise Testing

The studies that have evaluated beta-blockade in HF have also had mixed results in terms of their effect on exercise capacity. Few studies have evaluated the gas exchange response to exercise in a controlled fashion after beta-blockade. Metra et al[70] did not observe any difference in peak VO_2 despite marked hemodynamic benefits after 3 months of

carvedilol therapy. In a more recent study from these investigators, neither carvedilol nor metoprolol had any effect on peak VO_2, although carvedilol resulted in a greater increase in exercise time.[71] Our own studies suggest that beta-blockade has minimal effects on peak VO_2 in patients with HF, although we did observe a 24% increase in peak watts achieved ($P < 0.05$) and a 25% increase in exercise time.[72] Given these results and the mixed observations of others,[73,74] the benefits of beta-blockade on exercise capacity appear to be positive but relatively small. We also noted a 28% improvement in VO_2 at the lactate threshold. Why beta-blockade would delay the lactate threshold specifically is unclear, but this observation concurs with some studies showing improvements in submaximal measures of exercise tolerance (e.g., 6-minute walk test) after beta-blockade in patients with HF.[75,76] Other studies have shown that beta-blockade with metoprolol or carvedilol has no effect on 6-minute walk performance.[77-80] Some of the major trials assessing the effects of beta-blockade on exercise test responses in HF are presented in Table 10-4.

TABLE 10-4. Major trials on the effect of beta blockers on exercise test responses in heart failure

Study	Year	Number of subjects	Beta blocker	Mode/Protocol	Effect on exercise response versus placebo
Dubach	2002	28	Bisoprolol	Ramp bicycle	No difference in peak VO_2, but trend for higher work rate and exercise time on bisoprolol
CIBIS	1994	641	Bisoprolol	Bicycle	21% improved NYHA class on bisoprolol versus 15% on placebo
MERIT-HF	2000	3991	Metoprolol	Treadmill	No increase in peak VO_2, but improvement in submaximal exercise performance. Exercise time and HF-related symptoms improved with metoprolol
RESOLVD	2000	426	Metoprolol	6MW	No increase in peak VO_2 or submaximal exercise performance while on metoprolol, but exercise time and HF-related symptoms improved
MDC	1993	383	Metoprolol	Bicycle	No change in peak VO_2, but improvement in submaximal exercise performance, exercise duration, and HF-related symptoms on metoprolol
ANZ	1997	415	Carvedilol	Treadmill	No effect on treadmill performance
PRECISE	1996	278	Carvedilol	6MW, 9MTM	No improvement in exercise performance
Colucci et al	1996	366	Carvedilol	9MTM	No improvement in exercise performance
MOCHA	1996	345	Carvedilol	6MW, 9MTM	No effect on exercise performance
Metra et al	2000	150	Metoprolol versus carvedilol	6MW	No difference in exercise tolerance, QoL, or sub-maximal exercise performance

HF, heart failure; 6MW, 6-minute walk test; 9MTM, 9-minute treadmill; QoL, quality of life.

Cardiac-Resynchronization Therapy Evaluation by Exercise Testing

CRT has been demonstrated to result in favorable ventricular remodeling, increased exercise capacity, and improved survival in HF patients. Dyssnchrony appears to contribute at least in part to the left ventricular dysfunction in HF, and by pacing dyssynchronous areas, the normal activation pattern of the ventricle can be achieved. Some of the studies using exercise testing to evaluate CRT follow.

Four hundred fifty-three patients with HF, an EF less than 35%, and a QRS interval greater than 130 msec were randomly assigned to a CRT group (228 patients) or to a control group (225 patients) for 6 months.[81] As compared to the control group, patients assigned to cardiac resynchronization experienced an improvement in distance walked in 6 minutes, quality of life, exercise time on the treadmill, and EF.

Auricchio et al[82] aimed to provide a detailed analysis of the changes in metabolic, ventilatory parameters, and heart rate profiles in patients with HF and ventricular conduction delay following implantation with resynchronization devices. They performed a retrospective review on 50 HF patients evaluated by cardiopulmonary exercise testing before and after CRT. Following CRT, peak VO_2 increased significantly from 14 to 17 mL/kg/min, and VO_2 at the ventilatory threshold increased from 9 to 12 mL/kg/min. All ventilatory and metabolic parameters significantly improved following CRT. Patients with more depressed metabolic and ventilatory parameters and higher heart rate at baseline appeared to benefit most from CRT.

The Multicenter InSync ICD Randomized Clinical Evaluation II (MIRACLE ICD II) was a randomized, double-blind, parallel-controlled clinical trial of CRT in HF patients with NYHA class II, EF less than or equal to 35%, and a QRS duration greater than or equal to 130 msec.[83] One hundred eighty-six patients were randomized: 101 to a control group (ICD activated, CRT off) and 85 to a CRT group (ICD activated, CRT on). Endpoints included peak VO_2, peak VE/VCO_2, NYHA class, quality of life, 6-minute walk distance, LV volumes and EF, and a composite clinical response. Compared with the control group at 6 months, no significant improvement was noted in peak VO_2, yet there were significant improvements in ventricular remodeling indices. CRT patients also showed statistically significant improvements in peak VE/VCO_2 and NYHA class. No significant differences were noted in 6-minute walk distance or quality of life scores.

In recent years, a number of other multicenter and single-center trials have assessed the effects of CRT on a variety of functional measures, including cardiopulmonary exercise responses, 6-minute walk performance, and quality of life.[84-87] Virtually all of these studies have shown the effects of CRT to be favorable. Therefore, a significant proportion of patients with HF appear to derive clinical benefits from CRT. While early studies suggested that the improvement in exercise tolerance after CRT was due to hemodynamic changes, other adaptations may include a better chronotropic response to exercise, reverse left ventricular remodeling, improved skeletal muscle metabolism, and more efficient regulation of vascular beds.[86,88] A summary of some of the major studies evaluating exercise test responses to CRT is presented in Table 10-5.

SUMMARY

HF represents the one category of patients with cardiovascular disease that is increasing in prevalence. Although the exercise test was once considered only a tool to diagnose coronary disease, it is now recognized that it has major applications for assessing functional capabilities, therapeutic interventions, and estimating prognosis in HF. Numerous hemodynamic abnormalities underlie the reduced exercise capacity commonly observed in chronic HF, including impaired heart rate responses, inability to distribute cardiac output normally, abnormal arterial vasodilatory capacity, abnormal cellular metabolism in skeletal muscle, higher than normal systemic vascular resistance, higher than normal pulmonary pressures, and ventilatory abnormalities that increase the work of breathing and cause exertional dyspnea.[54] Intervention with ACE-inhibition, beta-blockade, CRT, or exercise training can improve many of these abnormalities. However, although ACE inhibitors and beta-blockers are now widely used in HF because of their well-documented effects on survival, their effect on exercise capacity has been inconsistent. This is in part due to differences in methodology; for example, differences in study design, exercise protocols, functional endpoints used, and absence of gas exchange data. Submaximal exercise responses (e.g., the ventilatory threshold, the VE/VCO_2 slope, 6-minute walk performance) have shown marked improvements in some studies, but these responses are underutilized among studies assessing these interventions.

Over the last 15 years, exercise testing with ventilatory gas exchange responses has been demonstrated to have a critical role in the risk

TABLE 10–5. Summary of studies on the effects of resynchronization therapy on exercise capacity in patients with heart failure

Study (Year)	N	Inclusion criteria	Effect on exercise capacity
Auricchio (2004)	86	NYHA class II QRS > 150 msec	Improved peak VO_2 Higher ventilatory threshold Improved 6-minute walk distance
Chan (2003)	63	Consecutive CRT Patients with HF	Improved NYHA class Improved 6-minute walk distance Reduced LVEDD Improved LVEF
MIRACLE-ICD (2003)	636	NYHA class 2-4 LVEF < 35% QRS > 120 msec	Improved 6-minute walk distance
MUSTIC (2003)	58	NYHA class 3 LVEF < 35% QRS > 150 msec	Improved peak VO_2 Improved 6-minute walk distance Elevated AT Reduction in VE/VCO2 Improved QOL
Gras (2002)	103	Consecutive CRT Patients with HF	Improved NYHA class Improved QOL Improved 6-minute walk distance Improved LVEDD Improved mitral regurgitation and LV filling time
INSYNC (2002)	81	Symptomatic HF EF < 35% QRS > 130 msec	Improved NYHA class Improved 6-minute walk distance Improved LV dimensions Improved fractional shortening
MIRACLE (2002)	453	NYHA class 3-4 LVEF > 35% QRS > 130 msec	Improved peak VO_2 Improved 6-minute walk distance Improved QOL
Molhoek (2002)	40	NYHA class III or IV EF < 35% QRS > 120 msec	Improved NYHA class Improved QOL Improved 6-minute walk distance
PATH-CHF (2002)	53	NYHA class 3-4 QRS > 120 msec "Severe cardiomyopathy" PR interval > 150 msec	Improved peak VO_2 Improved 6-minute walk distance Elevated AT Reduction in VE/VCO2 Improved QOL Effect greater with lower baseline VO_2
CONTAK CD (2001)	490	NYHA class 2-4 LVEF > 35% QRS < 120 msec	Improved peak VO_2 Improved 6-minute walk distance Improved QOL

AT, anaerobic threshold; CM, cardiomyopathy; CRT, cardiac resynchronization therapy; HF, heart failure; LVEDD, left ventricular end-diastolic dimension; LVEF, left ventricular ejection fraction; NYHA, New York Heart Association; QOL, quality of life; VE/VCO$_2$, slope of minute ventilation/CO$_2$ production; VO$_2$, oxygen uptake.

paradigm in HF. In many studies, peak VO_2 has been shown to be a stronger predictor of risk then established clinical markers such as symptoms, clinical signs, EF, and other invasive hemodynamic data. However, these studies have also been confounded by differences in the approach to the exercise test, in addition to the use of different endpoints in the various studies (e.g., transplant listing, change in listing status, and hospitalization in addition to mortality). Recent studies have been consistent in the demonstration that the VE/VCO$_2$ slope is an even stronger predictor of

risk than peak VO_2. These studies have also suggested that other cardiopulmonary exercise test responses, for example, oxygen kinetics, oxygen uptake in recovery, and the OUES, are important risk markers. These may evolve to have a greater role in establishing risk in HF.

REFERENCES

1. Zile MR, Baicu CF, Gaasch WH: Diastolic heart failure—Abnormalities in active relaxation and passive stiffness of the left ventricle N Engl J Med 2004;350:1953-1959.

2. Gottdiener JS, McClelland RL, Marshall R, et al: Outcome of congestive heart failure in elderly persons: Influence of left ventricular systolic function. The Cardiovascular Health Study. Ann Intern Med 2002;137:631-639.

3. Kannel WB, Belanger AJ: Epidemiology of heart failure. Am Heart J 1991;121:951-957.

4. Leor J, Cohen S: Myocardial tissue engineering: Creating a muscle patch for a wounded heart. Ann N Y Acad Sci 2004;1015:312-319.

5. Myers J, Gullestad L: The role of exercise testing and gas exchange measurement in the prognostic assessment of patients with heart failure. Curr Opin Cardiol 1998;13:145-155.

6. Myers J: Applications of cardiopulmonary exercise testing in the management of cardiovascular and pulmonary disease. Int J Sports Med 2005;26(suppl 1):S49-S55.

7. Costanzo MR, Augustine S, Bourge R, et al: Selection and treatment of candidates for heart transplantation. A statement for health professionals from the Committee on Heart Failure and Cardiac Transplantation of the Council on Clinical Cardiology, American Heart Association. Circulation 1995;92:3593-3612.

8. Mudge GH, Goldstein S, Addonizio LJ, et al: Twenty-fourth Bethesda conference: Cardiac transplantation: Task Force 3: Recipient guidelines/prioritization. J Am Coll Cardiol 1993;22:21-31.

9. Wasserman K, Hansen JE, Sue DY, et al: Principles of Exercise Testing and Interpretation, 3rd ed. Philadelphia, Lippincott, Williams & Wilkins, 1999.

10. Stewart S, Marley JE, Horowitz JD: Effects of a multidisciplinary, home-based intervention on planned readmissions and survival among patients with chronic congestive heart failure: A randomized controlled trial. Lancet 1999;354:1077-1083.

11. Szlachcic J, Massie BM, Kramer BL, et al: Correlates and prognostic implication of exercise capacity in chronic congestive heart failure. Am J Cardiol 1985;55:1037-1042.

12. Likoff MJ, Chandler SL, Kay HR: Clinical determinants of mortality in chronic congestive heart failure secondary to idiopathic dilated or to ischemic cardiomyopathy. Am J Cardiol 1987;59:634-638.

13. Willens HJ, Blevins RD, Wrisley D, et al: The prognostic value of functional capacity in patients with mild to moderate heart failure. Am Heart J 1987;114:377-382.

14. Mancini DM, Eisen H, Kussmaul W, et al: Value of peak exercise oxygen consumption for optimal timing of cardiac transplantation in ambulatory patients with heart failure. Circulation 1991;83:778-786.

15. Stevenson LW, Couper G, Natterson B, et al: Target heart failure populations for newer therapies. Circulation 1995;92(suppl II): II-174-II-181.

16. Opasich C, Pinna GD, Bobbio M, et al: Peak exercise oxygen consumption in chronic heart failure: Toward efficient use in the individual patient. J Am Coll Cardiol 1998;31:766-775.

17. Haywood GA, Rickenbacher PR, Trindade PT, et al: Analysis of deaths in patients awaiting heart transplantation: Impact on patient selection criteria. Heart 1996;75:455-462.

18. Saxon LA, Stevenson WG, Middlekauff HR, et al: Predicting death from progressive heart failure secondary to ischemic or idiopathic dilated cardiomyopathy. Am J Cardiol 1993;72:62-65.

19. Cohn JN, Johnson GR, Shabetai R, et al: Ejection fraction, peak exercise oxygen consumption, cardiothoracic ratio, ventricular arrhythmias, and plasma norepinephrine as determinants of prognosis in heart failure. Circulation 1993;87[suppl VI]:VI-16.

20. Myers J, Gullestad L, Vagelos R, et al: Clinical, hemodynamic, and cardiopulmonary exercise test determinants of outcome in patients referred for evaluation of heart failure. Ann Intern Med 1998;129: 286-293.

21. Osada N, Chaitman BR, Miller LW, et al: Cardiopulmonary exercise testing identifies low risk patients with heart failure and severely impaired exercise capacity considered for heart transplantation. J Am Coll Cardiol 1998;31:577-582.

22. Roul G, Moulichon M-E, Bareiss P, et al: Exercise peak VO2 determination in chronic heart failure: is it still of value? Eur Heart J 1994;15:495-502.

23. Kao W, Winkel EM, Johnson MR, et al: Role of maximal oxygen consumption in establishment of heart transplant candidacy for heart failure patients with intermediate exercise tolerance. Am J Cardiol 1997;79:1124-1127.

24. Gitt A, Wasserman K, Kilkowski C, et al: Exercise anaerobic threshold and ventilatory efficiency identify heart failure patients for high risk of early death. Circulation 2002;106:3079-3084.

25. Arena R, Myers J, Aslam S, et al: Peak VO2 and VE/VCO2 slope in patients with heart failure: A prognostic comparison. Am Heart J 2004;147:354-360.

26. Wada O, Asanoi H, Miyagi K, et al: Importance of abnormal lung perfusion in excessive exercise ventilation in chronic heart failure. Am Heart J 1992;125:790-798.

27. Corra U, Mezzani A, Bosimini E, et al: Ventilatory response to exercise improves risk stratification in patients with chronic heart failure and intermediate functional capacity. Am Heart J 2002;143: 418-426.

28. Coats AJS: Grading heart failure and predicting survival: Slope of VE versus VCO2. In: Wasserman K, Cardiopulmonary Exercise Testing and Cardiovascular Health. Armonk, NY, Futura, 2002, pp 53-62.

29. Kleber FX, Vietzke G, Wernecke KD, et al: Impairment of ventilatory efficiency in heart failure: Prognostic impact. Circulation 2000; 101:2803-2809.

30 Robbins M, Francis G, Pashkow FJ, et al: Ventilatory and heart rate responses to exercise: Better predictors of heart failure mortality than peak oxygen consumption. Circulation 1999;100:2411-2417.

31. Arena R, Myers J, Aslam SS, et al: Technical considerations related to the minute ventilation/carbon dioxide output slope in patients with heart failure. Chest 2003;124:720-727.

32. Chua TP, Ponikowski P, Harrington D, et al: Clinical correlates and prognostic significance of the ventilatory response to exercise in chronic heart failure. J Am Coll Cardiol 1997;29:1585-1590.

33. Francis DP, Shamim W, Davies LC, et al: Cardiopulmonary exercise testing for prognosis in chronic heart failure: Continuous and independent prognostic value from VE/VCO2 slope and peak VO2. Eur Heart J 2000;21:154-161.

34. Bol E, de Vries WR, Mosterd WL, et al: Cardiopulmonary exercise parameters in relation to all-cause mortality in patients with chronic heart failure. Int J Cardiol 2000;72:255-263.

35. Rickli H, Kiowski W, Brehm M, et al:Combining low-intensity and maximal exercise test results improves prognostic prediction in chronic heart failure. J Am Coll Cardiol 2003;42:116-122.

36. Schalcher C, Rickli H, Brehm M, et al: Prolonged oxygen uptake kinetics during low-intensity exercise are related to poor prognosis in patients with mild-to-moderate congestive heart failure. Chest 2003;124:580-586.

37. Brunner-La Rocca HP, Weilenman D, Schalcher C, et al: Prognostic significance of oxygen uptake kinetics during low level exercise in patients with heart failure. Am J Cardiol 1999;84:741-744.

38. Baba R, Tsuyuki K, Kimura Y, et al: Oxygen uptake efficiency slope as a useful measure of cardiorespiratory functional reserve in adult cardiac patient. Eur J Appl Physiol 1999;80:397-401.

39. Baba R, Nagashima M, Goto M, et al: Oxygen uptake efficiency slope: A new index of cardiorespiratory functional reserve derived from the relation between oxygen uptake and minute ventilation during incremental exercise. J Am Coll Cardiol 1996;28:1567-1572.

40. Van Laethem C, Bartunek J, Goethals M, et al: Oxygen uptake efficiency slope, a new submaximal parameter in evaluating exercise capacity in chronic heart failure patients. Am Heart J 2005;149: 175-180.

41. Mourot L, Perrey S, Tordi N, Rouillon JD: Evaluation of fitness level by the oxygen uptake efficiency slope after a short-term intermittent endurance training. Int J Sports Med 2004;25:85-91.

42. Pichon A, Jonville S, Denjean A: Evaluation of the interchangeability of VO2MAX and oxygen uptake efficiency slope. Can J Appl Physiol 2002;27:589-601.

43. Pardaens K, Van Cleemput J, Vanhaecke J, Fagard RH: Peak oxygen uptake better predicts outcome than submaximal respiratory data in heart transplant candidates. Circulation 2000;101:1152-1157.

44. de Groote P, Millaire A, Decoulx E, et al: Kinetics of oxygen consumption during and after exercise in patients with dilated cardiomyopathy. J Am Coll Cardiol 1996;28:168-175.

45. Hayashida W, Kumada T, Kohno F, et al: Post-exercise oxygen uptake kinetics in patients with left ventricular dysfunction. Int J Cardiol 1993;38:63-72.

46. Pavia L, Myers J, Cesare R: Recovery kinetics of oxygen uptake and heart rate in patients with coronary artery disease and heart failure. Chest 1999;116:808-813.

47. Cohen-Solal A, Laperche T, Morvan D, et al: Prolonged kinetics of recovery of oxygen consumption after maximal graded exercise in patients with chronic heart failure. Circulation 1995;91:2924-2932.

48. Sietsema KE, Ben-Dov I, Zhang YY, et al: Dynamics of oxygen uptake for submaximal exercise and recovery in patients with chronic heart failure. Chest 1994;105:1693-1700.

49. Scrutinio D, Passantino A, Lagioia R, et al: Percent achieved of predicted peak exercise oxygen uptake and kinetics of recovery of oxygen uptake after exercise for risk stratification in chronic heart failure. Int J Cardiol 1998;64:117-124.

50. Myers J, Gullestad L, Vagelos R, et al: Cardiopulmonary exercise testing and prognosis in severe heart failure: 14 mL/kg/min revisited. Am Heart J 2000;139:78-84.

51. Myers J, Geiran O, Simonsen S, et al: Clinical and exercise test determinants of survival after cardiac transplantation. Chest 2003;124:2000-2005.

52. Madsen BK, Hansen JF, Stokholm KH, et al: Chronic congestive heart failure. Description and survival of 190 consecutive patients with a diagnosis of chronic congestive heart failure based on clinical signs and symptoms. Eur Heart J 1994;15:303-310.

53. Dec GW: Idiopathic dilated cardiomyopathy. N Engl J Med 1994;331:1564-1575.

54. Myers J, Froelicher VF: Hemodynamic determinants of exercise capacity in chronic heart failure. Ann Intern Med 1991;115:377-386.

55. Wilson JR, Rayos G, Keoh TK, Gothard P: Dissociation between peak exercise oxygen consumption and hemodynamic dysfunction in potential heart transplantation candidates. J Am Coll Cardiol 1995;26:429-435.

56. Chomsky DB, Lang CC, Rayos GH, et al: Hemodynamic exercise testing: A valuable tool in the selection of cardiac transplantation candidates. Circulation 1996;94:3176-3183.

57. Metra M, Faggiano P, D'Aloia A et al: Use of cardiopulmonary exercise testing with hemodynamic monitoring in the prognostic assessment of ambulatory patients with chronic heart failure. J Am Coll Cardiol 1999;33:943-950.

58. Isnard R, Pousset F, Chafirovskaia O, et al: Combination of B-type natriuretic peptide and peak oxygen consumption improves risk stratification in outpatients with chronic heart failure. Am Heart J 2003;146:729-735.

59. de Groote P, Dagorn J, Soudan B, et al: B-type natriuretic peptide and peak exercise oxygen consumption provide independent information for risk stratification in patients with stable congestive heart failure. J Am Coll Cardiol 2004;43:1584-1589.

60. Stelken AM, Younis LT, Jennison SH, et al: Prognostic value of cardiopulmonary exercise testing using percent achieved of predicted peak oxygen uptake for patients with ischemic and dilated cardiomyopathy. J Am Coll Cardiol 1996;27:345-352.

61. Aaronson KD, Mancini DM: Is percentage of predicted maximal exercise oxygen consumption a better predictor of survival than peak exercise oxygen consumption for patients with severe heart failure? J Heart Lung Transplant 1995;14:981-989.

62. Richards DR, Mehra MR, Ventura HO, et al: Usefulness of peak oxygen consumption in predicting outcome of heart failure in women verses men. Am J Cardiol 1997;80:1236-1238.

63. Scrutinio D, Passantino A, Lagioia R, et al: Percent achieved of predicted peak exercise oxygen uptake and kinetics of recovery of oxygen uptake after exercise for risk stratification in chronic heart failure. Int J Cardiol 1998;64:117-124.

64. Myers J: Essentials of Cardiopulmonary Exercise Testing. Champaign: Human Kinetics, 1996.

65. Kiowski W, Sutsch G, Dossegger L: Clinical benefit of angiotensin-converting enzyme inhibitors in chronic heart failure. J Cardiovasc Pharmacol 1996;27(Suppl 2):S19-24.

66. Abdulla J, Burchardt H, Z Abildstrom S, et al: The angiotensin converting enzyme inhibitor trandolapril has neutral effect on exercise tolerance or functional class in patients with myocardial infarction and reduced left ventricular systolic function. Eur Heart J 2003;24:2116-2122.

67. Russell SD, Selaru P, Pyne DA, et al: Rationale for use of an exercise end point and design for the ADVANCE (A Dose evaluation of a Vasopressin ANtagonist in HF patients undergoing Exercise) trial. Am Heart J 2003;145:179-186.

68. Narang R, Swedberg K, Cleland JG: What is the ideal study design for evaluation of treatment for heart failure? Insights from trials assessing the effect of ACE inhibitors on exercise capacity. Eur Heart J: 1996;17:120-134.

69. Cooke GA, Williams SG, Marshall P, et al: A mechanistic investigation of ACE inhibitor dose effects on aerobic exercise capacity in heart failure patients. Eur Heart J 200223:1360-1368.

70. Metra M, Nardi M, Giubbini R, Cas LD: Effects of short- and long-term carvedilol administration on rest and exercise hemodynamic variables, exercise capacity and clinical conditions in patients with idiopathic dilated cardiomyopathy. J Am Coll Cardiol 1994;24:1678-1687.

71. Metra M, Giubbini R, Nodari S, et al: Differential effects of β-blockers in patients with heart failure. Circulation 2000;102:546-551.

72. Dubach P, Myers J, Bonetti P, et al: Effects of bisoprolol fumarate on left ventricular size, function, and exercise capacity in patients with heart failure: analysis with magnetic resonance myocardial tagging. Am Heart J. 2002;143(4):676-83.

73. Sackner-Bernstein JD, Mancini DM: Rationale for treatment of patients with chronic heart failure with adrenergic blockade. J Am Coll Cardiol 1995;274:1462-1467.

74. Hjalmarson A, Kneider M, Waagstein F: The role of beta-blockers in left ventricular dysfunction and heart failure. Drugs 1997;54:501-510.

75. Packer M, Colucci WS, Sackner-Bernstein JD et al: Double-blind, placebo-controlled study of the effects of carvedilol in patients with moderate to severe heart failure. The PRECISE Trial. Circulation 1996;94:2793-2799.

76. Sanderson JE, Chan SK, Yu CM, et al: Beta blockers in heart failure: A comparison of a vasodilating beta blocker with metoprolol. Heart 1998;79:86-92.

77. Colucci WS, Packer M, Bristow MR, et al: Carvedilol inhibits clinical progression in patients with mild symptoms of heart failure. US Carvedilol Heart Failure Study Group. Circulation 1996;94:2800-2806.

78. Packer M, Colucci WS, Sackner-Bernstein JD, et al: Double-blind, placebo-controlled study of the effects of carvedilol in patients with moderate to severe heart failure. The PRECISE Trial. Prospective randomized evaluation of carvedilol on symptoms and exercise. Circulation 1996;94:2793-2799.

79. The RESOLVED Investigators: Effects of metoprolol CR in patients with ischemic and dilated cardiomyopathy: The randomized evaluation of strategies for left ventricular dysfunction pilot study. Circulation 2000;101:378-384.

80. Bristow MR, Gilbert EM, Abraham WT, et al: Carvedilol produces dose-related improvements in left ventricular function and survival in subjects with chronic heart failure. MOCHA Investigators. Circulation 1996;94:2807-2816.

81. Abraham WT, Fisher WG, Smith AL, et al: Multicenter InSync Randomized Clinical Evaluation. Cardiac resynchronization in chronic heart failure. N Engl J Med 2002;346:1845-1853.

82. Auricchio A, Kloss M, Trautmann SI, et al: Exercise performance following cardiac resynchronization therapy in patients with heart failure and ventricular conduction delay. Am J Cardiol 2002;89:198-203.

83. Abraham WT, Young JB, Leon AR, et al: Effects of cardiac resynchronization on disease progression in patients with left ventricular systolic dysfunction, an indication for an implantable cardioverter-defibrillator, and mildly symptomatic chronic heart failure Circulation 2004;110:2864-2868. Epub 2004 Oct 25.

84. Molhock SG, Bax JJ, van Erven L, et al: Comparison of benefits from cardiac resynchronization therapy in patients with ischemic cardiomyopathy versus idiopathic dilated cardiomyopathy. Am J Cardiol 2004;93:860-863.

85. Chan KL, Tang AS, Achilli A, et al: Functional and echocardiographic improvement following multisite biventricular pacing for congestive heart failure. Can J Cardiol 2003;19:387-390.

86. Gururaj AV: Cardiac resynchronization therapy: Effects on exercise capacity in the patient with chronic heart failure. J Cardiopulm Rehabil 2004;24:1-7.

87. Kuhlkamp V; InSync 7272 ICD World Wide Investigators. Initial experience with an implantable cardioverter-defibrillator incorporating cardiac resynchronization therapy. J Am Coll Cardiol 2002;39:790-797.

88. Khaykin Y, Saad E, Wilkoff B: Pacing in heart failure: The benefit of revascularization. Cleve Clin J Med 2003;70:841-865.

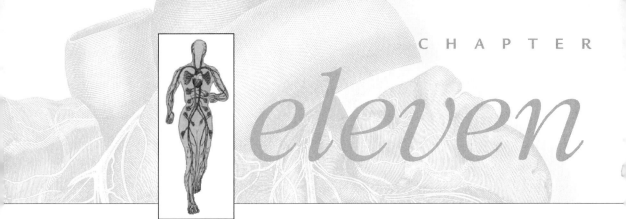

Special Applications: Screening Apparently Healthy Individuals

INTRODUCTION

Definition of Screening

Screening can be defined as the presumptive identification of unrecognized disease by the utilization of procedures that can be applied rapidly. The relative value of techniques for identifying individuals who have asymptomatic or latent coronary heart disease (CHD) should be assessed to optimally and cost-effectively direct secondary preventive efforts towards those with disease.

Criteria for Selecting a Screening Procedure

Eight criteria have been proposed for the selection of a screening procedure:

1. The procedure is acceptable and appropriate
2. The quantity and/or quality of life can be favorably altered
3. The results of intervention outweigh any adverse effects
4. The target disease has an asymptomatic period during which its outcome can be altered
5. Acceptable treatments are available
6. The prevalence and seriousness of the disease justify the costs of intervention
7. The procedure is relatively easy and inexpensive
8. Sufficient resources are available

Guides for Deciding if Screening Should be Performed

In addition, seven guides have been recommended for deciding whether a community screening program does more harm than good and they are as follows:

1. Has the program's effectiveness been demonstrated in a randomized trial, and if so,
2. Are efficacious treatments available?
3. Does the current burden of suffering warrant screening?
4. Is there a good screening test?
5. Does the program reach those who could benefit from it?
6. Can the healthcare system cope with the screening program?
7. Will those who had a positive screening comply with subsequent advice and interventions?

Screening Efficacy

These criteria will be resolved and the questions will be answered relative to the exercise test in this chapter. However, true demonstration of the effectiveness of a screening technique requires randomizing the target population, one half receiving the screening technique, standardized action being taken in response to the screening test results, and then outcomes being assessed. For the screening technique to be effective, the screened group must have lower mortality and/or morbidity. Such a study has been completed for mammography but not for any cardiac testing modalities. The next best validation of efficacy is to demonstrate that the technique improves the discrimination of those asymptomatic individuals with higher risk for events over that possible with the available risk factors. Mathematical modeling makes it possible to determine how well a population will be classified if the characteristics of the testing method are known.

PREVENTION OF CORONARY ARTERY DISEASE

Risk Factor Scores

Targeting asymptomatic individuals with early disease could facilitate the process of primary prevention of CHD. Thus, it is advisable to evaluate screening methods for detection of coronary artery disease (CAD) prior to death or disability. For a screening test to be worth the additional expense it must add significantly to the ability of the standard risk factors to identify asymptomatic individuals with subclinical disease. The method with which the risk is estimated with the risk factors must also be considered for such a comparison. Simple adding of risk factors, as recommended by JNC or NCEP, is not as accurate as using the logistic regression equations developed from the Framingham data.[1] In an asymptomatic population, the Framingham score calculates an estimate of the 5-year incidence of cardiovascular events using age, smoking, diabetes, standing systolic blood pressure, ECG-left ventricular hypertrophy (LVH), and the levels of high density lipoprotein (HDL) and total cholesterol.[2] The most recent version of the Framingham score removed ECG-LVH, since its prevalence has declined with the improved treatment of high blood pressure.[3]

The Framingham group evaluated its risk score, designed to estimate the 10-year risk of CHD. The score was assessed to see if it also predicted lifetime risk for CHD.[4] All subjects in the Framingham Heart Study examined from 1971 to 1996 who were free of CHD were included. Subjects were stratified into age- and gender-specific tertiles of Framingham risk score (FRS), and lifetime risk for CHD was estimated. They followed 2716 men and 3500 women; 939 developed CHD and 1363 died free of CHD. At 40 years of age, in risk score tertiles 1, 2, and 3, respectively, the lifetime risks for CHD were 38%, 42%, and 51% for men and

12%, 25%, and 33% for women. At age of 80 years, risks were 16%, 17%, and 39% for men and 13%, 22%, and 27% for women, respectively. The FRS stratified lifetime risk well for women at all ages. It performed less well in younger men but improved at older ages as remaining life expectancy approached 10 years. Lifetime risks contrasted sharply with shorter term risks: at age 40 years, the 10-year risks of CHD in tertiles 1, 2, and 3, respectively, were 0%, 2%, and 12% for men and 0%, 0.7%, and 2% for women. The Framingham 10-year CHD risk prediction model discriminated short-term risk well for men and women. However, it may not identify subjects with low short-term but high lifetime risk for CHD, likely due to changes in risk factor status over time. The serial use of multivariate risk models is most likely the only way to reliably predict lifetime risk for CHD; the Framingham score can also be calculated yearly as a motivational tool to keep patients aware of their risk factor status.

Baseline levels of C-reactive protein (CRP) were evaluated among 27,939 apparently healthy women who were followed up for myocardial infarction (MI), stroke, coronary revascularization, or CV death.[5] Crude and FRS-adjusted relative risks of incident CV events were calculated across a full range of CRP levels. CV risks increased linearly from the very lowest (referent) to the very highest levels of CRP. Crude relative risks for those with baseline CRP levels of less than 0.5 to greater than 20.0 mg/L trended from one to eight times. After adjustment for FRS, these risks trended from one to three times. All risk estimates remained significant in analyses stratified by FRS and after control for diabetes. Of the total cohort, 15% had CRP less than 0.50 mg/L, and 5% had CRP more than 10.0 mg/L. Both very low (<0.5 mg/L) and very high (>10 mg/L) levels of CRP provide important prognostic information on CV risk. Whether or not CRP lowers cardiovascularly risk with statins and acetylsalicylic acid has not been demonstrated, but this marker certainly can be used along with the Framingham score to screen for CAD risk.

The SCORE project was initiated to develop a risk scoring system for use in the clinical management of CV risk in European clinical practice that would be more appropriate for Europeans than the American population-derived Framingham score (http://www.escardio.org/initiatives/prevention/SCORE+Risk+Charts.htm).[6] The project assembled a pool of datasets from 12 European cohort studies, mainly carried out in general population settings. There were 205,178 persons (88,080 women and

117,098 men) representing 2.7 million person-years of follow-up. There were 7934 CV deaths, of which 5652 were deaths from CHD. Ten-year risk of fatal CV disease was calculated using a Weibull model in which age was used as a measure of exposure time to risk rather than as a risk factor. Separate estimation equations were calculated for CHD and for noncoronary CV disease. These were calculated for high- and low-risk regions of Europe. Two parallel estimation models were developed, one based on total cholesterol and the other on total cholesterol/HDL cholesterol ratio. The risk estimations were displayed graphically in simple risk charts. Predictive value of the risk charts was examined by applying them to subjects aged 45 to 64 years; areas under receiver operating characteristics curves ranged from 0.71 to 0.84.

Data from two population studies (The Glostrup Population Studies, n = 4757, the Framingham Heart Study, n = 2562) were used to examine three different levels of cross-validation.[7] The first level of examination was whether a risk score developed from one sample adequately ordered the risk of participants in the other sample, using the area under a receiver operating characteristic curve. The second level compared the magnitude of coefficients in logistic models in the two studies; while the third level tested whether the level of risk of CHD death in one sample could be estimated based on a risk function from the other sample. CHD mortality was 515 per 100,000 person-years in Framingham and 311 per 100,000 person-years in Glostrup. The area under curve was between 0.75 and 0.77 and regardless of which risk score was used. Logistic coefficients did not differ significantly between studies. The FRS significantly overestimated the risk in the Glostrup sample and the Glostrup risk score underestimated the Framingham sample. Using a Framingham risk-score on a Danish population led to a significant overestimation of coronary risk. The validity of risk-scores developed from populations with different incidences of the disease should preferably be tested prior to their application.

Non-Exercise Test Measurements

Other non-exercise test measurements that have been recommended as screening techniques include the resting ECG, cardiac fluoroscopy, digital radiographic imaging carotid ultrasound measurements of intimal thickening (i.e., >1mm), the ankle-brachial index, and electron beam computed tomography (EBCT). Various add-on techniques have been recommended to improve the diagnostic characteristics of exercise ECG testing. These include ECG criteria, other exercise test responses, cardiac radionuclide procedures, cardiokymography (CKG), echocardiography (ECHO), and the computerized application of Bayesian statistics. We will provide a cursory look at some of these while we concentrate on the standard exercise test and its combination with risk factors.

TEST PERFORMANCE

In order to evaluate the value of any screening test, sensitivity, specificity, predictive value, and relative risk must be demonstrated. Although discussed in depth elsewhere, these terms will be presented here briefly. *Sensitivity* is the percentage of times a test gives an abnormal response when those with disease are tested. *Specificity* is the percentage of times a test gives a normal response when those without disease are tested—a definition quite different from the conventional use of the word "specific." These two values are inversely related and are determined by the discriminant values or cutpoints chosen for the test that separate abnormal from normal subjects and the intrinsic ability of the test to separate those with disease from those without disease. The predictive value of an abnormal test is the percentage of individuals with an abnormal test who have disease. The relative risk or odds ratio of an abnormal test response is the relative chance of having disease if the test is abnormal compared to having disease if the test is normal. The values for these last two terms are dependent upon the prevalence of disease in the population being tested.

A basic step in applying any testing procedure for the separation of normal subjects from patients with a disease is to determine a test value that best separates the two groups. One problem is that there is usually a considerable overlap of measurement values of a test in groups with and without disease. Consider two bell-shaped normal distribution curves, one representing a normal population and the other representing a population with disease, with a certain amount of overlap of the two curves (see Fig. 7-1). Along the vertical axis is the number of patients and along the horizontal axis could be the value for measurements such as Q-wave size, exercise-induced ST-segment depression, or troponin. The optimal test would be able to achieve the most marked separation of these two bell-shaped curves and minimize the overlap. Unfortunately, most tests have a considerable overlap of the range of measurements for the normal population and for those with heart disease. Therefore, problems arise when a certain value is used to separate these two groups (i.e., Q-wave amplitude or width, 0.1 mV of ST-segment depression, <5 METs exercise capacity, three ventricular beats). If the value is set far to the right (i.e., 0.2 mV of ST-segment depression) in order to identify nearly all the normal subjects as being free of disease, the test will have a high specificity. However, a substantial number of those with disease will be called normal. If a value is chosen far to the left (i.e., 0.05 mV ST-segment depression) to identify nearly all those with disease as being abnormal, giving the test a high sensitivity, then many normal subjects will be identified as abnormal. If a cutpoint value is chosen that equally mislabel the normal subjects and those with disease, the test will have its highest predictive accuracy.

However, there may be reasons for wanting to adjust a test to have a relatively higher sensitivity or relatively higher specificity than possible when predictive accuracy is optimal. For instance, sensitivity should be highest in the emergency room and the specificity the highest when doing insurance exams. Remember that sensitivity and specificity are inversely related. That is, when sensitivity is the highest, specificity is the lowest and vice versa. Any test has a range of inversely related sensitivities and specificities that can be chosen by selecting a certain discriminant or diagnostic value. Attempts have been made to use a series of tests to improve diagnostic power, but test interaction is complex. Usually the highest sensitivity and the lowest specificity of the tests represent their combined performance.

RESTING ECG AS A SCREENING TECHNIQUE

As part of the Copenhagen City Heart Study, nearly 20,000 men and women, 20 years of age or older, had a resting 12-lead ECG done.[8] The Minnesota Code was used to classify the electrocardiograms (ECGs). The prevalence of all electrocardiographic findings, with the exception of axis deviation, high-amplitude R waves, minor Q-wave abnormalities, and prolonged or short PR interval, was very low below the age of 40 in men and 50 in women. Rates for Q-wave abnormalities, left axis deviation, ST depression, premature beats, and atrial fibrillation increased with age and were higher for men than for women. A strong association between total mortality and major ST depression and T-wave abnormalities, Q-wave patterns, and left bundle branch block existed. During a period from 1976 to 1980, 489 subjects died, but there were only a few deaths among those under the age of 50. As a result, and because the prevalence of ECG abnormalities was low in the young, relative risk was only significant in those 50 years or older. Over 50% of the deaths were due to non-CV-specific deaths. The relative risk of ST-segment depression was as high as five times. Some Q-wave abnormalities carried a relative risk of about three times.

Rose et al[9] performed limb lead ECGs on 8403 male civil servants aged 40 to 64 and coded them using the Minnesota Code.[9] CHD mortality rates were established over the ensuing 5 years (657 men died). Q waves, left axis deviation, ST depression, T-wave changes, ventricular conduction defects, and atrial fibrillation were related to mortality. However, there was little significance to increased R-wave amplitude, QT interval, premature beats, or heart rate extremes. Among the 6% of men with patterns suggesting ischemia, the subsequent CHD mortality was little more than 1% per year and even lower in those who were asymptomatic when screened. However, a five times risk ratio was found.

As part of the Busselton City, Australia Study, 2119 unselected subjects had a 12-lead ECG performed and coded according to the Minnesota Code.[10] In addition, all subjects completed the Rose chest pain questionnaire. Subjects were between the ages of 40 and 79 and included both male and female. Between 1967 and 1979, mortality in this group was determined and the 13-year mortality from CV disease was significantly higher in those with an initial ECG that showed Q wave and QS patterns, left axis deviation, ST-segment depression, and T-wave abnormalities, atrial fibrillation, or premature ventricular beats. In subjects free of angina and other ECG abnormalities, ventricular extrasystoles were associated with a significantly higher mortality from CV disease compared with controls. Q-wave patterns had the highest risk ratio (3.7×), whereas the other abnormalities had about a two times risk ratio.

As part of the Manitoba Study, a cohort of 3983 men with a mean age of 30 years at entry were followed with annual examinations, including ECG, since 1948.[11] During the 30-year observation period, 70 cases of sudden death occurred in men without previous clinical manifestations of heart disease. The prevalence of ECG abnormalities before sudden death was 71%. The frequencies of these abnormalities was 31% for major ST and T-wave abnormalities, 16% for ventricular extra beats, 13% for LVH, and 7% for left bundle branch block. Left bundle branch block had a 14 times risk for sudden death, while ST and T-wave abnormalities, increased R-wave and premature beats had a relative risk as high as five times. It must be remembered that this was a serial ECG study with ECGs being obtained usually each year and thus specificity was not determined.

In 2000 Framingham Study participants, the 12-lead ECG failed to correctly classify over half of the persons with clinically definite heart disease.[12] The sensitivity was about 50% and specificity 90%. The utility of the ECG for assessing prior infarction can be evaluated by comparing results with post-mortem findings or by comparing results with survivors of a previously documented infarction. Levine and Phillips[13] found that only 20% of old infarcts found at autopsy were correctly identified by the ECG. ECG abnormalities may not persist in patients with a previously documented MI. In the Framingham Study, 18% of the infarction patients had no ECG abnormalities on subsequent examination. Other studies have reported a 10% to 15% loss of diagnostic Q waves in the year following an MI. However, the ECG has a much stronger prognostic value in survivors of a CHD event than in apparently healthy populations.

The independent contributions of baseline major and minor ECG abnormalities to subsequent 11.5-year risk of death were explored among 9643 white men and 7990 white women aged 40 to 64 years without definite prior CHD in the Chicago Heart Association Detection Project in Industry by Liao et al.[14] At baseline, prevalence rates of major ECG abnormalities were higher in women than in men, with age-adjusted rates of 12.9% and 9.6%, respectively. Minor ECG abnormalities were more common in men than in women (7.3% versus 4.5%). Both major and minor ECG abnormalities were associated with an increased risk of death from CHD, all CV diseases, and all causes. The strength of these associations was greater in men than in women. When baseline age and other risk factors were taken into account, major ECG abnormalities continued to be significantly related to each cause of death in both genders with much larger adjusted absolute excess risk and relative risk for men than for women. In multivariate analyses, minor ECG abnormalities contributed independently to risk of death in men, but not clearly so in women.

The aim of an Italian project was to determine the predictive power on 6-year mortality of ECG findings in asymptomatic subjects.[15] The cohorts were spread throughout Italy. ECGs were coded for five categories of abnormalities: Q-QS abnormalities, ST-T abnormalities, increased R waves, major arrhythmias, and blocks. Some clinically relevant ECG combinations were also analyzed. Most ECG findings on most occasions were associated with an excess mortality from the three endpoints. The strongest predictors of fatal events were Q-QS items and blocks. Combinations of ECG findings were associated with relative risks over three times.

To determine the prevalence of silent myocardial ischemia, 925 non-insulin-dependent diabetic outpatients (333 women and 592 men), aged 40 to 65 years, asymptomatic, free from known CAD or complications of their diabetes, underwent a rest and exercise ECG.[16] Multivariate analysis showed that in the whole population, and in the men, the associated independent risk factors were age, total cholesterol, proteinuria, and ST-T abnormalities at rest. To examine the relation between resting ECG abnormalities and risk of CHD[17] a prospective study of 7735 men aged 40 to 59 years was performed (British Regional Heart Study). At baseline assessment each man completed a chest pain questionnaire, gave details of his medical history and had an ECG. Symptomatic CHD included history of anginal chest pain and/or a prolonged episode of chest pain. To evaluate the long-term prognostic value of ST-segment depression in the ECG of patients with acute MI,[18] 1234 patients who survived with acute Q wave ($n = 896$) or non-Q wave ($n = 338$) changes were followed for 4 years and resting ST-segment depression was an independent predictor of mortality.

To evaluate the prognostic value and clinical characteristics associated with ST-T changes among men without other manifestations of CHD, 9139 men born in the years 1907 to 1934 were followed up for 4 to 24 years.[19] On initial visit they were assigned to different categories of CHD on the basis of Rose chest pain questionnaire, hospital records, 12-lead ECG, history, and physical examination. The prevalence of silent ST-T changes among men without overt CHD was strongly influenced by age, increasing from 2% at 40 years of age to 30% at 80 years. Men with such ST-T changes were older and had higher serum triglyceride levels and worse glucose tolerance than men without such changes or other evidence of CHD. Their blood pressure was higher, and they more often had an enlarged heart or LVH and more often took antihypertensive medication, digitalis, or diuretic drugs. Serum cholesterol levels were not different between the two groups. After adjustment for other risk factors, these silent ST-T changes had a risk ratio of 2.0 for death from CHD and 1.6 for subsequent MI or angina pectoris. Silent ST-T changes that are ischemic as per the Minnesota code are probably both a marker of silent CHD and high blood pressure. They define a distinct group of patients with highly abnormal risk factor profile. Although not specific for CHD and often transient, these silent ST-T changes are associated with the development of every clinical manifestation of CHD and are independent predictors of reduced survival.

Spatial QRS-T Wave Measurements

Numerous studies support the value of repolarization measures[20–22] as determined by the spatial QRS-T angle as a tool for risk stratification (Fig. 11-1). Kors et al[23] investigated the prognostic importance of the frontal T axis, using ECGs from 5781 men and women aged 55 years and older from a prospective population-based study.[23] Participants with an abnormal frontal plane T axis, defined as those in the range of 105° to 180° and −180° to −15° (11%) had an increased risk of cardiac events and death. Rautaharju et al[24] focused on the spatial T-axis deviation in 4173 subjects considered free of CV disease.[24] The prevalence of marked T-axis deviation (>45° from the reference vector) was 12%. Adjusting for clinical risk factors and other ECG abnormalities, there was a nearly twofold excess risk of CV death and an approximate 50% excess risk of CV and all-cause mortality for those with marked T-axis deviation. Investigators from the Netherlands demonstrated the spatial QRS-T angle to be a strong and independent predictor of cardiac death.[25] The 6134 men and women aged >55 years and above in the prospective Rotterdam

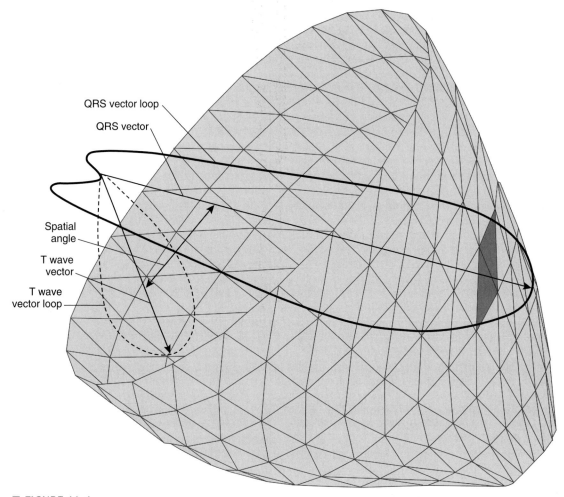

QRS vector loop

QRS vector

Spatial angle

T wave vector

T wave vector loop

FIGURE 11–1

Illustration of QRS-T spatial angle.

Study were categorized as having normal (0° to 105°), borderline (105° to 135°) or abnormal (135° to 180°) spatial QRS-T angles. Abnormal angles independently predicted multiple cardiac endpoints, including sudden death, the latter with an impressive *hazard ratio of 5.2.*

Criteria for Left Ventricular Hypertrophy

Extensive studies of ECG and LVH have been carried out[26–28] but recent studies provide the potential to better identify patients with pathophysiologic findings. Obesity is associated with the presence of LVH and, conversely, with decreased sensitivity of the ECG for LVH due to attenuating effects on QRS amplitudes.[29] Okin et al[30] examined the test accuracy of the criteria for LVH in relation to body mass index in 250 patients and confirmed the need to consider body mass index in LVH estimates. Also confirming this finding was an analysis of ECG and ECHO measurements taken from 3351 adults in the Framingham Heart Study.[31,32] The voltage sum of the R wave in lead aV_L and the S wave in lead V_3, alone and in combination with QRS duration, had a sensitivity at 95% specificity of 32% and 39%, respectively, in men and 46% and 51%, respectively, in women. Incorporation of obesity and age in ECG algorithms consistently improved the detection of hypertrophy.

Crow et al[33] studied the association between eight ECG criteria and ECHO-LVH estimates in men and women with mild hypertension. The ECGs and echocardiograms were recorded at baseline, 3 months, and annually for 4 years. The ECGs were computer-processed to define eight different criteria. This was a negative study that found a poor correlation between the ECG and ECHO but it was marred by poorly reproducible ECHO measurements. This emphasizes the need for clinical outcomes that will be available in our study.

Siscovick et al[34] conducted a population-based case-control study among patients who were free of clinically recognized heart disease and who received care at a health maintenance organization. Resting ECGs were reviewed to estimate the severity of LVH, myocardial injury, and QT-interval prolongation. These ECG indexes were directly related to the risk of primary cardiac arrest among hypertensive patients without clinically recognized heart disease.

The Hypertension Detection and Follow-up Program followed 10,940 hypertensive adults for 5 years.[35] ECGs were compared between stepped care and the referred care groups. In those with tall R wave by ECG at baseline, who survived the 5-year follow-up, incidence of LVH by ECG criteria was 4% and 9% in the stepped care and referred care group, respectively. With respect to ECG evidence of tall R wave or LVH at baseline, the rate of regression toward normal was 54% and 43% in the stepped care and referred care group, respectively. Antihypertensive treatment tended to reverse LVH.

In a sentinel prognostic study, the value of ECG criteria for LVH in patients with essential hypertension was evaluated.[36] Six methods were compared. A total of 1717 white hypertensive subjects were prospectively followed-up for mean of 3.3 years. At entry, the prevalence of LVH was highest with the Perugia score (18%) and lowest with the Framingham (4%). During follow-up there were 159 major CV events (33 fatal). The event rate was higher in the subjects with than in those without LVH. The Perugia score best predicted CV events, accounting for 16% of all cases, while the others only accounted for 7%. LVH diagnosed by the Perugia score was also associated with an increased risk of CV mortality (4×) and outperformed the classic LVH criteria.

ECG Abnormalities on Serial Resting ECGs

As part of the Manitoba Study, a cohort of 3983 men with a mean age of 30 years at entry, were followed with annual ECG from 1948 till 1978.[11] There were 70 cases of sudden death in men without previous clinical manifestations of heart disease. The prevalence of ECG abnormalities before sudden death was 71%. The frequencies of these abnormalities was 31% for major ST and T-wave abnormalities, 16% for ventricular extra beats, 13% for LVH, and 7% for left bundle branch block. The evolution of Q waves on serial ECGs was strongly and independently associated with total and coronary disease mortality in the MRFIT trial.[37]

Summary of Outcome Prediction with the ECG Studies

The outcome prediction of studies reviewed above are summarized in Table 11-1 and the prevalence of ECG abnormalities for age groups by gender are illustrated in Figure 11-2. The studies summarized have all been accomplished in asymptomatic individuals have shown the predictive power of ECG abnormalities for CV death and morbidity.

TABLE 11-1. The outcome prediction of studies using the resting ECG in asymptomatic individuals showning the predictive power of the ECG abnormalities for cardiovascular death and morbidity by relying on visual analysis

Study	Pop size	Age (yr)	Q wave RR	St DEPR RR	LBBB RR	LVH RR	Atrial FIB RR	Duration	Endpts
Copenhagen Heart Study	20,000 men/women	20–80	3×	5×	5×			4 years	489 deaths
Rose (England)	8403 male	40–64	2×	2×				5 years	657 deaths
Busselton, Australia	2119 men/women	40–79	4×	2×	2×		2×	12 years	
Italian RIFLE pooling project	12,180 men; 10,373 women	30–69	10×	4×	4×		2×	6 years	
Chicago Health Study	9643 men; 7990 women	40–64	2×	2×	2×			11 years	
British Regional Heart Study	7735 men	40–59	2.5×	2×		2×			611 major CHD; 243 deaths
Italian HBP Study	1717 hypertensives					4×		3.3 years	159 major CHD; 33 deaths
MISAD (Diabetics)	333 women 592 men	40–65		10×					
Manitoba Study	3983 men	30		5×	14×			30 years	70 deaths
MRFIT trial	2000 men	35–55	4×	2×				16 years	

Atrial fib, atrial fibrillation; Endpts, endpoints; LBBB, left bundle branch block; LVH, left ventricular hypertrophy; POP, population; RR, relative risk; ST depr, ST depression.

In general, routine screening with ECG is not indicated but ECG is ingrained as part of the health evaluation and so is frequently available.

Angiographic Findings in Asymptomatic Men with Resting ECG Abnormalities

Cardiac catheterization was used to evaluate 298 asymptomatic, apparently healthy aircrew men with ECG abnormalities.[38] These men were identified from annual ECGs and exercise tests used to screen them for latent heart disease (Fig. 11-3). Data from 27 additional symptomatic aircrew men who underwent cardiac catheterization because of mild angina pectoris were also included. The men were grouped according to the major reason for cardiac catheterization. The order of groups by increasing prevalence of significant CAD was as follows: abnormal ST response to exercise in a vertical lead (4% prevalence of CAD), supraventricular tachycardia (14%), right bundle branch block (20%), left bundle branch block (24%), abnormal exercise-induced ST depression (31%), ventricular irritability (38%), probable infarct (56%), and angina (70%). Approximately 60% of the men were completely free of angiographically significant coronary disease. The ECG abnormalities studied

had a poorer predictive value for CAD in asymptomatic, apparently healthy men than they did in a hospital or clinical population. A hypothesis based on the USAFSAM data is that a first tier of serial screening with the resting ECG could identify a subpopulation that could be more effectively screened with a next tier of testing, that is, exercise testing.

RECOMMENDATIONS FROM THE ACC/AHA GUIDELINES REGARDING EXERCISE TESTING AS A SCREENING PROCEDURE

The *1997* ACC/AHA guidelines were *updated in 2002* and had the following specific recommendations regarding this special application of the exercise test.[39]

Class I. Conditions for which there is evidence and/or general agreement that the standard exercise test is useful and helpful for screening asymptomatic individuals *(definitely use)*.

1. None

Class II a. Conditions for which there is conflicting evidence and/or a divergence of opinion that the

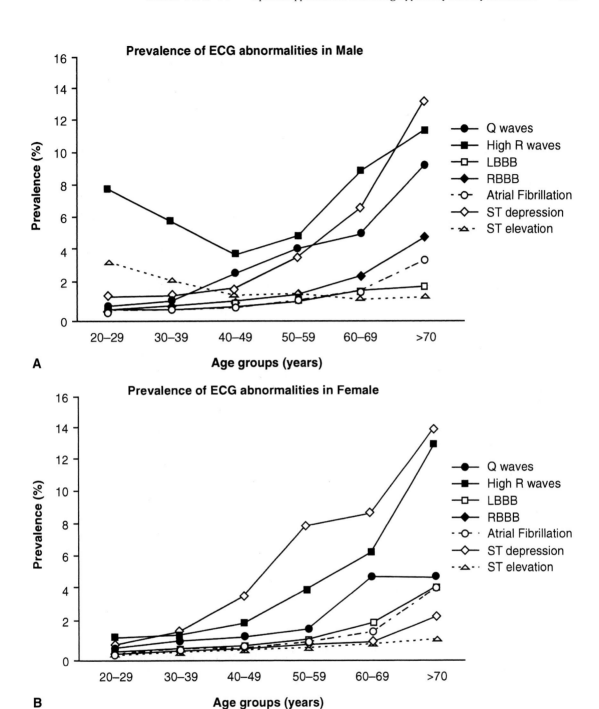

■ FIGURE 11–2

Plots of prevalence of ECG abnormalities for age groups by gender: *A* (males) and *B* (females).

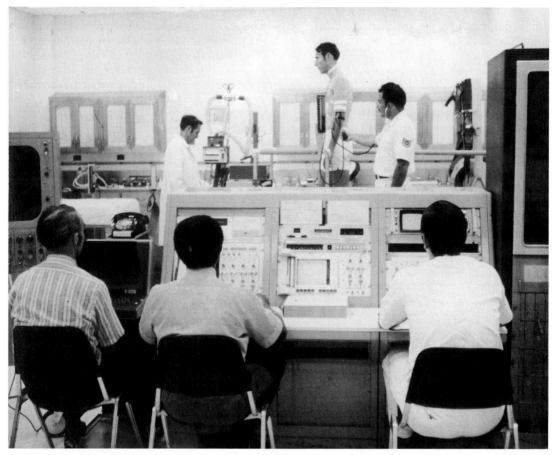

■ **FIGURE 11–3**
Picture from 1972 of the USAFSAM exercise testing laboratory showing the ECG recording and expired gas analysis systems used for gathering the data for many of the early studies presented in this book.

standard exercise test is useful and helpful for screening, but the weight of evidence for usefulness or efficacy is in favor of the exercise test *(probably use)*.

1. Evaluation of asymptomatic diabetic patients who plan to start vigorous exercise *(Evidence level: C)*

Class II b. Conditions for which there is conflicting evidence and/or a divergence of opinion that the standard exercise test is useful and helpful for screening asymptomatic individuals but the usefulness/efficacy is less well established *(maybe use)*.

1. Evaluation of individuals with multiple risk factors as a guide to risk factor reduction
2. Evaluation of asymptomatic men and women above 45 and 55 years of age, respectively:
   a. Who plan to start vigorous exercise (especially if sedentary)

b. Involved in occupations where impairment may impact on public safety
c. At high risk of CAD due to other diseases (such as peripheral vascular disease and chronic renal disease)

Class III. Conditions for which there is evidence and/or general agreement that the standard exercise test is not useful and helpful for screening and in some cases may be harmful *(do not use)*.

1. Routine screening of asymptomatic men or women

Multiple risk factors defined (113 here) by hypercholesterolemia (>240 mg/dl), hypertension (systolic blood pressure >140 mmHg or diastolic BP >90 mmHg), smoking, diabetes, family history of heart attack or sudden cardiac death in a first degree relative less than 60 years of age. An alternate approach might be to select individuals with a Framingham risk score consistent with at least a moderate risk of a greater than 2% chance of serious cardiac events within 5 years.

Logic for the Guidelines

The purpose of screening for possible CAD in individuals without known CAD is either to prolong the individual's life or improve its quality because of early detection of disease. In asymptomatic individuals with severe CAD, data from the Coronary Artery Surgery Study and Asymptomatic Cardiac Ischemia Pilot studies suggest that revascularization may prolong life. The detection of ischemia may identify individuals for risk factor modification. Although risk factor reduction should be attempted in all individuals, the identification of exercise capacity less than expected for age or increased risk may motivate individuals to be more compliant with risk factor modification.

The prediction of MI and death are considered the most important endpoints of screening in asymptomatic individuals. In general, the relative risk of a subsequent event is increased in individuals with an abnormal exercise test, although the absolute risk of a cardiac event in an asymptomatic individual remains low. The annual rate of MI and death in such individuals is only approximately 1%, even if ST-segment changes are associated with risk factors. A positive exercise test is more predictive of a later development of angina than the occurrence of a major event. Even when angina is taken into account, fewer individuals with a positive test suffer cardiac events than those individuals with a normal test. Unfortunately, those subjects with abnormal tests can suffer from being labeled as "at risk of CAD."

General population screening programs, for example, attempting to identify young individuals with early disease, have the limitation that severe CAD that requires intervention in asymptomatic individuals is exceedingly rare. While the physical risks of exercise testing are negligible, false-positive test results usually cause anxiety, and have serious consequences related to work and insurance. For these reasons, the use of exercise testing in healthy, asymptomatic persons is not recommended.

Selected individuals with multiple risk factors for CAD are at greater absolute risk for subsequent MI and death. Screening may be potentially helpful in those individuals who are at least at moderate subsequent risk (0.5% annual risk of death and nonfatal MI). Such individuals may be identified from the available data in asymptomatic individuals from the Framingham study (point system chart). These criteria could be utilized to stratify the highest risk individuals for CAD screening. Alternatively, screening may be performed in individuals with multiple risk factors. For these purposes, risk factors should be very strictly defined. Attempts to extend screening to individuals with lower degrees of risk, and lesser risk factors, are not recommended, since they are unlikely to improve individual outcome.

FOLLOW-UP STUDIES THAT HAVE UTILIZED A SCREENING EXERCISE TEST

Next we discuss the follow-up studies that utilized maximal or near-maximal exercise testing to screen asymptomatic individuals for latent CHD. The populations in these studies were tested and followed for the CHD endpoints of angina, acute MI, and sudden death. Later distinction will be made as to the results of these studies by the endpoints utilized and they will be divided into two groups: angina included as an endpoint (Table 11-2) and "hard" endpoints (Table 11-3). Table 11-4 lists the endpoints in all of the studies for comparison. As we will see later, the controversy over whether or not in the absence of conventional risk factors, exercise testing provides additional prognostic information has been resolved in the affirmative. Another concern is whether the knowledge of having an abnormal exercise test makes an individual more likely to report angina.

Bruce and McDonough[40] studied 221 clinically normal men in Seattle who were 35 to 82 years of age. A CB5 bipolar lead was used and 0.1 mV or more of ST-segment depression was the criterion for an abnormal response. The patients were monitored in the sitting position postexercise. Ten percent of them had abnormal ST-segment responses to the symptom-limited maximal treadmill test.

Aronow and Cassidy[41] tested 100 normal men in Los Angeles, aged 38 to 64 years, and followed them up for 5 years.[42] Risk-factor analysis was not performed, but all subjects were normotensive. A V_5 lead was used and 0.1 mV or more of ST-segment depression was the criterion for an abnormal response. The patients were monitored in the supine position after exercise.

Cumming et al[42] reported their 3-year follow-up for CHD endpoints in 510 asymptomatic men 40 to 65 years of age.[42] Maximal or near-maximal effort was performed and a CM_5 lead was monitored. The criterion for abnormal was 0.2 mV or more of

TABLE 11-2. Screening studies that included angina as an endpoint

Investigator	Number	Years followed	Incidence of CHD (%)	Sens (%)	Spec (%)	Positive predictive value (%)	Risk ratio
Bruce	221	5	2.3	60	91	14	14X
Aronow	100	5	9.0	67	92	46	14X
Cumming	510	3	4.7	58	90	25	10X
Froelicher	1390	6	3.3	61	92	20	14X
Allen	356	5	9.6	41	79	17	2.4X
Manca	947	5	5.0	67	84	18	10X
	508 (w)	5	1.6	88	73	5	15X
MacIntyre	578	8	6.9	16	97	26	4X
McHenry	916	13	7.1	14	98	39	6X
			Averages*	48	90	26	9X

*Averages do not include women.
CHD, coronary heart disease; Sens, sensitivity; Spec, specificity; w, women.

TABLE 11-3. Four screening studies with hard endpoints only (not angina)

Study	Number	Years followed	Incidence of CHD (%)	Sens (%)	Spec (%)	Positive predictive value (%)	Risk ratio
Seattle Heart Watch	2365	6	2.0	30	91	5	3.5X
MRFIT (SI)	6217	6-8	1.7	17	88	2.2	1.4X
(UC)	6205		1.9	34	88	5.2	3.7X
LRC (Gordon)	3630	8	2.2	28	96	12	6X
(Ekelund)	3806	7	1.8	29	95	7	5X
			Averages	27	91	6	4X

CHD, coronory heart disease; LRC, Lipid Research Clinics Coronary Primary Prevention Trial; MRFIT, Multiple Risk Factor Intervention Trial; Sens, sensitivity; SI, special intervention group; Spec, specificity; UC, usual care group.

TABLE 11-4. Events used as endpoints for follow-up studies

	Number	Events	Total deaths	Cardiovascular deaths	MI	CABS	AP
Aronow	100	9	3	3	4	1	1
Bruce	221	5	NR	1	1		3
Cumming	510	26	5	3	8		13
McHenry	916	65	8	8	26		30
MacIntyre	548	38	NR	10	16	6	6
Allen	888	48	NR	?	?	NR	?
Froelicher	1390	65	47	25	82	35	11
Seattle Heart Watch	2365	65	47	25	82	35	11
MRFIT (SI)	6427	265	115	NR	NR	NR	NR
(UC)	6438	260	124	NR	NR	NR	NR
LRC	3630	NR	151	75	NR	NR	NR

AP, Angina pectoris; CABS, coronary artery bypass surgery; LRC, Lipid Research Clinics Coronary Primary Prevention Trial; MI, myocardial infarction; MRFIT, Multiple Risk Factor Intervention Trial; NR, not reported; SI, special intervention group, UC, usual care group; ?, used as endpoint.

ST-segment depression and the patients were monitored in the supine position postexercise. Twelve percent had an initial abnormal response to a bicycle exercise test. Subjects with an abnormal response had a higher prevalence of hypertension and hypercholesterolemia.

At USAFSAM (see Fig. 11-3), 1390 asymptomatic men aged 20 to 54 years, who did not have any of the known causes for false-positive treadmill tests, were screened for latent CHD by maximal treadmill testing and followed-up for a mean of 6.3 years.[43] A CC_5 lead was mainly used, but additional leads were obtained in the supine position postexercise. The criterion for abnormal was 0.1 mV or more horizontal or downsloping ST-segment depression.

In Italy, Manca et al[44] studied 947 men and 508 women who were referred for exercise testing because of atypical chest pain. Those with typical symptoms of angina pectoris, valvular disease, hypertension, bundle branch block, dysrhythmias, Wolff-Parkinson-White syndrome, LVH with strain, significant resting repolarization abnormalities, and previous MI were excluded. No patient received drugs, such as digitalis, beta-blockers, antidysrhythmics, or diuretics, in the 2 weeks preceding exercise testing. Exercise was carried out after routine hyperventilation, using a supine bicycle, until at least 85% of the predicted maximal heart rate was reached. The conventional 12-lead ECG was recorded during and after the exercise test. The criterion for an abnormal response was 0.1 mV or more of horizontal or downsloping ST-segment depression. Eighteen percent of the men and 28% of the women had an abnormal ECG response. The endpoints for coronary disease were MI or sudden death, and there was a mean follow-up of 5.2 years. The overall incidence of coronary disease was 5% in the men and 1.6% in the women. The sensitivity was 67% in the men versus 88% in the women. The specificity of the test in the men was 84% versus 73% in the women. The predictive value of a positive test was 18% in men, but only 5% in women. Men with positive tests had a relative risk of 10 for developing clinical manifestations of CHD; the relative risk for women with positive tests was 15. This study clearly shows how predictive value is influenced by the prevalence of CHD in the population under study, and that the specificity of the exercise test is lower in women.

Allen et al[45] recently reported a 5-year follow-up of 888 asymptomatic men and women without known CHD who had initially undergone maximal treadmill testing. When tested, none of the subjects were on medications that would affect the ECG.

None had pathologic Q-waves or other abnormalities. None had clinical evidence of pulmonary disease or vascular disease. No subject that was included developed serious dysrhythmias, conduction abnormalities, or chest pain in conjunction with the exercise test. Maximal treadmill testing was performed using the Ellestad protocol, and leads CM_5, V_1, and a bipolar vertical lead were recorded. Subjects were exercised until they reached 100% of predicted maximal heart rate, fatigue, or marked dyspnea. Flat ST-segment depression of 0.1 mV or greater and downsloping of the ST segment were considered a positive response. Subjects with major ST-segment changes at rest were excluded. If there were minor changes in the ST segment before exercise, an additional 0.15 mV of depression at 80 msec from the J point were required to indicate an abnormal exercise test. R-wave amplitude was measured for an average of six beats during a control period and immediately after exercise, and an increase or no change in the R wave immediately after exercise compared with control was defined as an abnormal response. A decrease in R-wave amplitude was defined as a normal response. Ten percent were lost to follow-up. There was a 1.1% incidence of CHD per year manifested as angina pectoris, MI, or sudden cardiac death.

Only 2 of 221 men 40 years of age or less developed heart disease endpoints, and neither of the two had ST-segment abnormalities, abnormal R-wave response, or exercise duration of 5 minutes or less. Hence, in this study, abnormal results did not correlate with subsequent CHD in asymptomatic men 40 years of age or younger. These results contrast with those of the USAFSAM study of 563 men of 30 to 39 years of age that found a 1.4% incidence of coronary disease. The exercise ECG was found to have 50% sensitivity, 95% specificity, 13% predictive value, and a risk ratio of 17. Allen et al[45] concluded that the exercise test was only of value in men older than 40 years of age. Of the 311 women whom Allen et al followed, 10 developed CHD endpoints. Incomplete follow-up and the low incidence of coronary disease endpoints in women and in men younger than 40 years of age are limitations of this study.

Bruce et al[46] reported a 6-year follow-up of 2365 clinically healthy men (mean age 45 years) who were exercise tested as part of the Seattle Heart Watch. They underwent symptom-limited maximal treadmill testing using neither ST depression or target heart rates as endpoints of maximal exercise. The Bruce protocol was used, and the ECG was monitored with a bipolar CB_5 lead. Conventional risk factors were assessed at the time of the initial examination in a subset of the population. Follow-up was obtained by questionnaire, with morbidity defined as hospital admission. Forty-seven men (2%) experienced CHD morbidity or mortality. Univariate analysis of the individual conventional risk factors (positive family history, hypertension, smoking, and hypercholesterolemia) did not show a statistically significant increase in the 5-year probability of primary CHD events. Only when the sum of risk factors in an individual were assessed did conventional risk factors become statistically significant in relation to the event rate. Four variables from treadmill testing were predictive:

1. Exercise duration less than 6 METS
2. 0.1-mV ST depression during recovery
3. Greater than 10% heart rate impairment
4. Chest pain at maximal exertion

The ST-segment criteria had a sensitivity of 30%, specificity of 89%, predictive value of 5.3%, and a risk ratio of 3.3. Angina and exercise duration each had sensitivities of about 6%. Heart rate impairment had a sensitivity of 19% and was comparable to ST-segment depression for the other parameters.

Table 11-5 summarizes the performance of the exercise test predictors and conventional risk factors. The presence of two or more of the exercise test predictors identified men in all age groups who were at increased risk. Furthermore, it was found that in the presence of one or more conventional risk factors and as the prevalence of exertional risk predictors rose from none to any three, the relative risk rose from 1 to 30. The group that had one or more conventional risk factors and two or more exertional risk predictors was found to have the highest 5-year probability of primary CHD.

The striking finding is the increase in risk ratio when conventional risk factors are considered with the exercise test responses as well as the importance of exercise capacity in these three screening studies.

MacIntyre et al[47] performed maximal exercise tests on 548 fit, healthy, middle-aged, former aviators at the Naval Aerospace Medical Laboratory. Subjects that were included had to have no clinical evidence of heart or lung disease as determined by history, physical examination, chest x-ray, and a completely normal resting ECG. Leads XYZ and V_5 were analyzed only after exercise for 0.1 mV or more of horizontal depression 80 msec after QRS end. Criteria for coronary disease after an 8-year follow-up were sudden death, MI, coronary artery bypass surgery, or angina. The predictive value of the test was not significantly greater in those with the cardinal risk factors. An abnormal exercise ECG generated a higher risk ratio than the risk factors.

McHenry et al[48] reported the results of an 8- to 15-year follow-up of 916 apparently healthy men between the ages of 27 and 55 (mean 37 years) who underwent serial medical and exercise test evaluations.[48] In 1968, the Indiana University School of Medicine entered into an agreement with the Indiana State Police Department to provide employees with periodic medical evaluations, including treadmill tests. This report covers their experience with the first male employees who underwent initial medical evaluations between July 1968 and June 1975 and includes a follow-up for all subjects through to June 1983. A CC_5 lead was monitored and 1 mm or more horizontal or downsloping ST-segment depression during or after exercise was considered abnormal. A modified Balke protocol was used for all treadmill tests and

TABLE 11–5. Performance of exercise test variables and risk factors in detecting asymptomatic coronary artery disease

First author	Abnormal response	Sensitivity (%)	Specificity (%)	Predictive (%)	Risk ratio
Allen	ST depression	41	79	17	2
	METs <6	27	96	43	6
	ST depr and METs <6	24	99	71	11
Bruce	ST depr	30	91	5	4
	Angina during test	6	99	15	8
	METs <66	99	19	10	
	HRI	19	93	7	4
	≥1 RF and ≥2 Ex RP	19	–	46	18
Uhl	≥0.3 mV ST depr	36	79	38	2
	METs <8	46	92	67	4
	Persistent ST depr 28	87	43	6	
	≥1 RF and ≥2 Ex RP	55	86	84	4

Ex RP, Exercise risk predictor; HRI, heart rate impairment; RF, risk factor; ST depr, abnormal ST-segment depression; TM, treadmill test.

was mostly symptom-limited. Serial evaluations were planned at 2- to 5-year intervals; however, about 15% of subjects elected not to return after their initial evaluation. During the initial evaluation, there were 23 subjects with an abnormal ST-segment response. During follow-up, there were nine coronary events in this group: eight cases of angina and one of sudden death. With serial testing, additional 38 subjects experienced conversion to abnormal ST-segment response. During follow-up there were 12 coronary events in this group; 10 cases of angina, one MI and one "other". There were 833 subjects with normal ST-segment responses to exercise with all tests. In this group, there were 44 coronary events; 25 MI, 7 sudden deaths, and 12 diagnosed as having angina. They concluded that an abnormal ST-segment response to exercise predicted angina pectoris but not other coronary events.

McHenry et al[48] did not present sensitivity/specificity calculations, but the data they reported enabled the calculations shown in Table 11-2. The surprisingly low sensitivity from initial testing is probably due to the long follow-up period. An abnormal test indicates obstructive coronary disease that was most likely not present initially in most subjects who developed endpoints but which developed later during the 12 years. An analysis of the treadmill test performance at 5 years, a time frame similar to the prior studies reporting a higher sensitivity, would be most informative, but it is probable that the treadmill test is much less sensitive in asymptomatic men than previously demonstrated. They found that serial testing did not improve the predictive value of the test and that angina was the main cardiac event predicted. Sudden death was actually more common in the individuals with normal test results. The USAF-SAM study also had angina as its most common endpoint, both supporting the concept that the knowledge of an abnormal exercise test makes an individual more likely to report angina. McHenry et al also performed serial exercise tests on 900 presumably healthy men and identified 14 men with labile ST-T changes with standing or hyperventilation and abnormal ST-segment depression at exercise. At 7-year follow-up, none had manifested a coronary event while in 24 men with exercise-induced ST changes, but no labile ST-T wave phenomena pre-exercise, 10 (42%) had a coronary event.

The Multiple Risk Factor Intervention Trial (MRFIT), a CHD primary prevention trial, examined the effect of a special intervention (SI) program to reduce cholesterol, high blood pressure, and cigarette smoking in men whoever 35 to 57 years old.[49] Half of the 12,866 participants were randomly assigned to usual care (UC) in the community. During a 6- to 8-year follow-up, the CAD mortality rate was 7% lower in the SI than in the UC group, a nonsignificant difference. A prior subgroup hypothesis proposed that men with an abnormal exercise ECG would particularly benefit from intervention. An abnormal ST integral measured by computer of −16 μV-sec, was observed in 12.5% of the men at baseline, and was associated with a three times risk of CAD death within the UC group. In the subgroup with a normal ECG, there was no significant SI-UC difference in the CAD mortality rate. In contrast, there was a 57% lower death rate among men in the SI group with an abnormal test compared with men in the UC group. The relative risks (SI/UC) in these two strata were significantly different. These findings suggest that men with elevated risk factors that have an abnormal exercise ECG benefit from risk factor reduction. This study certainly is the largest and probably the most reliable for demonstrating the predictive accuracy of exercise testing in an asymptomatic population since only cardiac deaths were considered the endpoint as opposed to angina in most of the other studies.

Rautaharju et al[50] presented the prognostic value of the exercise ECG in the 6438 men of the MRFIT UC group in relation to fatal and nonfatal CHD events, resting ECG abnormalities and CHD risk factors. An abnormal response to exercise, defined as an ST depression integral of −16 −V-sec or more, was observed in 12.2% of the men. There was a nearly fourfold increase in the 7-year coronary mortality among men with an abnormal response to exercise compared with men with a normal ST segment in exercise (risk ratio 4). The risk ratio for coronary death, adjusted for age, diastolic blood pressure, serum cholesterol, and smoking status at baseline was 3.5, and the corresponding adjusted risk ratio for death from all causes was 1.6. A similar trend toward excess coronary events was seen for angina pectoris (risk ratio of 1.6). The trend was not significant for nonfatal MI. Multivariate analyses indicated that the ST-depression integral was a strong independent predictor of future coronary death. Men with an abnormal resting ECG (mainly high-amplitude R waves) and with an abnormal ST response to exercise had an over sixfold relative risk for coronary death compared with men with an abnormal resting ECG and a normal ST response to exercise.

Gordon et al[51] presented one of many interesting analyses of the Lipid Research Clinics Mortality

Follow-Up Study. More than 3600 white men, from 30 to 79 years of age and without a history of MI, underwent submaximal treadmill tests as part of their baseline elevation. The exercise test was conducted according to a common protocol and coded centrally; depression of the ST segment by at least 1 mm (visual coding) and/or 10 μV-sec (ST integral, computer coding) signified a positive test. Concurrent measurements of age, blood pressure, history of cigarette smoking, and plasma levels of lipids, lipoproteins, and glucose, as well as other coronary risk factors, were obtained. Cumulative CV mortality was 11.9% (22/185) over 8 years mean follow-up among men with a positive exercise test versus 1.2% (36/2993) among men with a negative test. Three quarters (43) of these deaths were due to CHD. The relative risk for CV mortality associated with a positive exercise test was nine times before and five times after age adjustment. CV mortality rates were especially elevated (relative risk 16 before and 5 after age adjustment) among the 82 men whose exercise tests were adjudged "strongly" positive based on degree and timing of the ischemic ECG response. A positive exercise test was also moderately associated with non-CV mortality; the relative risk for all-cause mortality was seven times before and three times after age adjustment. The relative risk for CV mortality associated with an abnormal exercise test was not appreciably altered by covariance adjustment for known coronary risk factors other than age. An abnormal exercise test was a stronger predictor of CV death than were increased levels of low-density lipoprotein cholesterol, decreased levels of HDL cholesterol, smoking, hyperglycemia, or hypertension. Its impact on risk of CV death was equivalent to that of a 17-year increment in age.

Ekelund et al[52] attempted to predict CHD morbidity and mortality in hypercholesterolemic men from an exercise test performed as part of The Lipid Research Clinics Coronary Primary Prevention Trial. To study whether the test was more predictive for hypercholesterolemic men (i.e., thus increasing the pretest probability for disease), data from 3806 asymptomatic hypercholesterolemic men were analyzed. All the men had performed a submaximal treadmill test at baseline, before they were assigned to the cholestyramine or placebo treatment group. A test was abnormal if the ST segment was displaced by 1 mm or more (visual code) or there was 10-uV-sec or more change in the ST integral (computer code), or both. The prevalence of an abnormal test was 8.3%. During the 7- to 10-year (mean 7.4) follow-up period, the mortality rate from CHD was 6.7% (21 of 315) in men with an abnormal test and 1.3% (46 of 3460) in men with a negative

test (placebo and cholestyramine groups combined). The age-adjusted rate ratio for an abnormal test, compared with a negative test, was 6.7 in the placebo group and 4.8 in the cholestyramine group. Cox's proportional hazards models, demonstrated that the risk of death from CHD associated with an abnormal test was 5.7 times higher in the placebo group and 4.9 times higher in the cholestyramine group after adjustment for age, lipids, and other risk factors. An abnormal test was not significantly associated with nonfatal MI.

Josephson et al[53] analyzed the results of serial exercise tests performed at two to four intervals in 726 male and female volunteers, aged 22 to 84 years (mean, 55.1 years), from the Baltimore Longitudinal Study of Aging. All subjects were free of CV disease at entry by history, physical examination, and resting 12-lead ECG. Over a mean overall follow-up of 7.4 years, coronary events occurred in 34 of 178 (19.1%) of those with an abnormal ST response to exercise versus 30 of 548 (5.5%) in those with a normal response (P = 0.001). Angina pectoris was the most common presenting coronary event regardless of ST-segment exercise response. Among individuals with an abnormal ST-segment response, the incidence of events was virtually identical between those with an initially abnormal response (group 1) and those who converted from a normal to an abnormal response (group 2), 19.8% versus 18.5%, respectively. After adjustment for standard coronary risk factors by proportional hazards regression analysis, the risk of a coronary event relative to subjects with persistently normal ST-segment responses (group 3) remained nearly identical in the two groups, 2.72 in group 1 (P < 0.003) and 2.80 in group 2 (P < 0.002). Thus, in asymptomatic individuals, conversion from a normal to an abnormal exercise ST-segment response is associated with a prognosis similar to an initially abnormal response and is not a more specific marker for future coronary events.

Gordon et al[54] analyzed smoking, physical activity, and other predictors of endurance and heart rate response to exercise in asymptomatic hypercholesterolemic men. The association of known coronary risk factors with progressive submaximal treadmill exercise test performance was studied in 6238 asymptomatic, white, 34- to 60-year-old hypercholesterolemic men screened between 1973 and 1976 for the Lipid Research Clinics Coronary Primary Prevention Trial. Cigarette smoking and habitual physical inactivity were each associated with a doubling of the rate of symptom-related discontinuation of the exercise test; the tests of sedentary smokers were discontinued at four times the rate observed for active nonsmokers. Smaller increases in heart rate were observed during exercise testing in physically active men and in smokers than in their sedentary and nonsmoking counterparts. Thus, smoking, like habitual physical activity, reduced the heart rate required to sustain a given external workload. However, the heart rates of smokers tended to remain elevated after exercise, while those of physically active men returned more rapidly toward resting levels. Age, Quetelet index, and low plasma levels of GDL cholesterol were also strong predictors of decreased exercise capacity, while resting heart rate and blood pressure levels were significant predictors of heart rate response.

Endpoint Considerations in These Screening Studies

The Seattle Heart Watch study was the first study that reported quite different results from previous studies. These results were different from Bruce's earlier findings. The explanation became apparent when considering the endpoints used. The earlier studies all considered angina pectoris as one of the cardiac events or endpoints. In the Seattle Heart Watch, the angina endpoint had to be associated with a hospital admission diagnosis of angina making it a more definite cardiac endpoint. The other recent studies considered only hard endpoints such as death or MI and not angina.

When the studies are separated by those that used angina as an endpoint (see Table 11-2) the average sensitivity was 50%, predictive value was 26%, and risk ratio was nine times. This means that 26% or one out of four with ST depression would have a cardiac event, including angina, during approximately 5 years of follow-up. However, when the studies that used only hard endpoints were considered (see Table 11-3), much poorer results were obtained. The sensitivity was 27% and the predictive value was 6%. Only 6% or 1 out of 17 with ST-segment depression would have a hard endpoint during follow-up. Rather than one cardiac event out of four with ST-segment depression, it turns out to be 1 out of 17. This means that 16 out of 17 abnormal responses are false positives. This must be considered since these studies are being cited as showing the dangers of silent ischemia. Silent ischemia induced by exercise testing in apparently healthy men is not as predictive of a poor outcome as once thought. In addition, the use of the exercise test for screening is even more misleading than previously appreciated because of the higher false-positive rate. The earlier better results can be explained by the cardiac concerns caused by an abnormal exercise test. Individuals with abnormal tests would be more likely to report chest pain and doctors would be more likely to diagnose it as angina given the exercise test results. In the only Holter study of its kind, Hedblad et al[55] obtained similar results using ambulatory Holter monitoring. Table 11-6 demonstrates his findings in the asymptomatic and symptomatic subjects he studied.

The nonselective utilization of exercise testing for screening apparently healthy individuals should be discouraged because of the poor predictive value of only 1mm of ST-segment depression. Unfortunately, this "abnormal" response leads to psychologic and vocational disability as well as unnecessary medical expenses and risks. When this response is no longer equated with disease, then perhaps the test could be used in such individuals for setting exercise prescriptions and for motivational purposes.

CV mortality should be the ideal endpoint, but it is usually determined from death certificates. While death certificates have their limitations, in general they classify those with accidental, GI, pulmonary, and cancer deaths accurately so that the remaining deaths are most likely to be of CV causes. This endpoint is more appropriate for a test for CV disease and certainly when screening for CV risk. While all-cause mortality is a more important endpoint for intervention studies, CV mortality is more appropriate for evaluating a CV test.

EXERCISE TESTING AND CORONARY ANGIOGRAPHY IN ASYMPTOMATIC POPULATIONS

In the USAFMC, we used cardiac catheterization to evaluate 111 asymptomatic men with abnormal exercise test-induced ST depression. Only one

TABLE 11-6. The holter study of Hedblad reporting results of screening in both asymptomatic and symptomatic population

History of CAD	ST depression on holter	Number	MI/deaths	Risk ratio
Yes	No	34	2 (5.9%)	2.6×
	Yes	19	7 (39%)	16×
No	No	262	6 (2.3%)	1×
	Yes	79	8 (10.8%)	4.4×

CAD, Coronary heart disease, previous myocardial infarction (MI), or positive Rose questionnaire result.
From Hedblad B: Eur Heart J 1989;10:149-158.

third of the subjects had at least one lesion equal to or greater than 50% lumenal narrowing of a major coronary artery. Resting mild ST-segment depression that appears on serial ECGs and persists increases the predictive value of an abnormal exercise test. Borer et al[56] reported angiographic findings in 11 asymptomatic individuals with hyperlipidemia and an abnormal exercise test. Only 37% were found to have coronary artery occlusions.

Barnard et al[57] used near-maximal treadmill testing to screen randomly selected Los Angeles firefighters. Ten percent had abnormal exercise-induced ST depression despite few risk factors for coronary disease. Six men with an abnormal exercise test elected to undergo cardiac catheterization. One had severe three-vessel disease, and another had a 50% obstruction of the left circumflex coronary artery. The other four men had normal studies.

Uhl et al[58] have reported their findings in 255 asymptomatic men who underwent coronary angiography for an abnormal ST-segment response to exercise testing over a 7-year period at the USAFSAM. None of the clinical or ECG variables were able to detect those with significant diseases. The three exercise test responses with high likelihood ratio were: (1) at least 0.3-mV depression, (2) persistence of ST depression 6 minutes postexercise, and (3) an estimated oxygen uptake of less than 9 METS. However, because of their low sensitivity and predictive value, it was necessary to combine them with risk factors. A combination of any risk factor and two exercise responses was highly predictive (89%) but insensitive (39%) for any coronary disease. However, this combination had a sensitivity of 55% and a predictive value of 84% for two- or three-vessel diseases.

Erikssen et al[59] reported angiographic findings in 105 men aged 40 to 59 of a working population with one or more of the following criteria: (1) a questionnaire for angina pectoris positive on interview or either (2) typical angina or (3) ST depression as responses to a near-maximal bicycle test. The exercise test had a predictive value of 84% if a slowly ascending ST segment was included. The higher predictive value in this study may be due to the older age of their population and inclusion of men with angina. Of the 36 who were found to have normal coronary arteries, a 7-year follow-up revealed that three died of sudden death, four received a diagnosis of cardiomyopathy, and one had developed aortic valve disease.[60] They had a relative decline in their physical performance over the follow-up period. Thallium studies were normal but the radionuclide ventriculogram revealed a subnormal increase in ejection fraction during exercise in half of them.

Kemp et al[61] evaluated 7-year survival in patients having normal or near normal coronary angiograms using data from the CASS registry of 21,487 consecutive coronary angiograms taken in 15 clinical sites. Of these, 4051 angiograms were normal or near normal, and the patients had normal left ventricular function as judged by absence of a history of congestive heart failure, no reported segmental wall motion abnormality and an ejection fraction of at least 50%; 3136 angiograms were entirely normal and the remaining 915 revealed mild disease with less than 50% stenosis in one or more segments. Of the total number, 843 patients had exercise tests and of these, 195 had abnormal ST depression. The 7-year survival rate was 96% for the patients with a normal angiogram and 92% for those whose study revealed mild disease. They noted that the ECG response to exercise was not a predictive variable. This is in contrast to the 7-year follow-up study of only 36 apparently healthy middle-aged men with a positive exercise test and normal coronary angiograms reported by Erikssen et al.[59] They concluded that patients with an abnormal exercise test could not be assured of a good prognosis on the basis of a normal coronary angiogram. The CASS data do not support this conclusion. There were 195 subjects with abnormal ST-segment depression and Kemp et al[61] were unable to show any predictive value of even marked amounts of depression. If exercise-induced ST-segment depression is due to ischemia in patients with normal coronaries, it is not related to a disease process that has an impact on mortality over 7 years of follow-up. In general, these angiographic studies confirm the low predictive value of an abnormal exercise test response also found in the epidemiological studies of populations with a low prevalence of CHD.

TECHNIQUES TO IMPROVE SCREENING

Numerous techniques have been recommended to improve the sensitivity and specificity of exercise testing. Various computerized criteria for ischemia have been proposed, as well as new standard visual ST criteria. In addition, there are ancillary techniques that could possibly improve the discriminating power of the exercise test. These methods are listed in Table 11-7.

TABLE 11–7. Ancillary techniques discussed that have been used to screen for asymptomatic CHD

Nuclear perfusion imaging
Intimal thickening of carotid arteries
Imaging coronary artery calcification with cardiac
  fluoroscopy or electron beam computed tomography
Cardiokymography
Total cholesterol/HDL ratio, conventional risk factors
ECG-gated chest x-ray pre- and postexercise
Computerized multifactorial risk prediction using
  Bayesian statistics
Digital subtraction angiography with intravenous
  injection of contrast to visualize the coronary arteries
Echocardiography
Biomarkers

Electrocardiographic Criteria

Hollenberg et al[62] has applied his computerized treadmill score in an asymptomatic Army population with success. Okin et al[63] compared the dST/HR index and the rate-recovery loop with standard ECG criteria for prediction of CHD events in 3168 asymptomatic men and women in the Framingham Offspring Study who underwent treadmill testing. These individuals were free of clinical and ECG evidence of heart disease. After a mean follow-up of 4.3 years, there were 65 new CHD events: four sudden deaths, 24 new MIs, and 37 new cases of angina pectoris. When a Cox proportional hazards model with adjustment for age and sex was used, an abnormal exercise ECG by standard criteria ($\geq$0.1 mV of horizontal or downsloping ST-segment depression) was not predictive of new CHD events. In contrast, stratification according to the presence or absence of an abnormal dST/HR index ($\geq$1.6 μV per beat per minute) and an abnormal (counterclockwise) rate-recovery loop was associated with CHD event risk and separated subjects into three groups with varying risks of coronary events: high risk, when both tests were abnormal (relative risk 4$\times$); intermediate risk, when either the dST/HR index or the rate-recovery loop was abnormal (relative risk, 2$\times$); and low risk, when both tests were negative. After multivariate adjustment for age, sex, smoking, total cholesterol level, fasting glucose level, diastolic blood pressure, and ECG-LVH, the combined dST/HR index and rate-recovery loop criteria remained predictive of coronary events. The problem with this study is that actual visual interpretation of the exercise ECGs was not available and the computer criteria were too rigorous. To match visual analysis, the computer measurement threshold must be set at 0.75-mm depression and 1 mV/sec

slope since the eye flattens out the ST slope and rounds off depression. The results obtained did not justify screening asymptomatic individuals, because of the high false-positive rate. Angina was included as an endpoint and this is a problem as previously noted.

Exercise-Induced Dysrhythmias

Studies in asymptomatic subjects have evaluated exercise-induced ventricular premature beats for detecting coronary disease. In USAFSAM study of 1390 men, only 39 men (2.1%) of the population developed "ominous" dysrhythmias. The risk ratio of developing coronary disease over 6 years of follow-up with these dysrhythmias was three times; however, the predictive value was only 10%, and sensitivity only 7% (a more recent research in this area has been covered in greater detail elsewhere in this book). Controversy exists regarding the meaning of these findings since they appear to be associated with later risk than other responses and no preventive or therapeutic strategy has been developed for them. Exercise-induced premature atrial contractions appear to be benign, except that they may predict a risk for atrial fibrillation.

Nuclear Perfusion Exercise Testing

Caralis et al[64] used thallium exercise testing and coronary angiography to evaluate asymptomatic individuals with abnormal ST-segment responses to exercise testing. Of 3496 consecutive treadmill exercise tests performed primarily on asymptomatic individuals, 22 developed 0.2 mV or more of asymptomatic horizontal ST-segment depression. These individuals had physical examinations, routine laboratory studies, chest x-rays, and resting ECGs, all of which were normal. Fifteen of these 22 patients agreed to be evaluated further with thallium and coronary angiography. Once subjects were selected on the basis of an abnormal exercise test, the thallium exercise scans classified 13 of 15 patients properly.

Nolewajka et al[65] performed thallium treadmill tests on 58 asymptomatic men as part of a screening study. The risk for CHD was determined using the Framingham risk equation. The risk calculation was greater in those with abnormal exercise studies compared with those who had normal studies. However, classification results were very disappointing.

Uhl et al[66] performed thallium exercise tests on 119 aircrewmen prior to undergoing coronary angiography for abnormal treadmill tests or serial ECG changes. Of these, 41 men had significant angiographic disease (≥50% occlusion) for a predictive value of the ECG screening procedures of 21%. There were mixed results in the 10 men who had minimal angiographic disease (less than 50% occlusion); 10 had abnormal scans and five had normal scans. The high sensitivity and specificity of the computer-enhanced thallium exercise test in this population of apparently healthy men is a strong support for its use as a second-line screening procedure. If both an abnormal exercise ECG and abnormal nuclear perfusion scan had been required before angiography was performed, 136 of those free of coronary disease would not have needed to undergo angiography.

To examine whether perfusion scintigraphy improved the predictive value of exercise-induced ST-segment depression, Fleg et al[67] performed maximal treadmill tests and thallium scans on 407 asymptomatic volunteers, 40 to 96 years of age (mean = 60), from the Baltimore Longitudinal Study on Aging. The prevalence of exercise-induced silent ischemia, defined by concordant ST-segment depression and a thallium perfusion defect, increased more than sevenfold from 2% in the fifth and sixth decades to 15% in the ninth decade. Over a mean follow-up period of 4.6 years, cardiac events developed in 9.8% of subjects and consisted of 20 cases of new angina pectoris, 13 MIs, and seven deaths. Events occurred in 7% of individuals with both negative thallium scan and ECG, 8% of those with either test positive, and 48% of those in whom both tests were positive ($P < 0.001$). By proportional hazards analysis, age, hypertension, exercise duration, and a concordant positive ECG and thallium scan result were independent predictors of coronary events. Furthermore, those with positive ECG and thallium scan had a 3.6-fold relative risk for subsequent coronary events, independent of conventional risk factors.

Cardiokymography

The cardiokymograph (CKG) is an electronic device that produces a representation of regional left ventricular wall motion noninvasively. It generates an electromagnetic field, and motion within the field causes a change in the frequency of an oscillator.

A change in frequency is converted into a change in voltage proportional to the motion. The CKG produces a recording similar to the apexcardiogram and the kinetocardiogram. The advantage of the CKG is that it records absolute cardiac motion without chest motion, thus eliminating the distortion problem inherent in both the apexcardiogram and kinetocardiogram. There is considerable tissue penetration, so the CKG responds to deeper cardiac motion as well as precordial surface movement. CKG recordings have been shown to be associated with ventriculographic wall motion abnormalities.

Silverberg et al[68] reported their use of the CKG after exercise in 157 patients, including 27 apparently healthy volunteers and 130 patients with suspected CHD who underwent coronary angiography. The subjects performed a progressive symptom-limited maximal treadmill test. The CKG was recorded within 2 minutes of termination of exercise, and every minute thereafter for 10 minutes. Two sets of empiric criteria for an abnormal CKG pattern were defined in relation to known effects of ischemia on regional wall motion. The first abnormality was defined as paradoxical systolic outward motion. The second abnormality was defined as development of total absence of inward motion, a resultant holosystolic outward motion, or systolic outward motion occurring for less than the entire period of ejection but not preceded by inward motion. For detecting CHD in atypical chest pain patients, the CKG had a higher sensitivity, specificity, and predictive value than did the electrocardiogram. However, no statistical difference existed between the ECG and the CKG in asymptomatic patients. Exercise-induced CKG abnormalities persisted longer during recovery than ECG changes.

A multicenter study has demonstrated the diagnostic accuracy of CKG recorded 2 to 3 minutes after exercise in 617 patients undergoing cardiac catheterization.[69] Of these patients, 29% had prior MI. There were 12 participating centers using a standardized protocol. Adequate CKG tracings, which were obtained in 82% of patients, were dependent on the skill of the operator and on certain patient characteristics. Of the 327 patients without prior MI who had technically adequate CKG and ECG tracings, 166 (51%) had coronary disease. Both the sensitivity and specificity of CKG (71% and 88%, respectively) were significantly greater than the values for the exercise ECG (61% and 76%, respectively). CAD and multivessel disease were present in 98% and 68%, respectively, of the 70 patients with both abnormal CKG and

ECG results, and in 15% and 5%, respectively, of the 132 patients with both studies normal. The CKG was most helpful in those patients in whom the post-test probability of coronary disease was between 21% and 72% after the exercise ECG. In these patients, an abnormal concordantly positive CKG result increased the probability of coronary disease to between 67% and 100%, whereas a normal response decreased it to between 12% and 15%. In the subgroup of 102 patients undergoing concomitant exercise thallium testing, the sensitivity and specificity for the nuclear perfusion scans (81% and 80%, respectively) were similar to the values for CKG (72% and 84%, respectively).

Although this study confirmed that CKG improves the diagnostic accuracy of the exercise test even without significant numbers of asymptomatic patients, unfortunately, this device is no longer available commercially. The technical skills and need for breath holding after exercise were impediments in the widespread acceptance of this procedure, but failure to obtain generalized reimbursement is the more likely explanation. Several German companies have resolved some of the difficulties by signal averaging and using multiple transducers but have not brought a product to the market.

Coronary Artery Calcification

Calcification of the coronary arteries has been noted on radiographic studies for some time. Newer technologies have renewed interest in using this marker for screening for asymptomatic CAD. The following is a summary of the AHA statement on the pathophysiology, epidemiology, imaging methods, and clinical implications of coronary artery calcification.[70]

Atherosclerotic calcification is an organized, regulated process similar to bone formation that occurs only when other aspects of atherosclerosis are also present. Nonhepatic Gla-containing proteins like osteocalcin, which are actively involved in the transport of calcium out of vessel walls, are suspected to have key roles in the pathogenesis of coronary calcification. Osteopontin, other chemicals, and osteoblastic and osteoclastic cells, also involved in bone mineralization, have been identified in calcified atherosclerotic lesions. Arterial calcification is an active process and not simply a passive precipitation of calcium phosphate crystals. Although calcification is found more frequently in advanced lesions, it may also occur in

small amounts in earlier lesions that appear in the second and third decades of life. Histopathologic investigation has shown that plaques with microscopic evidence of mineralization are larger and associated with larger coronary arteries than are plaques or arteries without calcification. The relation of arterial calcification to the probability of plaque rupture is unknown. Although the amount of coronary calcium correlates with the amount of atherosclerosis in different individuals and to a lesser extent in segments of the coronary tree in the same individuals, it is not known if the quantity of calcification tracks the quantity of atherosclerosis over time in the same individuals. Calcification could even stabilize plaque and prevent rupture. In vivo epidemiologic evidence and postmortem studies show that the prevalence of coronary calcium deposits in a given decade of life is 10 to 100 times higher than the expected 10-year incidence of CHD events for individuals of the same age. This disparity is less evident in the elderly and symptomatic than in the young and asymptomatic. Coronary calcium content (such as the calcium score determined by EBCT can be taken as an estimate of atherosclerotic burden.

Fluoroscopy, electron beam, and helical computed tomography (CT) can identify calcific deposits. Only EBCT can quantitate the amount or volume of calcium. The absence of calcific deposits on an EBCT scan strongly predicts the absence of angiographically significant coronary narrowing; however, it does not imply the absence of atherosclerosis, including unstable plaque. Similarly, calcification may frequently be seen in the absence of significant angiographic narrowing and before there has been sufficient plaque build-up to narrow the vessel to the extent that ischemia would be apparent on exercise ECGs or stress-nuclear perfusion determinations.

Calcium Deposition in Coronary Artery Disease

Atherosclerotic calcification begins as early as the second decade of life, just after fatty streak formation. Calcific deposits are found more frequently and in greater amounts in elderly individuals and more advanced lesions. They appear not to be due to passive adsorption but instead part of a regulated process like bone formation that is genetically controlled. Coronary arterial calcification can be viewed as a natural attempt to protect threatened myocardium by strengthening weakened atherosclerotic plaque prone to rupture.

Coronary calcification can be stabilizing, minimizing the risk of plaque rupture.

In Vivo Imaging Methods

Coronary artery calcification can be detected by standard chest x-rays; coronary arteriography; fluoroscopy, including digital subtraction fluoroscopy; cinefluorography; conventional, helical, and EBCT; intravascular ultrasound; and transthoracic and transesophageal ECHO. Fluoroscopy and EBCT are most commonly used to detect coronary calcification noninvasively.

Fluoroscopy

Langou et al[71] reported the use of cardiac fluoroscopy as a prescreening tool in asymptomatic men prior to exercise tests. In one study, 129 healthy men (average age 49) were evaluated with cardiac fluoroscopy to detect coronary artery calcification, followed by a submaximal exercise test. Of the 108 subjects who completed the exercise test, 37%, or 34%, had at least one fluoroscopically detected calcified coronary artery. Of this group of subjects with positive fluoroscopic findings, 13 (35%) had an abnormal ST-segment response to the exercise test. Of the 68 subjects with normal fluoroscopy, only three (4%) had an abnormal exercise response. Consequently, those with calcification of at least one coronary artery had a ninefold increased risk of having an abnormal exercise ECG test. Of the 16 subjects with an abnormal exercise test, 81% had calcification of at least one coronary artery. The location of the calcified deposit conferred greater risk for exercise-induced ischemic changes than did multivessel involvement with left anterior descending artery disease, most often positive.

Detrano and Froelicher[72] summarized seven studies examining fluoroscopic detection of coronary calcification in 2670 patients undergoing coronary angiography. To further evaluate variability in the reported accuracy of fluoroscopically detected coronary calcific deposits for predicting angiographic disease, Gianrossi et al[73] applied meta-analysis to 13 consecutively published reports comparing the results of cardiac fluoroscopy with coronary angiography. Population characteristics and technical and methodologic factors were analyzed. Sensitivity and specificity for predicting serious coronary disease compare quite well with those from the literature on the exercise ECG and thallium perfusion scan. Sensitivity for

any disease averaged 58% and specificity 82% and for severe disease, sensitivity averaged 87% and specificity 59%. Sensitivity increases and specificity decreases more significantly with patient age, and sensitivity is paradoxically lower in laboratories testing patients with more severe disease, as well as when 70% rather than 50% diameter narrowing is used to define angiographic disease. Work-up and test review bias was also significantly related to reported accuracy.

In a fluoroscopic study of 613 asymptomatic male aircrew members who underwent coronary angiography because of one or more abnormal screening tests,[74] coronary artery calcification had a 66% sensitivity and a 78% specificity in determining angiographically significant coronary stenosis. The positive predictive value was 38% and negative predictive value was 92%; for disease with greater than 10% stenosis, sensitivity was 61% and specificity 86%.

Data were retrospectively obtained from 778 patients who had been referred for angiography.[75] Patients with a previous MI, a previous abnormal angiogram, and unstable angina were excluded. The crude likelihood ratio of a positive and negative test result, with 95% confidence intervals, was 6 and 0.5, respectively, but was dependent on the clinical variables.

Electron Beam Computed Tomography

EBCT (cine or ultrafast) uses an electron gun and a stationary tungsten "target" rather than a standard x-ray tube to generate x-rays, permitting very rapid scanning times. The scans, which are usually acquired during one or two separate breath-holding sequences, are triggered by the ECG signal at 80% of the RR interval, near the end of diastole and before atrial contraction, to minimize the effect of cardiac motion. The rapid image acquisition time virtually eliminates motion artifact related to cardiac contraction. The unopacified coronary arteries are easily identified by EBCT because the lower CT density of periarterial fat produces marked contrast to blood in the coronary arteries, while the mural calcium is evident because of its high CT density relative to blood. Additionally, the scanner software allows quantification of calcium area and density. A study for coronary calcium can be completed within 10 or 15 minutes, requiring only a few seconds of scanning time.

Comparison with Coronary Angiography

One hundred sixty men and women with coronary disease (45 to 62 years of age), of whom 138 had obstructive CAD and 22 had normal coronary arteries, and 56 age-matched healthy control subjects underwent double-helix CT.[76] Double-helix CT findings indicated that calcification was significantly more prevalent in patients with CAD than in patients with normal coronary arteries or in healthy control subjects. Sensitivity in detecting obstructive CAD was high (91%); however, specificity was low (52%) because of calcification in nonobstructive lesions.

Using the volume mode of EBCT, 251 consecutive patients who underwent elective coronary angiography because of suspected CAD had results with those of ECG and thallium exercise tests compared.[77] Calcification was first noted in women in the fourth decade of life, approximately 10 years later than its occurrence in men. Among patients with advanced atherosclerosis, calcification scores were uniformly high in women but ranged widely in men. Nine percent of patients with significant stenoses had no calcification. The calcification scores of patients with significant stenosis in at least one vessel were significantly higher than those of patients without significant stenosis in the study group as a whole and in most patient subgroups classified according to age and gender. A cut-off calcification score for prediction of significant stenosis, determined by receiver operating characteristic curve analysis, showed high sensitivity (0.77) and specificity (0.86) in all study patients; sensitivity was similarly high even in older patients (≥70 years) and was enhanced in middle-aged patients (40 to ≤60 years).

A multicenter investigational study reported on the relative prognostic value of coronary calcific deposits and coronary angiographic findings for predicting CHD-related events in patients referred for angiography.[78] Four hundred ninety-one symptomatic patients underwent coronary angiography and EBCT at five different centers between 1989 and 1993. A cardiologist with no knowledge of the coronary angiographic and clinical data interpreted the EBCTs. Receiver operating characteristic curves were constructed to determine the relation between EBCT and coronary angiographic findings. The area under the receiver operating characteristic curve was 0.75 for the coronary calcium score, indicating moderate discriminatory power for this score for predicting angiographic findings. In this group, sensitivity of any detectable calcification by EBCT as an indicator of significant stenosis (>50% narrowing) was 92%, and specificity 43%. However, when these CT images were reinterpreted in a blinded and standardized manner, specificity was only 31%. Thirteen CHD-related deaths and eight nonfatal acute infarctions occurred over 30 months. Scores were sorted in ascending order and divided into quartiles of equal size. One patient in the first quartile had a fatal MI; two in the second quartile, eight in the third quartile, and 10 in the fourth quartile had a CHD-related event.

In another multicenter study[79] of 710 enrolled patients, 427 had significant angiographic disease, and coronary calcification was detected in 404, yielding a sensitivity of 95%. Of the 23 patients without calcification, 83% had single-vessel disease on angiography. Of the 283 patients without angiographically significant disease, 124 had negative EBCT studies (for a 44% specificity).

Thus, three of the four studies demonstrated a high sensitivity and a low specificity with a predictive accuracy of about 68%. While the cutpoint for calcium density can be adjusted to provide a high sensitivity, the EBCT is not more diagnostic for angiographic CAD than the standard exercise test. Similarly, the exercise ECG criteria could be set at 0.5 mm to heighten sensitivity but both tests lose considerable specificity when sensitivity is increased.

Costs and Risks of Scanning

Assessment of coronary calcification by EBCT can be done in virtually any subject and provides anatomic rather than physiologic information. Thus, no preparation or discontinuation of medications is required prior to testing, which is totally noninvasive, involves minimal patient cooperation, and produces results available for qualitative evaluation on an immediate basis. Quantitative review of calcium scoring using EBCT requires additional analysis but is available generally within 10 to 20 minutes. The current total charge for an EBCT examination (limited CT of the chest) and interpretation averages between $300 and $400.

The Cardiology group at Walter Reed constructed a decision tree to determine the marginal cost per additional patient who was "at risk" (>10% 10-year risk of CHD) identified with the addition of EBCT to the Framingham Risk Index in a screening population with no cardiac symptoms.[80] They also determined the marginal cost per quality adjusted life-year (QALY) saved, assuming a 30% improvement in life expectancy associated with primary prevention. A consecutive screening cohort of 39- to 45-year-old men and women was used for demographic and risk factor data. Estimates of the relevant input costs were made on the basis of published literature when available. The results showed that compared with using Framingham Risk Index alone, the strategy of incorporating EBCT detects patients who are "at risk" at a cost of $9,789 per additional case and a marginal cost of $86,752 per QALY. The marginal cost per QALY is highly sensitive to the gain in life expectancy from early intervention ($10,000 to $1,700,000 per QALY for a relative risk reduction in mortality of 50% or 25%, respectively), the utility of being "at risk" ($18,000 per QALY to dominated for a utility of 1.0 to less than 0.98, similar to other asymptomatic chronic illnesses), and the added prognostic value of EBCT ($60,000 per QALY to dominated in a wide range). The use of EBCT to improve CV risk prediction in a population with no cardiac symptoms who are at low absolute risk is expensive, even using favorable assumptions. If the utility of being "at risk" is comparable with other asymptomatic disease states, EBCT may, in aggregate, have a detrimental effect on the quality of life of screening populations.

Radiation dosimetry for a single screening EBCT scan for coronary calcium has an effective (integrated over thorax) radiation dose of 82 mrem for males and approximately 150 mrem for females (accounting for breast irradiation). Although it is difficult to make direct comparisons due to differences in dose delivery and localization, a chest x-ray combination involves approximately 10 mrem and a screening two-view mammogram about 35 mrem. A nuclear perfusion scan delivers a highly localized dose of approximately 1 rem to the thorax and abdomen; conventional coronary angiography results in radiation doses two to three orders of magnitude or greater than that from EBCT coronary calcium scan.

Epidemiology of Coronary Calcification

Atherosclerotic plaque is present in 50% of individuals aged 20 to 29 years, rising to 80% in individuals aged 30 to 39. Calcification is present in 50% of individuals aged 40 to 49 and 80% of individuals aged 60 to 69, whereas significant stenosis is present in only 30% of individuals aged 60 to 69. For individuals aged 30 to 39 with symptomatic CAD, calcification may be present in 72% and stenosis in 60%. In autopsy studies a modest correlation has been observed between percent coronary stenosis and extent of calcification. More calcified sites are associated with nonstenotic than stenotic disease. Because area varies by the square of the radius, histologically estimated coronary stenosis is considerably greater than that provided by coronary angiography; thus, 50% and 75% area stenosis on histopathology may correlate with 15% and 30% to 50% diameter stenosis by angiography, respectively.

A summary of the literature relating coronary calcification to clinical disease is complicated by the evolution of technology for identifying calcification. In an early study using fluoroscopy, prevalence of calcium in patients with and without symptoms was, respectively, 28% and 2% in persons aged 30 to 40 years and 95% and 56% in persons aged 60 to 70. More recent studies using EBCT have prevalences of 100% and 25% in younger persons and 100% and 74% in older persons with and without symptoms, respectively.

Follow-Up After Electron Beam Computed Tomography of Symptomatic Patients

Although the presence or absence of calcification is related to overall atherosclerotic plaque burden, it is event data (angina, MI, and interventions) that are important in determining the clinical significance of coronary artery calcification. While acute occlusions resulting in MI often occur in vessels with less than 50% angiographic stenosis, these patients frequently have other severe angiographic stenoses. In 800 patients referred for cardiac catheterization for angina pectoris, symptomatic patients with calcification demonstrated on conventional fluoroscopy had a 5-year survival rate of 58% versus 87% in those without detectable calcium.[81]

A multicenter EBCT calcium study[78] looked at event data in 501 symptomatic patients who were studied with both EBCT for calcium and coronary angiography. The majority of these patients had symptoms of CAD. In this group, 1.8% died and 1.2% had nonfatal MIs during a mean follow-up period of 31 months. A threshold of 100 or greater in the calcium score was shown to be highly predictive in separating patients with cardiac events at follow-up from those without events and calcium scores of less than 100. In this study, logistic regression, which included, in addition to calcium score, age, gender, and coronary angiographic findings as independent variables, showed that only log calcium score predicted events. It did not add much to the discrimination of disease using the Framingham risk score.

Follow-Up After Electron Beam Computed Tomography of Asymptomatic Individuals

Detrano et al[82] studied survival in asymptomatic, high-risk subjects with coronary artery calcification detected on fluoroscopy. These investigators followed 1461 subjects with a greater than 10% risk of having a coronary event within 8 years. (A coronary event was defined as angina, documented MI, myocardial revascularization, or death from CHD.) Events at 1 year occurred in 5.4% of 691 subjects with coronary calcification versus 2.1% of the 768 subjects without fluoroscopic calcium. One-vessel calcification incurred an event risk of 5.4%; two-vessel, 5.6%; and three-vessel, 6.2%. Detrano et al[82] found that radiographically detectable calcium was associated with a risk for having an event 2.7 times greater compared with the group with no calcification. They also found that the presence of calcification was an independent predictor of at least one coronary event when controlled for age, gender, and other risk factors. However, it should be emphasized that three deaths due to CHD and two nonfatal MIs occurred in subjects without detectable coronary calcium. Their conclusions were that the presence of coronary calcium detected fluoroscopically identified an increased risk of a cardiac event in asymptomatic high-risk subjects at 1 year, and this increased risk was independent of that incurred by standard risk factors.

Arad et al[83] followed 1173 initially asymptomatic individuals for an average of 19 months. Nineteen patients had 27 CV events, including one death, seven MIs, and one nonhemorrhagic stroke. In addition, 18 patients developed symptoms requiring coronary bypass surgery or percutaneous coronary angioplasty. EBCT coronary calcium scores were correlated with subsequent events, depending on the threshold for the lower limit of calcium score. For coronary artery calcium score thresholds of 100, 160, and 680, EBCT had sensitivities of 89%, 89%, and 53%, and specificities of 77%, 82%, and 95%, respectively. Negative predictive values were greater than 99%, and odds ratios ranged from 22:1 to 36:1 for these thresholds. Other risk factors, such as presence of hypercholesterolemia, low HDL cholesterol, hypertension, diabetes, and family history failed to predict subsequent events. There were only eight major coronary events (death or MI) and patients were self-selected for entry into the study.

The goal of CT scanning for coronary artery calcification has been to overcome the limited sensitivity of using scores for screening.[84] The location and extent of calcification correlate closely with pathologic and angiographic abnormalities, but whether such calcification predicts clinical events, especially in younger individuals, is equivocal. Most data on coronary calcification have been obtained with electron-beam CT, but recently multislice CT, which is more versatile, less expensive, and available in most large hospitals, has been increasingly used. The increasing use of multislice CT scanners should generate more data for comparison with those obtained from electron-beam CT. Radiation dose, which is higher with multi-slice than with electron-beam procedures, needs to be reduced, and calcification in scans needs to be quantified more accurately than with existing computer-based analyses. Further studies are needed to establish the predictive power of the coronary calcification score for clinical events and the effects of therapeutic intervention on both these outcomes. It would also be worth investigating the relation between coronary calcification and risk factors not quantified in Framingham-based estimates, including familial and racial predisposition to premature CHD.

Shaw et al[85] developed risk-adjusted multivariable models, including risk factors and coronary calcium scores determined with EBCT, in asymptomatic patients for the prediction of all-cause mortality. They followed a cohort of 10,377 asymptomatic individuals undergoing cardiac risk factor evaluation and coronary calcium screening with electron-beam CT. Multivariable Cox proportional hazards models were developed to predict all-cause mortality. Risk-adjusted models incorporated traditional risk factors for CAD and coronary calcium scores. Cardiac risk factors such as family history of CAD (69%), hypercholesterolemia (62%), hypertension (44%), smoking (40%), and diabetes (9%) were prevalent. The frequency of coronary calcium scores was 57% for scores of 10 or less, 20% for 11 to 100, 14% for 101 to 400, 6% for 401 to 1000, and 3% for greater than 1000. During a mean follow-up of 5.0 years, the death rate was 2.4%. In a risk-adjusted model (model chi-square = 388.2, $P < 0.001$), coronary calcium was an independent predictor of mortality ($P < 0.001$). Risk-adjusted relative risk values for coronary calcium were 1.6, 1.7, 2.5, and 4 for scores of 11 to 100, 101 to 400, 401 to 1000, and greater than 1000, respectively, as compared with that for a score of 10 or less. Five-year risk-adjusted survival was 99% for a calcium score of 10 or less and 95.0% for a score of greater than 1000. With a receiver operating characteristic curve, the concordance index increased from 0.72 for cardiac risk factors alone to 0.78 when the calcium score was added to a multivariable model for prediction of death.

Greenland et al[86] sought to determine whether calcium score assessment combined with Framingham Risk score (FRS) in asymptomatic adults provides prognostic information superior to either method alone and whether the combined approach can more accurately guide primary preventive strategies in patients with CHD risk factors. They performed a prospective observational population-based study of 1461 asymptomatic adults with coronary risk factors. Participants with at least one coronary risk factor (>45 years) underwent EBCT, were screened between 1990 and 1992, contacted yearly for up to 8.5 years after CT scan, and were assessed for CHD. This analysis included 1312 participants with calcium score results; excluded were 269 participants with diabetes and 14 participants with either missing data or who had had a coronary event before EBCT was performed. During a median of 7.0 years of follow-up, 84 patients experienced MI or CHD death; 70 patients died of any cause. There were 291 (28%) participants with an FRS of more than 20% and 221 (21%) with a calcium score of more than 300. Compared with an FRS of less than 10%, an FRS of more than 20% predicted the risk of MI or CHD death (hazard ratio [HR] 14). Compared with a calcium score of zero, calcium score more than 300 was predictive (HR 4). Across categories of FRS, calcium score was predictive of risk among patients with an FRS higher than 10% ($P < 0.001$) but not with an FRS less than 10%. Their findings support the hypothesis that high calcium score can modify predicted risk obtained from FRS alone, especially among patients in the intermediate-risk category in whom clinical decision-making is most uncertain.

Kondos et al[87] examined the association between EBCT and cardiac events in initially asymptomatic low- to intermediate-risk individuals, with adjustment for the presence of hypercholesterolemia, hypertension, diabetes, and a history of cigarette smoking. The study was performed in 8855 initially asymptomatic adults 30 to 76 years old (26% women) who self-referred for screening. Conventional CAD risk factors were elicited by use of a questionnaire. After 3 years, information on the occurrence of cardiac events was collected and confirmed by use of medical records and death certificates. In men, events ($n = 192$) were associated with the presence of calcium ([relative risk] RR = 10.5), diabetes (RR = 2), and smoking (RR = 1.4), whereas in women, events ($n = 32$) were linked to the presence of calcium (RR = 3) and not

risk factors. EBCT provided incremental prognostic information in addition to age and other risk factors.

The societal question to be answered is: is this modest gain in risk prediction worth the cost of this test? But an even more basic question is: is this test better than the available tests, such as exercise testing? We think not. As we will see later, the test characteristics of exercise test scores exceed EBCT.

Conclusions Regarding Electron Beam Computed Tomography

Atherosclerotic calcification is an organized, regulated process similar to bone formation that occurs only when other aspects of atherosclerosis are also present. Nonhepatic Gla-containing proteins like osteocalcin, which are actively involved in the transport of calcium out of vessel walls, are suspected to have key roles in the pathogenesis of coronary calcification. Osteopontin, which is involved in bone mineralization, is present in calcified atherosclerotic lesions. Calcification is an active process and not simply a passive precipitation of calcium phosphate crystals. Although calcification is found more frequently in advanced lesions, it may also occur in small amounts in earlier lesions, which appear in the second and third decades of life. Histopathological investigation has shown that plaques with microscopic evidence of mineralization are larger and associated with larger coronary arteries than plaques or arteries without calcification. The relation of arterial calcification to the probability of plaque rupture is unknown. Although the amount of coronary calcium correlates with the amount of atherosclerosis in different individuals and to a lesser extent in segments of the coronary tree in the same individuals, it is not known if the quantity of calcification tracks the quantity of atherosclerosis over time in the same individuals. Epidemiological evidence and postmortem studies show that the prevalence of coronary calcium deposits in a given decade of life is 10 to 100 times higher than the expected 10-year incidence of CHD events for individuals of the same age. This disparity is less evident in the elderly and symptomatic than in the young and asymptomatic.

Electron Beam Computed Tomography for Screening Asymptomatic Subjects. There are insufficient data to determine whether the relation between coronary calcium and CHD risk warrants the use of calcium screening in low-risk, asymptomatic subjects. Experience from the studies using exercise testing suggest that hard endpoints must be used and certainly not interventions. The ACC/AHA recommendations state that EBCT is a research tool and is not to be recommended for screening for CAD.[88] The EBCT researchers should examine the experience of workers in the exercise test arena and avoid the same mistakes. The rules of Feinstein should be considered in evaluating this exciting new procedure.

MULTIVARIABLE PREDICTION TECHNIQUES WITH EXERCISE TESTING FOR SCREENING

Angiographic Studies

Uhl et al[89] measured fasting total cholesterol and HDLs in 572 asymptomatic aircrewmen. Of these, 132 had an abnormal treadmill test and underwent coronary angiography. Coronary disease, defined as a lesion of 50% or greater diameter narrowing, was found in 16 subjects, with the rest having minimal or no CAD ($N = 102$). The 14 men with minimal CAD had TC-HDL ratios that differed from the normal men ($P < 0.001$). Two of the 16 with angiographically determined CAD had TC-HDL ratios of less than six, whereas four of the 102 angiographic normal subjects had a ratio of greater than six times. Only 42 of 440 (9.5%) with a normal treadmill test had a TC-HDL ratio greater than six; 87% of those with CHD had TC-HDL ratios greater than six. This ratio generated a risk of 172. A limitation of this study is that true sensitivity cannot be determined because only those with an abnormal treadmill test underwent coronary angiography.

At the USAFSAM, 255 totally asymptomatic men underwent cardiac catheterization because of at least 0.1 mV of ST depression. Sixty-five men had at least 50% coronary artery narrowing. Thus, the predictive value of ST-segment changes was only 24%. Five risk factors were studied (smoking, hypertension, hypercholesterolemia, family history, and glucose intolerance) and univariate analysis did not increase the predictive value. However, 41 men had no abnormal risk factors and the odds ratio was over 3:1 with hypercholesterolemia alone or the presence of three risk factors. The presence of at least one risk factor and two or more exercise variables identified as predictive (including 0.3 mV of ST depression early, persistent ST depression postexercise, or exercise duration under 10 minutes) identified over half the cases of two- or three-vessel disease with a predictive value of 84%.

Follow-up Studies

From the Cooper Clinic comes the largest screening study of the exercise test to predict CV death in a self-selected population of asymptomatic men.[90] It was a prospective study performed between 1970 and 1989, with an average follow-up of 8.4 years. There were 25,927 healthy men, 20 to 82 years of age at baseline (mean 43 years) who were free of CV disease and who were evaluated in the Cooper preventive medicine clinic (i.e., self-selected and willing to pay). During follow-up there were 612 deaths from all causes and 158 deaths due to CV disease. The sensitivity of an abnormal exercise test to predict coronary death was 61%. The age-adjusted relative risk of an abnormal exercise test for CV death was 21× in those with no risk factors, 27× in those with one risk factor, 54× in those with 2 risk factors, and 80× in those with three or more factors. This elegant study, summarized in Table 11-8, supports the incredible risk generated by the standard exercise test as found in the earlier studies but it adds support to the additive value of considering risk factors.

At the Cleveland Clinic, the validity for prediction of all-cause mortality of the FRS and the European Global Scoring System Systematic Coronary Risk Evaluation (SCORE) was evaluated.[91] This was done in asymptomatic individuals evaluated in a clinical setting, which included an exercise test. A prospective cohort of 3554 asymptomatic adults between the ages of 50 and 75 years who underwent exercise testing as part of an executive health program between October 1990 and December 2002 were followed up for a mean of 8 years. Global risk was calculated using the FRS and the European SCORE. The primary endpoint

TABLE 11-8. The results of the Cooper Clinic screening study using exercise testing and conventional risk factors

Testing results	Age-adjusted relative risk for cardiovascular disease-related death
Abnormal ETI-ST depression only	21×
Abnormal ETI-ST depression plus one risk factor	27×
Abnormal ETI-ST depression plus two risk factor	54×
Abnormal ETI-ST depression plus three risk factor	80×

ETI-ST, exercise test-induced ST depression.

was all-cause mortality; there were 114 deaths. The c-index, which corresponds to area under the receiver operating characteristics curves, and the Akaike Information Criteria found that the European SCORE was superior to the FRS in estimating global mortality risk. In a multivariable model, independent predictors of death were a higher SCORE (RR, 1.07), impaired functional capacity (RR 3), and an abnormal heart rate recovery (RR 1.6). ST-segment depression did not predict mortality. Among patients in the highest tertile from the SCORE, an abnormal exercise test, defined as either impaired functional capacity or an abnormal heart rate recovery, identified a mortality risk of more than 1% per year. Hopefully our friends at Cleveland will repeat this analysis using CV event data, which is a more appropriate endpoint for a study attempting to evaluate means of predicting CV risk.

Using Framingham data, Balady et al[92] evaluated the usefulness of exercise testing in asymptomatic persons in predicting CHD events over and above the FRS. Included were 3043 members of the Framingham Heart Study offspring cohort without CHD (1431 men and 1612 women; mean age 45 years, SD ± 9 years) who were followed-up for 18 years. The risk of developing CHD was evaluated considering three exercise test variables: (1) ST-segment depression equaling 1 mm or more, (2) failure to achieve target heart rate of 85% predicted maximum, and (3) exercise capacity. In multivariable analyses that adjusted for age and Framingham CHD risk score, among men, ST-segment depression or failure to achieve target heart rate doubled CHD risk, whereas a greater exercise capacity predicted lower CHD risk. Although similar hazard ratios were seen in women, those results were not statistically significant. Among men with 10-year predicted risk greater than 20%, failure to reach target heart rate and ST-segment depression both more than doubled the risk of an event, and each MET increment in exercise capacity reduced risk by 13%. In this random sample of asymptomatic men, ST-segment depression, failure to reach target heart rate, and exercise capacity provided additional prognostic information in age- and FRS-adjusted models, particularly among those in the highest risk group (10-year predicted CHD risk of greater than 20%).

Erikssen et al[93] compared the accuracy of CV risk assessment based on classical risk factors (CRFs) with an assessment also based on multiple exercise test parameters. In 1972 to 1975, 2014 apparently healthy men aged 40 to 60 years had a symptom-limited exercise test during a CV survey. Their average maximal heart rate was 162 beats per minute and their average systolic blood pressure at a submaximal load of 100 watts was 180 mmHg. The prognostic exercise test variables included the ST response, submaximal systolic blood pressure (>1 SD [25 mmHg]), and exercise capacity. There were 300 CV deaths during 26 years of follow-up. Compared to Cox regression models solely including CRF, models also including multiple exercise test parameters (CRF + ExTest) were clearly superior. Risk scores were computed based on the models. CRF and CRF + ExTest risk scores often differed markedly; CRF+ ExTest scores were generally most reliable in both the high- and low-risk range. In smokers with elevated cholesterol ($n = 470$), the CRF and CRF + ExTest models identified 67 versus 110 men at the highest CV risk level according to European guidelines (34% versus 32% CV mortality). This study demonstrates that integration of multiple exercise test parameters and conventional risk factors can improve CV risk assessment substantially, especially in smokers with high cholesterol.

These three important contemporary studies are summarized in Table 11-9.

Computer Probability Estimates

Diamond and Forrester[94] performed a literature review to estimate pretest likelihood of disease by age, sex, symptoms, and the Framingham risk equation. In addition, they have considered the sensitivity and specificity of four diagnostic tests (the exercise test, CKG, nuclear perfusion, and cardiac fluoroscopy) and applied Bayes's theorem. CADENZA is the acronym for the computer program that calculates these estimates. The biggest weakness of this approach is that the sensitivities and specificities of the secondary tests is uncertain, and it is not clear how they interact because of similar inadequacies. In addition, a step approach that uses risk markers to identify a high-risk group excludes the majority of individuals who will

TABLE 11–9. Three contemporary screening studies that considered multiple exercise test response and risk factors together with 8-year follow-up or more for hard endpoints

Study	Sample size	Years of follow-up
Cooper Clinic	26,000 men	8
Norway	2000 men,	26
Framingham	3000 men	18

eventually get coronary disease. This approach concentrates the preventive impact on the small, high-risk group, while ignoring the majority of individuals in the moderate-risk range who will contribute larger numbers but at a lesser rate to disease endpoints.

PROGNOSIS IN ASYMPTOMATIC PATIENTS WITH ANGIOGRAPHICALLY SIGNIFICANT CORONARY DISEASE

Hammermeister et al[95] reported the effects of coronary artery bypass surgery on asymptomatic or mildly symptomatic angina patients who were studied as part of the Seattle Heart Watch. The report was based on 227 medically treated and 392 surgically treated patients who were nonrandomly assigned to medical or surgical therapy. Cox's regression analysis was used to correct for the differences in baseline characteristics. Patients with three-vessel disease who underwent surgery had significantly improved survival, but surgically treated patients with one- and two-vessel disease did not. The results of this study suggest that surgery may be indicated in the asymptomatic or mildly symptomatic patient with three-vessel disease, moderate impairment of left ventricular function (ejection fraction 31% to 50%), good distal vessels, and no other major medical illness. Asymptomatic patients with normal left ventricular function had an excellent prognosis regardless of the treatment.

Hickman et al[96] at USAFSAM followed-up for 5 years 90 men aged 45 to 54 years with asymptomatic angiographically determined coronary disease without previous MI. Sixteen patients developed angina, four had MIs, and two died suddenly. The events were not significantly different in those with one-, two-, or three-vessel disease. They concluded that in asymptomatic patients with angiographically determined coronary disease, the 5-year prognosis was good even in those with high-risk lesions. Conventional risk factors predicted risk more than the angiographic severity of disease did. Angina, a soft endpoint, was the most common initial event.

Kent et al[97] have reported 147 asymptomatic or mildly symptomatic patients with CHD who were followed prospectively for an average of 2 years. None had significant one-vessel, 31% had two-vessel, and 41% had three-vessel coronary disease. The ejection fraction was 55% or greater in 70% of the patients. Thirty-five percent of the patients

had a normal ECG, while 30% had evidence of a previous MI. During the follow-up period there were eight deaths for an annual mortality of 3% for the entire group, 1.5% for patients with single- and double-vessel disease, and 6% for those with triple-vessel disease. In those with triple-vessel disease, exercise testing enabled better identification of high- and a low-risk groups. In spite of a history of mild symptoms, 25% of the patients with triple-vessel disease exhibited poor exercise tolerance; of these, 40% either died (for an annual mortality of 9%), or had progressive symptoms requiring an operation. In those with good exercise capacity, only 22% died or had progressive symptoms, giving an annual mortality of 4%. The prognosis is excellent in patients with absent or mild symptoms with one- or two-vessel disease. In those with three-vessel disease and good exercise capacity, there was an annual mortality of 4%, versus 9% in those with three-vessel disease and poor exercise capacity.

EXERCISE TESTING FOR SPECIAL SCREENING PURPOSES

Exercise Testing for Exercise Programs

The optimal exercise prescription, based on a percentage of an individual's maximal heart rate or oxygen consumption (50% to 80%) or exceeding the gas exchange anaerobic threshold, can only be written after performing an exercise test. The best way to assess the risk of an adverse reaction during exercise is to observe the individual during exercise. The level of exercise training then can be set at a level below that at which adverse responses or symptoms occur. Some individuals motivated by popular misconceptions about the benefits of exercise may disregard their natural "warning systems" and push themselves into dangerous levels of ischemia.

An individual with a good exercise capacity and only 0.1 mV ST-segment depression at maximal exercise, has a relatively low risk of CV events in the next several years compared to an individual with marked ST-segment depression at a low heart rate and/or systolic blood pressure. Most individuals with an abnormal test can be put safely into an exercise program if the level of intensity of the exercise at which the response occurs is considered. Such patients can be followed with risk factor modification rather than being excluded from exercise or their livelihood.

Siscovick et al[98] determined whether the exercise ECG predicted acute cardiac events during moderate or strenuous physical activity among 3617 asymptomatic, hypercholesterolemic men (age range, 35 to 59 years) who were followed up in the Coronary Primary Prevention Trial. Submaximal exercise test results were obtained at entry and at annual follow-up visits in years 2 through 7. ST-segment depression or elevation was considered to be an abnormal result. The cumulative incidence of activity-related acute cardiac events was 2% during a mean follow-up period of 7 years. The risk was increased 2.6-fold in the presence of clinically silent, exercise-induced ST-segment changes at entry after adjustment for 11 other potential risk factors. Of 62 men who experienced an activity-related event, 11 had an abnormal test result at entry (sensitivity, 18%). The specificity of the entry exercise test was 92%. The sensitivity and specificity were similar when the length of follow-up was restricted to 1 year after testing. For a newly abnormal test result on a follow-up visit, the sensitivity was 24%, and the specificity was 85%; for any abnormal test result during the study (six tests per subject), the sensitivity was 37%, and the specificity was 79%. They concluded that the test was not sensitive when used to predict the occurrence of activity-related events among asymptomatic, hypercholesterolemic men. For this reason, the utility of the submaximal exercise test to assess the safety of physical activity among asymptomatic men at risk of CHD appeared limited.

Exercise testing is indicated prior to entering an exercise program for individuals with a strong family history of coronary disease (i.e., family members aged <60 with a coronary event), the presence of increased risk factors (particularly serum cholesterol), or any symptoms suggestive of myocardial ischemia currently or in the past. In addition, there are clearly a group of patients who self-select themselves for exercise testing. They may request the test because of symptoms even though they deny having any symptoms.

Military Fitness

The U.S. Army Program to Screen for Coronary Artery Disease

The U.S. Army evaluated a program of serial testing to detect latent CHD. Screening was considered necessary before initiating a mandatory exercise program for all personnel older than 40 years. The screening tests were applied in a sequential manner in an attempt to eliminate low-risk patients from further testing and to enhance the pretest likelihood of disease in the remaining subset. Initial history, physical examination, and resting ECGs were performed on 285 men and two women over 40 years of age (mean age 44 years). A fasting biochemical profile was obtained and a risk factor index based on the Framingham database was calculated. All subjects underwent maximal exercise testing. All were encouraged to exercise to exhaustion and the average METs was 10 (range 7 to 18). Pre- and postexercise CKGs were performed. A risk factor index over 5.0 was considered abnormal. An abnormal ST-segment response occurred in four men and an "abnormal non-diagnostic" response, defined as upsloping ST changes, occurred in 15 men. Six men had frequent exercise-induced premature ventricular contractions. These 26 men underwent cardiac fluoroscopy and thallium scintigraphy. Seven men had abnormal thallium scintigraphic findings, six underwent cardiac catheterization, and one died of a MI. One man with a low risk index and normal treadmill test, CKG, and fluoroscopic findings had a MI after 6 months of follow-up. No patient had coronary calcification. An abnormal ST-segment response was insensitive and not highly predictive of coronary disease. CKG had 63% sensitivity, 74% specificity, a predictive value of 50% and was the most accurate individual test. Risk factor analysis was not predictive and screening accuracy improved only when there were two or more risk factors and an abnormal CKG.

Zoltick et al[99] reported preliminary results with application of the United States Army CV Screening Program. A two-tier-staged approach was initiated for a CV screening program for all active-duty army personnel over the age of 40 years. Criteria for primary CV screen failure include any one of the following abnormalities: (1) Framingham risk index equaling or greater than 5%; (2) abnormal CV history or examination; (3) abnormal ECG; and (4) fasting blood sugar equal to 115 mg/dl or more. Failure of the primary screen requires the taking of a secondary screening test, which includes an internal medicine or cardiology consultation, a maximum treadmill test, and/or further sequential follow-up. During the follow-up, recommendations were made for risk factor modification and exercise programs. Between June 1981 and August 1983, 42,752 individuals were screened. Of these, 23,428 (55%) cleared the primary screen, 7279 (17%) cleared the secondary screen, and 1040 (2.4%) did not pass the secondary screen. Hopefully, the long-term results of this important study will be published soon.

The ability of atherosclerosis imaging to overcome limitations of clinical risk screening with coronary risk factors is being explored in a study called the Prospective Army Coronary Calcium Project (PACC). The goals of the PACC Project are to determine the utility of EBCT for the detection of coronary calcium as a screening test for CAD and as an intervention for risk factor modification among young, asymptomatic, active-duty personnel undergoing the United States Army's CV Screening Program.[100] Three study designs will be used to address the objectives of this investigation: (1) a cross-sectional study of 2000 unselected, consecutive participants to determine the prevalence and extent of coronary calcification in the 40- to 50-year-old Army population, (2) a randomized, controlled trial with a 2×2 factorial design involving 1000 participants to assess the impact of EBCT information on several dimensions of patient behavior, with and without intensive risk factor case management, and (3) a prospective cohort study of 2000 participants followed for at least 5 years to establish the relation between coronary calcification and CV events in an unselected, "low-risk" (by conventional standards) Army population. From these aims, data from the PACC project support that subclinical coronary calcium is prevalent in asymptomatic individuals, even those with optimal risk factor profiles.[101] In the PACC Project, 22.4% of asymptomatic men have identifiable foci of subclinical atherosclerosis. Emerging data from this study show that, after adjusting for coronary risk factor levels and family history, this finding is associated with an 11-fold risk of coronary events over the following 5 years, compared to those with no detectable coronary artery calcium.[102] Thus, with the finding of calcified subclinical atherosclerosis, careful focus by the clinician on modifiable coronary risk factors is warranted. An appropriate starting point in low-clinical risk populations is behavioral lifestyle change. Interestingly, a randomized clinical trial performed in the PACC Project failed to show that the demonstration of coronary calcium alone motivates heart healthy lifestyle and behavioral changes.[103] Thus, healthcare providers are encouraged to focus on motivating patients towards healthy lifestyles in traditional ways, such as education and continuous care.

Flying Fitness

Unfortunately, politics and economic factors are two of the strongest factors influencing the use of exercise testing in subjects with flying responsibilities.[104] The pool of available pilots is obviously an important national resource. If there are many pilots available, society is more likely to be stricter with regulations regarding flying standards.

Clearly, physicians must be concerned with public safety. Allowing an individual with an increased health risk to take responsibility for many other peoples' lives could result in a tragedy. The presence of a back-up pilot and the impact of modern technology on flying do not lessen the stresses of this occupation. There are numerous situations of very high stress, such as takeoffs and landings, where it might not be possible for other cockpit personnel to take over control of the aircraft, and a disaster not averted if the key pilot was to have a cardiac event. In general, pilots are a highly motivated, intelligent group of men who feel a high level of responsibility for the performance of their work. Flying is their livelihood, however, and most of them love it so dearly that they may conceal medical information that could endanger their flying status. In addition, the stress of work often leaves them unable to maintain a healthy lifestyle. The stress of altering one's circadian cycle and trying to navigate in and out of today's busy airports, leaves many of them overweight, deconditioned, and smoking heavily. Whenever possible, health professionals should recommend that these men and women have the full benefits of modern preventive medicine, including the periodic assessment of exercise capacity, response to stress, and the probability of coronary atherosclerosis.

DOES SCREENING MOTIVATE PATIENTS TO ALTER THEIR RISK?

Exercise testing may prove to have value in asymptomatic populations other than for screening. Bruce et al[105] examined the motivational effects of maximal exercise testing for modifying risk factors and health habits.[105] A questionnaire was sent to nearly 3000 men, 35 to 65 years of age, who had undergone symptom-limited treadmill testing at least 1 year earlier. Individuals were asked if the treadmill test motivated them to stop smoking (if already a smoker), increase daily exercise, purposely lose weight, reduce the amount of dietary fat, or take medication for hypertension. There was a 69% response to this questionnaire, and 63% of the responders indicated that they had modified one or more risk factors and health habits and that they attributed this change to the exercise test. In fact, a greater percentage of patients with decreased exercise capacity, compared with normal subjects reported a modification of risk factors or health habits.

The Army Cardiology Research group studied the effects of incorporating EBCT as a motivational factor into a CV screening program in the context of either intensive case management (ICM) or usual care by assessing its impact over 1 year on a composite measure of projected risk.[103] They performed a randomized controlled trial, with a 2×2 factorial design and 1 year of follow-up, involving a consecutive sample of 450 asymptomatic active-duty U.S. Army personnel, aged 39 to 45 years, stationed within the Washington, DC, area and scheduled to undergo a periodic Army-mandated physical examination, and who were enrolled between January 1999 and March 2001 (mean age, 42 years; 79% male; 66 [15%] had coronary calcification; predicted 10-year coronary risk was 6%). Patients were randomly assigned to one of four intervention arms: EBT results provided in the setting of either ICM ($n = 111$) or usual care ($n = 119$) or withheld in the setting of either ICM ($n = 124$) or usual care ($n = 96$). The primary outcome measure was change in a composite measure of risk, the 10-year FRS. Comparing the groups who received EBT results with those who did not, the mean absolute risk change in 10-year FRS was +0.30 versus +0.36. Comparing the groups who received ICM with those who received usual care, the mean absolute risk change in 10-year FRS was −0.06 versus +0.74. Improvement or stabilization of CV risk was noted in 157 patients (40%). In multivariable analyses predicting change in FRS, after controlling for knowledge of coronary calcification, motivation for change, and multiple psychological variables, only the number of risk factors (odds ratio, 1.4× for each additional risk factor) and receipt of ICM (odds ratio, 1.6×) were associated with improved or stabilized projected risk. Using coronary calcification screening to motivate patients to make evidence-based changes in risk factors was not associated with improvement in modifiable CV risk at 1 year. Case management was superior to usual care in the management of risk factors.

SUMMARY

Screening has become a controversial topic because of the incredible efficacy of the statins even in asymptomatic individuals.[106] We now have agents that can cut the risk of cardiac events almost in half. The first step in screening asymptomatic individuals for preclinical coronary disease should be using global risk factor equations such as the Framingham score. This is available as nomograms that are easily applied by healthcare professionals, or it can be calculated as part of a computerized patient record. Additional testing procedures with

promise include the simple ankle-brachial index (particularly in the elderly), CRP, carotid ultrasound measurements of intimal thickening, and the resting ECG (particularly spatial QRS-T wave angle). Despite the promotional concept of atherosclerotic burden, EBCT does not have test characteristics superior to the standard exercise test. If any screening test could be used to decide on statin therapy and not affect insurance or occupational status, this would be helpful. However, the screening test should not lead to more procedures.

True demonstration of the effectiveness of a screening technique requires randomizing the target population, one half receiving the screening technique, standardized action taken in response to the screening test results, and then outcomes assessed. For the screening technique to be effective, the screened group must have lower mortality and/or morbidity. Such a study has been completed for mammography but not for any cardiac testing modalities. The next best validation of efficacy is to demonstrate that the technique improves the discrimination of those asymptomatic individuals with higher risk for events over that possible with the available risk factors. Mathematical modeling makes it possible to determine how well a population will be classified if the characteristics of the testing method are known.

Additional follow-up studies and one angiographic study from the CASS population (where 195 individuals with abnormal exercise-induced ST depression and normal coronary angiograms were followed for 7 years) improve our understanding of the application of exercise testing as a screening tool. No increased incidence of cardiac events was found. The concerns raised the findings of Erikssen et al[60] in 36 subjects that those with abnormal ST depression and normal coronary angiograms were still at increased risk have not been substantiated.

The later follow-up studies (MRFIT, Seattle Heart Watch, Lipid Research Clinics, and Indiana State police) have shown different results compared to prior studies, mainly because hard cardiac endpoints, and not angina, were required. The first 10 prospective studies of exercise testing in asymptomatic individuals included angina as a cardiac disease endpoint. This led to a bias for individuals with abnormal tests to subsequently report angina or to be diagnosed as having angina. When only hard endpoints (death or MI) were used, as in the MRFIT, Lipid Research Clinics, Indiana State Police, or the Seattle Heart Watch studies, the results were less encouraging. The test could only identify one third of the patients with hard events and 95% of abnormal responders were false positives; that is, they did not die or have a MI. The predictive value of the abnormal maximal exercise ECG ranged from 5% to 46% in the studies reviewed. However, in the studies using appropriate endpoints (other than angina pectoris) only 5% of the abnormal responders developed CHD over the follow-up period. Thus, more than 90% of the abnormal responders were false positives. Actually though, the exercise test's characteristics as a screening test probably lie in between the results with hard or soft endpoints because some of the subjects who develop chest pain really have angina and CAD. The sensitivity is probably between 30% and 50% (at a specificity of 90%) but the critical limitation is the predictive value (and risk ratio), which depends on the prevalence of disease (which is low in the asymptomatic population).

Some of these individuals have CAD that has yet to manifest itself, but angiographic studies have supported this high false-positive rate when using the exercise test in asymptomatic populations. Moreover, the CASS study indicates that such individuals have a good prognosis. In a second Lipid Research Clinics study, only patients with elevated cholesterol's were considered, and yet only a 6% positive prediction value was found. If the test is to be used to screen, it should be done in groups with a higher estimated prevalence of disease using the Framingham score and not just one risk factor. The iatrogenic problems resulting from screening must be considered. Hopefully, using a threshold from the Framingham score would be more successful in identifying asymptomatic individuals that should be tested.

Some individuals who eventually develop CAD will change on retesting from a normal to an abnormal response. However, McHenry et al[48] and Fleg et al[67] have reported that a change from a negative to a positive test is no more predictive than is an initially abnormal test. One individual has even been reported who changed from a normal to an abnormal test but was free of angiographically significant disease.[107] In most circumstances an add-on imaging modality (ECHO or nuclear) should be the first choice in evaluating asymptomatic individuals with an abnormal exercise test.

The motivational impact of screening for CAD is not evidence-based with one positive study for exercise testing and one negative study for EBCT. Further research in this area is certainly needed.

While the risk of an abnormal exercise test is apparent from these studies, the iatrogenic problems resulting from screening must be considered (i.e., employment, insurance, etc.). The recent

U.S. Preventive Services Task Force statement states that "false-positive tests are common among asymptomatic adults, especially women, and may lead to unnecessary diagnostic testing, overtreatment and labeling." This statement summarizes the current U.S. Preventive Services Task Force (USPSTF) recommendations on screening for CHD and the supporting scientific evidence and updates the 1996 recommendations on this topic. The complete information on which this statement is based, including evidence tables and references, is available in the background article and the systematic evidence review, available through the USPSTF Web site (http://www.preventiveservices.ahrq.gov) and through the National Guideline Clearinghouse (http://www.guideline.gov).[108] In the majority of asymptomatic people, screening with any test or test add-on, is more likely to yield false positives than true positives. This is the mathematical reality associated with all of the available tests.

However, if screening could be performed in a logical way with test results helping to decide on therapies (and more powerful therapeutics are on the way, particularly those raising HDL) and not leading to invasive interventions, insurance, or occupational problems, recent results summarized in this chapter should be applied. *Here is our strongest variance from the guidelines:* we feel that exercise testing should be used in a logical way for screening healthy, asymptomatic individuals along with risk factor assessment. The following reasons support this position:

1. Three contemporary studies have demonstrated incredible risk ratios for the combination of the standard exercise test results and risk factors.
2. Other modalities without the favorable test characteristics of the exercise test are being promoted for screening.
3. Physical inactivity has reached epidemic proportions and what better way to make our patients conscious of their deconditioning than having them do an exercise test which can also "clear them" for exercise and provide a baseline.
4. A MET increase in exercise capacity equates with a 10% to 20% improvement in survival in almost any population studied.

The data from the Cooper Clinic (26,000 men, 8-year follow-up), Norway (2000 men, 26-year follow-up) and Framingham (3000 men, 18-year follow-up) are convincing in demonstrating the additional risk classification power of adding the exercise test to the screening process. Furthermore, the exercise capacity itself has enormous prognostic predictive power. Given the epidemic of physical inactivity we are experiencing, including the exercise test in the screening process sends a strong message to our patients that we consider their exercise capacity as important.

REFERENCES

1. Grover SA, Coupal L, Hu XP: Identifying adults at increased risk of coronary disease. How well do the current cholesterol guidelines work? JAMA 1995;274:801–806.
2. Anderson P: An updated Risk factor profile. Circulation 1991;83: 356–362.
3. Wilson PW, D'Agostino RB, Levy D, et al: Prediction of coronary heart disease using risk factor categories. Circulation 1998;97: 1837–1847.
4. Lloyd-Jones DM, Wilson PW, Larson MG, et al: Framingham risk score and prediction of lifetime risk for coronary heart disease. Am J Cardiol 2004;94:20–24.
5. Ridker PM, Cook N: Clinical usefulness of very high and very low levels of C-reactive protein across the full range of Framingham Risk Scores. Circulation 2004;109:1955–1959. Epub 2004 Mar 29.
6. Conroy RM, Pyorala K, Fitzgerald AP, et al: Estimation of ten-year risk of fatal cardiovascular disease in Europe: the SCORE project. Eur Heart J 2003;24:987–1003.
7. Thomsen TF, McGee D, Davidsen M, Jorgensen T: A cross-validation of risk-scores for coronary heart disease mortality based on data from the Glostrup Population Studies and Framingham Heart Study. Int J Epidemiol 2002;31:817–822.
8. Ostor E, Schnohr, Jensen G, et al: Electrocardiographic findings and their association with mortality in the Copenhagen City Heart Study. Eur Heart J 1981;2:317–328.
9. Rose G, Baxter PJ, Reid DD, McCartney P: Prevalence and prognosis of electrocardiogram findings in middle-aged men. Br Heart J 1978;15:636–643.
10. Cullen K, Stenhouse NS, Wearne KL, Cumpston GN: Electrocardiograms and 13 year cardiovascular mortality in Busselton study. Br Heart J 1982;47:209–212.
11. Rabkin SW, Mathewson FAL, Tate RB: The electrocardiogram in apparently healthy men and the risk of sudden death. Br Heart J 1982;47:546–552.
12. Dawber TR, Kannel WB, Love DE, Streeper RB: The Framingham Study. Circulation 1952;5:559–566.
13. Levine HD, Phillips E: The electrocardiogram and MI. N Engl J Med 1951;245:833–842.
14. Liao Y, Liu K, Dyer A, Schoenberger JA, et al: Major and minor electrocardiographic abnormalities and risk of death from coronary heart disease, cardiovascular diseases and all causes in men and women. J Am Coll Cardiol 1988;12:1494–1500.
15. Menotti A, Seccareccia F: Electrocardiographic Minnesota code findings predicting short-term mortality in asymptomatic subjects. The Italian RIFLE Pooling Project (Risk Factors and Life Expectancy). G Ital Cardiol 1997;27:40–49.
16. Milan Study on Atherosclerosis and Diabetes (MiSAD) Group: Prevalence of unrecognized silent myocardial ischemia and its association with atherosclerotic risk factors in noninsulin-dependent diabetes mellitus. Am J Cardiol 1997;79:134–139.
17. Whincup PH, Wannamethee G, Macfarlane PW, et al: Resting electrocardiogram and risk of coronary heart disease in middle-aged British men. J Cardiovasc Risk 1995;2:533–543.
18. Krone RJ, Greenberg H, Dwyer EM Jr, et al: Long-term prognostic significance of ST segment depression during acute myocardial infarction. The Multicenter Diltiazem Postinfarction Trial Research Group. J Am Coll Cardiol 1993;22:361–367.
19. Sigurdsson E, Sigfusson N, Sigvaldason H, Thorgeirsson G: Silent ST-T changes in an epidemiologic cohort study—a marker of hypertension or coronary heart disease, or both: the Reykjavik study. J Am Coll Cardiol 1996;27:1140–1147.
20. Kors JA, van Herpen G, van Bemmel JH: QT dispersion as an attribute of T-loop morphology. Circulation 1999;99:1458–1463.
21. Lee KW, Kligfield P, Dower GE, Okin PM: QT dispersion, T-wave projection, and heterogeneity of repolarization in patients with coronary artery disease. Am J Cardiol 2001;87:148–151.
22. Okin PM, Devereux RB, Fabsitz RR, et al: Principal component analysis of the T wave and prediction of cardiovascular mortality in American Indians: the Strong Heart Study. Circulation 2002;105: 714–719.
23. Kors JA, de Bruyne MC, Hoes AW, et al: T axis as an indicator of risk of cardiac events in elderly people. Lancet 1998;352:601–605.
24. Rautaharju PM, Nelson JC, Kronmal RA, et al: Usefulness of T-axis deviation as an independent risk indicator for incident cardiac events in older men and women free from coronary heart disease (the Cardiovascular Health Study). Am J Cardiol 2001;88:118–123.
25. Kardys I, Kors JA, van der Meer IM, et al: Spatial QRS-T angle predicts cardiac death in a general population. Eur Heart J 2003;24: 1357–1364.
26. Murphy ML, Thenabadu PN, de Soyza N, et al: Sensitivity of electrocardiographic criteria for left ventricular hypertrophy according to type of cardiac disease. Am J Cardiol 1985;55:545–549.
27. Murphy ML, Thenabadu PN, de Soyza N, et al: Reevaluation of electrocardiographic criteria for left, right and combined cardiac ventricular hypertrophy. Am J Cardiol 1984;53:1140–1147.
28. Hutchins SW, Murphy ML, Dinh H: Recent progress in the electrocardiographic diagnosis of ventricular hypertrophy. Cardiol Clin 1987;5:455–468.
29. Rautaharju PM, Zhou SH, Park LP: Improved ECG models for left ventricular mass adjusted for body size, with specific algorithms for normal conduction, bundle branch blocks, and old myocardial infarction. J Electrocardiol 1996;29(suppl):261–269.
30. Okin PM, Roman MJ, Devereux RB, Kligfield P: ECG identification of left ventricular hypertrophy. Relationship of test performance to body habitus. J Electrocardiol 1996;29(suppl):256–261.
31. Norman JE, Levy D: Improved electrocardiographic detection of echocardiographic left ventricular hypertrophy: Results of a correlated data base approach J Am Coll Cardiol 1995;26:1022–1029.
32. Norman JE, Levy D: Adjustment of ECG left ventricular hypertrophy criteria for body mass index and age improves classification accuracy. The effects of hypertension and obesity. J Electrocardiol 1996;29 (suppl):241–247.
33. Crow RS, Hannan P, Grandits G, Liebson P: Is the echocardiogram an appropriate ECG validity standard for the detection and change in left ventricular size? J Electrocardiol 1996;29 (suppl): 248–255.
34. Siscovick DS, Raghunathan TE, Rautaharju P, et al: Clinically silent electrocardiographic abnormalities and risk of primary cardiac arrest among hypertensive patients. Circulation 1996;94:1329–1333.
35. Hypertension Detection and Follow-up Program Cooperative Group: Five-year findings of the Hypertension Detection and Follow-up Program. Prevention and reversal of left ventricular hypertrophy with antihypertensive drug therapy. Hypertension 1985;7: 105–112.
36. Verdecchia P, Schillaci G, Borgioni C, et al: Prognostic value of a new electrocardiographic method for diagnosis of left ventricular hypertrophy in essential hypertension. J Am Coll Cardiol 1998;31:383–390.
37. Crow RS, Prineas RJ, Hannan PJ, et al: Prognostic associations of Minnesota Code serial electrocardiographic change classification with coronary heart disease mortality in the Multiple Risk Factor Intervention Trial. Am J Cardiol 1997;80:138–144.
38. Froelicher VF, Thompson AJ, Wolthuis R, et al: Angiographic findings in asymptomatic aircrewmen with electrocardiographic abnormalities. Am J Cardiol 1977;39:32–39.
39. Gibbons RJ, Balady GJ, Timothy Bricker J, et al: ACC/AHA 2002 Guideline Update for Exercise Testing: Summary Article: A Report of the American College of Cardiology/American Heart Association Task Force on Practice Guidelines (Committee to Update the 1997 Exercise Testing Guidelines). Circulation 2002;106:1883–1892.
40. Bruce RA, McDonough JR: Stress testing in screening for cardiovascular disease. Bull NY Acad Med 1969;45:1288–1295.
41. Aronow WS, Cassidy J: Five year follow-up of double Master's test, maximal treadmill stress test, and resting and postexercise apexcardiogram in asymptomatic persons. Circulation 1975;52: 616–622.

42. Cumming GR, Samm J, Borysyk L, et al: Electrocardiographic changes during exercise in asymptomatic men: 3-year follow-up. Can Med Assoc J 1975;112:578–585.

43. Froelicher VF, Thomas M, Pillow C, et al: An epidemiological study of asymptomatic men screened with exercise testing for latent coronary heart disease. Am J Cardiol 1975;34:770–779.

44. Manca C, Barilli AL, Dei Cas L, et al: Multivariate analysis of exercise ST depression and coronary risk factors in asymptomatic men. Eur Heart J 1982;3:2–8.

45. Allen WH, Aronow WS, Goodman P, Stinson P: Five-year follow-up of maximal treadmill stress test in asymptomatic men and women. Circulation 1980;62:522–531.

46. Bruce RA, Fisher LD, Hossack KF: Validation of exercise-enhanced risk assessment of coronary heart disease events: Longitudinal changes in incidence in Seattle community practice. J Am Coll Cardiol 1985;5:875–881.

47. MacIntyre NR, Kunkler JR, Mitchell RE, et al: Eight-year follow-up of exercise electrocardiograms in healthy, middle-aged aviators. Aviat Space Environ Med 1981;52:256–259.

48. McHenry PL, O'Donnell J, Morris SN, Jordan JJ: The abnormal exercise electrocardiogram in apparently healthy men: A predictor of angina pectoris as an initial coronary event during long-term follow-up. Circulation 1984;70:547–551.

49. Multiple Risk Factor Intervention Research Group: Exercise electrocardiogram and coronary heart disease mortality in the multiple risk factor intervention trial. Am J Cardiol 1985;55:16–24.

50. Rautaharju PM, Prineas RJ, Eifler WJ, et al: Prognostic value of exercise electrocardiogram in men at high risk of future coronary heart disease: Multiple risk factor intervention trial experience. J Am Coll Cardiol 1986;8:1–10.

51. Gordon DJ, Ekelund LG, Karon JM, et al: Predictive value of the exercise tolerance test for mortality in North American men: The Lipid Research Clinics Mortality Follow-Up Study. Circulation 1986;74:252–261.

52. Ekelund LG, Suchindran CM, McMahon RP, et al: Coronary heart disease morbidity and mortality in hypercholesterolemic men predicted from an exercise test: The Lipid Research Clinics Coronary Primary Prevention Trial. J Am Coll Cardiol 1989;14:556–563.

53. Josephson RA, Shefrin E, Lakatta EG, et al: Can serial exercise testing improve the prediction of coronary events in asymptomatic individuals? Circulation 1990;81:20–24.

54. Gordon DJ, Leon AS, Ekelund LG, et al: Smoking, physical activity, and other predictors of endurance and heart rate response to exercise in asymptomatic hypercholesterolemic men. Am J Epidemiol 1987;125:587–600.

55. Hedblad B, Juul-Moller S, Svensson K, et al: Increased mortality in men with ST segment depression during 24 h ambulatory long-term ECG recording. Results from prospective population study 'Men born in 1914', from Malmo, Sweden. Eur Heart J 1989;10:149–158.

56. Borer JS, Brensike JF, Redwood DR, et al: Limitations of the electrocardiographic response to exercise in predicting coronary artery disease. N Engl J Med 1975;193:367–375.

57. Barnard RJ, Gardner GW, Diaco NV, Kattus AA: Near-maximal ECG stress testing and coronary artery disease risk factor analysis in Los Angeles City fire fighters. J Occupational Med 1975;18:818–827.

58. Uhl GS, Hopkirk AC, Hickman JR, et al: Predictive implications of clinical and exercise variables in detecting significant coronary artery disease in asymptomatic men. J Cardiac Rehabil 1984;4:245–252.

59. Erikssen J, Enge I, Forfang K, Storstein O: False positive diagnostic tests and coronary angiographic findings in 105 presumably healthy males. Circulation 1976;54:371–376.

60. Erikssen J, Dale J, Rottwelt K, Myhre E: False suspicion of coronary heart disease: A 7 year follow-up study of 36 apparently healthy middle-aged men. Circulation 1983;68:490–497.

61. Kemp HG, Kronmal RA, Vlietstra RE, Frye RL: Seven year survival of patients with normal and near normal coronary arteriograms: A CASS registry study. J Am Coll Cardiol 1986;7:479–483.

62. Hollenberg M, Zoltick JM, Go M, et al: Comparison of a quantitative treadmill exercise score with standard electrocardiographic criteria in screening asymptomatic young men for coronary artery disease. New Engl J Med 1985;313:600–606.

63. Okin PM, Anderson KM, Levy D, Kligfield P: Heart rate adjustment of exercise-induced ST segment depression. Improved risk stratification in the Framingham Offspring Study. Circulation 1991;83:866–874.

64. Caralis DG, Bailey I, Kennedy HL, Pitt B: Thallium-201 myocardial imaging in evaluation of asymptomatic individuals with ischemic ST segment depression on exercise electrocardiogram. Br Heart J 1979;42:562–571.

65. Nolewajka AJ, Kostuk WJ, Howard J, et al: 201 Thallium stress myocardial imaging: An evaluation of fifty-eight asymptomatic males. Clin Cardiol 1981;4:134–142.

66. Uhl GS, Kay TN, Hickman JR: Computer-enhanced thallium-scintigrams in asymptomatic men with abnormal exercise tests. Am J Cardiol 1981;48:1037–1046.

67. Fleg JL, Gerstenblith G, Zonderman AB, et al: Prevalence and prognostic significance of exercise-induced silent myocardial ischemia detected by thallium scintigraphy and electrocardiography in asymptomatic volunteers. Circulation 1990;81:428–436.

68. Silverberg RA, Diamond GA, Vas R, et al: Noninvasive diagnosis of coronary artery disease: The cardiokymographic stress test. Circulation 1980;61:579–589.

69. Weiner DA: Accuracy of cardiokymography during exercise testing: Results of a multicenter study. J Am Coll Cardiol 1985;6:502–509.

70. Wexler L, Brundage B, Crouse J, et al: Coronary artery calcification: Pathophysiology, epidemiology, imaging methods, and clinical implications. A statement for health professionals from the American Heart Association. Writing Group. Circulation 1996;94:1175–1192.

71. Langou RA, Huang EK, Kelley MJ, et al: Predictive accuracy of coronary artery calcification and abnormal exercise test for coronary artery disease in asymptomatic man. Circulation 1981;62:1196–1202.

72. Detrano R, Froelicher V: A logical approach to screening for coronary artery disease. Ann Intern Med 1987;106:846–852.

73. Gianrossi R, Detrano R, Colombo A, Froelicher VF: Cardiac fluoroscopy for the diagnosis of coronary artery disease: A meta analytic review. Am Heart J 1990;120:1179–1188.

74. Loecker TH, Schwartz RS, Cotta CW, Hickman JR, Jr: Fluoroscopic coronary artery calcification and associated coronary disease in asymptomatic young men. J Am Coll Cardiol 1992;19:1167–1172.

75. de Korte PJ, Kessels AG, van Engelshoven JM, Sturmans F: Usefulness of cinefluoroscopic detection of coronary artery calcification in the diagnostic work-up of coronary artery disease. Eur J Radiol 1995;19:188–193.

76. Shemesh J, Apter S, Rozenman J, et al: Calcification of coronary arteries: Detection and quantification with double-helix CT. Radiology 1995;197:779–783.

77. Kajinami K, Seki H, Takekoshi N, Mabuchi H: Noninvasive prediction of coronary atherosclerosis by quantification of coronary artery calcification using electron beam computed tomography: Comparison with electrocardiographic and thallium exercise stress test results. J Am Coll Cardiol 1995;26:1209–1221.

78. Detrano R, Hsiai T, Wang S, et al: Prognostic value of coronary calcification and angiographic stenoses in patients undergoing coronary angiography. J Am Coll Cardiol 1996;27:285–290.

79. Budhoff MJ, Georgiou D, Brody A, et al: Ultrafast computed tomography as a diagnostic modality in the detection of coronary artery disease: A multicenter study. Circulation 1996;93:898–904.

80. O'Malley PG, Greenberg BA, Taylor AJ: Cost-effectiveness of using electron beam computed tomography to identify patients at risk for clinical coronary artery disease. Am Heart J 2004;148:106–113.

81. Margolis JR, Chen JT, Kong Y, et al: The diagnostic and prognostic significance of coronary artery calcification: A report of 800 cases. Radiology 1980;137:609–616.

82. Detrano RC, Wong ND, Tang W, et al: Prognostic significance of cardiac cinefluoroscopy for coronary calcific deposits in asymptomatic high risk subjects. J Am Coll Cardiol 1994;24:354–358.

83. Arad Y, Spadaro LA, Goodman K, et al: Predictive value of electron beam CT of the coronary arteries: 19-month follow-up of 1173 asymptomatic subjects. Circulation 1996;93:1951–1953.

84. Thompson GR, Partridge J: Coronary calcification score: The coronary-risk impact factor. Lancet 2004 Feb 14;363:557–559.

85. Shaw LJ, Raggi P, Schisterman E, et al: Prognostic value of cardiac risk factors and coronary artery calcium screening for all-cause mortality. Radiology 2003;228:826–833. Epub 2003 Jul 17.

86. Greenland P, LaBree L, Azen SP, et al: Coronary artery calcium score combined with Framingham score for risk prediction in asymptomatic individuals. JAMA 2004;291:210–215.

87. Kondos GT, Hoff JA, Sevrukov A, et al: Electron-beam tomography coronary artery calcium and cardiac events: a 37-month follow-up of 5635 initially asymptomatic low- to intermediate-risk adults. Circulation 2003;107:2571–2576. Epub 2003.May 12.

88. O'Rourke RA, Brundage BH, Froelicher VF, et al: American College of Cardiology/American Heart Association Expert Consensus Document on electron-beam computed tomography for the diagnosis and prognosis of coronary artery disease. J Am Coll Cardiol 2000;36:326–340 and Circulation 2000;102:126–140.

89. Uhl GS, Troxler RG, Hickman JR, Clark D: Angiographic correlation of coronary artery disease with high density lipoprotein cholesterol in asymptomatic men. Am J Cardiol 1981;48:903–911.

90. Gibbons LW, Mitchell TL, Wei M, et al: Maximal exercise test as a predictor of risk for mortality from coronary heart disease in asymptomatic men. Am J Cardiol 2000;86:53–58.

91. Aktas MK, Ozduran V, Pothier CE, et al: Global risk scores and exercise testing for predicting all-cause mortality in a preventive medicine program. JAMA 2004;292:1462–1468.

92. Balady GJ, Larson MG, Vasan RS, et al: Usefulness of exercise testing in the prediction of coronary disease risk among asymptomatic persons as a function of the Framingham Risk Score. Circulation 2004;110:1920–1925.

93. Erikssen G, Bodegard J, Bjornholt JV, et al: Exercise testing of healthy men in a new perspective: From diagnosis to prognosis. Eur Heart J 2004;25:978–986.

94. Diamond GA, Forrester JS: Analysis of probability as an aid in the clinical diagnosis of coronary artery disease. N Engl J Med 1979; 300:1350–1359.

95. Hammermeister KE, DeRouen TA, Dodge HT: Effect of coronary surgery on survival in asymptomatic and minimally symptomatic patients. Circulation 1980;62:98–104.

96. Hickman JR, Uhl GS, Cook RL, et al: A natural history study of asymptomatic coronary disease. Am J Cardiol 1980;45:422–430.

97. Kent KM, Rosing DR, Ewels CJ, et al: Prognosis of asymptomatic or mildly symptomatic patients with coronary artery disease. Am J Cardiol 1982;49:1823–1831.

98. Siscovick DS, Ekelund LG, Johnson JL, et al: Sensitivity of exercise electrocardiography for acute cardiac events during moderate and strenuous physical activity. Arch Intern Med 1991;151:325–330.

99. Zoltick JM, McAllister HA, Bedynek JL: The United States Army Cardiovascular Screening Program. J Cardiac Rehabil 1984;4: 530–535.

100. O'Malley PG, Taylor AJ, Gibbons RV, et al: Rationale and design of the Prospective Army Coronary Calcium (PACC) Study: Utility of electron beam computed tomography as a screening test for coronary artery disease and as an intervention for risk factor modification among young, asymptomatic, active-duty United States Army Personnel. Am Heart J 1999;137:932–941.

101. Taylor AJ, Feuerstein IM, Wong H, et al: Do conventional risk factors predict subclinical coronary artery disease? Results from the Prospective Army Coronary Calcium Project. Am Heart J 2001;141:463–468.

102. Taylor AJ, Bindeman J, Feuerstein I, et al: The independent prognostic value of coronary calcium over measured cardiovascular risk factors in an asymptomatic male screening population: 5 year outcomes in the Prospective Army Coronary Calcium Project. J Am Coll Cardiol 2005;46:807–814.

103. O'Malley PG, Feuerstein IM, Taylor AJ: Impact of electron beam tomography, with or without case management, on motivation, behavioral change, and cardiovascular risk profile: A randomized controlled trial. JAMA 2003;289:2215–2223.

104. Bruce RA, Fisher LD: Clinical medicine: Exercise-enchanced risk factors for coronary heart disease vs. age as criteria for mandatory retirement of healthy pilots. Aviat Space Environ Med 1987;11:792–798.

105. Bruce RA, DeRouen TA, Hossack KF: Pilot study examining the motivational effects of maximal exercise testing to modify risk factors and health habits. Cardiology 1980;66:111–119.

106. Downs JR, Clearfield M, Weis S,et al: Primary prevention of acute coronary events with lovastatin in men and women with average cholesterol levels: Results of AFCAPS/TexCAPS. Air Force/Texas Coronary Atherosclerosis Prevention Study. JAMA 1998;279: 1615–1622.

107. Thompson AJ, Froelicher VF: Normal coronary angiography in an aircrewman with serial test changes. Aviat Space Environ Med 1975;46:69–73.

108. U.S. Preventive Services Task Force: Screening for coronary heart disease: Recommendation statement. Ann Intern Med 2004;140: 569–572.

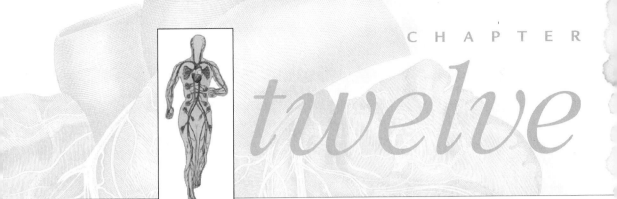

Miscellaneous Applications of Exercise Testing

INTRODUCTION

Earlier chapters dealt with the diagnostic and prognostic applications of the standard exercise test as well as its use after myocardial infarction (MI), patients with heart failure, and for screening. This chapter will present the applications of the test for evaluating treatments and therapeutic interventions, patients with valvular heart disease or arrhythmias, and as part of the preoperative workup for noncardiac surgery. The ACC/AHA Guidelines are included indicating the 2002 changes.

EVALUATION OF TREATMENTS

The exercise test can be used to evaluate the effects of both medical and surgical treatment. The effects of various medications, including antianginal agents, digoxin, and antihypertensive agents, have been evaluated by exercise testing. The test has also been used to evaluate patients before and after coronary artery bypass surgery and coronary angioplasty, and at one time, it was considered necessary to evaluate patients for these procedures. As discussed in earlier chapters, a common problem with using treadmill time or workload rather than measuring maximal oxygen uptake in is that individuals tend to perform treadmill walking more efficiently with repeat testing. Treadmill time or workload can increase during serial studies without any improvement in cardiovascular function. Thus, it is important to include the measurement of ventilatory oxygen uptake when the effects of medical or surgical treatments are being evaluated by treadmill testing or to insure a stable baseline.

Evaluation of Antianginal Agents

Reproducibility

Since studies using standard exercise testing are frequently required by the Food and Drug Administration prior to approval of antianginal and other pharmacologic agents, it is important to know the reproducibility of exercise variables in patients with angina. There have been numerous studies over the years assessing the reproducibility of exercise tolerance, as well as dyspnea or angina responses to exercise. Sullivan et al[1] from our laboratory studied 14 angina patients on 3 separate days of treadmill testing. A random effects analysis of variance model was used to measure reliability and to determine any trends in the test responses. The intraclass correlation coefficient (ICC; standard deviation divided by the mean $\times$ 100), a generalization of the Pearson product-moment correlation coefficient for bivariate data, along with the coefficient of variation were used to quantify reproducibility. The results are summarized in Table 12-1. A coefficient of variation of 6% for peak treadmill time was observed. This agreed closely with an earlier study by Smokler et al[2] using moderately severe angina as an endpoint, who observed coefficients of variation of approximately 5% for total treadmill time. However, when Sullivan et al[1] determined the ICC to test for reproducibility of

TABLE 12-1. Standard deviation of change of two measurements (SD), intraclass correlation (ICC), coefficient of variation (CV) at peak exercise, onset of angina, and ventilatory threshold

Variable	Peak exercise			Onset of angina			Ventilatory threshold		
	SD	ICC	CV (%)	SD	ICC	CV (%)	SD	ICC	CV (%)
Time (sec)	58	0.70	6 ± 6	65	0.70	11 ± 6	65	0.70	15 ± 9
VO_2 (L/min)	0.15	0.88	6 ± 4	0.15	0.85	6 ± 4	0.11	0.83	7 ± 4
Double product ($\times 10^3$)	2.6	0.90	9 ± 5	2.0	0.75	8 ± 5	2.2	0.75	8 ± 6
Heart rate (beats/min)	7	0.94	4 ± 2	6	0.89	4 ± 2	8	0.83	4 ± 4
ST_{60} X (mV)	0.06	0.80	34 ± 25	0.03	0.79	31 ± 25	0.03	0.78	45 ± 29
ST_{60} GD (mV)	0.05	0.83	23 ± 21	0.04	0.65	25 ± 16	0.05	0.65	53 ± 34

X, Lead X; GD, lead with greatest depression.
From Sullivan, et al: Chest 1984;86:374-382.

exercise time, a rather low value of r equaling 0.70 was obtained. The lack of reproducibility is attributable to the fact that patients increase their exercise time with repeat testing. This phenomenon has been observed repeatedly in the past in studies among normal subjects, patients with angina, and patients with heart failure. Importantly however, better reproducibility has been consistently reported for measured oxygen uptake compared with treadmill time. In our study, the ICC improved to 0.88 at peak exercise for measured VO_2, and better reproducibility was also observed at the onset of angina and the ventilatory threshold for measured VO_2 compared to exercise time.

The ability to reproducibly determine anginal pain or other endpoints during exercise testing is critical to the evaluation of therapeutic interventions. Many previous investigations have included a baseline exercise test in which the patient becomes familiar with the exercise testing equipment and staff; the inclusion of a "learning" test such as this improves the reproducibility of subsequent tests, and can also be used to individualize the protocol. Studies by Redwood et al[3] more than 30 years ago, along with many subsequent researchers have stressed the importance of a properly designed exercise test protocol when evaluating patients with stable angina pectoris. They suggested that exercise capacity and the onset of angina can be optimally evaluated using a progressive exercise test that elicits anginal pain within 3 to 6 minutes. In addition, increments in work should be relatively small (e.g., ≈1.0 MET) and evenly incremented. As outlined in Chapter 2, the advantage of an individualized protocol over one protocol for all patients is that it provides a gradual increase in work and is specific for each patient's exercise capacity or onset of symptoms. This is particularly important when studying angina responses to exercise, which are

subjective and depend on the patient's ability to express their perception of pain.

The criterion for stopping the exercise test is usually the patient's subjective anginal pain corresponding to that level of pain at which they would normally stop activities or take a sublingual nitroglycerin tablet. Many of the angina trials have used a 1 to 4 scale for this purpose, in which a rating of 3 represents this endpoint.[4] It would appear that there is a great deal of individual variation in the amount of tolerable anginal pain prior to stopping an activity. We observed that the reproducibility (ICC) of the double product, a noninvasive estimate of myocardial oxygen demand, was quite high at peak exercise (ICC = 0.90), but somewhat lower at the onset of angina and the ventilatory threshold (ICC = 0.75 for both). The poorer reproducibility at the onset of angina and the ventilatory threshold may be explained by the fact that blood pressure was measured every 2 minutes. The observed improvement in the ICC for the heart rate when compared to double product at the onset of angina (ICC = 0.89) and the ventilatory threshold (ICC = 0.83) and a slight increase at peak exercise (ICC = 0.94) supports this contention. Thus, when systolic blood pressure is difficult to obtain, heart rate may be used as a reproducible noninvasive estimate of myocardial oxygen demand. Heart rate, double product, or both, at the onset of ischemia (angina or occurrence of 1.0-mm ST depression) have frequently been used in angina trials as secondary analysis points.

Previous studies involving angina patients have reported high coefficients of variation for the amount of ST-segment displacement. When considering the ICC for lead X (a 3-dimensional lateral lead), the reproducibility is high at peak exercise, the onset of angina, and the ventilatory threshold (ICC ≈ 0.80); however, the coefficients of variation ranged from 31% to 45% (see Table 12-1). Although not nearly as reproducible at the onset of angina or ventilatory threshold (ICC = 0.65), the lead with the greatest ST-segment displacement is reproducible at peak exercise (ICC = 0.83). Table 12-2 provides a list of recommendations regarding exercise test reproducibility for drug evaluations.

Variable Anginal Threshold

Waters et al[5] investigated the frequency and mechanism of variable threshold angina by performing seven treadmill tests in each of 28 patients with stable effort angina and exercise-induced ST-segment depression. Each patient had tests at 8 AM on 4 days within a 2-week period and on one of these days had three additional tests at 9 AM, 11 AM, and 4 PM Time to 0.1-mV ST depression increased from 277 ± 172 seconds on day 1 to 319 ± 186 seconds on day 2, 352 + 213 seconds on day 3, and 356 ± 207 seconds on day 4. Rate-pressure product at 0.1-mV ST depression remained constant. Similarly, time to 0.1-mV ST depression increased from 333 ± 197 seconds at 8 AM to 371 ± 201 seconds at 9 AM and 401 ± 207 seconds at 11 AM and decreased to 371 ± 189 seconds at 4 PM. Again, rate-pressure product at 0.1-mV ST depression remained constant. The standard deviation for time to 0.1-mV ST depression was 22 ± 11%. The standard deviation for rate-pressure product at 0.1-mV ST depression was significantly less at 8.4 ± 2.8%. In 78 (40%) of the 196 tests, time to 0.1-mV ST depression was less than 80% or greater than 120% of the patient's mean; in contrast, rate-pressure product at 0.1-mV ST depression was less than 80% or greater than 120% of the patient's mean in only three tests (1.5%). Considerable variability was observed in exercise tolerance in patients with effort angina, even when rate-pressure product at the onset of ischemia remained fixed. This means that a history of variable threshold angina does not necessarily imply variations in coronary tone. This study also underscores the fact that patients increase their exercise time with repeat testing without any change in their cardiovascular status.

Evaluation of Long-Acting Nitrates

Nitrates have a very long history in the treatment of angina and are a good medium with which to evaluate the use of exercise testing for the treatment of symptomatic coronary disease. The use of organic nitrates in the treatment of angina dates back to the 19th century when the English physician Thomas Lauder-Brunton discovered the vasodepressor activity of amyl nitrate, by inhalation, and noted the immediate, but transient, relief of anginal pain. Subsequent findings by William Murrell, in 1879, established the use of sublingual nitroglycerin for the treatment of anginal pain as well as its use as a prophylactic agent prior to exertion.

Symptoms of effort angina are produced by a transient imbalance between the supply and demand of myocardial oxygen. The deficiency in myocardial oxygen is a result of increased myocardial demand in the face of restricted myocardial blood flow. Effort angina pectoris must be distinguished from spontaneous angina pectoris, in which coronary spasm plays an important role. Typical effort angina is highly predictive of obstructive coronary artery disease (CAD). It has been noted, however, that only one third of all patients examined at necropsy with significant coronary atherosclerosis have a history of angina pectoris. It is not clear why some patients with obstructive CAD have pain, and others having the same degree of obstruction do not manifest this symptom. The chest pain associated with angina is usually relieved promptly by sublingual nitroglycerin.

Most studies evaluating antianginal agents have relied on changes in treadmill time to assess drug efficacy. Peak VO_2, which is more reproducible than exercise time, has been rarely performed in these studies. Endpoints in angina patients are often very subjective, and the careful grading of angina to arrive at a consistent endpoint has not resolved this problem. Therefore, researchers have used submaximal endpoints as measures of change.

TABLE 12–2. Recommendations regarding exercise test reproducibility when evaluating drugs

Measured oxygen uptake should be used instead of total exercise time because it is a more reproducible measure of exercise capacity

The ventilatory threshold is a reproducible submaximal exercise variable in which to evaluate myocardial ischemia and myocardial oxygen demand

A pretrial exercise test allows the patient to become familiar with the exercise testing staff, the equipment, and the nature of his/her anginal endpoints

The treadmill protocol should be individualized for each patient, with small (≈1 MET) increments per stage

Computerized techniques for ECG analysis provide reproducible measurements of ST-segment displacement

Statistical methods based on the estimate of the measurement error associated with a particular variable can be used by the clinician and/or investigator to better plan and evaluate an intervention

These have included the onset of ST-segment depression, the anginal threshold, heart rate and blood pressure responses to exercise, and the ventilatory anaerobic threshold. Patients are also frequently able to walk longer on the treadmill because of delayed lactate accumulation due to improved cardiac performance during exercise after an anti-anginal medication. An additional methodology is to assess ST-segment changes using computer methodology and determine if anti-anginal agents alter this objective estimate of myocardial ischemia.

Given this background, measurements should be made at the following points when evaluating interventions[6]:

1. Supine and sitting heart rate and blood pressure—the rationale for this is that the action of anti-anginal therapy has been shown to occur through a decrease in blood pressure. Previous studies have found a relationship between the change in VO_2 and decrease in blood pressure. If this is demonstrated, a nitrate effect could be documented or titrated in the office by changes in resting blood pressure.
2. Standard workload—a modest work rate such as 3.0 mph/5% grade represents a "standard" submaximal workload that most angina patients can achieve. Hemodynamic and symptom responses can be assessed at this matched work rate while on versus off therapy.
3. Submaximal heart rate and double product—these are chosen specifically for each individual using the baseline test. The heart rate and the double product where definite abnormal ST depression is first seen is the value used for subsequent comparisons.
4. Ventilatory anaerobic threshold—submaximal point chosen by gas analysis techniques.
5. Onset of angina—patients' first appreciation of usual angina.
6. Maximal exercise—to optimize the evaluation of an intervention, this would include measured VO_2. As mentioned above, exercise times can only be compared if the same protocol is used. When expressing exercise capacity in predicted METs, a MET level should only be ascribed to a patient who completes more than half a given stage.

Transdermal Nitrates. The variable response to this once-popular therapy has generated a significant amount of controversy. Some of the reasons for the disparate results are listed in Table 12-3. Many investigators have described "nitrate tolerance," in which the drug's effect is lessened over time.[7–10,11] In the 1990s, this was addressed by the Nitrate Cooperative Study Group, in which a total of 562 patients who were responders to sublingual nitroglycerin were studied.[12] Patients received either placebo or nitrate patches delivering low (15 to 30 mg/24 hours), moderate, or large (75 and 105 mg/24 hours, respectively) amounts of nitrate. Four hours after the initial application, nitrate patches increased exercise duration compared to placebo, but this beneficial effect had disappeared by 24 hours. In addition, after 8 weeks of continuous therapy, none of the nitrate patches were superior to placebo, whether patients were or were not taking concomitant beta-blockers. Parker et al[7] has demonstrated partial tolerance to the hemodynamic effects of isosorbide dinitrate within 48 hours of initiating therapy. Thadani et al[8] demonstrated that acute resting hemodynamic and exercise variables in angina patients are attenuated during chronic therapy. Resting hemodynamic changes that persisted for 8 hours during acute therapy were demonstrable for only 4 hours during chronic therapy. Similarly, significant increases in exercise capacity were observed for 8 hours after acute and only 2 hours during chronic therapy.

Thompson[9] observed significant increases in treadmill time at 2 and 26 hours after application of individually titrated patches. In contrast, other investigators have been unable to document significant changes in exercise capacity 24 hours after application of the patches, although increases in exercise time were observed at intervals up

TABLE 12–3. Some of the explanations for controversy and disparate results with clinical studies on the use on the long-acting nitrates

Acute (single dose) effects can be demonstrated for the long-acting preparations but when the agents are given chronically, tolerance can develop

There is a placebo effect involved in the treatment of angina

Nitrate blood levels are difficult to measure but some modes of delivery clearly do not result in effective blood levels

Acute peaks of nitrates in the blood may be more effective than a chronic level

Treadmill time or workload is not a reproducible measurement

More objective measurements using cardiopulmonary exercise testing and computerized ST-segment analysis have rarely been used to 8 hours. We studied 16 patients with stable angina in a double-blind crossover manner utilizing treadmill exercise testing with the direct measurement of ventilatory oxygen uptake, 1 and 24 hours after application of a 20-cm^2 transdermal nitrate system and identical placebo.[13] Testing was performed after a 3-day lead in period on either an active patch or placebo. No statistically significant differences were observed between nitrate and placebo in any of the resting hemodynamic or peak angina variables at 1 or 24 hours. A significant increase in double product at a matched submaximal workload was observed 1 hour after nitrates relative to placebo. However, no significant differences were observed in any of the other measured variables at the submaximal workload.

The current opinion is that continuous therapy with nitrate patches produces pharmacologic tolerance and is ineffective. Pharmacologic tolerance can be minimized when patches are applied every morning and removed at night. Intermittent therapy with patches may lead to rebound nocturnal angina in some patients. In addition, intermittent therapy with patches has been associated with worsening of exercise performance in the morning prior to the patch renewal. Other explanations for the inconsistent findings among studies include the timing of the initial test, and differences between patients in the development of tolerance. Regarding the latter, 24 hours after transdermal application, blood nitroglycerin concentrations have been observed to be similar to concentrations obtained at 2 and 8 hours. However, changes in exercise capacity recorded at 2 and 8 hours after transdermal application rarely persist up to 24 hours.

Relationship of Changes in Resting Systolic Blood Pressure with Exercise Capacity

Although the effectiveness of nitrates for the long-term prophylaxis of exertional angina is controversial, investigations utilizing large doses have demonstrated persistent physiologic effects. During a titration period, the observation of a 10 mmHg decrease in resting systolic blood pressure and/or a 10-beats per min (bpm) increase in resting heart rate has been used in studies attempting to demonstrate an increase in exercise capacity following nitrate administration. These criteria have served a dual purpose of documenting physiologic changes in variables known to affect myocardial oxygen demand and to identify subjects nonresponsive to nitrates prior to inclusion in a study. If after nitrate administration, changes in blood pressure and/or heart rate are correlated with changes in exercise capacity, the utilization of these variables by the clinician could identify patients expected to improve exercise tolerance during nitrate therapy.

In order to determine if these practical criteria could predict improved exercise capacity in angina patients treated with nitrates, both nitrate responsive and nonresponsive subjects were included in a study performed in our lab. Nineteen patients with stable angina pectoris were studied in a double-blind placebo-controlled manner. Significant increases in resting heart rate and peak oxygen uptake and decreases in resting systolic blood pressure were observed 1-hour postnitrate relative to placebo. Changes in peak oxygen uptake and total treadmill time during nitrate administration relative to placebo correlated with changes in resting supine systolic and diastolic blood pressure ($r = -0.54$ to -0.62), but not to changes in resting heart rate. The multiple regression correlation coefficient utilizing the changes in supine systolic and diastolic blood pressures during nitrate administration as independent variables to predict changes in peak oxygen uptake was $R = 0.66$. This suggests that during administration of nitrates, a decrease in resting systolic and diastolic blood pressure is essential to insure increases in exercise capacity. Improvement in oxygen uptake and treadmill time was noted in 10 out of 11 patients with a greater than 5 mmHg drop in supine systolic blood pressure. Conversely, a lack of blood pressure response to nitrates was indicative of no improvement in exercise tolerance.

Studies demonstrating the positive effects of nitrates on exercise capacity have utilized a titration criterion of a 10-mmHg fall in resting systolic blood pressure or a 10-bpm increase in heart rate. The increased heart rate criterion is based on the baroreceptor-mediated rise in heart rate due to decreased arterial pressure. Standard doses of nitrates produced variability in the hemodynamic and exercise response. These results suggest that clinicians should document changes in resting systolic and diastolic blood pressure in angina patients receiving nitrate therapy. It would appear that the greater the decreases in blood pressure, the greater the benefit. The magnitude of this change in blood pressure may be limited by symptoms of headaches, hypotension, or possible nitrate tolerance during chronic administration. On the other hand, a lack of blood pressure response after nitrate administration suggests little or no therapeutic effect and warrants a reevaluation of therapy.

Meta-Analysis of Antianginal Agents

Because it is not known which drug is most effective as a first-line treatment for stable angina, Heidenreich et al[14] performed a meta-analysis to compare the relative efficacy and tolerability of treatment with beta-blockers, calcium antagonists, and long-acting nitrates for patients who have stable angina. They identified English-language studies published between 1966 and 1997 by searching the MEDLINE and EMBASE databases and reviewing the bibliographies of identified articles to locate relevant studies. Randomized or crossover studies comparing antianginal drugs from two or three different classes (beta-blockers, calcium antagonists, and long-acting nitrates) lasting at least 1 week were reviewed. Studies were selected if they reported at least one of the following outcomes: cardiac death, MI, study withdrawal due to adverse events, angina frequency, nitroglycerin use, or exercise duration. Ninety (63%) of 143 identified studies met the inclusion criteria. They combined results using odds ratios for discrete data and mean differences for continuous data. Studies of calcium antagonists were grouped by duration and type of drug (nifedipine versus non-nifedipine). Rates of cardiac death and MI were not significantly different for treatment with beta-blockers versus calcium antagonists (i.e., neither increased or decreased). There were fewer episodes of angina per week with beta-blockers than with calcium antagonists. Too few trials compared nitrates with calcium antagonists or beta-blockers to draw firm conclusions about relative efficacy. Beta-blockers provide similar clinical outcomes and are associated with fewer adverse events than calcium antagonists in randomized trials of patients who have stable angina. No significant differences in time to ischemia were found between the agents.

Evaluation of the Latest Antianginal Agent

Since antianginal monotherapy with ranolazine, a drug believed to partially inhibit fatty acid oxidation, increased treadmill performance, its long-term efficacy and safety in combination with beta-blockers or calcium antagonists in a large patient population with severe chronic angina was studied.[15] A randomized, three-group parallel, double-blind, placebo-controlled trial of 823 eligible adults with symptomatic chronic angina, who were randomly assigned to receive placebo or one of two doses of ranolazine, was carried out. Patients treated at the 118 participating ambulatory outpatient settings in several countries were enrolled in the Combination Assessment of Ranolazine In Stable Angina (CARISA) trial from 1999 to 2001 and followed for 1 year. Patients received twice-daily placebo or 750 mg or 1000 mg of ranolazine. Trough exercise duration increased by nearly 2 minutes from baseline in both ranolazine groups versus 1.5 minutes in the placebo group. The times to angina and to ST depression also increased in the ranolazine groups, at peak more than at trough. The increases did not depend on changes in blood pressure, heart rate, or background antianginal therapy and persisted throughout 3 months. Twice-daily doses of ranolazine increased exercise capacity and provided additional antianginal relief to symptomatic patients with severe chronic angina taking standard doses of atenolol, amlodipine, or diltiazem, without survival consequences over 1 to 2 years of therapy.

Myocardial Laser Revascularization

Transmyocardial revascularization (TMR) and percutaneous myocardial revascularization (PMR) are recently studied operative treatments for refractory angina pectoris when bypass surgery or percutaneous transluminal angioplasty is not indicated or possible. There have been at least 10 large, multicentric randomized trials of TMR or PMR that have addressed the effect of this modality on exertional symptoms and exercise capacity. These studies are summarized in Table 12-4. Our lab was the exercise testing core center for the ATLANTIC study (Angina Treatments—Lasers and Normal Therapies in Comparison), a prospective randomized trial comparing TMR to continued medication.[16] The study included 182 patients from 16 U.S. centers with Canadian Cardiovascular Society Angina (CCSA) score III (38%) or IV (62%), reversible ischemia, and incomplete response to other therapies. Patients were randomly assigned TMR and continued medication ($n = 92$) or continued medication alone ($n = 90$). Baseline assessments were angina class, exercise tolerance, Seattle Angina Questionnaire for quality of life, and stress perfusion scans. Patients were reassessed at 3, 6, and 12 months, with independent masked angina assessment at 12 months. At 1 year, total exercise time increased by 1 minute in the TMR group compared with nearly a minute decline in the medication-only group. Independent CCSA score was II or lower in half of the TMR group. Using the Seattle Angina Questionnaire, there was an improvement in symptoms in the TMR group compared to the medication-only group. It appears that TMR can lower angina scores, increase exercise time, and

TABLE 12-4.   Randomized clinical trials of laser revascularization versus medical therapy

Transmyocardial revascularization studies

Author	Number of patients	Percentage of patients with a decrease of ≥2 CCS angina classes: TMR versus control (p value)	Improvement in exercise time (seconds): TMR versus control (p value)	Survival TMR versus control (p value)
Allen et al	275	76 versus 32 ($p < 0.001$)	+5.0 versus + 3.9 METs ($p = 0.05$)*	84% versus 89% ($p = $ NS)
Frazier et al	192	72 versus 13 ($p < 0.001$)	NA	85% versus 79% ($p = $ NS)
Schofield et al	188	25 versus 4 ($p < 0.001$)	NA†	89% versus 96% ($p = $ NS)
Burkhoff et al	182	48 versus 14 ($p < 0.001$)	+65 versus –46 ($p < 0.0001$)	95% versus 90% ($p = $ NS)
Aaberge et al	100	39 versus 0 ($p < 0.01$)	+8 versus –10‡ ($p = $ NS)	88% versus 92% ($p = $ NS)
Jones et al	86	NA§	+119 versus –85 ($p = 0.0001$)	NA

*Post-treatment results for 81 patients only who underwent Naughton testing; †Exact data not available, however, the difference in exercise times between the two groups was 40 seconds (in favor of TMR) at 12 months ($p = $ NS); ‡time to chest pain during exercise increased by 66 seconds in the TMR group and decreased by 3 seconds in the control group ($p < 0.01$); §Mean CCS class at the conclusion of the 12-month follow-up period was 1.7 among patients treated with TMR and 3.8 among the medically treated group ($p < 0.0001$).
CCS, Canadian Cardiovascular Society; MET, metabolic equivalent; NA, data not available; NS, statistically not significant; TMR, transmyocardial laser revascularization.

Percutaneous myocardial revascularization studies

Author	Number of patients	Percentage of patients with a decrease of ≥2 CCS angina classes: PMR versus control (p value)	Improvement in exercise time (seconds): PMR versus control (p value)
Leon	298	65 versus 56 ($p = $ NS)	+27 versus +31 ($p = $ NS)
Oesterle et al	221	30 versus 12 (–0.002)	+89 versus +13 ($p = 0.008$)
Stone et al	141	49 versus 37 ($p = $ NS)	+62 versus +54 ($p = $ NS)
Salem et al	82	41 versus 13 ($p = 0.006$)	NA*

*No statistically significant difference in exercise time between the two groups; however, the time to chest pain increased by 76 seconds in the laser group and decreased by 12 seconds in the control group ($p < 0.05$).
CCS, Canadian Cardiovascular Society; NA, data not available; NS, statistically not significant; PMR, percutaneous myocardial revascularization.

improve patients' perceptions of quality of life and can provide clinical benefits in patients with no other therapeutic options.

Interestingly, however, the results of the studies using TMR or PMR presented in Table 12-4 on the response to exercise are mixed; although several of the studies using TMR or PMR showed a significant improvement in exercise time compared to controls, others showed no difference.[17-19] In addition, although the follow-up times were relatively short (1 to 2 years), none showed a difference in survival. The major benefit of laser revascularization is probably alleviation of angina symptoms; most of the studies have observed decreases in CCSA Class and some trials reported an increase in the anginal onset time. A number of mechanisms have been proposed to explain why laser revascularization might alleviate angina symptoms. In addition to improved perfusion directly through laser-created channels, mechanisms that have been suggested include angiogenesis, myocardial denervation, and the placebo effect.[15-17] Several additional trials are currently underway to further explore the effects of laser revascularization on functional and symptomatic responses to exercise.

Safety of Placebo in Studying Angina

The safety of withholding standard therapy and enrolling patients with stable angina in placebo-controlled trials has long been a controversial issue in angina trials. Glasser et al[20] identified all events leading to dropout from trials of 12 antianginal drugs submitted in support of new drug applications to the U.S. Food and Drug Administration. Subjects who dropped out of the trials were classified as occurring due to adverse cardiovascular events or other causes without knowledge of drug assignment. There were a combined 3161 subjects who entered any randomized, double-blind phase of placebo-controlled protocols; 197 (6.2%) withdrew because of cardiovascular events. There was no difference in risk of adverse events between drug and placebo groups. A prospectively defined subgroup analysis showed that groups who received calcium antagonists were at an increased risk of dropout compared with placebo groups, primarily because of a disproportionate number of adverse events in studies of one drug. These investigators concluded that there were few adverse experiences associated with short-term placebo use. Withholding active treatment for treatment of angina did not increase the risk of serious cardiac events.

Pre- and Postrevascularization (ACC/AHA Exercise Test Guidelines)

The following summarizes the ACC/AHA Guidelines regarding recommendations for exercise testing of patients pre- and postrevascularization procedures (no changes were made in 2002 from the 1997 Guidelines).[21]

Class I. Conditions for which there is evidence and/or general agreement that the standard exercise test is useful and helpful for evaluating patients pre- and postrevascularization.

Definitely Use the Exercise Test:
1. To demonstrate the presence of ischemia in patients prior to revascularization.
2. Evaluation of patients with recurrent symptoms suggesting ischemia after revascularization.

Class II a. Conditions for which there is conflicting evidence and/or a divergence of opinion that the standard exercise test is useful and helpful for evaluating patients pre- and postrevascularization but the weight of evidence for usefulness or efficacy is in favor of the exercise test.

Probably Use the Exercise Test:
1. After discharge for activity counseling and/or exercise training as part of cardiac rehabilitation in patients who have undergone a coronary revascularization procedure.

Class II b. Conditions for which there is conflicting evidence and/or a divergence of opinion that the standard exercise test is useful and helpful for

evaluating patients pre- and postrevascularization but the usefulness/efficacy is less well established.

Maybe Use the Exercise Test For:
1. Detection of restenosis in asymptomatic patients within the first months after angioplasty.
2. Routine monitoring on a periodic basis of asymptomatic patients after revascularization for restenosis, graft occlusion, or disease progression.

Class III. Conditions for which there is evidence and/or general agreement that the standard exercise test is not useful and helpful for evaluating patients pre- and postrevascularization and in some cases may be harmful.

Do Not Use the Standard Exercise ECG Test:
1. To localize ischemia for determination of the site for intervention (which is better done with an imaging study).

Patients who undergo myocardial revascularization should have documented ischemic or viable myocardium, especially if they are asymptomatic. The exercise ECG is useful in these circumstances, particularly if the patient has multivessel disease and the culprit vessel does not need to be defined. However, in the setting of single-vessel disease, the sensitivity of the exercise ECG is frequently suboptimal, especially if the revascularized vessel supplies the posterior wall. Moreover, imaging studies preclude the use of the exercise ECG in situations where the culprit vessel needs to be defined.

Exercise testing after revascularization has different goals depending upon the time postrevascularization. Early on, the goal of exercise testing is to determine the immediate result of revascularization. After six months or more, the goal of exercise testing is to assist in the evaluation and management of patients.

In symptomatic patients after coronary artery bypass surgery, exercise testing may be used to discriminate cardiac and noncardiac causes of recurrent chest pain, which is often atypical after surgery. If a management decision is to be based on the presence of ischemia, the exercise ECG is sufficient. However, if a management decision is to be based on the site and extent of ischemia, the exercise ECG is less desirable than an imaging test. In asymptomatic patients after coronary artery bypass surgery, the development of silent graft disease, especially with venous conduits, is clearly a major concern. The value of the exercise ECG for the detection of silent graft disease is not well established. Stress imaging tests are more favored in this group because of their ability to document the site of ischemia, and their increased sensitivity.

In symptomatic patients after PCI, an abnormal exercise test is predictive of restenosis. However, the value of a negative exercise test is reduced by the limited sensitivity of exercise testing, particularly for single-vessel disease. In asymptomatic patients following PCI, silent restenosis is a common clinical manifestation. Some authorities have advocated routine exercise testing, as restenosis is frequent. The alternative approach is to perform exercise testing in selected patients considered to be particularly at high risk. Regardless of the strategy utilized, the exercise ECG is an insensitive predictor of restenosis with a sensitivity of about 50%, reflecting the high prevalence of single-vessel disease in this population.

Evaluation of Percutaneous Coronary Interventions

One important application of the exercise test is to assess the effects of PCI on physical function, ischemic responses, and symptoms in the immediate and longer period following the various interventions which now fall under the general term "PCI." The exercise test has been used for this purpose in numerous trials of PCI, and a few notable examples are described in the following. Berger et al[22] reported follow-up data in 183 patients who had undergone PCI at least 1 year earlier. The duration of follow-up ranged from 1 to 5 years. Subjective clinical information was obtained in all patients and exercise testing in 91. PCI was initially successful in 141 patients (79%). Of the 42 patients in whom PCI was unsuccessful, 26 underwent CABG, while 16 were maintained on medical therapy. When compared to the medical patients at time of follow-up, successful PCI patients experienced less angina (13% versus 47%), used less nitroglycerin (25% versus 73%), were hospitalized less often for chest pain (8% versus 31%), and subjectively felt their condition had improved (96% versus 20%). During exercise testing, the prevalence of angina was less (9% versus 43%), and exercise duration was greater (8.2 versus 5.8 minutes) among PCI patients. However, there were no significant differences in ST depression (26% PCI patients versus 55% medical patients). Although no pre-PCI exercise testing results were reported, there were no significant differences in the incidence of subsequent MI, mortality, or need for CABG.

Vandormael et al[23] reported the safety and short-term benefit of multilesion PCI in 135 patients, 66 of whom had a minimum of 6 months of follow-up.[23] Primary success, defined as successful dilation of the most critical lesion or all lesions attempted, occurred in 87% of the 135 patients. Complete revascularization was achieved in 46% of the 117 patients with a primary success. Of the 66 patients eligible for 6-month follow-up, 80% had an uncomplicated course and required no further procedures. Clinical improvement by at least one angina functional class was observed in 90% of the patients. Cardiac events, including a second revascularization procedure, were significantly more common in patients who had incomplete versus complete revascularization. All patients who had a primary success demonstrated clinical improvement with a reduction in symptoms or improved exercise tolerance. Exercise-induced angina occurred in 11 (12%) and an abnormal exercise ECG in 30 (32%) of the 95 patients with post-PCI exercise test data. Exercise-induced angina occurred in 1 (2%) of 46 patients with complete revascularization versus 10 (20%) of 49 patients with incomplete revascularization; an abnormal exercise ECG occurred in 9 versus 21 patients, respectively. Of 57 patients who had paired exercise test data before and after angioplasty, exercise-induced angina occurred in 56% of patients before the procedure, compared with only 11% of patients after angioplasty. Exercise-induced ST-segment depression of more than 0.1 mV occurred in 75% of patients before PCI versus 32% after the procedure. When patients were stratified according to completeness of revascularization, the number of patients with exercise-induced angina was reduced to zero when complete revascularization was obtained; the difference was less marked in the patients who had incomplete revascularization. Abnormal exercise-induced ST-segment depression was significantly reduced in patients who had complete and incomplete revascularization compared with before angioplasty.

Rosing et al[24] reported that exercise testing after successful PCI exhibited improved ECG and symptomatic responses, as well as improved myocardial perfusion and global and regional left ventricular function. Sixty-six patients were studied before and after successful PCI. Surprisingly, only 33% had abnormal ST-segment depression, while 68% had angina during initial treadmill testing. Follow-up studies an average of 8 months after the successful procedure showed 7% to have ST-segment depression or angina during treadmill studies and there were no abnormal studies with scintigraphy. Radionuclide results demonstrated similar ejection fraction (EF) at rest before and after PCI, but an improvement of 9% ± 10% in the exercise EF at follow-up. However, 52% of patients with paired data still had an abnormal nuclear study after successful PCI, most likely due to a false-positive result.

From the Netherlands came the results of follow-up of 25 patients who underwent PCI.[25] All patients had subjective and objective evidence of CAD mainly due to proximal discrete one-vessel disease. Patients were studied prior to, within 14 days after, and at 4 to 8 months later. History, exercise ECG, scintigraphy, and EF were performed at rest and maximal exercise. The mean stenosis of a dilated vessel decreased significantly from 83% to 38%. The functional status of the patients improved as reflected by a decrease in anginal complaints, an increase in negative exercise ECGs, exercise level, and EF response. The EF response to exercise was the most reliable way to discover a possible restenosis in the late follow-up period.

Prediction of Restenosis with the Exercise Test

To determine whether a treadmill test could predict restenosis after angioplasty, Honan et al[26] studied 289 patients 6 months after a successful emergency angioplasty of the infarct-related artery for acute MI. After excluding those with interim interventions, medical events, or medical contraindications to follow-up testing, both a treadmill test and a cardiac catheterization were completed in 144 patients; 88% of those eligible for this assessment. Of six clinical and treadmill variables examined by multivariable logistic analysis, only exercise ST deviation was independently correlated with restenosis. The clinical diagnosis of angina at follow-up, although marginally related to restenosis, did not add significant information once ST deviation was known. The sensitivity of ST deviation of 0.10 mV or greater for detecting restenosis was only 24% (13 of 55 patients), and the specificity was 88% (75 of 85 patients). Extent or severity of wall motion abnormalities at follow-up did not affect the sensitivity of exercise-induced ST deviation for detection of restenosis, by the timing of thrombolytic therapy or of angioplasty, or by the presence of collateral blood flow at the time of acute angiography. A second multivariable analysis evaluating the association of the same variables with number of vessels with significant coronary disease at the 6-month catheterization found an association with both exercise ST deviation and

exercise duration. Angina symptoms and exercise test results in this population had limited value for predicting anatomic restenosis 6 months after emergency angioplasty for acute MI.

Bengtson et al[27] studied 303 consecutive patients with successful PCI and without a recent MI.[27] Among the 228 patients without interval cardiac events, early repeat revascularization, or contraindications to treadmill testing, 209 (92%) underwent follow-up angiography, and 200 also had a follow-up treadmill test and formed the study population. Restenosis (>75% luminal diameter stenosis) occurred in 50 patients (25%). Five variables were individually associated with a higher risk of restenosis: recurrent angina, exercise-induced angina, a positive treadmill test, greater exercise ST deviation, and a lower maximum exercise heart rate. However, only exercise-induced angina, recurrent angina, and a positive treadmill test were independent predictors of restenosis. Using these three variables, patient subsets could be identified with restenosis rates ranging from 11% to 83%. The exercise test added independent information to symptom status regarding the risk of restenosis after elective PCI. Nevertheless, 20% of patients with restenosis had neither recurrent angina nor exercise-induced ischemia at follow-up.

At the Thorax Center, exercise nuclear perfusion testing was used to predict recurrence of angina and restenosis after a primary successful PCI.[28] In 89 patients, a symptom-limited exercise test was performed 4 weeks after PCI. Patients were followed for 6 months or until recurrence of angina. All underwent a repeat coronary angiography at 6 months or earlier if symptoms recurred. PCI was considered successful if the patients had no symptoms and if the stenosis was reduced to less than 50% of the luminal diameter. Restenosis was defined as an increase of the stenosis of more than 50% luminal diameter. The ability of a reversible defect to predict recurrence of angina was 66% versus 38% for the exercise ECG (ST-segment depression or angina at peak workload). Restenosis was predicted in 74% of patients by nuclear perfusion but only in 50% of patients by the exercise ECG. Nuclear perfusion was highly predictive, but the ECG was not. Restenosis had already occurred to some extent at 4 weeks after the PCI in most patients in whom it was going to occur.

The ROSETTA (Routine versus Selective Exercise Treadmill Testing after Angioplasty) registry was studied to demonstrate the effects of routine post-PCI functional testing on the use of follow-up cardiac procedures and clinical events.[29] The ROSETTA registry is a prospective multicenter observational study examining the use of functional testing after PCI. A total of 788 patients were enrolled in the registry at 13 clinical centers in five countries. The frequencies of exercise testing, cardiac procedures and clinical events were examined during the first 6 months following a successful PCI. Patients were predominantly elderly men (mean age, 61 ± 11 years; 76% male) who underwent single-vessel PCI (85%) with stent implantation (58%). During the 6-month follow-up, a total of 237 patients underwent a routine exercise testing strategy (100% having exercise testing for routine follow-up), while 551 patients underwent a selective (or clinically driven) strategy (73% having no exercise testing and 27% having exercise testing for a clinical indication). Patients in the routine testing group underwent a total of 344 exercise tests compared with 165 tests performed in the selective testing group (mean, 1.45 versus 0.3 tests per patient). However, clinical events were less common among those who underwent routine exercise testing, for example, unstable angina (6% versus 14%), MI (0.4% versus 1.6%), death (0% versus 2%), and composite clinical events (6% versus 16%). After controlling for baseline clinical and procedural differences, routine exercise testing had a persistent independent association with a reduction in the composite clinical event rate. This association may be attributable to the early identification and treatment of patients at risk for follow-up events, or it may be due to clinical differences between patients who are referred for routine and selective exercise testing.

Acampa et al[30] performed a study to determine the long-term prognostic value of nuclear perfusion scans in predicting cardiac events after PCI in symptomatic and symptom-free patients. Exercise scans were performed in 206 patients about 1 year after PCI. All patients were followed for a mean period of 3 years. Myocardial ischemia per scan was detectable in 44 patients. During follow-up, 24 patients experienced events (four died, 10 had MIs, and 10 had coronary interventions). The summed stress score and summed difference score were significant predictors of cardiac events. Event-free survival curves showed a higher event rate in patients with than without ischemia. The occurrence of cardiac events was higher in the presence of perfusion defects in symptomatic and symptom-free patients.

A group of investigators from the Mayo Clinic evaluated the long-term (7-year) prognostic value of exercise nuclear perfusion imaging after PCI in a series of 211 patients 1 to 3 years after PCI.[31] Most (73%) had one- or two-vessel CAD and normal left ventricular function and 193 (91%) had successful PCI. Two thirds of the patients were symptomatic at the time of testing. The mean Duke score was 5, and 125 (60%) patients had a low-risk Duke score. The 5-year overall survival was 95%, yielding a low annual mortality rate of 1% per year. The summed stress score exhibited a significant association with cardiac death or MI as endpoints. The Duke score was predictive of the combination endpoint of hard and soft cardiac events. This study demonstrated that exercise perfusion imaging performed 1 to 3 years after PCI can be predictive of cardiac events.

After myocardial perfusion imaging, 114 diabetic patients were followed for 2 years.[32] PCI-related events were studied after exercise testing and included major cardiac events (cardiovascular death, MI) and revascularization. Stress perfusion scans were performed 5 months after PCI and ischemia was considered as present if at least two contiguous segments were showing reversible defects. Persistent silent ischemia was found in 43%. No difference was observed between the two groups. In contrast, 15 (31%) among the ischemic patients and 4 (6%) among the nonischemic patients underwent iterative revascularization. The relative risk of revascularization for patients with significant ischemia was six times that of nonischemic patients.

Evaluation of Patients Who Underwent Coronary Artery Bypass Grafting

Hultgren et al[33] analyzed the 5-year effects of medical versus surgical treatment on symptoms and exercise performance in patients with stable angina who entered the Veterans Administration Cooperative Study from 1972 to 1974. Exercise testing revealed comparable changes to symptoms and physical performance. At 1 year, surgical patients had fewer tests stopped by angina compared to medically treated patients (28% versus 64%) and a higher MET level (7.4 versus 6.0). Other measures of exercise performance improved comparably between groups. At 5 years, exercise performance of surgical patients remained superior to that of medical patients, but the treatment difference was smaller. The beneficial effect of surgical treatment in patients with stable angina was maintained, with only a modest increase in symptoms and a slight decrease in exercise performance at 5 years compared with 1 year. Benefits of surgery were still substantially superior to medical treatment at 5 years.

The group at the Cleveland Clinic sought to determine the independent and incremental prognostic value of exercise thallium perfusion scans for prediction of death and nonfatal MI in post-CABG patients.[34] Analyses were based on 873 symptom-free patients undergoing symptom-limited exercise thallium tests between 1990 and 1993. All had undergone CABG and none had recurrent angina or other major intercurrent coronary events. Exercise and thallium-perfusion variables were analyzed to determine their prognostic importance during 3 years of follow-up. Myocardial-perfusion defects were noted in 508 (58%) patients. There were 57 deaths and 72 patients had major events (death or nonfatal MI). Patients with thallium-perfusion defects were more likely to die (9% versus 3%) or suffer a major event (11% versus 4%). Reversible defects were also predictive of death (12% versus 5%) and major events (13% versus 7%). The exercise variable with the strongest predictive power was an impaired exercise capacity (= 6 METs); poor exercise capacity was predictive of both death (18% versus 4%) and death or nonfatal MI (19% versus 5%). After adjusting for baseline clinical variables, surgical variables, time elapsed since CABG, and standard cardiovascular risk factors, perfusion defects remained predictive of death (adjusted relative risk 2.8) and major events (adjusted relative risk 2.6). Similarly, impaired exercise capacity remained strongly predictive of death (four times) and major events (3.6 times) after adjusting for confounders. In this group of patients who were symptom free after CABG, thallium-perfusion defects and impaired exercise capacity were strong and independent predictors of subsequent death or nonfatal MI.

The Coronary Artery Surgery Study (CASS) group reported the results of exercise testing performed in 81% of the 780 patients randomized at entry.[35] The cumulative survival at the end of the 7-year follow-up was 90% for those assigned to surgical treatment and 88% for those assigned to medical therapy. The survival rates did not differ significantly from either those of the entire randomized cohort or those of the 149 patients who did not have a qualifying exercise test at baseline. No differences in important baseline characteristics existed between those who were exercised and not exercised at entry. Stratification of patients according to the degree of ST-segment depression and final exercise stage achieved during a Bruce treadmill test failed to show any significant differences in 7-year survival rates between medically and surgically assigned patients. Additionally, no differences in survival were noted within either the medical

or surgical groups regardless of the degree of ST-segment depression or the final stage achieved. The presence of exercise-induced angina, however, identified patients who had a survival advantage if assigned to surgical therapy, with a 7-year survival rate of 94% compared with 87% of medically assigned patients. This advantage was observed primarily in the subset of patients with three-vessel CAD and impaired left ventricular function. These mortality rates were quite low, consistent with the selection of a low-risk population.

In Germany, a study was performed of exercise responses in patients with different angiographically defined degrees of revascularization with serial exercise tests in 435 patients 1 to 6 years after CABG.[36] All patients had undergone postoperative angiography 2 to 12 months after CABG to determine the degree of revascularization achieved. Revascularization was complete in 182, sufficient in 176 and incomplete in 57 patients. Twenty patients had all grafts occluded. Exercise capacity, angina threshold, maximal double product, prevalence of greater than 0.1 mV exercise-induced ST-segment depression, and the prevalence of the combination of ST-segment depression plus angina were determined in serial supine bicycle tests. Patients with complete, sufficient, and incomplete revascularization showed improvement of all exercise parameters for 6, 4, and 1 year after CABG, respectively. In those with the best result, the prevalence of ST depression preoperatively was 76%, and was 20%, 22%, 20%, 27%, 34%, and 33% in successive years. The prevalence also decreased in patients whose grafts occluded. Patients with all grafts occluded had improvement of only some exercise parameters. Exercise capacity had improved by 50% in patients with complete and sufficient revascularization at 1 year, and had still improved by 30% at 5 years. Surprisingly, it was also improved in patients with incomplete revascularization or with all grafts occluded.

To determine whether preoperative exercise testing adds important independent prognostic information in patients undergoing CABG, Weiner and the CASS group analyzed 35 variables in 1241 enrolled patients.[37] All patients underwent a treadmill test before CABG and were followed-up for 7 years. Survival in this surgical cohort was 90.6%. Multivariate stepwise discriminant analysis identified a left ventricular score and the final exercise stage achieved as the two most important independent predictors of postoperative survival. In a subgroup of 416 patients with three-vessel coronary disease and preserved left ventricular function, the probability of postoperative survival at 7 years ranged from 95% for those patients able to exercise to 10 METs to 83% for those whose exercise capacity was less than 5 METs. Exercise capacity was found to be an important independent predictor of postoperative survival.

Comparison of PCI and CABG

CABG is an accepted procedure in the management of angina pectoris refractory to medical treatment. It has also been documented to improve survival in selected patients.[37-39] PCI has become a widely used alternative to CABG. Gruntzig et al[40] initially advocated the use of PCI only for patients with a discrete stenosis of a single coronary artery, but the application of coronary angioplasty to narrowing in more than one coronary artery has had excellent results. The usefulness of exercise testing before and after PCI and CABG interventions to document their efficacy has been made clear by many studies for more than 3 decades. Since PCI is now routinely applied in multivessel disease, a comparison between the effects of PCI and CABG on the exercise response can be very helpful in the clinical choice of revascularization procedures. Dubach et al[41] performed a retrospective assessment of Veterans who were treated at the Long Beach VA Medical Center. All patients identified as having undergone exercise testing before and after PCI and CABG were considered for selection according to medication status and timing of exercise tests. Twenty-eight patients formed the CABG group and 38 patients formed the PCI group. Since the timing of the tests was determined by usual clinical practices, the exercise tests were performed an average of 2.5 weeks after PCI and 5 months after CABG. The medication status was comparable, but there were significantly more patients with multivessel disease in the CABG group than in the PCI group. CABG was found to be significantly more effective in decreasing signs and symptoms of ischemia than PCI, but there were no significant differences in estimated aerobic capacity; both procedures improved exercise capacity by about 2 METs.

In this report, Dubach et al[41] also reviewed the literature on exercise responses in patients who had clinically successful revascularizations. This included studies reporting exercise testing both before and after revascularization with CABG or PCI. Twenty-seven reports were found and their results are summarized in Table 12-5. Medication status, percent with multivessel disease, and methods of exercise capacity measurement differed

between studies. However, the results could be tabulated to permit comparison. As shown in Table 12-5, more than twice as many patients had multivessel disease in the CABG studies than in the PCI studies. Hemodynamic improvements and lessening of ischemia during exercise testing were comparable in both groups.

Efficacy of an intervention can be assessed noninvasively by exercise testing since signs and symptoms of ischemia can be demonstrated and exercise capacity can be measured. Table 12-5 summarizes the important points of the most complete studies that compared the pre- and postexercise test variables in patients who underwent either PCI or CABG. As can be appreciated, there is great variability in the results reported, especially in the reduction of angina and normalization of the ST segment. This is due to the problems inherent in such comparisons, including differences in medications, percentage of patients with multivessel disease, the interval between intervention and testing, and the experience of the individuals performing the revascularization procedures. Despite the much lower percentage of patients with multivessel disease included in the PCI groups (28% versus 80% in CABG group), the average reduction in angina and in ST-segment depression in the pooled studies was similar: 49% reduction in angina and 40% reduction in ST-segment depression after PCI, and 50% and 35% reductions after CABG, respectively. Meier et al[42] have performed one of the few studies comparing exercise test results in patients who have undergone PCI to those who have undergone CABG. However, their CABG group was composed of patients in whom PCI failed. Thus, the patients were not primarily assigned to CABG. Those patients who underwent PCI had a higher work capacity 1, 2, and 3 years after revascularization compared to the CABG group. It is difficult to generalize their results or contrast them with other studies.

Ideally, exercise test variables would be obtained immediately after CABG or PCI in order to have comparable situations. It has been demonstrated that within 5 to 6 months after PCI, 30% to 35% of the dilated vessels reocclude.[43] After CABG, about 10% to 15% of the grafts are occluded in the first 6 months. However, whereas patients after PCI will be able to perform a symptom-limited exercise test within days after the procedure,[44] patients after CABG will only be able to do so weeks or months after the operation, during which time the highest rate of early graft occlusions is reported.[45] While the Dutch have reported a 5% incidence of acute occlusion in patients with intimal dissection,[46]

TABLE 12–5. Review of studies that included exercise testing both before and after either PCI or CABG

Author	No. Patients	Medication	Multivessel disease (%)	Exercise capacity Before	Exercise capacity Change (%)	Mean maximal heart rate (BPM) Before	After	Maximal double product Before	After	Angina pectoris during ET Before	After	Abnormal ST-segment response (%) Before	After
PCI (percutaneous coronary intervention)													
Rod	14	BB and Dig NR	0%	6.2 METs	10%	138	149	27	30	71%	7%	(1.0 mm, 0.2 mm)	
Suzuki	14	Off BB, Dig, Nit	0%	14 min	14%	122	145	20	25	57%	21%	36%	7%
Rousing	45	Off BB, Dig, Nit	6%	7.6 min	38%					67%	7%	33%	7%
Kent	32	Off BB, Nit	14%	7 ± 2 min	143%					28%	1%	—	
Scholl	36	Off Dig, Nit	17%	7.5 min	37%			21	31	NA	8%	56%	20%
Meier	132	NA	41%	74 watts	86%					97%	23%	72%	21%
Gruenzig	133	NA	42%	47% APN	67%					100%	33%	79%	10%
Bandormael	57	Off medications	84%	6.2 min	35%					56%	11%	75%	32%
Dubach	38	Usual medications	50%	6.8 METs	27%	126	142	21	25	71%	39%	36%	47%
TOTAL	501	Average	28%		51%	128	145	22	28	68%	19%	61%	21%
CABG (coronary artery bypass graft)													
Guiney	40	Off Dig, BB	85%	NA	61%					95%	8%	95%	38%
Gohlke	467	NA	87%	62 watts	47%			19	24	54%	5%	79%	28%
Hultgren	190	NA	48%	5.0 min	40%			21	24	71%	28%	38%	25%
Bartel	123	Dig and BB NR	80%	NA	NA	130	142			100%	32%	67%	36%
Kloster	38	NA	84%	388 kpm/min	63%	130	142			100%	107%	71%	56%
Lapin	46	NA	64%	NA	16%	107	119			85%	20%	73%	26%
Frick	45	BB and Nit NR	100%	569 kpm/min	26%	124	135	21	24	40%	Decrease	—	
Meier	28	NA	41%	68 watts	79%			21	24	89%	29%	82%	14%
Dubach	28	Used medications	93%	6.0 METs	37%	122	134	12	14	50%	7%	61%	29%
TOTAL	1005	Average	80%		41%	123	134	19	22	67%	17%	69%	34%

APN, age-predicted exercise capacity; BB, beta-blocker; bpm, beats per minute; Dig, digoxin; ET, exercise test; kpm/min, kilogram-meters/minute; maximal double product, systolic blood pressure × heart rate at maximal × 10³; METs, 3.5 cc (or ml) of O_2/kg/min; NA, not available; Nit, nitrates; NR, not restricted.
From Dubach, P et al: J Cardiopulm Rehabil 1990;10:120–125.

a group from Switzerland has demonstrated the safety of exercise testing the day after coronary stenting.[47] In the latter study, 1000 patients were randomized to a symptom-limited exercise test the day after coronary stenting or to no exercise test. The primary endpoint was the incidence of clinical stent thrombosis at 14 days. The secondary endpoint was the occurrence of access site complications. Clinical stent thrombosis occurred in five patients (1%) undergoing the exercise test and in five patients (1%) randomized to no exercise test. Access site complications were detected in 4% and 5.2% of cases, respectively.

The evaluation of success of a therapeutic procedure is related to the technical and clinical goals set for that procedure and this may be different for PCI and CABG. In a patient with stable angina pectoris for instance, the goal is the elimination of exertional pain. In an elderly patient with associated noncardiac disease in whom CABG would be too hazardous, the goal may be to reduce the severity of angina to acceptable levels. When PCI is used for treating unstable angina, baseline exercise test data is usually not available. Overall, the available data suggest that CABG and PCI result in a similar decrease in the signs and symptoms of exercise-induced ischemia. However, the severity of coronary disease was milder in those who underwent PCI.

ACC/AHA GUIDELINES FOR PERIOPERATIVE CARDIOVASCULAR EVALUATION FOR NONCARDIAC SURGERY

The ACC/AHA guidelines provide a framework for considering cardiac risk of noncardiac surgery in a variety of patient and surgical situations.[48] The overriding message from the guidelines is that intervention is rarely necessary simply to lower the risk of surgery unless such intervention is indicated irrespective of the preoperative context. In addition, risk can be lowered by the administration of beta-blockers. Rather than to "clear the patient" for surgery, the preoperative evaluation is an evaluation of the patient's current medical status. It should result in recommendations concerning the risk of cardiac problems over the entire perioperative period, and provide a clinical risk profile that the patient, physician, anesthesiologist, and surgeon can use in making decisions. No test should be performed unless it is likely to influence patient treatment and the preoperative evaluation should include the rational, cost-effective use of testing.

A careful history is crucial to the discovery of cardiac and associated diseases that would place the patient in a high surgical risk category. The history should also seek to determine the patient's exercise capacity using specific questions. A patient classified as high risk due to age or known CAD, but who is asymptomatic and runs for 30 minutes daily, may need no further evaluation. In contrast, a sedentary patient without a history of cardiovascular disease but with clinical factors that suggest increased perioperative risk may benefit from a more extensive preoperative evaluation. The importance of an appropriate medical history is apparent from a prospective study of 878 consecutive patients performed by Paul et al.[49] A preoperative clinical index (diabetes mellitus, prior MI, angina, age older than 70 years, and congestive heart failure) was used to stratify patients. A gradient of risk for severe disease was seen with increasing numbers of clinical markers. The following prediction rules were developed: The absence of severe coronary disease was predicted with a positive predictive value of 96% for patients who had no: (1) history of diabetes, (2) prior angina, (3) previous MI, or (4) history of congestive heart failure. The absence of critical coronary disease was predicted with a positive predictive value of 94% for those who had no: (1) prior angina, (2) previous MI, or (3) history of congestive heart failure.

The goal of this section is to help the reader determine the indications for recommending exercise testing as part of the preoperative evaluation of patients seen in consultation. The guidelines should be referred to for more details with regard to the preoperative evaluation. Table 12-6 provides a shortcut to those who require an exercise test or pharmacologic stress test before an operation.

Table 12-7 stratifies the risk of various types of noncardiac surgical procedures. This risk stratification is based on several reported studies.[50] It is clear that major emergency operations in the elderly, that is, those involving opening of a visceral cavity and those likely to be accompanied by

TABLE 12–6. **Shortcut indicators for noninvasive testing (two of the three must be present)**

Poor functional capacity by questionnaire or specific questioning (<4 METs)
High surgical risk procedure
Intermediate clinical risk predictors are present (Canadian class I or II angina, prior MI by ECG or history, CHF, diabetes, or renal insufficiency)

TABLE 12-7. Cardiac risk stratification for noncardiac surgical procedures

High (reported cardiac risk often >5% with combined incidence of cardiac death and nonfatal MI)
  Major emergency operations, particularly in the elderly
  Aortic and other major vascular surgery
  Peripheral vascular surgery
  Anticipated prolonged surgical procedures associated with large fluid shifts and/or blood loss
Intermediate (reported cardiac risk generally <5%)
  Carotid endarterectomy
  Head and neck surgery
  Intraperitoneal and intrathoracic surgery
  Orthopedic surgery
  Prostate surgery
Low (reported cardiac risk generally <1%; no further testing)
  Endoscopic procedures
  Superficial procedures
  Cataract surgery
  Breast surgery

major bleeding or fluid shifts, place patients at highest risk. Vascular procedures appear particularly risky, and primarily because of the likelihood of associated coronary disease, they justify careful preoperative screening for myocardial ischemia in many instances.

Preoperative Evaluation of Patients with Known CAD

In some patients, the presence of coronary disease is established, such as an acute MI, bypass grafting, coronary angioplasty, or abnormal coronary angiogram. On the other hand, many patients without cardiac symptoms may have severe disease that is not clinically obvious because severe arthritis or peripheral vascular disease limits the patients. Such patients may benefit from noninvasive testing for diagnosis if the patient is a candidate for myocardial revascularization. The first choice for testing is the standard exercise test. In patients with known CAD the issues are:

- How much of the myocardium is in jeopardy?
- What level of stress will produce ischemia?
- What is the patient's ventricular function?

Resolution of these issues is an important goal of the preoperative history, physical examination, and selected noninvasive testing. Many patients with known CAD do not require noninvasive testing, particularly if they are not candidates for myocardial revascularization.

The use of preoperative exercise ECG testing to estimate coronary disease presence and risk of perioperative events in patients undergoing major noncardiac surgery was reviewed through a Medline search of the English literature on exercise and peripheral vascular disease from 1975 to 1994. In most series, very high-risk patients (recent MI, unstable angina, heart failure, and serious ventricular arrhythmia) were excluded. McPhail et al[51] reported on preoperative exercise treadmill testing and supplemental arm ergometry in 100 patients undergoing surgery for peripheral vascular disease or abdominal aortic aneurysm. Of the 100 patients, 30 were able to reach 85% of age-predicted maximum heart rate, and only two had cardiac complications (6%). In contrast, 70% of the population was unable to reach 85% of age-predicted maximal heart rate or had an abnormal exercise ECG. In the latter group the cardiac complication rate (MI, death, heart failure, or ventricular arrhythmia) was 24% (17 patients). A peak exercise heart rate greater than 75% of age-predicted maximum can be expected in approximately half of patients who undergo treadmill exercise, with supplemental arm ergometry when necessary for patients limited by claudication.[52] The frequency of an abnormal exercise ECG response is dependent on prior clinical history. In patients without a cardiac history and with a normal resting ECG, approximately 20% to 25% of patients will have an abnormal exercise ECG. The frequency is greater (35% to 50%) in patients with a prior history of MI or an abnormal rest ECG. The risk of perioperative cardiac events and long-term risk is significantly increased in patients with an abnormal exercise ECG at low workloads.

In contrast to the above studies of patients with vascular disease, Carliner et al[53] reported abnormal exercise-induced ST-segment depression in 16% of 200 patients older than 40 years (mean age, 59 years) being considered for elective surgery. Their prospective study was in a general population of patients in whom less than a third had peripheral vascular disease and were undergoing noncardiac surgery. Only two patients (1%) had a markedly abnormal exercise test. The patients were followed with serial pre- and postoperative ECGs and determinations of creatine kinase and creatine kinase-MB. Of the 32 patients with an abnormal exercise test, five (16%) died or had a nonfatal MI. Of 168 patients with a negative test, 157 (93%) did not die or have an MI. In this series, however, the results of preoperative exercise testing were not statistically significant independent predictors of cardiac risk. Events were more common in patients aged 70 years or older. Events were also more common in patients with an abnormal (positive or equivocal) exercise test response than in those with a negative response (27% versus 14%); however, preoperative exercise results were not statistically significant independent predictors of cardiac risk. Using multivariate analysis, the only statistically significant independent predictor of risk was the preoperative ECG. The finding that endpoint events were more common in patients with an abnormal than in those with a normal ECG (23% versus 7%) is consistent with another study of the resting ECG.[54]

Non–Exercise Stress Testing

The two main techniques used in preoperative evaluation of patients undergoing noncardiac surgery who cannot exercise are to increase myocardial oxygen demand (pacing, intravenous dobutamine) and to induce hyperemic responses by pharmacological vasodilators such as intravenous dipyridamole or adenosine. The two most common methodologies presently in use are dobutamine stress echocardiography and intravenous dipyridamole myocardial perfusion imaging. Adenosine can also be used as an alternative to dipyridamole and arbutamine as an alternative to dobutamine in these types of studies.

Myocardial Perfusion Imaging Methods

A computerized search of the English literature from 1975 to 1994 identified 23 publications describing the use of dipyridamole nuclear perfusion scans in the preoperative evaluation of patients before both vascular and nonvascular surgery. Included were mostly prospectively recruited patient studies that predominantly involved patients undergoing vascular surgery. Cardiac events in the perioperative period were defined as only MI or death from cardiac causes, and information about events and scan results had to be available. The percentage of patients with evidence of ischemic risk as judged by perfusion redistribution ranged from 23% to 69%. The positive predictive value of redistribution ranged from 4% to 20% in reports that included more than 100 patients. The negative predictive value of a normal scan remains uniformly high at approximately 99% for MI and/or cardiac death. Although the risk of a perioperative cardiac event in patients with fixed defects is higher

than in patients with a normal scan, it is still significantly lower than the risk in patients with thallium redistribution.

The need for caution in routine screening with a dipyridamole nuclear perfusion scans of all patients before vascular surgery has been raised by Baron et al.[55] In this review of 457 patients undergoing elective abdominal aortic surgery, the presence of definite CAD and age greater than 65 years were better predictors of cardiac complications than perfusion imaging. The scoring or quantification of scan abnormalities had a significant impact on improving risk assessment and positive predictive value. The data suggest that as the size of the defect increases, cardiac risk significantly increases.[56]

Dobutamine Stress Echocardiography

The use of dobutamine stress echocardiography in preoperative risk assessment was evaluated in six studies, all published since 1991 and identified by a computerized search of the English language literature. Dobutamine stress echocardiography can be performed safely and with acceptable patient tolerance. The range of positive test results was 23% to 50%. The predictive value of a positive test ranged from 17% to 43% for all events and 7% to 23% for hard events (MI or death). The negative predictive value ranged from 93% to 100%. In the series by Poldermans et al,[57] the presence of a new wall motion abnormality was a powerful determinant of an increased risk for perioperative events after multivariable adjustment for different clinical and echocardiographic variables. Several studies suggest that the degree of wall motion abnormalities and/or wall motion change at low infusion rates of dobutamine is especially important.

Ambulatory Electrocardiographic Monitoring

The use of preoperative ambulatory ECG monitoring to estimate coronary disease presence and risk of perioperative events in patients undergoing major noncardiac surgery was reviewed through a Medline search of the English literature on preoperative and myocardial ischemia and surgeries from 1976 to September 1994. The predictive value of preoperative ST changes on 24- to 48-hour ambulatory electrocardiography for cardiac death or MI in patients undergoing vascular and nonvascular noncardiac surgery has been reported by several investigators. The frequency of abnormal ST-segment changes observed in 869 patients reported in seven series was 25% (range, 9% to 39%). In two studies, it had a predictive value similar to dipyridamole thallium imaging.[58,59]

Recommendations: Which Test?

In most ambulatory patients, the test of choice is the standard exercise ECG, which provides exercise capacity and detects myocardial ischemia. In patients with important abnormalities on their resting ECG (left bundle branch block, left ventricular hypertrophy with strain pattern, digitalis effect), other techniques such as exercise echocardiography or exercise myocardial perfusion imaging should be considered. In patients unable to perform adequate exercise, a nonexercise stress test should be used. In this regard, dipyridamole nuclear perfusion imaging and dobutamine echocardiography are the most common. Intravenous dipyridamole should be avoided in patients with significant bronchospasm, critical carotid disease, or in patients with a condition that prevents their being withdrawn from theophylline preparations. Dobutamine should not be used as a stressor in patients with serious arrhythmias or severe hypertension or hypotension. For patients in whom echocardiographic image quality is likely to be poor, a myocardial perfusion study is more appropriate. Soft tissue attenuation can also be a problem with myocardial perfusion imaging. If there is an additional question about valvular dysfunction, the echocardiographic stress test is favored. In many instances, either stress perfusion or stress echocardiography is appropriate. In a meta-analysis of dobutamine stress echocardiography, ambulatory electrocardiography, radionuclide ventriculography, and dipyridamole nuclear perfusion scans in predicting adverse cardiac outcome after vascular surgery, all tests had a similar predictive value, with overlapping confidence intervals.[60] The expertise of the local laboratory in identifying advanced coronary disease is probably more important than the particular type of test.

For certain patients at high risk, it may be appropriate to proceed with coronary angiography rather than perform a noninvasive test. For example, preoperative consultation may identify patients with unstable angina or evidence of residual ischemia following recent MI for whom coronary angiography is indicated.

Indications for Coronary Angiography in Perioperative Evaluation for Noncardiac Surgery (ACC/AHA Guidelines)

Class I. There is evidence for and/or general agreement that a cardiac catheterization is of benefit.

Definitely Send the Following Patients to Cardiac Catheterization
- Patients with suspected or proven CAD:
- High-risk results during noninvasive testing
- Angina pectoris unresponsive to adequate medical therapy
- Most patients with unstable angina pectoris
- Nondiagnostic or equivocal noninvasive test in a high-risk patient undergoing a high-risk noncardiac surgical procedure

Class II. There is a divergence of evidence and/or opinion that a cardiac catheterization is of benefit.

Probably Send the Following Patients to Cardiac Catheterization
- Intermediate-risk results during noninvasive testing
- Nondiagnostic or equivocal noninvasive test in a lower-risk patient undergoing a high-risk noncardiac surgical procedure
- Urgent noncardiac surgery in a patient convalescing from acute MI
- Perioperative MI

Class III. There is evidence and/or general agreement that cardiac catheterization is not necessary.

Do Not Send the Following Patients to Cardiac Catheterization
- Low-risk noncardiac surgery in a patient with known CAD and low-risk results on noninvasive testing
- Screening for CAD without appropriate noninvasive testing
- Asymptomatic after coronary revascularization, with excellent exercise capacity (>7 METs)
- Mild stable angina in patients with good left ventricular function, low-risk noninvasive test results

- Patient is not a candidate for coronary revascularization because of concomitant medical illness
- Prior technically adequate normal coronary angiogram within 5 years
- Severe left ventricular dysfunction (e.g., EF less than 20%) and patients not considered candidate for revascularization procedure
- Patient unwilling to consider coronary revascularization procedure

Summary of the Recommendations Specifically for Preoperative Exercise Testing

Who Should Undergo an Exercise Test Prior to Noncardiac Surgery?

Is the Noncardiac Surgery an Emergency? If an emergency, there is no time for further evaluation and the patient should proceed to surgery. *Exercise testing is not indicated!*

Has the Patient Undergone Coronary Revascularization in the Past 5 Years? If the patient has had complete surgical revascularization in the past 5 years or coronary angioplasty from 6 months to 5 years ago, and if his or her clinical status has remained stable without recurrent signs or symptoms of ischemia in the interim, the likelihood of perioperative cardiac death or MI is extremely low and exercise testing would not lead to another intervention. *Exercise testing is not indicated!*

Has the Patient Undergone a Coronary Evaluation in the Past 2 Years? If an individual has undergone extensive coronary evaluation with either noninvasive or invasive techniques within 2 years and if the findings indicate that coronary risk has been adequately assessed with favorable findings, repeat stress testing is usually unnecessary. An exception to this rule is the patient who has experienced a definite change or new symptoms of coronary ischemia since the prior coronary evaluation. *Exercise testing is not indicated!*

Does the Patient Have One of the Unstable Coronary Syndromes or Major Clinical Predictors of Risk (Unstable Coronary Disease, or Decompensated HF, Hemodynamically Significant Arrhythmias, and/or Severe Valvular Heart Disease)? Stabilization then non-invasive (*possibly exercise testing*) or invasive testing is required prior to surgery.

Does the Patient Have Intermediate Clinical Predictors of Risk (Angina Pectoris, Prior MI by History or ECG, Compensated or Prior HF, or Diabetes Mellitus)? If such a patient has an estimated exercise capacity of less than 4 METs (unable to do normal activities) or if a high-risk surgical procedure is to be done (aortic and other major vascular, peripheral vascular, or prolonged surgical procedures associated with large fluid shifts and/or blood loss), then an *exercise test or another stress test is indicated.* The first choice for noninvasive testing is the standard exercise test. If the patient cannot exercise, then a nonexercise stress test is indicated.

Does the Patient Have None or Only the Minor Clinical Predictors of Risk? Noncardiac surgery is generally safe for patients with minor or none of the clinical predictors of clinical risk who exhibit moderate or excellent exercise capacity (≥4 METs), regardless of surgical type. Patients with poor exercise capacity facing higher-risk operations (vascular, anticipated long and complicated thoracic, abdominal, and head and neck) *should be considered for an exercise or another stress test.* The first choice for testing is the standard exercise test. It is almost never appropriate to recommend CABG or other invasive interventions, such as coronary angioplasty, that would not otherwise be indicated in an effort to reduce the risk of noncardiac surgery.

Is the Patient Scheduled For a High-Risk Surgical Procedure? All patients with intermediate clinical predictors and all patients with none or minor predictors with a low estimated exercise capacity *should undergo an exercise or nonexercise stress test.* The first choice for testing is the standard exercise test.

The results of noninvasive testing can then be used to determine further perioperative management. Such management may include intensified medical therapy or cardiac catheterization, which may lead to coronary revascularization or potential cancellation or delay of the elective noncardiac operation. Alternatively, results of the noninvasive test (usually a standard exercise test) may lead to a recommendation to proceed directly with surgery. In some patients, the risk of coronary angioplasty or corrective cardiac surgery may approach or even exceed the risk of the proposed noncardiac surgery.

EVALUATION OF PATIENTS WITH HIGH BLOOD PRESSURE

The exercise test has been considered as a tool to evaluate the treatment of high blood pressure, and to identify patients at risk for developing hypertension. Abnormal blood pressure responses to exercise were detailed in Chapter 5. In the following, the applications of the exercise test in the identification and treatment of hypertension is discussed. Franz[61] has investigated the blood pressure response during and after exercise in 552 males to determine if an exercise test can differentiate normotensive and hypertensive subjects. Patients with mild hypertension showed significantly higher blood pressures at 100 watts and after exercise than age-matched normotensive subjects and significantly lower values than stable hypertensive subjects. In addition, the systolic pressure response to bicycle exercise was significantly influenced by age. Using the upper limits of blood pressure during and after exercise, 50% of the patients with borderline hypertension could be classified as hypertensives. Their blood pressure response at 100 watts did not significantly differ from patients with mild hypertension. In contrast, in the 50% who responded negatively to exercise testing, the systolic blood pressure response at 100 watts was significantly lower than that of those demonstrating a positive response. They had exactly the same diastolic pressure value as the normotensive subjects. This study suggests that the assessment of blood pressure during exercise is useful in distinguishing between normotensive and hypertensive patients and in making estimates of blood pressure responses to daily stress.

The new guidelines have added the following with regard to blood pressure. Exercise testing has been used to identify patients with abnormal blood pressure responses destined to develop high blood pressure. Identification of such patients may allow for preventive measures. In asymptomatic normotensive subjects, an exaggerated exercise systolic and diastolic blood pressure during exercise, peak systolic greater than 214 mmHg, or the presence of an elevated systolic pressure at 3 minutes in recovery is associated with long-term risk of high blood pressure. Exercise capacity is reduced in patients with poor blood pressure control, and markedly high blood pressure has been suggested to cause false-positive ST responses. In the following, we provide a review of the important citations the guidelines utilized for this addition.

From the Framingham study, the relations of systolic blood pressure and diastolic blood pressure during the exercise and recovery periods of a graded treadmill test to the risk of developing new-onset hypertension was studied in normotensive subjects.[62] Blood pressure data from exercise testing in 1026 men and 1284 women (mean age, 42 ± 10 years) from the Framingham Offspring Study who were normotensive at baseline were related to the incidence of hypertension 8 years later. New-onset hypertension, or the initiation of antihypertensive drug treatment, occurred in 228 men (22%) and 207 women (16%). Exaggerated systolic blood pressure and diastolic blood pressure responses to exercise and delayed recovery of blood pressures were defined as age-adjusted values greater than the 95th percentile during the second stage of exercise and third minute of recovery, respectively. After multivariable adjustment, exercise testing was highly predictive of incident hypertension in both men (odds ratio = 4) and women (odds ratio = 2). Recovery systolic blood pressure was predictive of hypertension in men using a multivariable model that included exercise duration and peak exercise blood pressure (odds ratio = 2). Baseline resting systolic and diastolic blood pressures had stronger associations with new-onset hypertension than exercise diastolic blood pressure and recovery systolic blood pressure responses. The authors concluded that an exaggerated diastolic blood pressure response to exercise was predictive of new-onset hypertension in normotensive men and women while elevated recovery systolic blood pressure was predictive of hypertension only in men.

At the Mayo Clinic, the prognostic significance of exercise hypertension was studied in 150 healthy, asymptomatic subjects with normal resting blood pressures and exercise systolic blood pressures greater than 214 mmHg (90th percentile) on Bruce treadmill tests.[63] They were age- and gender-matched with subjects having normal exercise systolic blood pressures. Subjects were contacted by survey 8 years after the index treadmill test. Among the 93% that responded, there were 12 deaths, including eight in the exercise hypertension group. A major cardiovascular event, defined as cardiovascular death, MI, stroke, or coronary intervention occurred in 5 controls and 10 subjects with exercise hypertension. At follow-up, 13 controls and 37 subjects with exercise hypertension were diagnosed as having resting hypertension. In multivariate analysis, exercise hypertension was not a significant predictor for death or any individual cardiovascular event, but was for total cardiovascular events and new resting hypertension. The multivariate risk ratio for exercise hypertension was 3.6 for predicting a major cardiovascular event. Other significant predictors included body mass index and age. For predicting new resting hypertension, the multivariate odds ratio for exercise hypertension was two times. Their data suggest that exercise hypertension carries a small but significant risk for major cardiovascular events in asymptomatic normotensive subjects.

Another study from Mayo Clinic sought to determine if a history of hypertension or an exaggerated rise in exercise systolic blood pressure was associated with a false-positive exercise ECG.[64] Retrospective analysis was performed of the associations between exercise-induced ST-segment depression and a history of hypertension, exercise systolic blood pressure, and several other clinical and exercise test variables. Among 20,097 patients referred for exercise nuclear imaging, 1873 patients met the inclusion criteria, which included no history of MI or coronary artery revascularization, a normal resting ECG, and normal exercise thallium images. False-positive ST-segment depression occurred in 20% of the population. A history of hypertension was actually associated with a 30% decreased risk of ST-segment depression. A higher peak exercise systolic blood pressure was associated with a higher likelihood of ST-segment depression (8% increase for each 10-mmHg increase in systolic blood pressure). However, the association between peak exercise systolic blood pressure and ST-segment depression was so weak that this measurement could not be predictive in the individual patient. For every 20-mmHg increase in peak exercise systolic blood pressure, the percentage of patients with ST-segment depression increased by only 3%. In patients with normal resting ECGs, they concluded the following: (1) a history of hypertension is not a cause of a false-positive exercise test and (2) higher exercise systolic blood pressure is a significant but weak predictor of ST-segment depression.

Lim et al[65] reviewed information on exercise testing in hypertensive patients and persons at risk for developing hypertension to determine whether the test was valuable for diagnosis, prognosis, or assessment of the effect of therapy. A Medline search of English language articles published between 1985 and 1995 and reviews of the bibliographies of textbooks was performed. Primary research articles on exercise testing in patients with hypertension were included, with an emphasis on methods, diagnosis, prognosis, and assessment of drug therapy. Study design and quality were assessed, with particular attention paid to methods and aims. Relevant data on hemodynamic responses in hypertensive patients and persons at risk for developing hypertension and correlations to end-organ damage, mortality, and exercise

tolerance were analyzed. The exercise capacity of hypertensive patients was found to be reduced by as much as 30% compared with age-matched controls. This exercise impairment increased with age and end-organ damage, and its origin was traced back to adolescence. Total peripheral resistance also progressively increased with age. These changes were associated with functional and structural involvement of the cardiovascular system. Diastolic dysfunction was a prominent factor in this exercise limitation. Blood pressure responses to exercise were suggested to have prognostic value for the future development of hypertension, end-organ damage, and death. The adequacy of antihypertensive treatment should therefore be evaluated in terms of normalizing these stress-related blood pressure responses. They concluded that exercise testing is a simple procedure that has great potential for assessing and treating hypertensive patients.

Erikssen et al[66] compared the accuracy of coronary heart disease risk assessment based on classical risk factors with an assessment also based on multiple exercise test parameters. From 1972 to 1975, 2014 apparently healthy men aged 40 to 60 years had a symptom-limited exercise test during a cardiovascular survey. Their average maximal heart rate was 162 bpm and their average systolic blood pressure at a submaximal load of 100 watts was 180 mmHg. The exercise test variables that predicted risk for coronary heart disease included the ST response, submaximal systolic blood pressure (greater than one standard deviation above the norm [25 mmHg]) and exercise capacity. The submaximal systolic blood pressure exceeding one standard deviation carried a similar hazard as the other predictors of the exercise test.

EVALUATION OF CARDIAC RHYTHM DISORDERS

The following is a summary of the ACC/AHA Guidelines regarding recommendations for use of exercise testing in patients with cardiac rhythm disorders which were modified in the 2002 update.

Class I. Conditions for which there is evidence and/or general agreement that the standard exercise test is useful and helpful for evaluating patients with cardiac rhythm disorders.

A Standard Exercise Test is Definitely Appropriate for the Following Patients:

1. Identification of optimal pacemaker settings in patients with rate-adaptive pacemakers

2. Evaluation of congenital complete heart block in patients considering increased physical activity or competitive sports (Level of evidence: class C)

Class II a. Conditions for which there is conflicting evidence and/or a divergence of opinion that the standard exercise test is useful and helpful for patients with cardiac rhythm disorders but the weight of evidence for usefulness or efficacy is in favor of the exercise test.

A Standard Exercise Test is Probably Appropriate for the Following Patients:
1. Patients with known or suspected exercise-induced arrhythmia
2. Medical, surgical, or ablative therapy in patients with exercise-induced arrhythmia (including atrial fibrillation [AF])

Class II b. Conditions for which there is conflicting evidence and/or a divergence of opinion that the standard exercise test is useful and helpful for evaluating patients with cardiac rhythm disorders but the usefulness/efficacy is less well established.

A Standard Exercise Test May be Appropriate for the Following Patients:
1. Isolated ventricular premature beats in middle-aged patients without other evidence of CAD.
2. Investigation of prolonged first-degree AV block or type I second degree Wenkebach, bundle branch block, or isolated premature ventricular contractions (PVCs) in young patients considering participation in competitive sports (Level of evidence: class C)

Class III. Conditions for which there is evidence and/or general agreement that the standard exercise test is not useful and helpful for patients with cardiac rhythm disorders and in some cases may be harmful.

A Standard Exercise Test is Definitely Not Appropriate for the Following Patients:
1. Investigation of isolated premature beats in young patients
2. Exercise testing has a well-established role in the identification of the appropriate settings for adaptive-rate pacemakers using various physiologic sensors. A number of studies have compared different pacing modes with respect to their influence on exercise capacity. A formal exercise test may not always be necessary since the required data can often be obtained using a simple walk

Exercise testing may be employed in the evaluation of patients with symptoms that suggest exercise-induced arrhythmias, such as exercise-induced syncope. The utility of exercise testing in such patients is variable, depending on the arrhythmia in question. Exercise testing may also be used to evaluate medical therapy in patients with exercise-induced arrhythmias. A common, specific example of this indication is the use of exercise testing to assess the control of the ventricular response to exercise in patients with AF.

Exercise testing has been employed to investigate isolated ventricular premature beats in middle-aged patients without other clinical evidence of CAD. This is a special case about the problem of screening of asymptomatic individuals, which was covered earlier. An exercise test can also be used to evaluate patients with dysrhythmias or to induce dysrhythmias in patients with the appropriate symptoms. The dysrhythmias that can be evaluated include PVCs, sick sinus syndrome, and various degrees of heart block. Ambulatory monitoring or isometric exercise often detects a higher prevalence of dysrhythmias, including more serious dysrhythmias than does dynamic exercise testing. The findings from each of these tests, however, may have different significance.

Evaluation of Ventricular Arrhythmias

Lown et al[67] has expressed the opinion that maximal exercise testing is useful for detection of arrhythmias and assessment of antiarrhythmic drug efficacy. Because few reports had documented the safety of exercise testing in patients with malignant ventricular arrhythmias, Lown et al reviewed complications associated with symptom-limited exercise in 263 patients with such arrhythmias who underwent a total of 1377 maximal treadmill tests. Seventy-four percent of the population studied had a history of ventricular fibrillation or hemodynamically compromising ventricular tachycardia and the remainder had experienced ventricular tachycardia in the setting of either recent MI or poor left ventricular function. A complication was defined as the occurrence of arrhythmias during exercise testing—ventricular fibrillation, ventricular tachycardia, or bradycardia that mandated immediate medical treatment. Complications were noted in 24 patients (9.1%) during 32 tests (2.3%), whereas 239 patients (90.9%) were free of complications during 1345 tests (97.7%). There were no deaths, MIs, or lasting morbid events.

Clinical descriptors associated with complications included male gender, presence of CAD, and a history of exertional arrhythmias. Clinical variables previously considered to confer increased risk during exercise, such as poor left ventricular function, high-grade ventricular arrhythmias before or during exercise, exertional hypotension, and ST depression, were not predictive of complications. Occurrence of a complication was also unaffected by the use of antiarrhythmic drugs at the time of exercise. Complication frequency in their study group was compared with that in a reference population of 3444 cardiac patients without histories of symptomatic arrhythmias who underwent 8221 exercise tests. Of these, four subjects (0.12%) developed ventricular fibrillation (0.05% of tests) without fatality or lasting morbidity. They concluded that maximal exercise testing can be conducted safely in patients with malignant arrhythmias, and clinical variables previously considered to confer risk during exercise were not predictive of complications.

Lown et al[67] also compared the provocation of PVCs in a standard exercise test with provocation of PVCs in an abbreviated form of testing that seemed to approximate more closely the demands of daily activities. The abbreviated protocol was as follows: the treadmill was kept at 12% elevation and speed began at 1.7 mph and was increased every 15 seconds to the following speeds: 2.5, 3.4, 4.2, 5.5, and 6.0 mph. It was then kept at 6.5 mph until the test was completed. The study involved 52 patients with known or suspected history of ventricular arrhythmias—42 men and 10 women, average age 49 years. Hemodynamic and ST-segment changes were similar during both forms of testing. Thirty-seven patients (71%) undergoing a standard exercise test exhibited PVCs, whereas 32 (62%) did so during abbreviated testing. Of 13 patients with repetitive PVCs, standard as well as abbreviated exercise testing provoked the same degree of PVCs in 10. In two patients, the yield of these complex forms of PVCs was higher with the abbreviated testing and in one patient with standard exercise testing. This abbreviated protocol may be useful for patients undergoing serial exercise studies to assess drug efficacy for the suppression of PVCs.

Woelfel et al[68] studied 14 patients with exercise-induced ventricular tachycardia (ventricular tachycardia) with serial treadmill testing.[68] Those with reproducible ventricular tachycardia were treated with a beta-blocking agent and later with verapamil. In 11 patients (79%), ventricular tachycardia of similar rate, morphologic characteristics and duration was reproduced on two consecutive treadmill tests performed 1 to 14 days apart. Beta-blockade prevented recurrent ventricular tachycardia during acute testing in 10 of 11 patients and during chronic therapy in nine. Eight patients had a consistent relation between a critical sinus rate and the onset of ventricular tachycardia. In these patients, successful therapy correlated with preventing achievement of the critical sinus rate during maximal exercise. They also found verapamil to be effective in this group.

Evaluation of Patients with Atrial Fibrillation

The reported prevalence of AF has varied widely, but it is directly related to age. Kannel et al,[59] in a 22-year analysis from the Framingham Study, described the onset of chronic AF in 49 of 2325 males and 49 of 2,866 females. This represents an overall 2% chance of developing AF in 20 years. They noted a direct relationship between the incidence of AF and age, ranging from approximately 0.2% of individuals between 25 and 34 years to greater than 3% at 55 to 64 years. Only 30 men and 18 women had no history of concomitant cardiovascular disease, and the other 50 cases were preceded more frequently than controls by congestive heart failure and rheumatic heart disease; in addition, males had stroke and hypertension as precursors. Stroke was an antecedent predictor of AF, suggesting transient or intermittent AF as a possible cause of cerebral emboli. There was an increased mortality associated with the onset of AF; within 6 years, 60% of males and 45% of females died. In a 30-year follow-up of 43 individuals with AF but without cardiovascular disease, Framingham researchers found them to have an increased risk for strokes. In a similar study from the Mayo Clinic, individuals with "lone AF" were found to have a good prognosis. Rose et al[69] screened 18,403 male civil servants and found the prevalence of AF to be 0.2%, 0.4%, and 1% in those 40 to 49, 50 to 59, and 60 to 64 years of age, respectively. Those with AF had a mortality rate more than three times that of age-matched peers. Cullen et al[70] studied 2254 subjects over the age of 65 and found the prevalence of AF to be 2%. They also noted a higher prevalence (5%) in subjects over the age of 75 years. These studies document that AF is an important clinical problem that increases in prevalence as the population grows older. One problem regarding management of patients with chronic AF has been how to achieve the optimal medical control of their cardiovascular response to exercise.

Response to Exercise in patients with Atrial Fibrillation

Many authors have noted that patients in AF have an inordinately fast ventricular response during the first stage of an exercise test. This is important because it suggests that control of the ventricular rate, a primary goal of therapy in AF, is poorly controlled during low-level daily activities. For example, Aberg et al[71] noted that the largest increment in the ventricular rate occurred during the first stage of exercise and was greater than 45% of the total increase in heart rate. Likewise, Hornsten and Bruce[72] reported an increase in the ventricular response from 83 to 152 bpm during stage I of the Bruce protocol and a maximal response of 176 bpm at least two stages later. In fact, most studies evaluating pharmacologic efficacy of heart rate control have used only a submaximal exercise level, and few studies have addressed exercise capacity. We have also observed a rapid increase in heart rate during the lowest workloads with smaller incremental changes approaching maximal exercise.[71] This contrasts with the linear relationship between heart rate and workload in subjects in normal sinus rhythm.

Table 12-8 summarizes the results of studies on maximal testing in patients with AF. Only the more recent studies included measured oxygen uptake. Functional aerobic impairment is calculated by the formula: estimated peak VO_2 (from workload performed) minus predicted peak VO_2 (from age) divided by estimated peak VO_2. Aerobic capacity differed depending upon the extent to which patients with underlying conditions were included (valvular heart disease, chronic heart failure, coronary disease). In fact, functional aerobic impairment ranges considerably, from 10% to 60%, likely depending upon the extent to which these underlying conditions were present. Interestingly, studies have shown that patients with "lone AF" achieve roughly the same exercise capacity as age-matched subjects in normal sinus rhythm.

The Effect of Drugs on Exercise Performance in Patients with Chronic AF

In patients with chronic AF, the primary goal of therapy is to control the rapid heart rate response

TABLE 12–8. Summary of studies assessing maximal heart rate and exercise capacity in patients with atrial fibrillation

Parameter	Hornsten	Aberg	Aberg	Aberg	Khalsa	Davidson	Lang	Molajo	Dibianco
Year	1968	1972	1972	1977	1979	1979	1983	1984	1984
No. of patients	65	179	24	15	11	11	20	10	20
Mean age	50	47	45	45	56	55	59	52	60
Exercise protocol	Bruce	Bike	Bike	Bike	Bike	Bruce	Bike	Bruce	Modified Bruce
Max HR	176	134	157	138	142	176	169	162	175
Est METs	5	3.5	3.5	4	5.7	6.5	4.5	5	7
Est VO_2	18	12	12	13	20	23	15	18	25
FAI	35%	60%	60%	55%	30%	50%	50%	55%	40%
Measured VO_2	—	—	—	—	—	—	—	—	—

Parameter	Atwood	Roth	Steinberg	Lundstrom	Ueshima	Vanhees	Levy
Year	1986	1986	1987	1990	1993	2000	2001
No. of patients	34	12	14	13	79	19	18
Mean age	66	48	66	65	64	63	69
Exercise protocol	Modifid B-W	Modified Bruce	Modified Bruce	Bike	Modified B-W	Bike	CAEP
Max HR	171	170	163	179	175	135	148
Est METs	8	—	7	6.5	—	—	—
Est VO_2	27	—	—	22.3	—	—	—
FAI	14%				22%	38%	32%
Measured VO_2	21				21	17	17

B-W, Balke-Ware protocol; CAEP, chronotropic assessment exercise protocol; Est, estimated; FAI, functional aerobic impairment; HR, heart rate; Max, maximal; MET, 3.5 ml O_2/kg/min; VO_2, ventilatory oxygen uptake in ml O_2/kg/min.

at rest and during exercise. For many years, digoxin was a drug of choice to control resting heart rate. However, digoxin has limited effectiveness in controlling heart rates during exercise or other stresses. The concomitant use of beta-adrenergic or calcium channel-blocking agents with digoxin has been recommended as better for controlling heart rate. More recently, the AV nodal-blocking effect of amiodarone has been applied.

A concern with beta-adrenergic blockade therapy is the possible reduction in cardiac output resulting not only from a reduced maximal heart rate but also from the depression of myocardial function. If a significant reduction in cardiac output occurs, maximal oxygen uptake would be decreased causing a reduction in exercise capacity. Studies in normal subjects have provided conflicting results as to the effect of beta-adrenergic-blocking agents on maximal oxygen uptake and other ventilatory variables associated with aerobic capacity. Similarly, in studies of patients with AF, the effects of beta-adrenergic blockade on maximal exercise capacity have been inconclusive, and few of the studies have included measurements of ventilatory parameters.

To investigate the effect of maximum dose (600 mg) celiprolol, a beta-1 selective adrenergic blocker, on hemodynamic and respiratory gas exchange variables in patients with chronic AF during maximal exercise testing, Atwood et al[73] studied a group of patients with chronic AF in a randomized, double-blind crossover trial. A significant decrease in heart rate and systolic blood pressure at the submaximal workload of 3.0 mph per 0% grade was observed during celiprolol administration. These reductions were similar to previous data obtained in normal subjects and patients in AF. Celiprolol did not alter gas exchange variables such as minute ventilation, oxygen uptake, and respiratory exchange ratio at this submaximal work rate, but oxygen uptake at the ventilatory threshold and maximal exercise were significantly reduced.

In the few studies that have addressed the effect of beta-adrenergic blockade on maximal exertion in AF, similar results have been reported. Di Bianco et al, in a multicentric trial involving 20 subjects in AF, studied the maximal exercise heart rate response to exercise while on placebo and digoxin versus nadolol and digoxin. They noted not only a reduction in heart rate and systolic pressure while on beta-blockade, but also a significant reduction in exercise capacity (a 23% reduction). Molajo et al[74] reported a reduction in maximal heart rate with administration of Corwin but also noted a significant (20%) increase in exercise time. These studies suggest that the effects of beta-blockade on

controlling heart rate in AF need to be balanced with its adverse effect or exercise capacity.

Segal et al[75] conducted a comprehensive review of the literature using the Cochrane database and Medline. English language articles describing randomized controlled trials of drugs used for heart rate control in adults with AF were included through 1998. Forty-five articles evaluating 17 drugs met the criteria for review. In the five trials of verapamil and five of diltiazem, heart rate was reduced significantly ($P < 0.05$), both at rest and with exercise, compared to placebo, with equivalent or improved exercise tolerance in six of seven comparisons. In 7 of 12 comparisons of a beta-blocker with placebo, the beta-blocker was efficacious for control of resting heart rate, with evidence that the effect was drug specific; nadolol and atenolol proved to be most efficacious. All nine comparisons demonstrated good heart rate control with beta-blockers during exercise, although exercise tolerance was compromised in three of nine comparisons. In seven of eight trials, digoxin administered alone slowed the resting heart rate more than placebo, but it did not significantly slow heart rate during exercise in four studies. The trials evaluating other drugs yielded insufficient evidence to support their use. Segal et al[75] concluded that the calcium channel blockers, verapamil or diltiazem, or select beta-blockers were efficacious for heart rate control at rest and during exercise for patients with AF without a clinically important decrease in exercise tolerance. Digoxin was useful only when rate control during exercise is less of a concern.

From a clinical standpoint, the addition of a beta-blocker for heart rate control in patients with chronic AF makes sense when the only goal is to reduce myocardial oxygen demand through reduction of heart rate such as in patients with concomitant angina. However, in adding beta-blocker therapy there is the risk of compromising exercise capacity because of the negative chronotropic and inotropic effects associated with these agents. In studies addressing this issue, maximum doses of beta-blockade have frequently led to decreased exercise capacity. However, use of lower, individualized doses of particular beta-blockers may perhaps normalize heart rate without reducing exercise tolerance.

Treatment with Diltiazem. Since a calcium antagonist may offer chronotropic control but has less of a negative inotropic effect, some have suggested it may be more advantageous in the treatment of AF. We and other groups have studied AF patients after stabilizing them on diltiazem.[76]

These studies have generally observed improvements in treadmill time and no decrease in peak VO_2 along with heart rate control.

Clinically, any intervention that decreases the ventilatory threshold or reduces oxygen uptake at higher workloads becomes important in patients who desire an active lifestyle. Since the patient perceives an equivalent amount of work as being harder during beta-adrenergic blockade, their motivation to engage in previous activities may be affected. The effective control of submaximal exercise heart rates must be weighed against the impairment in oxygen delivery at moderate to heavy workloads. The key to therapy in AF patients would appear to be normalizing the heart rate response to exercise without affecting exercise tolerance.

EVALUATION OF VALVULAR HEART DISEASE

The following is a summary of the ACC/AHA Guidelines regarding recommendations for exercise testing adults with valvular heart disease.

Class I. Conditions for which there is evidence and/or general agreement that the standard exercise test is useful and helpful for evaluating patients with valvular heart disease.

1. In chronic aortic insufficiency, assessment of exercise capacity and symptomatic responses in patients with equivocal symptoms.

Class II A. Conditions for which there is conflicting evidence and/or a divergence of opinion that the standard exercise test is useful and helpful for evaluating adults with valvular heart disease but the weight of evidence for usefulness or efficacy is in favor of the exercise test.

1. In chronic aortic insufficiency, evaluation of exercise capacity and symptomatic responses before participation in athletics
2. In chronic aortic insufficiency, prognostic assessment in asymptomatic or minimally symptomatic patients with left ventricular dysfunction

Class II B. Conditions for which there is conflicting evidence and/or a divergence of opinion that the standard exercise test is useful and helpful for evaluating adults with valvular heart disease but the usefulness/efficacy is less well established.

1. Evaluation of exercise capacity

Class III. Conditions for which there is evidence and/or general agreement that the standard exercise test is not useful and helpful for evaluating adults with valvular heart disease and in some cases may be harmful.

1. Do not use the standard exercise test to evaluate patient with symptomatic, severe critical aortic stenosis (AS)
2. Diagnosis of CAD in patients with moderate or severe valvular disease or with the baseline ECG abnormalities mentioned in the diagnostic section.

In symptomatic patients with documented valvular disease, the course of treatment is usually clear and exercise testing is not required. However, Doppler echocardiography has greatly increased the number of asymptomatic patients with defined valvular abnormalities. The primary value of exercise testing in valvular heart disease is to objectively assess exercise capacity and the extent of patient disability, both of which may have implications for clinical decision-making. This is particularly important in the elderly, who may not have symptoms because of their limited activity. The use of the exercise ECG for the diagnosis of CAD in these situations is limited by false-positive responses due to left ventricular hypertrophy and baseline ECG abnormalities. In patients with AS, the test should be directly supervised by a physician using a slowly progressive protocol with frequent manual blood pressure determinations. Exercise should be terminated in the absence of an appropriate increase in systolic blood pressure, slowing of the heart rate with increasing exercise, and premature beats.

Exercise testing has been used to qualify the amount of disability caused by valvular disease, to reproduce any exercise-induced symptoms, and to evaluate their response to medical and surgical intervention. The exercise ECG has been used as a means to identify concurrent CAD, but there is a high prevalence of false-positive responses (ST depression not due to ischemia) because of the frequent baseline ECG abnormalities and left ventricular hypertrophy. Some physicians have used the exercise test to help decide when surgery is indicated. Exercise testing has been utilized most in patients with AS, and so this section will emphasize evaluation of this valvular abnormality.[77,78]

Aortic Stenosis

Effort syncope is an important and well-appreciated symptom in patients with AS. Most guidelines on exercise testing list moderate to severe AS as a contraindication for exercise testing due to concern with syncope and cardiac arrest. The following discussion illustrates the potential danger of exercising adults with AS. In addition, the mechanisms responsible for effort syncope and the value and limits of exercise testing in patients with AS will be presented. Guidelines for monitoring patients with AS during exercise testing and clinical situations in which exercise testing may be of value in AS will be reviewed.

Physiological Mechanisms of Effort Syncope

From the time that syncope in AS was first described, with reduced systolic pressure during syncope, an absence of pulses and apical impulse, and the disappearance of murmurs, various mechanisms have been hypothesized for effort syncope in AS. Carotid artery hyper-reactivity and inadequate cardiac output leading to "cerebral anemia" and syncope have been proposed. An inability to increase cardiac output during exercise because of left ventricular failure or arrhythmias could also contribute to syncope in AS.

The most plausible explanation for syncope during exercise in patients with AS is that of left ventricular stretch baroreceptor stimulation or mechanoreceptor stimulation with concomitant arterial hypotension, reduced venous return, and bradycardia. Elevation of left arterial and left ventricular pressure in dogs can cause a decrease in venous return and a fall in systemic vascular resistance that is most prominent during extrasystoles. The abrupt elevation of left ventricular systolic pressure without a corresponding rise in aortic pressure could allow left ventricular baroreceptors to produce "a violent depressor reflex." This could lead to bradycardia, peripheral vasodilation, and hypotension, which would reduce coronary arterial flow and result in left ventricular dysfunction and arrhythmia.

Exercise Testing in Subjects with Aortic Stenosis

Although studies have delineated possible mechanisms for effort syncope in AS, a review of the literature (Table 12-9) demonstrates rare complications from exercise testing when performed with appropriate caution and monitoring. While predominantly used in pediatric cardiology to assess congenital AS and the need for surgical therapy, exercise testing has more recently been performed in adults. Appropriate caution and

monitoring must be applied, but the test can be used to resolve problems when there is a disparity between history and clinical findings. Since Doppler echocardiography has been available, asymptomatic AS in the elderly has been detected more frequently and treatment decisions in this group have become a clinical challenge.

Exercise testing in children with valvular stenosis has been used to distinguish who would benefit from surgery. However, this was before Doppler echocardiography was available. In children with congenital AS who were tested by bicycle exercise, those with gradients of 60 mmHg or greater had 2-mm or more ST depression. An exercise profile consisting of ST-segment depression of 2 mm or more, a decreased systolic blood pressure response of two standard deviation below normal, and a decreased total work capacity of two standard deviation below normal has been proposed. Two or more of these abnormal exercise responses occurred predominantly among those with a resting gradient greater than 70 mmHg.

Scandinavian cardiologists have reported no complications in over 600 tests in adults with AS. In a series of 50,000 exercise tests performed in Sweden, only two deaths were reported—one of the two deaths reported was in a patient with AS.[79] A "coronary insufficiency index score," expressed using the degree of ST depression relative to predicted exercise capacity, was predictive of CAD even in patients who had left ventricular hypertrophy and were receiving digitalis.

Exercise testing is a relatively safe test in both the pediatric and adult patient when appropriately performed. Attention should be focused on the minute-by-minute response of the blood pressure, the patient's symptoms, heart rate slowing, and premature ventricular and atrial arrhythmias. In the presence of an abnormal blood pressure response, a patient with AS should undergo at least a 2-minute cool-down walk to avoid the acute left ventricular volume overload that may occur when placed supine. As in the elderly, detrained, and CAD patients, when testing patients with AS, low-level protocols should be used.

Exercise testing plays an important role in the objective assessment of symptoms, hemodynamic responses, and functional capacity in AS. Whether ST-segment depression indicates significant CAD or not remains unclear. By performing exercise testing preoperatively and postoperatively, the benefits of surgery and baseline impairment can be quantified. Exercise testing offers the opportunity to evaluate objectively any disparities between history and clinical findings, for example, in the

TABLE 12–9. Review of studies using exercise testing in patients with aortic stenosis

	Halloran (1971)	Chandramouli (1975)	Aronow (1975)	Whitmer (1981)	James (1982)	Barton (1983)	Kveselis* (1985)	Linderholm† (1985)	Nylander (1986)	Amato (2001)	Das (2003)
No. Patients	31	44	19	23	65	11	12	20	91	66	19
Age (years)	(8–17)‡	(5–19)	(35–56)	11	12	12 (6–20)	13 ± 3	58 ± 14	65 (52–78)	44 ± 14	69
Mode	Bike	Treadmill	Treadmill	Bike	Bike	Treadmill	Bike	Bike	Bike	Treadmill	Treadmill
Mean valve area (cm²)	1.22 ± 0.74	NA	NA	NA	NA	NA	0.60 ± 0.16	NA	(0.48–1.63)	0.72 ± 0.16	1.01 ± 0.12
Mean valve gradient (mmHg)	50	(10–112)	(53–80)	86 (30–235)	(<30 –>70)	38 (14–80)	59 ± 18	57 ± 23	(18–64)	73 ± 25	NA
Maximal heart rate (beats/min)	(160–200)	NA	NA	NA	(183–194)	182	180 ± 17	NA	NA	NA	NA
Exercise capacity	NA	NA	NA	NA	NA	NA	800 kpm/min	500 kpm/min	NA	NA	4.6 METs
Angina (%)	0	0	0	0–29	6(38–89)	9	0	35	29	18	NA
>1.0 min ST-segment depression (%)	48	27	37	(71–100)	(0–32)	54	100	Mean = 1.33 ± 0.8	NA	20	NA
Abnormal blood pressure response (%)	NA	NA	NA	NA	NA	63	58	NA	NA	NA	28

*Selected subgroup with >1.0 min ST-segment depression; †Selected subgroup without CAD; ‡Parentheses denote range.
NA, Not available; kpm/min, kilogram-meters/minute.

elderly "asymptomatic subject" with physical and/or Doppler findings of severe AS. Often the echocardiographic studies are inadequate in such patients, particularly when they are smokers. When Doppler echocardiography reveals a significant gradient in the asymptomatic patient with normal exercise capacity, he/she could be followed closely until symptoms develop. In patients with an inadequate systolic blood pressure response to exercise or a fall in systolic blood pressure below the resting value with concomitant symptoms, surgery appears to be indicated.

SUMMARY

The studies evaluating antianginal agents have been greatly hampered by the increase in treadmill time that occurs merely by performing serial tests. This phenomenon of habituation or learning is not due to training but due to enhanced mechanical efficiency. For this reason, expired gas analysis is frequently being added to protocols evaluating therapeutic agents. Another common approach is to include only those individuals who show a minimal variation during a series of baseline tests in clinical trials. The review by Glasser et al[20] showing the safety for patients enrolled in antianginal drug studies is very important and reassuring. In terms of nitrate therapy, it would appear that the greater the decreases in rest and exercise blood pressure the greater the functional benefit. The magnitude of this change in blood pressure may be limited by symptoms of headaches, hypotension, or possible nitrate tolerance during chronic administration. On the other hand, a lack of resting blood pressure response after nitrate administration suggests little or no therapeutic effect and warrants a re-evaluation of therapy.

The studies of CABG and PCI are confounded by differences in medications before and after intervention and by the low rate of abnormal preintervention studies in the patients undergoing PCI who mostly have single-vessel disease. In addition, there have been considerable technological advances in both of these procedures. Standard exercise testing does not appear to be very helpful in predicting restenosis, but recent studies suggest that exercise perfusion studies provide prognostic information in patients who have undergone CABG. In the ROSETTA study, there was little difference in the rates of follow-up cardiac procedures among the patients undergoing the routine and selective exercise testing strategies.

The standard exercise test is the test of choice in patients requiring evaluation for possible ischemia or exercise intolerance prior to noncardiac surgery. The ACC/AHA guidelines emphasize the importance of exercise capacity in assessing the surgical risk. We have summarized the guidelines for this application.

Exercise testing has been used to identify patients with abnormal blood pressure responses to exercise likely to develop hypertension in the future. Identification of such patients may allow for preventive measures. In asymptomatic normotensive subjects, an exaggerated exercise systolic and diastolic blood pressure during exercise, or elevated blood pressure at 3 minutes in recovery is associated with long-term risk of hypertension. Exercise capacity is reduced in patients with poor blood pressure control. Although this has been controversial in the past, hypertension does not appear to cause false-positive ST responses. An excessive submaximal systolic blood pressure (> 200 mmHg at about 4 METs) carried a similar hazard as maximal exercise capacity and ST depression in a Norwegian study.

We have summarized the updated recommendations for use of exercise testing in patients with cardiac rhythm disorders. Other applications of exercise testing include its use for evaluating patients with valvular heart disease and AF. The updated guidelines focus on the evaluation of aortic insufficiency and we add our experience with AS. A summary of the literature addressing rate control in patients with AF underscores the controversy regarding the best therapy for this common arrhythmia; these studies indicate that exercise capacity is unchanged by the use of a calcium antagonist, while a beta-blocker can cause a decrease in exercise capacity.

REFERENCES

1. Sullivan M, Genter F, Savvides M, et al: The reproducibility of hemodynamic, electrocardiographic, and gas exchange data during treadmill exercise in patients with stable angina pectoris. Chest 1984;86: 375–382.
2. Smokler PE, MacAlpin RN, Alvaro A, Kattus AA: Reproducibility of a multi-stage near maximal treadmill test for exercise tolerance in angina pectoris. Circulation 1973;48:346–351.
3. Redwood DR, Rosing DR, Goldstein RE, et al: Importance of the design of an exercise protocol in the evaluation of patients with angina pectoris. Circulation 1971;43:618–28.
4. Myers JN: Perception of chest pain during exercise testing in patients with coronary artery disease. Med Sci Sports Exerc 1994;26: 1082–1086.
5. Waters DD, McCans JL, Crean PA: Serial exercise testing in patients with effort angina: Variable tolerance, fixed threshold. J Am Coll Cardiol 1985;6:1011–1015.
6. Myers JN, Froelicher VF: Optimizing the exercise test for pharmacological studies in patients with angina pectoris. In Ardissino D,

Savonitto S, Opie LH (eds): Drug Evaluation in Angina Pectoris. Norwell, Mass, Kluwer Academic Publishers, 1995, pp 41–52.

7. Parker JO, VanKoughnett KA, Fung HL: Transdermal isosorbide dinitrate in angina pectoris: effect of acute and sustained therapy. Am J Cardiol 1984;54:8–13.

8. Thadani U, Manyari D, Parker JO, Fung HL: Tolerance to the circulatory effects of isosorbide dinitrate: Rate of development and cross tolerance to glyceral trinitrate. Circulation 1980;61:526–535.

9. Thompson RH: The clinical use of transdermal delivery devices with nitroglycerin. Angiology 1983;34:23–31.

10. Thadani U: Nitrate tolerance, rebound, and their clinical relevance in stable angina pectoris, unstable angina, and heart failure. Cardiovasc Drugs Ther 1996;10:735–742.

11. Thadani U, Opie LH: Nitrates for unstable angina. Cardiovasc Drugs Ther 1994;8:719–726.

12. Steering Committee, Transdermal Nitroglycerin Cooperative Study: Acute and chronic antianginal efficacy of continuous twenty-four hour application of transdermal nitroglycerin. Am J Cardiol 1991;68:1263–1273.

13. Sullivan MA, Savvides M, Abouantoun S, et al: Failure of transdermal nitroglycerin to improve exercise capacity in patients with angina pectoris. J Am Coll Cardiol 1985;5:1220–1223.

14. Heidenreich PA, McDonald KM, Hastie T, et al: Meta-analysis of trials comparing beta-blockers, calcium antagonists, and nitrates for stable angina. JAMA 1999;281:1927–1936.

15. Chaitman BR, Pepine CJ, Parker JO, et al: Effects of ranolazine with atenolol, amlodipine, or diltiazem on exercise tolerance and angina frequency in patients with severe chronic angina: A randomized controlled trial. Combination Assessment of Ranolazine In Stable Angina (CARISA) JAMA 2004;291:309–316.

16. Burkhoff D, Schmidt S, Schulman SP, et al: Transmyocardial laser revascularization compared with continued medical therapy for treatment of refractory angina pectoris: A prospective randomized trial. ATLANTIC Investigators. Angina Treatments-Lasers and Normal Therapies in Comparison. Lancet 1999;354:885–890.

17. Saririan M, Eisenberg MJ: Myocardial laser revascularization for the treatment of end-stage coronary artery disease. J Am Coll Cardiol 2003;41:173–183.

18. Szatkowski A, Ndubuka-Irobunda C, Oesterle SN, Burkhoff D: Transmyocardial laser revascularization: A review of basic and clinical aspects. Am J Cardiovasc Drugs 2002;2:255–266.

19. Horvath KA: Mechanisms and results of transmyocardial laser revascularization. Cardiology 2004;101:37–47.

20. Glasser SP, Clark PI, Lipicky RJ, et al: Exposing patients with chronic, stable, exertional angina to placebo periods in drug trials. JAMA 1991;265:1550–1554.

21. Gibbons RJ, Balady GJ, Bricker JT, et al: ACC/AHA 2002 guidelines update for exercise testing: summary article. A report of the American College of Cardiology/American Heart Association Task Force on Practice Guidelines. J Am Coll Cardiol 2002;40:1531-1540.

22. Berger E, Williams DO, Reinert S, Most AS: Sustained efficacy of percutaneous transluminal coronary angioplasty. Am Heart J 1986;111:233–236.

23. Vandormael MG, Chaitman BR, Ischinger T, et al: Immediate and short-term benefit of multilesion coronary angioplasty: Influence of degree of revascularization. J Am Coll Cardiol 1985;6:983–991.

24. Rosing DR, Van Raden MJ, Mincemoyer RM, et al: Exercise, electrocardiographic and functional responses after percutaneous transluminal coronary angioplasty. Am J Cardiol 1984;53:36C–41C.

25. Ernst S, Hillebrand FA, Klein B, et al: The value of exercise tests in the follow-up of patients who underwent transluminal coronary angioplasty. Int J Cardiol 1985;7:267–279.

26. Honan MB, Bengtson JR, Pryor DB, et al: Exercise treadmill testing is a poor predictor of anatomic restenosis after angioplasty for acute myocardial infarction. Circulation 1989;80:1585–1594.

27. Bengtson JR, Mark DB, Honan MB, et al: Detection of restenosis after elective percutaneous transluminal coronary angioplasty using the exercise treadmill test. Am J Cardiol 1990;65:28–34.

28. Wijns W, Serruys PW, Simoons ML, et al: Predictive value of early maximal exercise test and thallium scintigraphy after successful percutaneous transluminal coronary angioplasty. Br Heart J 1985;53:194–200.

29. Eisenberg MJ, Schechter D, Lefkovits J, et al: Utility of routine functional testing after percutaneous transluminal coronary angioplasty: Results from the ROSETTA registry. J Invasive Cardiol 2004;16:318–322.

30. Acampa W, Petretta M, Florimonte L, et al: Prognostic value of exercise cardiac tomography performed late after percutaneous coronary intervention in symptomatic and symptom-free patients. Am J Cardiol 2003;91:259–263.

31. Ho KT, Miller TD, Holmes DR, et al: Long-term prognostic value of Duke treadmill score and exercise thallium-201 imaging performed one to three years after percutaneous transluminal coronary angioplasty. Am J Cardiol 1999;84:1323–1327.

32. L'Huillier I, Cottin Y, Touzery C, et al: Predictive value of myocardial tomoscintigraphy in asymptomatic diabetic patients after percutaneous coronary intervention. Int J Cardiol 2003;90:165–173.

33. Hultgren HN, P Peduzzik, Ketre K, Takoro T: The 5 year effect of bypass surgery on relief of angina and exercise performance. Circulation 1985;72:V79–V83.

34. Lauer MS, Lytle B, Pashkow F, et al: Prediction of death and myocardial infarction by screening with exercise-thallium testing after coronary-artery-bypass grafting. Lancet 1998;351:615–622.

35. Ryan TJ, Weiner DA, McCabe CH, et al: Exercise testing in the coronary artery surgery study randomized population. Circulation 1985;72:V31–V38.

36. Gohlke H, Gohlke-Barwolf C, Samek L, et al: Serial exercise testing up to 6 years after coronary bypass surgery: Behavior of exercise parameters in groups with different degrees of revascularization determined by postoperative angiography. Am J Cardiol 1983;51:1301–1306.

37. CASS Principal Investigators and Their Associates: Coronary Artery Surgery Study (CASS): A randomized trial of coronary artery bypass surgery—survival data. Circulation 1983;68:939–950.

38. Read RC, Murphy ML, Hultgren HN, Takaro T: Survival of men treated for chronic stable angina pectoris—A cooperative randomized study. J Thorac Cardiovasc Surg 1978;75:1–16.

39. European Coronary Surgery Study Group: Long-term results of prospective randomized study of coronary artery bypass surgery in stable angina pectoris. Lancet 1982;II:1173–1180.

40. Gruntzig AR, Senning A, Siegenthaler WE: Nonoperative dilatation of coronary artery stenosis: Percutaneous transluminal coronary artery. N Engl J Med 1979;301:61–68.

41. Dubach P, Froelicher V, Atwood JE, et al: A comparison of the exercise test responses pre/post revascularization: Does coronary artery bypass surgery produce better results than percutaneous transluminal coronary angioplasty? J Cardiopulm Rehab 1990;10:120–125.

42. Meier B, Gruentzig AR, Siegenthaler WE, Schlumpf M: Long-term exercise performance after percutaneous transluminal coronary angioplasty and coronary artery bypass grafting. Circulation 1983;68:796–802.

43. King SB, Talley JD: Coronary arteriography and percutaneous transluminal coronary angioplasty. Changing patterns of use and results. Circulation 1989;79(suppl I):I-19-I-23.

44. Deligonul U, Vandormael MG, Younis LT, Chaitman BR: Prognostic significance of silent myocardial ischemia detected by early treadmill exercise after coronary angioplasty. Am J Cardiol 1989;64:1–5.

45. Grondin CM, Campeau L, Thornton JC, et al: Coronary artery bypass grafting with saphenous vein. Circulation 1989;79(suppl I):I-24-I-29.

46. Sionis D, Vrolix M, Glazier J, et al: Early exercise testing after successful PTCA:A word of caution. Am Heart J 1992;123:530–532.

47. Roffi M, Wenaweser P, Windecker S, et al: Early exercise after coronary stenting is safe. J Am Coll Cardiol 2003;42:1569–1573.

48. Eagle KA, Berger PB, Calkins H, et al (Committee to Update the 1996 Guidelines on Perioperative Cardiovascular Evaluation for Noncardiac Surgery): ACC/AHA guideline update for perioperative cardiovascular evaluation for noncardiac surgery. Circulation 2002;105:1257–1267.

49. Paul SD, Eagle KA, Kuntz KM, et al: Concordance of preoperative clinical risk with angiographic severity of CAD in patients undergoing vascular surgery. Circulation 1996;94:1561–1566.

50. Rao TL, Jacobs KH, El-Etr AA: Reinfarction following anesthesia in patients with myocardial infarction. Anesthesiology 1983;59:499–505.

51. McPhail N, Calvin JE, Shariatmadar A, et al: The use of preoperative exercise testing to predict cardiac complications after arterial reconstruction. J Vasc Surg 1988;7:60–68.

52. Cutler BS, Wheeler HB, Paraskos JA, Cardullo PA: Applicability and interpretation of electrocardiographic stress testing in patients with peripheral vascular disease. Am J Surg 1981;141:501–506.

53. Carliner NH, Fisher ML, Plotnick GD, et al: Routine preoperative exercise testing in patients undergoing major noncardiac surgery. Am J Cardiol 1985;56:51–58.

54. Goldberger AL, O'Konski M: Utility of the routine electrocardiogram before surgery and on general hospital admission. Ann of Intern Med 1986;105:552–557.

55. Baron JF, Mundler O, Bertrand M, et al: Dipyridamole-thallium scintigraphy and gated radionuclide angiography to assess cardiac risk before abdominal aortic surgery. N Engl J Med 1994;330:663–669.

56. Younis L, Stratmann H, Takase B, et al: Preoperative clinical assessment and dipyridamole thallium-201 scintigraphy for prediction and prevention of cardiac events in patients having major noncardiovascular surgery and known or suspected CAD. Am J Cardiol 1994;74:311–317.

57. Poldermans D, Fioretti PM, Forster T, et al: Dobutamine stress echocardiography for assessment of perioperative cardiac risk in patients undergoing major vascular surgery. Circulation 1993;87:1506–1512.

58. McPhail NV, Ruddy TD, Barber GG, et al: Cardiac risk stratification using dipyridamole myocardial perfusion imaging and ambulatory ECG monitoring prior to vascular surgery. Eur J Vasc Surg 1993;7:151–155.

59. Kannel W, Abbott R, Savage D, McNamara PM: Epidemiologic features of chronic atrial fibrillation. N Engl J Med 1982;306:1018–1022.

60. Mantha S, Roizen MF, Barnard J, et al: Relative effectiveness of four preoperative tests for predicting adverse cardiac outcomes after vascular surgery: A meta-analysis. Anesth Analg 1994;79:422–433.

61. Franz IW: Ergometry in the assessment of arterial hypertension. Cardiology 1985;72:147–159.

62. Singh JP, Larson MG, Manolio TA, et al: Blood pressure response during treadmill testing as a risk factor for new-onset hypertension. The Framingham heart study. Circulation 1999;99:1831–1836.

63. Allison TG, Cordeiro MA, Miller TD, et al: Prognostic significance of exercise-induced systemic hypertension in healthy subjects. Am J Cardiol 1999;83:371-375.

64. Miller TD, Christian TF, Allison TG, et al: Is rest or exercise hypertension a cause of a false-positive exercise test? Chest 2000;117:226–232.

65. Lim PO, MacFadyen RJ, Clarkson PB, MacDonald TM: Impaired exercise tolerance in hypertensive patients. Ann Intern Med 1996;124:41–55.

66. Erikssen G, Bodegard J, Bjornholt JV, et al: Exercise testing of healthy men in a new perspective: From diagnosis to prognosis. Eur Heart J 2004;25:978–986.

67. Young DZ, Lampert S, Graboys TB, Lown B: Safety of maximal exercise testing in patients at high risk for ventricular arrhythmia. Circulation 1984;70:184–191.

68. Woelfel A, Foster JR, McAllister RG, et al: Efficacy of verapamil in exercise-induced ventricular tachycardia. Am J Cardiol 1985;56:292–297.

69. Rose G, Baxter PJ, Reid DD, McCartney P: Prevalence and prognosis of electrocardiogram findings in middle-aged men. Br Heart J 1978;15:636–643.

70. Cullen K, Stenhouse NS, Wearne KL, Cumpston GN: Electrocardiograms and 13 year cadiovascular mortality in Busselton study. Br Heart J 1982;47:209–212.

71. Aberg H, Strom G, Werner I: On the reproducibility of exercise tests in patients with atrial fibrillation. Ups J Med Sci 1977;82:27–30.

72. Hornsten TR, Bruce RA: Effects of atrial fibrillation on exercise performance in patients with cardiac disease. Circulation 1968;37:543–548.

73. Atwood JE, Sullivan M, Forbes S, et al: The effect of beta-adrenergic blockade on exercise performance in patients with chronic atrial fibrillation. J Am Coll Cardiol 1987;10:314–320.

74. Molajo AO, Coupe MO, Bennett DH: Effect of corwin on resting and exercise heart rate and exercise tolerance in digitalized patients with chronic atrial fibrillation. Br Heart J 1984;52:392–395.

75. Segal JB, McNamara RL, Miller MR, et al: The evidence regarding the drugs used for ventricular rate control. J Fam Pract 2000;49:47–59.

76. Atwood JE, Myers JN, Sullivan MJ, et al: Diltiazem and exercise performance in patients with chronic atrial fibrillation. Chest 1988;93:20–25.

77. Areskog NH: Exercise testing in the evaluation of patients with valvular aortic stenosis. Clin Physiol 1984;4:201–208.

78. Atwood JE, Kawanishi S, Myers J, Froelicher VF: Exercise and the heart. Exercise testing in patients with aortic stenosis. Chest 1988;93:1083–1087.

79. Atterhog JH, Jonsson B, Samuelsson R: Exercise testing: A prospective study of complication rates. Am Heart J 1979;98:572–579.

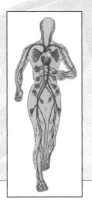

thirteen

Effect of Exercise on the Heart and the Prevention of Coronary Heart Disease

The protective effects of regular physical activity have been elucidated in many animal and human studies over the past 50 years. The overwhelming majority of these studies have demonstrated that habitual physical activity or physical fitness is associated with better cardiovascular health and improved survival. As a result, many international health organizations have put forth recommendations regarding the quantity and quality of exercise needed to improve the health of the public. In this chapter, the many research studies that have been performed over the last 5 decades are outlined, including animal and human studies, which document the effects of exercise on the heart and the prevention of coronary disease.

DEFINITION OF EXERCISE TRAINING

Exercise training can be defined as maintaining a regular habit of exercise at levels greater than those usually performed. An exercise program can be designed for increasing muscular strength, muscular endurance, or dynamic performance. The type of exercise that results in an increase in muscular strength involves short bursts of activity against a high resistance. *Isometric* exercise involves developing muscular tension against resistance with minimal or no external movement. Although this results in an increase in muscular mass along with strength, such exercise generally does not benefit the cardiovascular system. Isometric exercise causes a pressure load on the heart rather than a flow load because mean pressure is greatly elevated in proportion to the increase in cardiac output. Flow cannot be increased by much because of greater pressure within the active muscle groups. Exercise that is purely isometric should be considered differently from that of a typical resistance exercise program, which generally results in improvements in muscular strength *and* endurance. *Dynamic* exercise, also called isotonic, involves the rhythmic movement of large groups of muscles and requires an increase in cardiac output, ventilation, and oxygen uptake. It is this type of exercise that generally results in the most favorable cardiovascular changes.

The features of an aerobic exercise program that must be considered include the mode, duration, intensity, and frequency. In general, the mode of exercise must involve movement of large muscle groups such as is required by bicycling, walking, running, skating, cross-country skiing, swimming, and the like. Favorable training responses have generally been demonstrated when exercise is carried out in the course of at least three to five sessions a week. An optimal duration of an exercise session is considered to be in the range of 30 to 60 minutes. The intensity should be at least 50% of an individual's maximal oxygen uptake (typically ranging from 60% to 80%) and should involve at least 300 kilocalories (kcal) of energy expenditure per session. The percentage of maximal oxygen uptake required can be approximated by heart rate or by level of perceived exertion.

The changes that occur as a result of an aerobic exercise program can be classified as hemodynamic, morphologic, and metabolic (Table 13-1). The hemodynamic consequences of an exercise program include a decrease in resting heart rate, a decrease in the heart rate and systolic blood pressure at any matched submaximal workload, an increase in work capacity and maximal oxygen uptake, and a faster recovery from a bout of exercise. It is argued whether these changes are due to peripheral or cardiac adaptations. This is dependent upon age and other factors, but, at least to some extent, both peripheral and cardiac changes contribute to the response to training. Peripheral adaptations clearly are more important in older individuals and in patients with heart or lung disease, whereas cardiac adaptations are more likely to occur in younger individuals. Cardiac hemodynamic changes that have been observed in some instances include enhanced cardiac function and cardiac output, although these changes have not been observed in all studies.

It has become clear in recent years that the coronary arteries are not fixed channels but actually vary their diameter in response to various stimuli. Normal coronary arteries dilate in response to exercise, but these arteries can constrict in the presence of atherosclerosis.[1-3] The dynamic nature of the artery makes it possible for the heart to function more efficiently and to have greater perfusion during any stress. No studies have shown definitively that an exercise program alone decreases atherosclerotic plaques once they are present. However, animal studies have shown that exercise can offset the impact of an atherogenic diet by increasing the coronary artery's size, and exercise has been a component in some of the recent studies that have shown regression of atherosclerosis with intensive lipid-lowering therapy.

The morphologic changes that occur with an exercise program are age-related. These changes occur most definitely in younger individuals and may not occur in older individuals. The exact age limit at which chronic exercise causes morphologic changes is uncertain, but it would appear to be in the early 30s. Morphologic changes include an increase in myocardial mass and left ventricular end-diastolic volume. Paralleling these changes is an increase in the myocardial capillary-to-fiber ratio. The metabolic alterations secondary to an aerobic exercise program are summarized below. The total serum cholesterol level generally is not affected, but the level of high-density lipoproteins (HDL) is increased, particularly when weight loss accompanies the exercise. Serum triglyceride and fasting glucose levels are decreased. In addition, favorable alterations in insulin sensitivity occur. Membrane permeability to glucose improves with exercise, and this decreases an individual's resistance to insulin and increases insulin sensitivity. Thus, maintaining a regular exercise program is particularly important for diabetics. In addition, after an exercise program, blood catecholamine levels are lower in response to any stress. Studies have shown that the fibrinolytic system is enhanced, which is potentially beneficial in preventing myocardial infarction (MI).

The concept that exercise might enhance psychological well-being and reduce depression and anxiety has been the subject of numerous investigations.[4] However, randomized controlled trials in this area are lacking. Although evidence for both cross-sectional and prospective studies is generally consistent—that higher amounts of activity are associated with reductions in depression and anxiety—these studies are only observational. It would seem, however, that exercise does have a tranquilizing effect and increases pain tolerance, which may be beneficial in many individuals.

In the following, studies that have investigated the effects of chronic exercise on the heart—specifically in terms of animal and human studies of hemodynamics, the echocardiogram, and the electrocardiographic response to exercise testing—are presented. The available body of literature concerning the effects of chronic exercise on the hearts of humans and animals is now substantial. Several excellent and detailed reviews of this topic

TABLE 13-1. Physiologic adaptations to physical training in humans

Morphologic Adaptations
Myocardial hypertrophy
Hemodynamic Adaptations
Increased blood volume
Increased end-diastolic volume
Increased stroke volume
Increased cardiac output
Reduced heart rate for any submaximal workload
Metabolic Adaptations
Increased mitochondrial volume and number
Greater muscle glycogen stores
Enhanced fat utilization
Enhanced lactate removal
Increased enzymes for aerobic metabolism
Increased maximal oxygen uptake

are available.[5-9] In the following, only some of the classic articles are described to underscore each issue.

ANIMAL STUDIES RELATING EXERCISE TO CARDIAC CHANGES

Morphologic and Capillary Changes

Studies on the effects of exercise training on myocardial structure, function, and vasculature were widely performed in the U.S. and Europe in the 1960s and 1970s, and animals provided an ideal model to address many research questions not possible in humans. These studies provided some of the strongest evidence for the health benefits of regular exercise. It must be recognized, however, that animals and humans do not necessarily respond the same way to an exercise program, so it is always uncertain as to whether the results from these studies can be applied to humans. The many effects listed in Table 13-2 have been demonstrated using various animal models, methods of training, and techniques used to measure cardiac or vessel size. Vigorous exercise has been shown to induce cardiac hypertrophy in animals. Heart-to-body size ratios are invariably larger and the density of muscle cells and capillaries are greater in wild animals as compared with the domestic form of a given animal species. In young animals, cardiac hypertrophy is secondary to fiber hyperplasia (an increase in muscle cell number), whereas in older animals it appears to be secondary to cellular hypertrophy (an increase in muscle cell size).

TABLE 13-2. Results of animal studies investigating the effects of chronic exercise

Age-dependent myocardial hypertrophy
Myocardial microcirculatory changes (increased ratio of capillaries to muscle fibers)
Proportional increase in coronary artery size
Mixed results when studying changes in coronary collateral circulation
Improved cardiac mechanical and metabolic performance
Favorable changes in skeletal muscle mitochondria and enzyme changes
Little effect on established atherosclerotic lesions or risk factors
Improved peripheral blood flow during exercise
These observations provide strong support for the exercise hypothesis. Perhaps if people were as compliant as animals, the benefits of exercise to humans would be more apparent

The capillary bed responds most markedly to growth stimuli if applied at an early age.[10] There is an age-related response of the ventricular capillary bed and myocardial fiber width in rats. At autopsy, the myocardial fiber width is constant, whereas the capillary-to-fiber ratios are increased in trained rats when compared with controls in all age groups.[11] Experiments have been performed to study the effects of chronic exercise on the heart at different ages in rats. Although the response of the rat heart to chronic exercise appears to vary with age, the capillary-to-fiber ratio increases at all ages. Capillary proliferation in the heart and skeletal muscle has been studied by radioautography after injecting radioactive thymidine in rats exercised by swimming.[12] Swimming led to hypertrophy of the myocardium and in muscle fibers of the limbs. There was also new formation of myocardial capillaries in swimming-induced cardiac hypertrophy.

Coronary Artery Size Changes

The effects of exercise on the coronary tree of rats have been assessed in a classic study by the corrosion-cast technique. Tepperman and Pearlman[13] studied two groups of rats, one of the groups underwent a swimming program and the other, a running program. At autopsy, their hearts were weighed and the coronary arteries were injected with vinyl acetate. Compared with the controls, both exercise groups had an increased heart-to-body weight ratio and substantially increased coronary trees.

Coronary Collateral Circulation

Eckstein's[14] landmark 1957 study addressed the effects of exercise and coronary artery narrowing on coronary collateral circulation. He surgically induced constriction in the circumflex artery in approximately 100 dogs during a thoracotomy. After 1 week of rest, the dogs were put into two groups. One group was exercised on a treadmill 1 hour a day, 5 days a week, for 6 to 8 weeks. The other group remained at rest in cages. The extent of arterial anastomoses to the circumflex artery was then determined during a second thoracotomy. Moderate and severe arterial narrowing resulted in collateral development proportional to the degree of narrowing. Exercise led to even greater coronary collateral flow. This study provided the first evidence that exercise can improve coronary blood flow via collateral vessels.

Coronary blood flow was studied in trained and sedentary rats using labeled microspheres during hypoxemic conditions.[15] Even though cardiac hypertrophy was found in the trained rats, this increase in perfused mass accounted for only one third the increase in total coronary blood flow. Thus, there was a greater coronary blood flow per unit mass of the myocardium in the trained rats.

The effects of endurance exercise on coronary collateral blood flow has been studied in miniature swine.[16] Coronary collateral blood flow was measured in 10 sedentary control pigs and in seven pigs that ran 20 miles a week for 10 months. Ten months of endurance exercise training did not have an effect on the development of coronary collaterals, as assessed by microsphere blood flow measurements in the left ventricle of the pigs. When this was repeated after causing artificial partial occlusions in the coronary arteries of the pigs (i.e., ischemia present), exercise enhanced myocardial perfusion.

The effect of physical training on collateral blood flow in 14 dogs with chronic coronary occlusions revealed that myocardial blood flow to collateral dependent zones (measured using injected radionuclides) was increased by 39% in the dogs that underwent training.[17]

The effects of exercise training on the development of coronary collaterals in response to gradual coronary occlusion in dogs has been studied.[18] After placement of an amaroid constrictor on the proximal left circumflex coronary artery, 33 dogs were randomly assigned to exercise or sedentary groups. After 2 months, the exercised dogs developed greater epicardial collateral connections to the occluded left circumflex, as judged by higher blood flow and less of a distal pressure drop. However, no difference in collaterals was found angiographically. Injection of microspheres demonstrated that exercised dogs were not better protected against subendocardial ischemia. Exercise promoted coronary collateral development without improving perfusion of ischemic myocardium. Thus, even if collateral development does occur, the question remains as to whether it significantly influences myocardial perfusion.

Effects of Training on the Coronary Artery Endothelium

More recent studies have focused on coronary smooth muscle and the endothelium. An important advancement in this area has been the recognition that the coronary vasculature is not merely a series of fixed conduits, but that the endothelium responds significantly to the various relaxing and constricting factors that regulate blood flow. Important among these factors is nitric oxide, which is derived from the endothelium and produces dilation of the vessel. The first evidence that exercise training provides nitric oxide-mediated dilation of the coronary arteries was published by Wang et al.[19] Dogs were trained by treadmill running for 2 hours per day for 7 days. After training, the vasodilatory response of the left circumflex artery to acetylcholine was markedly greater in the trained dogs versus controls. The enhanced dilation was attributed to increased production and release of nitric oxide, because the response was eliminated in the presence of arginine analogs, which inhibit nitric oxide activity.

To assess whether training caused greater endothelium-mediated vasodilation in the coronary microcirculation, Muller et al[20] trained a group of pigs for 16 to 20 weeks on a treadmill. These investigators observed that training enhanced the sensitivity of the coronary arterioles to bradykinin, a potent vasodilator and nitric oxide stimulant. This enhanced sensitivity appeared to be mediated by increased production of nitric oxide, because the effect of training was blocked by nitric oxide inhibitors.

It is now well known that the coronary endothelium in both animals and humans adapts to a program of regular exercise. This adaptation is characterized by enhanced potential for endothelium-mediated vasodilation. Increases in blood flow caused by exercise and the periodic sheer stress at the surface of the endothelium appears to be a major stimulus for nitric oxide production, which leads to enhanced vasodilation. This is an important mechanism governing the supply and distribution of coronary blood flow, and is presently a fertile area for research on the effects of training on the heart.

Ventricular Fibrillation Threshold

Ventricular fibrillation threshold studies in rats and dogs have found increased resistance to ventricular fibrillation after regular running, possibly through mechanisms involving cyclic adenosine monophosphate and the slow calcium channel.[21] Marked increases in the fibrillation threshold also have been demonstrated in rats subjected to experimental infarction who underwent a running program.[22] Others have associated this phenomenon to marked changes in autonomic balance, including increases in baroreflex activity, heart rate variability, and vagal tone.[23] These observations in animals have been hypothesized as one explanation for the reduction in sudden death in the meta-analyses of cardiac rehabilitation.[7,24-27]

Mortality

Holloszy[28] reviewed the literature and his own data regarding the effects of exercise on longevity in rats and concluded that exercise increases the average lifespan and can prevent the adverse effects of overeating. Lundeberg et al[29] assessed the effects of training on survival in 80 rats randomly assigned to either a sedentary or trained group (7 days/week for 6 weeks), starting 2 weeks after coronary ligation. The animals were followed for 183 days. Size of MI was determined by planimetry of serial histologic sections of the left ventricle. Although training had no effect on survival in the total treatment group, rats with large MIs randomized to training had significantly better survival (50%) after 6 months than control rats (17%) with large infarctions. Powers et al[30] suggested that the better survival and protection against ischemic injury observed in rats that have undergone training is due to the higher levels of cardioprotective proteins, possibly including higher cardiac antioxidant capacity and higher myocardial levels of heat shock proteins. The latter are regulatory proteins that are induced by stress that have a strong antigenic effect.

Effects of Exercise on Atherosclerosis

Kramsch et al[31] randomly allocated 27 young adult male monkeys into three groups. Two groups were studied for 36 months and one group was studied for 42 months. Of the groups studied for 36 months, one was fed a vegetarian diet for the entire study, whereas the other was fed the vegetarian diet for 12 months and then an isocaloric atherogenic diet for 24 months. Both were designated as sedentary because their physical activity was limited to a single cage. The third group was fed the vegetarian diet for 18 months and then the atherogenic diet for 24 months. This group exercised regularly on a treadmill for the entire 42 months. Total serum cholesterol remained the same, but HDL cholesterol was higher in the exercise group. ST-segment depression, angiographic coronary artery narrowing, and sudden death were observed only in the

sedentary monkeys fed the atherogenic diet. In addition, postmortem examination revealed marked coronary atherosclerosis and stenosis in this group. Exercise was associated with substantially reduced overall atherogenic involvement, lesion size, and collagen accumulation. These results demonstrate that exercise in young adult monkeys increases heart size, left ventricular mass, and the diameter of coronary arteries. In addition, the subsequent experimental atherosclerosis induced by the atherogenic diet was reduced substantially in the trained group. Exercise before exposure to the atherogenic diet delayed the development of CHD. This study has been widely cited for more than 2 decades as the strongest evidence that exercise might favorably influence the atherosclerotic process. This study was also influential in that it was the only such study in primates, which represent the closest surrogate to humans.

HUMAN STUDIES SUPPORTING CARDIAC ADAPTATIONS

The effects of an exercise program can be studied by a cross-sectional approach, comparing athletes to normal individuals, and by a longitudinal approach, comparing individuals before and after a training program. Both of these approaches have limitations. The cross-sectional approach is the easier of the two because the difficulty and expense of organizing a training program can be avoided. However, athletes are endowed with biologic attributes and motivation that make them capable of superior performance. In addition, they undergo long periods of physical training that usually begins at a young age, when dimensional and morphologic changes are more apt to occur. This fact makes comparison with sedentary subjects questionable because most trained normal individuals cannot reach an athlete's level of cardiovascular function or performance. Besides the expense and difficulty in organizing and maintaining an exercise program, there are other problems encountered in longitudinal studies. Volunteers often are athletic and differ from randomly selected normal subjects. An exercise program can modify important variables such as body weight and smoking habits, and results can be biased by volunteer dropouts. In persons with CHD, a placebo effect on hemodynamic responses has been documented and a training program may select a healthier group.

The response to any training program depends on a number of factors. These include the initial level of fitness, physical endowment, previous physical training, age, gender, and health of the individual entering the program, along with the type, intensity, and duration of the training program. The changes are often greater in sedentary individuals compared with those who are somewhat physically fit, and are greater in younger rather than older individuals. In the following sections, exercise prescription is discussed initially, followed by a review of studies on the physiologic effects of training in normal subjects of different ages and in persons with cardiovascular disease.

Exercise Prescription

The structure of an exercise program is important when considering the potential benefits of regular exercise. Intensity and duration of the exercise periods must be considered, as well as the overall time an individual is engaged in exercise. Individuals with stable heart disease must be selected. The major ingredients of the exercise prescription are the *frequency, intensity, duration, mode,* and *rate of progression.*[32,33] Based on numerous studies performed over the last several decades, it is generally accepted that increases in maximal oxygen uptake are achieved if an individual exercises dynamically for a period ranging from 15 to 60 minutes three to five times per week at an intensity equivalent to 50% to 80% of their maximal capacity. Short periods for warm-up and cool-down are strongly encouraged, particularly for participants in cardiac rehabilitation programs. Physiologic benefits have been shown to occur from training programs lasting anywhere from 1 month to more than 1 year, with a typical program lasting 2–3 months.

Much of the art of exercise prescription involves individualizing the exercise intensity. Typically, exercise intensity is expressed as a percentage of the maximal capacity in absolute terms (i.e., workload or watts) or relative to the maximal heart rate, maximal oxygen uptake, or perceived effort. Training benefits have been shown to occur using exercise intensities ranging from 40% to 85% of maximal oxygen uptake, which usually are equivalent to 50% to 90% of maximal heart rate. Ordinarily, the most appropriate intensity for most patients in rehabilitation programs is 60% to 70% of maximal capacity. The actual prescribed exercise intensity for an individual patient depends on his or her goals, health status, proximity to infarction or surgery, symptoms, and initial state of fitness.

Training is a general phenomenon; there is no true "threshold" at which patients achieve benefits. As long as patients exercise safely, setting the exercise intensity has become a less rigid practice than it was years ago. Other factors—such as time of day, environment, and time since medications were taken—can influence the response to exercise, and the exercise prescription must be adjusted accordingly. It also is helpful to use a "window" when setting the intensity, such that it ranges roughly 10% above and below the desired level.

The graded exercise test is the foundation on which a safe and effective exercise prescription is based. To achieve a desired training intensity, oxygen uptake or some estimation of it must be measured during a maximal or symptom-limited exercise test. Because heart rate is measured easily and is related linearly to oxygen uptake, it has become a standard by which intensity is estimated during training sessions. The most useful method is known as the *heart rate reserve.* This method uses a percentage of the difference between maximum heart rate and resting heart rate, and adds this value to the resting heart rate. For example, for a patient who achieves a maximum heart rate of 150 beats per minute, has a resting heart rate of 70 beats per minute, and wishes to exercise at an intensity equivalent to 60% of maximum, the calculation is as follows:

Maximal heat rate = 150 beats/min	
− Resting heart rate	70
= Heart rate range	80
× Desired intensity	60%
=	48
+ Resting heart rate	70
= Training heart rate	118

A reasonable training heart rate range for this individual would be 115 to 125 beats per minute. This also is referred to as the *Karvonen formula* and is reliable in patients with normal sinus rhythm whose measurements of resting and maximal heart rates are accurate. An estimated target heart rate for exercise should be supplemented by considering the patient's MET level relative to his or her maximum, the patient's perceived exertion, and symptoms.

Resistance exercises (e.g., weight lifting) have historically been considered isometric rather than aerobic in nature, but recent studies clearly indicate that resistance exercise has benefits not just for muscular strength but also for endurance.

Thus, they are generally considered an integral component of rehabilitation programs today. In addition, strength training programs have been shown to have favorable effects on existing conditions such as hypertension, hyperlipidemia, obesity, and diabetes. However, weight training can be contraindicated for some patients with heart disease, such as those with dilated ventricles, because of the excessive level of myocardial pressure work associated with them. Modest resistance exercise programs for many cardiac rehabilitation patients are now accepted as a complement to aerobic activities, but guidelines issued by the American Association of Cardiovascular and Pulmonary Rehabilitation (AACVPR)[34] should be considered before recommending these activities to patients with heart disease. Improvements in muscular strength can facilitate return to vocational activities after a cardiac event. However, in healthy individuals, this type of exercise has less effect on improving cardiovascular function and aerobic fitness, as demonstrated by relatively normal hearts and unexceptional maximal oxygen uptakes in individuals who train only in this manner. For healthy individuals and some patients with stable heart disease, a recent increase in the popularity of "circuit" weight training has occurred, which involves high-repetition, low-resistance weight training at different stations interspersed with brief periods of rest, and aerobic benefits have been demonstrated.[35]

Echocardiography Before and After Exercise Training in Normal Subjects

The advent of echocardiography in the 1970s engendered the concept that exercise training could result in improvements in ventricular size and function, and numerous investigators addressed this issue both cross-sectionally and longitudinally over the next 2 decades. Summaries of some of the major studies in this area are provided in Tables 13-3, 13-4, and 13-5. Ehsani et al[36] reported rapid changes in left ventricular dimensions and mass in response to physical conditioning and deconditioning. Two groups of healthy young subjects were studied. The training group consisted of eight competitive swimmers who were studied serially for 9 weeks. Mean left ventricular end-diastolic dimension increased by a total of 3.3 mm and posterior wall thickness increased 0.7 mm by the ninth week of training. There was no significant change in ejection fraction. The deconditioned group consisted of six competitive runners who stopped training for 3 weeks. End-diastolic dimension decreased 4.7 mm

and posterior wall thickness decreased 2.7 mm by the end of the 3-week period. Deconditioning did not influence ejection fraction. Exercise training induced rapid adaptive changes in left ventricular dimensions and mimicked the pattern of chronic volume overload, and modest degrees of exercise-induced left-ventricular enlargement were reversible. Surprisingly, the change in left ventricular dimensions occurred early during endurance training, but there was no significant increase in measured left ventricular posterior wall thickness until the fifth week of training. Estimated left ventricular mass increased significantly after the first week of training.

DeMaria et al[37] reported the results of M-mode echocardiography in 24 young normal subjects before and after 11 weeks of endurance exercise training. After training, they exhibited an increased left ventricular end-diastolic dimension, a decreased end-systolic dimension, and both an increased stroke volume and fractional shortening. An increase in mean fiber shortening velocity was observed, as were increases in left ventricular wall thickness, ECG voltage, and left ventricular mass.

Stein et al[38] studied the effects of exercise training on ventricular dimensions at rest and during supine submaximal exercise. Fourteen healthy students were studied using M-mode echocardiography at rest and during the third minute of 300 kp supine bike exercise. They were studied before and after a 14-week training program that resulted in a 30% increase in maximal oxygen uptake. The authors concluded that exercise training was associated with an increased stroke volume mediated by the Frank-Starling effect (greater end-diastolic volume and enhanced contractility). Parrault et al[39] studied 14 middle-aged subjects with a chest x-ray, ECG, vectorcardiogram, and echocardiogram before and after 5 months of training. Maximal oxygen uptake increased by 20%. The echocardiograms showed no significant changes, in contrast to results reported by others in younger subjects. Wolfe et al[40] performed a similar study in 12 men with a mean age of 37 years who exhibited 14% and 18% increases in aerobic capacity after 3 and 6 months of training, respectively. They concluded that resting end-diastolic volume and stroke volume were increased, but that left ventricular structure and resting contractile status were not altered by 6 months of jogging in healthy, previously sedentary men.

Adams et al[41] noninvasively studied the effects of an aerobic training program on the hearts of healthy college-age men. Compared with a control group, echocardiography after training showed

TABLE 13-3. Cross-sectional echocardiographic studies comparing athletes to controls

Gilbert et al, 1977 (20 distance runners, 26 sedentary controls)	Controls	Athletes
LV PWT	9.8	10.9
LV VIED (ml)	62	72
VO_2 (mL/kg/min)	43	71
LVEF	72%	68%
Resting HR	62	51

Parker et al, 1978 (12 distance runners, 12 controls)	Controls	Athletes
LV PWT	9	11
LV EDD	52	57
LV ESD	37	34
MVCFS	0.9	1.2

Roeske et al, 1976 (10 professional basketball players, 10 controls)	Controls	Athletes
RV EDD	13	21
Septum	13	14
LV ID_d (mm)	49.9	53.7
IV ST_d (mm)	12.8	13.7
PWT_d (mm)	9.8	11.1
LV PWT	10	11
LV EDD	50	54
LV ESD	31	32
LVEF	76%	79%
LV Mass (g)	214	274
MVCFS	1.13	1.18

Seals et al, 1994 (9 male master athletes, mean age 64, 9 older sedentary healthy men, mean age 63)	Controls		Athletes	
	Rest	Exercise	Rest	Exercise
LV EDV (mL)	133 ± 4	153 ± 8	153 ± 6	173 ± 5
LV ESV (mL)	43 ± 2	42 ± 6	56 ± 4	42 ± 5
EF (%)	67 ± 1	73 ± 3	63 ± 2	76 ± 3
SV (mL/min)	90 ± 3	111 ± 6	97 ± 2	132 ± 6
Q (L/mL)	6.3 ± 0.4	16.7 ± 0.9	4.86 ± 0.1	19.10 ± 0.9
HR (bpm)	71 ± 3	151 ± 5	51 ± 4	146 ± 3
TPR (dynes/cm^2)	1262 ± 74	674 ± 50	1614 ± 41	580 ± 30

Macfarlane et al, 1991 (30 male subjects ≈24 years)	Controls (n = 10)	Endurance runners (n = 10)	Weight lifters (n = 10)
LV mass (g)	202.1 ± 5.75	283.4 ± 10.4	260.6 ± 8.77
LVMI (g/m^2)	104.1 ± 3.16	156.4 ± 5.97	138.6 ± 7.27
SWT (mm)	100 ± 3	118 ± 3	115 ± 4
PWT (mm)	88 ± 2	105 ± 3	106 ± 3
LV EDD (mm)	519 ± 9	572 ± 7	529 ± 9
Proportional wall thickness	0.36 ± 0.01	0.39 ± 0.01	0.42 ± 0.01
FS	35.7 ± 1.44	34.5 ± 2.6	35.7 ± 1.9

Morganroth et al, 1975 (56 athletes ≈21 years)	Aerobic athletes	Isometric athletes	Controls
LV PWT	11	13.7	10
Septum	10.8	13	10.3
LV EDD	55	48	46

TABLE 13-3.   Cross-sectional echocardiographic studies comparing athletes to controls—*cont'd*

Rubal et al, 1981 (19 female subjects, 19–24 years)	Controls ($n = 10$)	Athletes ($n = 9$) (softball)
IV ST$_d$ (mm)	7.5	8.9
PWT$_d$ (mm)	7.3	8.21
LV mass (g)	123	168
FS%	34	33
VO$_2$ Peak (mL/min/kg)	40	55

Van decker et al, 1989 (23 male subjects, ≈28 years)	Controls ($n = 11$)	Athletes ($n = 12$) (basketball)
HR (beats/min)	63	61
LV ID$_d$ (mm)	57	59
IV ST$_d$ (mm)	9.5	11.4
PWT$_d$ (mm)	9.3	11.4
LV mass (g)	201	284
LVEF (%)	54	52
FS%	34	34

Zeldis et al, 1978 (35 female subjects, ≈21 years)	Controls ($n = 11$)	Athletes ($n = 12$) (field hockey)
HR (beats/min)	71	59
LV ID$_d$ (mm)	42.3	47.3
IV ST$_d$ (mm)	8.7	8.3
PWT$_d$ (mm)	10.3	10.7
LV mass (g)	128	178
LVEF (%)	75	76
VO$_2$ peak (mL/min/kg)	41	52

Wolfe et al, 1985 (12 healthy trained subjects, 12 controls, ≈40 years)	Controls ($n = 12$)		Trained ($n = 12$)	
	Rest	Heavy exercise	Rest	Heavy exercise
HR (beats/min)	65 ± 11	144 ± 8	55 ± 7	142 ± 11
LVEF	0.72 ± 0.04	0.67 ± 0.07	0.72 ± 0.04	0.72 ± 0/09
LV EDV, % pre-exercise ESC (bc)	127 ± 31	110 ± 17	138 ± 39	124 ± 30
LV ESV	36 ± 13	89 ± 35	8 ± 11	94 ± 53
PSER EDC (bc)S^{-1}	3.3 ± 0.3	5.4 ± 1.3	3.3 ± 0.6	35.5 ± 1.1

Whalley et al, 2004 (58 males, ≈40 years)	Controls ($n = 28$)	Endurance athletes ($n = 30$)
LV EDD	52.5 ± 0.38	55.6 ± 0.62
LV ESD	34.5 ± 4.8	38.1 ± 3.8
LV Mass	162.1 ± 46.6	181.6 ± 40.9
IVS	8.6 ± 1.7	8.4 ± 1.5
PWT	8.5 ± 1.5	8.9 ±1.5

Note: differences between athletes and controls were not present when expressed relative to fat-free mass.

All dimensions are in millimeters unless indicated. DBP (SBP), diastolic (systolic) blood pressure; ED, end diastole; EDC(bc) or ESC(bc), expressed as % pre-exercise background corrected end-diastolic or end-systolic counts; EDD or ESD, end-diastolic or -systolic dimension; EDV or ESV, end-diastolic or -systolic volume; EF, ejection fraction; ES, end systole; ESA, endocardial surface area; FS, fractional shortening; HR, heart rate (beats/min); ID, internal dimension; IVS, intraventricular septum; LV, left ventricular; LV EDV or LV ESV, left ventricular end-diastolic or -systolic volume; LV VIED, left ventricular volume index at end-diastole; LVEF, left ventricular ejection fraction; LVEI, left ventricular expansion index; LVMI, left ventricular mass index; LVWMA, left ventricular wall motion abnormalities; MVCFS, mean ventricular circumferential fiber shortening (contractions per second); PSER, peak systolic ejection rate; PW, posterior wall; PWT, posterior wall thickness; Q, cardiac output; RV, right ventricular; SV, stroke volume; VIED, volume index at end diastole in mL; VO$_2$, peak oxygen consumption (mL of O$_2$/kg/min). Data are presented as mean value ± SD.

TABLE 13-4. Serial echocardiographic studies evaluating the cardiac effects of exercise training in normals

Ehsani et al, 1978 (14 college athletes)	Swimmers trained for 9 weeks (n = 8)		Runners detrained for 3 weeks (n = 6)	
	Before training	After training	Before detraining	After detraining
LV PWT	9.4	10.1	10.7	8.0
VO$_2$	52	60	62	57
Resting HR	70	63	57	64
EF	63%	63%	68%	63%

Demaria et al, 1978 (24 policemen, ≈26 years)	Before training	After training
LV EDD	48	50
LV ESD	30	29
LV PWT	9.1	10.1
Resting HR	69	63
VO$_2$	36	41
EF	75%	80%
MVCFS	1.21	1.28

Stein et al, 1978 (14 healthy subjects)	Before training		After training	
	Rest	300 Kpm	Rest	300 Kpm
LV EDD	46	50	50	—
LV ESD	32	21	32	30
EF	70%	90%	73%	78%

Parrault et al, 1978 (Normal men ≈40 years old)	Before training	After training
VO$_2$	34	41
Septum	12.5	12.7
LV PWT	10	9.8
LV EDD	47.8	48.2
	33	33

ADAMS et al, 1981 (25 men, mean age 22 years)	Before training	After training
Rest HR	63	54
VO$_2$	49	56
% Body fat	17.2	13.7
R-wave lead V$_5$	1.7 mV	2.0 mV
LV EDD	45.8	49.6
EF	62%	66%
LV PWT	10.9	10.3
LV ESD	32.3	33.5

Ehsani et al, 1991 (10 healthy men, mean age 64 yrs)	Rest		Exercise	
	Pre	Post	Pre	Post
EF (%)	66.3 ± 6.7	67 ± 4.8	70.6 ± 6.9	77.6 ± 7.5
LV ESV (mL)	46 ± 8	51 ± 12	43 ± 13	38 ± 13
LV EDV (mL)	138 ± 11	155 ± 26	153 ± 9	170 ± 27

Sadaniantz et al, 1996 (16 trained men, 6 controls, ≈39 years)	Exercise (n = 16)		Controls (n = 6)	
	Before training	Change after training	Baseline	Change
LV ED	550 ± 60	−10 ± 40	530 ± 50	−30 ± 50
LV ES	310 ± 40	−20 ± 60	280 ± 20	−20 ± 30
IVS ED	100 ± 10	00 ± 20	90 ± 20	20 ± 20
IVS ED	160 ± 30	00 ± 30	130 ± 20	10 ± 30
LV PWT ED	90 ± 10	20 ± 10	80 ± 10	20 ± 10

TABLE 13-4. Serial echocardiographic studies evaluating the cardiac effects of exercise training in normals—*cont'd*

Sadaniantz et al, 1996 (16 sedentary men, 6 controls, ≈39 years)	Exercise (*n* = 16)		Controls (*n* = 6)	
	Before training	Change after training	Baseline	Change
LVPW ES	190 ± 30	40 ± 50	190 ± 10	20 ± 20
AO	340 ± 40	00 ± 20	330 ± 30	00 ± 10
LA	370 ± 40	10 ± 30	390 ± 50	10 ± 20
RV (ED)	190 ± 50	20 ± 60	180 ± 50	00 ± 30
% FS	43.8 ± 7.0	3.1 ± 9.4	46.2 ± 4.4	0.33 ± 4.47
LV mass (g)	119.9 ± 20.4	5.1 ± 19.1	120.5 ± 15.3	7.8 ± 23.2
LV mass index	55.6 ± 8.0	2.5 ± 8.4	60.1 ± 2.9	4.2 ± 11.8
Resting HR	71 ± 8	−6 ± 11	65 ± 11	4 ± 12

All dimensions are in millimeters unless indicated. AO, aortic dimension; ED, end diastole; EDD or ESD, end-diastolic or -systolic dimension; EDV or ESV, end-diastolic or -systolic volume; EF, ejection fraction; ES, end systole; ESA, endocardial surface area; FS, fractional shortening; HR, heart rate (beats/min); IVS, intraventricular septum; IVSD, interventricular septal thickness; LA, left atrium; LV, left ventricular; PW, posterior wall; PWT, posterior wall thickness; RV, right ventricular; VO_2, peak oxygen consumption (mL of O_2/kg/min). Data are presented as mean value ± SD.

TABLE 13-5. Serial echocardiographic studies evaluating the cardiac effects of exercise training in patients with heart disease

Ehsani et al, 1982 (8 post-MI patients, 1 year of exercise)	Pre	Post		
LV EDD	51	56		
LV PWT	9	10		
Lead RV_5	1.7 mV	2.0 mV		
Dubach et al, 1997 (25 Patients post-MI with ↓ LV function, 2 months exercise, measured using MRI)	Exercise group (*n* = 12)		Control group (*n* = 13)	
	Pre	Post	Pre	Post
LV EDV (mL/m²)	98.4 ± 25	103.2 ± 18	99.4 ± 29	100.0 ± 28
LV ESV (mL/m²)	62.1 ± 22	63.7 ± 17	66.1 ± 30	64.4 ± 31
EF (%)	38.0 ± 9	38.2 ± 10	37.0 ± 10	38.3 ± 13
LV mass (ED) (g/m²)	96.6 ± 18	96.9 ± 17	91.1 ± 16	90.0 ± 18
Giannuzzi et al, 1993 (95 Patients with ↓ LV function, mean age 51 ± 8 years, 6 months training)	Exercise group (*n* = 49)			
	Pre	Post	Pre	Post
LV VIED (mL/m²)	60 ± 14	61 ± 16	63 ± 16	66 ± 20
LV VIED (mL/m²) (EF <40%, *n* = 31)	74 ± 11	77 ± 15	77 ± 14	85 ± 17
LV ESV (mL/m²)	31 ± 15	29 ± 16	35 ± 16	36 ± 20
LV EF (%)	51 ± 14[*]	54 ± 14	48 ± 13	50 ± 16
% LVWMA	30 ± 16[*]	26 ± 18	34 ± 15	31 ± 20
LVEI	1.08 ± 0.1[*]	0.98 ± 0.4	1.1 ± 0.12	0.98 ± 0.4

Continued

TABLE 13–5. Serial echocardiographic studies evaluating the cardiac effects of exercise training in patients with heart disease—*cont'd*

Giannuzzi et al, 1997 (78 post-MI patients with ↓ LV function, mean age 53 ± 9 years, 6 months Training)	Exercise group (*n* = 39)		Control group (n = 39)	
	Pre	Post	Pre	Post
LV EDV (mL/m²)	93 ± 28	92 ± 28	94 ± 26*	99 ± 27
LV ESV (mL/m²)	61 ± 22	57 ± 23	62 ± 20*	67 ± 23
EF (%)	34 ± 5	38 ± 8	34 ± 5*	33 ± 7
LV WMA (%)	49 ± 8	44 ± 10	50 ± 10*	51 ± 12
LV RD (%)	43 ± 18	45 ± 26	47 ± 18*	57 ± 22

Jette et al, 1991 (39 male patients with anterior MI, mean 51 ± 8 years, 4 weeks exercise)	Exercise group		Control group	
	Pre	Post	Pre	Post
EF <30%				
EDD	0.56 ± 0.04	0.55 ± 0.06	0.57 ± 0.08	0.54 ± 0.09
FS (%)	25.7 ± 4.9	30.3 ± 4.8	26.9 ± 11.6	27.3 ± 9.1
LVET (seconds)	0.272 ± 0.042	0.299 ± 0.010	0.264 ± 0.064	0.284 ± 0.023
LVEF (%)	23.9 ± 3.5	28.2 ± 7.7	25.3 ± 4.4	32.4 ± 10.9
EF > 30%				
EDD	0.53 ± 0.05	0.53 ± 0.05	0.50 ± 0.04	0.50 ± 0.04
FS (%)	34.2 ± 9.0	37.0 ± 6.4	34.6 ± 7.2	35.2 ± 6.5
LVET (seconds)	0.275 ± 0.031	0.293 ± 0.042	0.271 ± 0.043	0.351 ± 0.043
LVEF (%)	39.5 ± 5.7	41.3	40.0 ± 7.4	46.4 ± 8.4

Myers, et al, 2000 (12 exercise, 13 controls with CHF, 2 months training, 1-year follow-up, measured with MRI)	Exercise group		Control group	
	Pre	Post	Pre	1-Year
LV EDV, mL	172.0 ± 46	186.0 ± 46	158.3 ± 46	162.1 ± 46
LV ESV, mL	115.2 ± 47	119.2 ± 47	105.4 ± 47	102.5 ± 47
LVEF, %	35.3 ± 11	35.0 ± 11	36.0 ± 11	38.0 ± 11
SV	56.8 ± 16	66.2 ± 16	52.8 ± 16	59.6 ± 16

Cannistra, et al, 1999 (30 exercise, 30 controls, 12 weeks training, post-MI)	Exercise group		Control group	
	Pre	Post	Pre	Post
ESAI (cm²/mm²)	57.4 ± 13	57.8 ± 12	64.8 ± 11	64.0 ± 11
% AWM	19.3 ± 15	3020.1 ± 1657.8 ± 1220.1 57.8 ± 12	18.8 ± 14	16.7 ± 15

Hambrecht et al, 2000, 31 exercise, 33 controls (with CHF, 6 months training)	Exercise group		Control group	
	Pre	Post	Pre	Post
LV EDD	69 ± 10	66 ± 10	65 ± 9	66 ± 9
LV ESD	60 ± 10	55 ± 10	55 ± 9	56 ± 9
LV EDV	229 ± 75	207 ± 85	207 ± 66	218 ± 68
LV ESV	161 ± 65	137 ± 66	147 ± 56	148 ± 56
LV EF, %	30 ± 8	35 ± 9	30 ± 9	33 ± 9

TABLE 13–5. Serial echocardiographic studies evaluating the cardiac effects of exercise training in patients with heart disease—*cont'd*

Giannuzzi et al, 2003 (45 exercise, 45 controls with CHF, 6 months training)	Exercise group	(n = 14)	Control group	
	Pre	Post	Pre	Post
LV EDV, mL	142 ± 26	1 ± 135 / 135 ± 26	147 ± 41	156 ± 42
LV ESV, mL	107 ± 24	97 ± 24	110 ± 34	118 ± 34
EF, %	25 ± 4	29 ± 4	25 ± 4	25 ± 5

Otsuka et al, 2003 (126 post-MI patients with LV dysfunction, 3 months training)	LVEF ≥ 45%		LVEF ≥ 35 to < 45%		LVEF ≥ 45%	
	Pre	Post	Pre	Post	Pre	Post
LV EDD, mm	48 ± 5	49 ± 4	53 ± 8	52 ± 8	57 ± 5	57 ± 7

Belardinelli et al, 1995 (55 patients with DCM, mean age 55 ± 7 years, 2 months exercise)	Exercise group (n = 9)		Control group (n = 5)	
	Pre	Post	Pre	Post
PEFR, EDV/s	1.48 ± 0.6	1.68 ± 0.7	1.46 ± 0.6	1.41 ± 0.6[†]
PAFR, EDV/s	1.62 ± 0.5	1.1 ± 0.4*	1.71 ± 0.5	1.68 ± 0.7[†]
PFR, EDV/s	2.7 ± 0.3	3.0 ± 0.3*	2.8 ± 0.5	2.7 ± 0.9[†]
TPEFR, (ms)	168 ± 7	162 ± 7	171 ± 17	165 ± 12
TPAFR, (ms)	213 ± 60	260 ± 80*	202 ± 45	210 ± 66[†]
TPFR, (ms)	142 ± 8	133 ± 15	144 ± 11	139 ± 18
DFP (ms)	324 ± 55	532 ± 102*	330 ± 38	345 ± 92[†]
RFF (%)	51.0 ± 12	60.0 ± 16*	49.0 ± 6	50.0 ± 16[†]
AFF (ms)	39.1 ± 14	31.3 ± 15*	41.2 ± 12	40.4 ± 9[†]

*$p < 0.05$ versus before training; [†]$p < 0.05$, training versus control.

Jugdutt et al, 1988 (15 week training; all patients post-anterior MI)	Exercise group (n = 13)		Control group (n = 24)	
	Group 1 (n = 7) Asynergy <18%	Group 2 (n = 6) Asynergy >18%	Group 3 (n = 11) Asynergy >18%	Group 4 (n = 13) Asynergy >18%
Total asynergy (%)	6 ± 6	40 ± 9*	9 ± 5	26 ± 4*
Rest LVEF (%)	58 ± 7	30 ± 5*	48 ± 5	40 ± 5*
LV EI	1.55 ± 0.16	2.07 ± 0.28*	1.59 ± 0.15	1.77 ± 0.19*
LV anterior ESL (cm)	9.1 ± 1.0	14.6 ± 1.8*	9.9 ± 2.0	12.4 ± 1.5*
Thinning ratio	0.72 ± 0.11	0.51 ± 0.07*	0.71 ± 0.12	0.56 ± 0.10*
LV AW thickness (mm)	7.8 ± 1.0	5.8 ± 0.7*	8.4 ± 0.8	6.8 ± 1.0*
Peak distortion ($P_k$cm)	0.12 ± 0.28	2.09 ± 0.74*	0.08 ± 0.08	1.25 ± 0.81*
LV ID (mm)	47.1 ± 3.3	58.0 ± 6.2*	49.3 ± 3.8	52.0 ± 4.5

*$p ≤ 0.05$, comparing group 1 and 2, *$p ≤ 0.05$, comparing group 3 and group 4.

All dimensions are in millimeters unless indicated. AFF, atrial filling fraction; DFP, diastolic filling period; ED, end diastole; EDD or ESD, end-diastolic or -systolic dimension; EF, ejection fraction; ES, end systole; ESAI, ratio of endocardial surface area to body surface area; FS, fractional shortening; ID, internal dimension; LV, left ventricular; LVEI, left ventricular expansion index; LVRD, left ventricular regional dilation; LVWMA, left ventricular wall motion abnormalities; LV EDV or LV ESV, left ventricular end-diastolic or -systolic volume; MRI, magnetic resonance imaging; PAFR, peak atrial filling rate; PEFR, peak early filling rate; PFR, peak filling rate; PWT, posterior wall thickness; RFF, rapid filling fraction; RV, right ventricular; SV, stroke volume; TPAFR, time to PAFR; TPEFR, time to PEFR; TPFR, time to PFR; %AWM, percent abnormal wall motion. Data are presented as mean value ± SD.

an increase in left ventricular end-diastolic dimensions, but no significant change in wall thickness or in ejection fraction. Although there was no change in myocardial wall thickness, the increase in end-diastolic dimensions resulted in an increase in left ventricular mass.

Landry et al[42] evaluated 20 sedentary subjects and 10 pairs of monozygotic twins who engaged in a 20-week endurance exercise program. Maximal oxygen uptake increased significantly in both groups. Statistically significant increases in left ventricular diameter, posterior wall and septal thicknesses, as well as left ventricular end-diastolic volume and left ventricular mass were observed in the sedentary subjects, but not in the monozygotic twins. After training, twin pairs differed more from each other than at the start. Concomitantly, within-pair resemblance was greater after training than before. These results suggest that cardiac dimensions are amenable to significant modifications under controlled endurance training conditions and that the extent and variability of the response of cardiac structures to training may be genotype dependent.

Clearly, echocardiographic studies have demonstrated that the heart adapts morphologically to training and detraining in relatively young healthy individuals (younger than 35 to 40 years old). Ten percent to 20% increases in left ventricular posterior wall thickness and end-diastolic dimensions have been demonstrated repeatedly both cross-sectionally and after a period of training. The effects of training on measures of contractility (ejection fraction, fractional shortening) are less clear, but they appear to be relatively small. The distinction between younger and older subjects is an important one, given that the available evidence suggests these morphologic changes are less likely to occur in the elderly.

CARDIAC ADAPTATIONS IN PATIENTS WITH HEART DISEASE

Ehsani et al[43] reported results of 12 months of intense exercise in a highly selected group of 10 patients with CHD. Eight comparable men were considered as controls. The trained group completed 12 months in a high-level exercise program. After 3 months of exercise training at a level of 50% to 70% of maximal oxygen uptake, the level of training increased to 70% to 80%, with two to three intervals at 80% to 90% interspersed throughout the exercise session. This training regimen resulted in a 38% increase in maximal oxygen uptake. The sum of ECG voltages representing ventricular mass increased by 15%. Both left ventricular end-diastolic dimensions and posterior wall thickness were significantly increased after training. This resulted in an increase in left ventricular mass from 93 to 135 g/m^2 body surface area. These findings were provocative and illustrate the potential morphologic changes that could occur as a result of training in patients with heart disease; however, because this was a select group, the results may not be generalized to the typical cardiac population.

Ditchey et al[44] obtained echocardiograms on 14 coronary patients before and after an average of 7 months (range, 3 to 14 months) of supervised arm and leg exercise. Each echocardiogram was interpreted jointly by two blinded observers, using three different measurement conventions and a semi-automated method of analysis to minimize errors in interpretation. Exercise training led to subjective improvement in all 14 patients and a 2-MET increase in estimated exercise capacity. However, this was not accompanied by any significant change in left ventricular end-diastolic diameter or wall thickness. Likewise, left ventricular cross-sectional area—an index of left ventricular mass that corrects for altered ventricular volume and theoretically reflects directional changes in mass despite nonuniform wall thickness—did not change significantly after training.

During the 1990s, a great deal of interest in the effects of training among patients with heart failure evolved. Based on some animal studies and one study in humans, concern was raised regarding whether training could further harm an already damaged myocardium. The result of this concern was several well-designed randomized trials in patients with heart failure using echocardiography or magnetic resonance imaging (MRI) to assess ventricular adaptations to cardiac rehabilitation programs. These studies were consistent in their demonstration that training did not cause a worsening of the myocardial remodeling process in patients with reduced ventricular function after an MI. In fact, recent evidence suggests that training may attenuate abnormal remodeling.[45] This issue is addressed in detail in Chapter 14.

Exercise Electrocardiographic Studies

Because abnormal ST-segment shifts in coronary patients are most likely secondary to ischemia, lessening of such shifts would be consistent with improved myocardial perfusion. A valid comparison of ischemia is only possible at similar myocardial oxygen demands; therefore, only ST-segment measurements at matched double products should be compared. The product of heart rate and systolic blood pressure has been shown to be a reasonable noninvasive estimate of myocardial oxygen demand during exercise. The studies of the effect of an exercise program on the exercise ECG are summarized in Table 13-6. In all of the studies, training produced a lowering of heart rate for all submaximal exercise levels, permitting performance of more work before the onset of angina, ST-segment depression (which usually occurred at the same heart rate before and after training), or both. Although this is an important benefit of a training program, it says little about an improvement in myocardial oxygen supply per se, because few differences in ST depression were observed at matched rate-pressure products.

As part of a study to evaluate perfusion and function with exercise training in the PERFEXT trial,[46] 48 patients who exercised and 59 control patients had computerized exercise ECGs performed initially and 1 year later. Obvious changes in exercise-induced ST-segment depression could

not be demonstrated. It seems unlikely that the exercise ECG is sensitive enough to detect the type of subtle changes, if any, which might occur as a result of exercise training. Debate continues as to whether central cardiac changes can occur in patients with heart disease who undergo training.

Effect of Exercise on Risk Factors in Patients with Heart Disease

There have been a multitude of randomized controlled trials using multifactorial intervention to reduce cardiac risk. While these approaches have had varying degrees of success, it has been difficult to ascertain the independent effects of exercise on the major risk factors, including smoking cessation, blood lipids, blood pressure, or body weight. How these risk factors interact is a difficult issue to study, and compliance to exercise and other lifestyle changes in high-risk individuals is a chronic problem when attempting to address these issues. It should be noted that although the effect of an exercise program on any single risk factor may be modest, the overall effect of sustained physical activity on global risk scores (e.g., Framingham Risk Score) has been shown to be dramatic in

TABLE 13-6. Effect of chronic exercise on the exercise electrocardiogram in patients with coronary artery disease

Investigator	Year	Subjects	Training duration	Results
Salzman	1969	100 males	33 months	ST-segment changes correlated with changes in functional capacity
Detry	1971	14 males	3 months	No change in computerized ST-segment measurements at matched double products
Kattus	1972	13 males	5 months	13% improvement of ST segments in exercise and control groups
Costill	1974	24 males	3 months	No change in ST-segment response
Raffo	1980	12 males	6 months	Higher heart rate for similar degree of ST-segment depression
Ehsani	1981	10 males	12 months	Less ST-segment depression at matched double product and maximal exercise; higher double product at ischemic ST threshold (0.1 mV flat)
Watanabe	1982	14 males	6 months	Changes only in spatial analysis with CAD
Myers	1984	48 males	12 months	Less ST depression at matched workload; no differences at matched heart rate or double product versus controls

several studies.[9,47,48] It is also important to note that increases in fitness, physical activity, or both, have been repeatedly demonstrated to reduce morbidity and mortality *independent* of changes in other risk factors.[49-52]

Lipids. The results of multifactorial approaches to improving blood lipids, although generally favorable, have been mixed. Whereas the majority of available evidence suggests that an exercise program has favorable effects on lipids (raising HDL, lowering low-density lipoprotein [LDL], and triglyceride levels),[47,53-56] there are several studies demonstrating that exercise has no effect.[57-60] Evidence suggests that regular exercise has its greatest effect on lowering triglycerides and raising HDL. Recent studies also suggest that programs of regular exercise improve plasma inflammatory risk markers (C-reactive protein and homocysteine).[61-64] Studies on lipids are complicated by the confounding effects of patient compliance, and few data are available on concomitant weight loss, which can have an independent effect on lipids. Among the studies demonstrating favorable outcomes, most were multifactorial rehabilitation programs, that is, dietary and behavioral strategies, in addition to exercise. The combination of exercise, dietary intervention, and counseling does not appear to have as strong an effect as the statin lipid-lowering medications, which have demonstrated striking effects in recent years not only on lipids but also on atherosclerosis and cardiovascular events (see Table 14-13).

Smoking Cessation. The effects of exercise programs on tobacco smoking behavior have also been mixed. Several randomized trials have reported significant reductions in smoking rates that favor rehabilitation patients as compared with control groups,[55,65] whereas several other studies have reported no difference.[53,54,66,67] Most of these studies have used self-reported smoking rates among patients enrolled in multifactorial rehabilitation programs. Because smoking cessation has well-documented benefits on coronary risk, specific techniques with more proven value have been proposed, using standards of behavior change for addictive behavior.[68]

Body Weight. An individual who begins an exercise program increases his or her energy expenditure; because gains or losses in body weight reflect a balance between energy intake and expenditure, exercise training should promote weight loss. However, sustained weight loss is a complex issue that involves not just exercise and diet, but also metabolic, sociologic, and psychologic factors. Multifactorial intervention programs of 3 months to 1 year in duration generally have a beneficial effect on improving body weight, other measures of excess body mass, or percentage of body fat.[47,54,56,66,69,70] However, exercise training as a sole intervention has less consistent effects. Review papers and meta-analyses generally indicate that losses in body weight and percentage of body fat induced by training, although often significant, are generally small when no dietary restriction is applied.[71] Moreover, *sustained* weight loss has been difficult to achieve in several population studies.[71-73] Nevertheless, adding exercise to other interventions for weight loss (e.g., drugs, dietary counseling, behavior therapy) is consistently associated with greater weight loss in studies that have followed subjects for up to 3 years.[74]

Blood Pressure. Large cross-sectional studies that have controlled for age and anthropometric characteristics have demonstrated an inverse relationship between blood pressure and either habitual physical activity[75-78] or measured physical fitness.[79-82] Moreover, poorly fit individuals are three to six times more likely to develop hypertension over 15 years.[83] In assessing such a relationship, the potentially confounding effects of self-selection must be considered. There are over 60 controlled, longitudinal studies on the effects of training on systolic and diastolic blood pressure. These studies have varied considerably in terms of populations and the training stimulus used, but the majority of the studies involved middle-aged men participating in a training program lasting a median duration of 4 months. The change in systolic blood pressure in these studies ranged from +6 to −20 mmHg, with a mean of −5.3. The change in diastolic blood pressure ranged from +5 to −16 mmHg, with a mean of −4.8.[75] The degree of reduction in blood pressure is roughly twice these amounts among subjects who were hypertensive at the beginning of the training program.

Inflammatory Markers. The recent observation that inflammatory proteins, such as C-reactive protein and homocysteine, are powerful markers of cardiovascular risk has stimulated a number of studies on whether an exercise program can modify them. These studies are consistent in demonstrating that training markedly reduces high-sensitivity C-reaction protein, in the range of 30% to 40%.[61,62] Recent studies have also reported strong inverse associations between level of fitness and C-reactive protein.[84,85] However, the effects of training on plasma homocysteine are less clear. A 12% reduction in plasma homocysteine was observed after a standard outpatient cardiac rehabilitation program,[64] and reductions in serum homocysteine were observed after a 6-month program of resistance training in the elderly;[63] others have demonstrated slight increases in homocysteine after training among healthy subjects.[86,87]

EPIDEMIOLOGIC STUDIES OF PHYSICAL ACTIVITY/FITNESS

Studies Relating Physical Activity to Cardiac Events

It has been estimated that as many as 250,000 deaths per year in the United States are attributable to lack of regular physical activity[88,89] (roughly one-quarter of all preventable deaths annually). However, others have suggested that these figures may be significantly underestimated.[90] Ongoing longitudinal studies have provided consistent evidence of varying strengths that document the protective effects of activity for a number of chronic diseases, including CHD,[7,24-27,49,52,91,92] non-insulin dependent diabetes,[93-99] hypertension,[100,101] osteoporosis,[102,103] and site-specific cancer.[104,105] In contrast, low levels of physical fitness are associated consistently with higher cardiovascular and all-cause mortality rates.[50,106-111] Midlife increases in physical activity, through changes in occupation or recreational activities, are associated with a decrease in mortality.[49,112,113] Recently, expert panels, convened by organizations such as the Centers for Disease Control (CDC), American College of Sports Medicine(ACSM), and the American Heart Association (AHA),[106,114,115] along with the 1996 U.S. Surgeon General's Report on Physical Activity and Health,[107] have reinforced scientific evidence linking regular physical activity to various measures of cardiovascular health. In 1994, the AHA added a sedentary lifestyle to the list of "primary" risk factors for coronary disease, along with smoking, high blood pressure, hyperlipidemia, and obesity. The prevailing view in all of these reports is that more active or fit individuals tend to develop less CHD than their sedentary counterparts, and when they do develop heart disease, it occurs at a later age and tends to be less severe. Despite this evidence, however, the vast majority of adults in the United States remain effectively sedentary.[90,116]

Before reviewing the major studies relating exercise or fitness level and health, it is important to consider some of their limitations. First, although it is popular in the media to suggest that exercise can reverse heart disease, exercise alone (in the absence of lipid-lowering therapy or other risk factor interventions) has not been definitively shown to reverse the atherosclerotic process. There are also a number of inherent difficulties in studying physical inactivity as a risk factor. One important consideration is that people often leave active jobs with the onset of the first symptoms of heart disease, even without realizing the cause of the symptoms. That is, there may be a premorbid transfer from an active job to a less active job, biasing the relationship of inactivity to CHD. This is one reason why the majority of studies have limited the measurement of energy expenditure to recreational (non-occupation-related) activity. There are other difficulties in studying this question, including the uncertainty of what type and quantity of exercise is protective. Questionnaires have been the most commonly used tool for quantifying energy expenditure, but there are obvious limitations to their use, including subjects' recollection, and their reproducibility and reliability. The studies have used various health outcome measures, and the methods of diagnosing CAD have included death certificates, rest and exercise ECGs, medical records, medical evaluations, and autopsy. All these methods have their shortcomings in terms of accuracy.

With these limitations in mind, there are numerous studies that have been performed since the 1950s that relate measures of physical activity to reductions in cardiac events. Some of the major studies are reviewed here; these studies are summarized in Table 13-7.

Jeremy Morris[117] was a pioneer in this field, and was one of the first investigators to establish a link between physical activity and cardiovascular mortality. In the 1950s, data were gathered from occupation-related mortality records in England and Wales to investigate the hypothesis that occupational physical inactivity is a risk factor for CAD. Social class as used in these studies was based on the grading of occupation by its level of skill and role in production, and its general standing in the community. The level of activity was based on the independent evaluation of occupations by several industrial experts. The activity level of the last job held was found to be inversely related to mortality from CAD, as determined from death certificates.

Morris[118] also published a classic series of epidemiologic studies to support the hypothesis that "men in physically active jobs have a lower incidence of CHD than men in physically inactive jobs." One of the first of these studies dealt with drivers

TABLE 13-7. Sampling of epidemiologic studies on the relation between physical activity and mortality

Investigator	Year	Activity level	Subjects	Conclusions
Morris	1958	Determined by social class	White males	Physical inactivity relates to class and occupation mortality from CAD
Blackburn	1970	Questionnaire	Middle-aged males	No difference between physically active and sedentary males
Paffenbarger	1970	Job description	Longshoremen	Low physical activity level on the job doubles risk of fatal MI
Epstein	1976	Questionnaire	17,000 middle-aged white male executives	Rigorous weekend activity is protective
Costas	1978	Questionnaire	8171 middle-aged Puerto Rican males	Slight increase in mortality in the most inactive group
Paffenbarger	1978	Questionnaire	16,936 male Harvard alumni	Low physical activity (<2000 kcal/wk) increases risk of MI and death
Kannel	1986	Questionnaire	5000 middle-aged males/females	Low physical activity increases risk of cardiac mortality
Leon	1987	Questionnaire	12,138 middle-aged males	Low physical activity moderately increases risk of mortality
Slattery	1989	Questionnaire	3043 males railroad workers	Near 50% increase risk of death from CAD in sedentary men (<40 kcal/wk)
Lee	1995	Questionnaire	17,321 male Harvard Alumni	Total energy expenditure and energy expenditure from vigorous activities, but not nonvigorous activities, inversely related to all-cause mortality
Rosengren	1997	Questionnaire	7142 middle-aged men	Leisure time physical activity protects against cardiovascular, cancer, and all-cause deaths, independent of other risk factors
Lee	2000	Questionnaire	7307 male Harvard Alumni	Several shorter exercise sessions similar to single, larger sessions. In reducing CHD risk, as long as energy expenditure was similar
Tanansescu	2002	Interview	44,452 male health professionals	Total physical activity, running, weight training, and walking are each inversely associated with CHD risk. Average exercise intensity reduced risk independent of hours spent in activity
Manson	2002	Questionnaire	73,743 postmenopausal women	Walking and vigorous exercise associated with similar reductions in cardiac events
Hu	2004	Questionnaire	116,564 women	Higher physical activity reduced mortality at all levels of adiposity, but did not eliminate the higher mortality associated with obesity
Myers	2005	Questionnaire/Interview	6213 men referred for exercise testing	1000 kcal/wk higher energy expenditure and each 1-MET higher exercise capacity associated with 20% reductions in mortality

and conductors of the London public transport system. Thirty-one thousand white males, 35 to 64 years of age, were included for analysis over a period of 18 months from 1949 to 1950. The endpoints were coronary insufficiency, MI, and angina as reported on sick leave records, and listing of CAD on death certificates. The age-adjusted total incidence was 1.5 times higher in the more sedentary group of drivers as compared with the conductor group, and the sudden death and 3-month mortality rates were two times higher.

In his original study, Morris did not investigate differences in selection in the two groups, but did so in a subsequent study of postmen and clerks. The results of this study concurred with their hypothesis that those with more active professions had lower rates of cardiac events. In 1966, Morris also showed that the drivers had higher serum cholesterol levels and higher blood pressures than did the conductors. In addition, a subsequent study by Oliver[119] documented that for some unknown reason, even the recruits for the two jobs differed in lipid levels and weight, suggesting that there was a self-selection in which less healthy individuals chose more sedentary occupations. These differences put the drivers at increased risk for CAD.

In 1958, Stamler et al[120] began a prospective study of 1241 apparently healthy male employees of the Peoples Gas Company in Chicago. By 1965, there were 39 deaths due to coronary disease among the groups. They found that coronary disease mortality was higher in blue-collar workers (37 deaths per 1000 men) who had higher habitual activity at work than in the white-collar workers (20 deaths per 1000). However, the population in general had a low level of physical activity and lacked a gradient between the groups, which limited the possibility of demonstrating an association between physical activity and mortality.

The Seven Countries Coronary Artery Disease Study[121] included Japan, Yugoslavia, the United States, Finland, Italy, the Netherlands, and Greece and took place in the 1960s. This study minimized self-selection by complete coverage of all men aged 40 to 59 years in the geographically defined areas. Individuals were classified as sedentary, moderately active, or very active, as determined by a questionnaire for evaluating total physical activity. Data from 200,000 person-years of observation showed no difference in coronary disease incidence between physically active and sedentary men.

Epstein et al[122] studied the relationship between cardiac events and vigorous exercise during leisure time in approximately 17,000 middle-aged male executive civil servants whose work was sedentary.

On a randomly selected Monday morning, they recorded their leisure-time activities over the previous weekend. An 8½-year follow-up of this population demonstrated a 50% lower incidence of coronary events in those who maintained vigorous activity on the weekend.

Costas et al[123] reported a prospective study involving 8171 urban and rural men 45 to 64 years old participating in the Puerto Rico Heart Program. A physical activity index was based on the number of hours spent at five different levels of physical activity as assessed by questionnaire. A slight increase in risk was found in the least active group of urban men. The level of physical activity was not related to the incidence of CHD.

Paffenbarger et al[124] have reported numerous analyses of epidemiologic data from San Francisco longshoremen, who work at relatively high activity levels under conditions well governed and documented by the longshoremen union. In a 22-year follow-up of the longshoremen, one third of their energy expenditure was classified as high-energy work by analyzing their various jobs. An annual accounting was taken of job transfers so that the data on energy expenditure could be related to the occurrence of fatal MI. Deaths from MIs were assigned to the category in which the deceased had been employed 6 months prior to death to avoid selection bias due to premorbid job transfers. Age-adjusted frequencies of other risk factors among longshoremen were compared between the high- and low-energy expenditure groups, and little difference was found. Three parameters were associated with increased risk for fatal infarction: low physical activity level, cigarette smoking, and an elevated systolic blood pressure. The presence of each of these factors posed approximately a two times greater risk. Paffenbarger et al[124] concluded that higher physical activity was protective. The threshold of 5 kcal per minute seemed to hold for strenuous bursts more than for sustained activity.

Paffenbarger et al[125] also have extensively studied the association between mortality and physical activity among Harvard alumni. In one of these early analyses, 36,000 alumni who entered college between 1916 and 1950 were studied. Alumni offices and questionnaires were used to obtain information on adult exercise habits, morbidity, and mortality. A 6- to 10-year follow-up during the period of 1961 to 1972 totaled 117,680 person-years of observation after the first questionnaire, and apparently healthy men were classified with specific measures of energy expenditure. They remained under study until heart attack occurrence, death from any cause, age 75 years, or the end of observation in 1972. Weekly updating of death lists by the alumni office provided the means to obtain official death certificates. A physical activity index, devised to provide a composite estimate of total energy expenditure, was scaled in kilocalories per week and divided at 2000 kcal per week, which produced a 60% and 40% division of person-years of observation into low- and high-energy categories.

During the follow-up, 572 men had their first MI. Three high-risk characteristics were identified: low physical activity index (less than 2000 kcal/wk), cigarette smoking, and hypertension. Presence of any one characteristic was accompanied by a 50% increase in risk of MI, and the presence of two characteristics tripled the risk. Former varsity athletes retained a lower risk only if they maintained as high a physical activity index as other alumni. Maintenance of a high physical activity index reduced heart attack risk by 26%.

In a further analysis of Harvard alumni, Paffenbarger et al[126] examined physical activity and other lifestyle characteristics of 16,936 alumni, aged 35 to 74 years, for relations to rates of mortality from all causes and for influences on length of life. A total of 1413 alumni died during 12 to 16 years of follow-up (1962 to 1978). Exercise reported as walking, stair climbing, and sports play was inversely related to total mortality, primarily to death due to cardiovascular or respiratory causes. Death rates declined steadily as energy expended on such activity increased from less than 500 to 3500 kcal per week, beyond which rates increased slightly. Rates were one quarter to one third lower among alumni expending 2000 kcal per week or more than among less active men, when controlling for hypertension, cigarette smoking, obesity or gains in body weight, or early parental death. Relative risk of death for individuals was highest among smokers and sedentary men. In a third analysis, Paffenbarger et al[49] reported that a change from a sedentary to a more active lifestyle in these same men reduced their risk of cardiac events. A synopsis of data from Paffenbarger et al relating different energy expenditure levels to mortality is presented in Table 13-8.

TABLE 13–8. Rates and relative risks of death* among Harvard alumni, 1977–1985, by patterns of physical activity

Physical activity (weekly)		Man-years (%)	Number deaths	Deaths per 10,000 man-years	Relative risk of death		P of trend
Walking (km)	<5	26	228	86.2	1.00		
	5–14	42	275	67.4	0.78		<0.001
	15+	32	194	57.7	0.67		
Stair-climbing (floors)	<20	37	341	80.0	1.00		
	20–54	48	293	62.9	0.79		0.001
	55+	15	80	59.6	0.75		
	None	12	156	88.9	1.00		
All sportsplay	Light only†	10	152	97.4	1.10		<0.001
	Light and moderate	36	208	59.7	0.67		
	Moderate only‡	42	178	56.4	0.63		
Moderate sportsplay (hours)	<1	30	308	92.9	1.00		
	1–2	41	126	58.2	0.63		<0.001
	3+	29	64	43.6	0.47		
	<500	12	197	110.3	1.00		
	500–999	18	135	69.1	0.63		
Activity Index (kcal)§	1000–1499	15	58 · 111	68.9	78.9 · 0.62	1.00	
	1500–1999	13	73	61.4	0.56		
	2000–2499	10	51	52.4	0.48		<0.001
	2500–2999	8	44	64.6	0.59		
	3000–3499	6	42 · 36	74.7	55.4 · 0.68	0.70	
	3500+	18	82	48.1	0.44		

*Age-adjusted.
†<4.5 METs intensity.
‡4.5+ METs intensity.
§Sum of walking, stair climbing, and all sports play.
METs, metabolic equivalents.

More recent analyses from the Harvard Alumni follow-up studies have focused on the effects of exercise *intensity* on longevity, and also *duration* of physical activity and CHD risk. In terms of exercise intensity, it was demonstrated that there was a graded inverse relationship between total baseline energy intensity (based on individualized perceived levels of exertion) from physical activity and risk of CHD, even among subjects not satisfying current activity recommendations.[127] Sesso et al[128] assessed subjects from the Harvard Alumni follow-up and observed that vigorous activities (those ≥6 METs), but not nonvigorous activities, were associated with longevity. This suggests that, although numerous health benefits have been shown for moderate intensity activities (e.g., lipid and glucose profiles), vigorous activity may be required to increase longevity. The early work of Morris and Crawford[117] similarly observed that the incidence of heart disease was reduced only among British men who reported themselves to be engaged in vigorous sports. Similar observations were made among Finish men by Lakka et al.[129] However, Shaper and Wannamethee,[130] in an 8-year follow-up of 7735 British men, observed that the rate of MI was reduced even among men with higher versus lower physical activity patterns, but in the absence of vigorous activities. Decreased mortality rates have also been observed among U.S. railroad workers with increasing amounts of light to moderate activity who reported no vigorous activity.[131]

As part of the Harvard Alumni Health Study, Lee et al[132] assessed the *duration* of exercise episodes and their association with CHD risk among 7307 men. After age adjustment, those engaging in longer exercise periods had a lower incidence of CHD events. However, after total energy expended on physical activity and potential confounders were accounted for, duration no longer had an independent effect on CHD risk. Stated differently, longer sessions of exercise did not have a different effect on risk compared with shorter sessions, as long as the total energy expenditure was similar. However, higher levels of overall energy expenditure were associated with decreased CHD risk.

In the Women's Health Initiative Observational Study, a prospective, multicentric clinical trial designed to address the major causes of illness and mortality in postmenopausal women, the role of walking was compared with vigorous exercise in relation to cardiovascular events.[92] A total physical activity score, amount of walking, vigorous exercise, and hours spent sitting were assessed as predictors of coronary and total cardiovascular events among 73,743 women aged 50 to 79 years. An increasing physical activity score had a strong, graded, inverse association with the risk of both coronary events and total cardiovascular events. Women in increasing quintiles of energy expenditure in METs had age-adjusted relative risks of coronary events of 1.00, 0.73, 0.69, 0.68, and 0.47, respectively (*P* for trend, <0.001). In multivariate analyses, the inverse gradient between the total MET score and the risk of cardiovascular events remained strong (adjusted relative risks for increasing quintiles, 1.00, 0.89, 0.81, 0.78, and 0.72, respectively; *P* for trend, <0.001). Walking and vigorous exercise were associated with similar risk reductions, and the results did not vary substantially according to race, age, or body-mass index. A brisker walking pace and fewer hours spent sitting daily also predicted lower risk.

The Health Professionals' Follow-up Study, a prospective study of U.S. health professionals, addressed exercise *type* and *intensity* in relation to CHD in men.[52] A cohort of 44,452 U.S. men were followed at 2-year intervals from 1986 to 1998, to assess potential CHD risk factors, identify newly diagnosed cases of CHD, and assess levels of leisure-time physical activity. Total physical activity, running, weight training, and rowing were each inversely associated with risk of CHD. The relative risks corresponding to quintiles of MET hours for total physical activity adjusted for age, smoking, and other cardiovascular risk factors were 1.0, 0.90, 0.87, 0.83, and 0.70 (*P* for trend <0.001). Men who ran for an hour or more per week had a 42% risk reduction compared with men who did not run. Men who trained with weights for 30 minutes or more per week had a 23% risk reduction compared with men who did not train with weights. Rowing for 1 hour or more per week was associated with an 18% risk reduction. Average exercise intensity was associated with reduced CHD risk independent of the total volume of physical activity. The relative risks corresponding to moderate (4–6 METs) and high (6–12 METs) activity intensities were 0.94 and 0.83 compared with low-activity intensity (<4 METs) (*P* for trend = 0.02). A half hour per day or more of brisk walking was associated with an 18% risk reduction. Walking pace was associated with reduced CHD risk independent of the number of walking hours. This study confirms that CHD risk is lowered by engaging in any of a wide variety of physical activities, including resistance exercise. In addition, the average exercise intensity was associated with reduced risk independent of the number of MET-hours spent in physical activity.

In the Framingham Heart Study, approximately 5000 men and women, 30 to 62 years old and free of clinical evidence of coronary disease at the onset, have been examined regularly since 1949. Coronary disease mortality was subsequently found to be higher in cohorts with indices consistent with a sedentary lifestyle. However, physical inactivity did not have the predictive power of three other primary risk factors (smoking, hypertension, increased lipids). Kannel et al[133] reanalyzed the Framingham data for the effects of physical activity on overall mortality and cardiovascular disease mortality. The effect of being sedentary on mortality was rather modest compared with the other risk factors, but persisted when these other factors were taken into account. A low correlation was noted between physical activity level and the major risk factors.

The relationship between self-selected leisure-time physical activity to first major coronary disease events and overall mortality was studied in 12,138 middle-aged men participating in the Multiple Risk Factor Intervention Trial.[134] Total leisure-time physical activity over the preceding year was quantified in mean minutes per day at baseline by questionnaire, with subjects classified into tertiles (low, moderate, and high leisure-time physical activity). During 7 years of follow-up, moderate leisure-time physical activity was associated with a 37% reduction in fatal CHD events and sudden deaths, and a 30% reduction in total deaths compared with low leisure-time physical activity ($P < 0.01$). Mortality rates with high leisure-time physical activity were similar to those for moderate leisure-time physical activity; however, combined fatal and nonfatal major CHD events were 20% lower with high as compared with low leisure-time physical activity. Leisure-time physical activity had a modest inverse relation to CHD and overall mortality in middle-aged men at high risk for CHD. The relationship of leisure-time physical activity to mortality was investigated in 3043 American railroad workers who were followed-up for 20 years.[131] The Minnesota Leisure Time Physical Activity Questionnaire was used. After adjusting for age and other risk factors, the risk estimate for CHD deaths was 1.39 in men who were sedentary compared with the most active men who expended more than 2000 kcal per week.

Prospective Studies Relating Exercise Capacity to Cardiac Events or Mortality

It has been recognized for several decades that exercise capacity determined from an exercise test is a strong predictor of mortality in patients with known heart disease.[135,136] Historically, however, the strength of exercise capacity as a predictor of risk has not been given its appropriate due.[137,138] This is largely because clinicians have tended to focus on ECG changes in terms of risk stratification, even though many studies, particularly in recent years, have demonstrated that exercise capacity may be the strongest predictor of risk among clinical and exercise test variables. This topic was touched on in Chapter 8. In the following sections, studies published about men and women referred for exercise testing for clinical reasons and followed-up for both cardiac morbidity and all-cause mortality are reviewed. The major studies in this area are outlined in Table 13-9.

A growing number of studies have been published in which physical fitness, determined by standardized exercise testing, was analyzed among large samples of men and women who have been followed for the incidence of CHD morbidity and mortality for up to 20 years.[50,111,139-145] Each of these studies demonstrated that higher levels of fitness were associated with lower rates of CHD or all-cause mortality. Importantly, these associations appear to be independent of other CHD risk factors. Moreover, the low levels of fitness in these studies did not appear to be associated with subclinical disease.

Early studies in addressing this topic measured various risk factors for cardiovascular disease and studied their association with exercise tolerance. Leon et al[146] demonstrated that, in healthy men, the combination of resting measurements and questionnaire responses related to health correlated highly with treadmill time using a multivariate equation. One hundred and seventy-five apparently healthy men completed questionnaires about habitual physical activity, smoking, alcoholic beverage consumption, and sleep habits. Body mass index, heart rate and blood pressure at rest and during submaximal exercise, frequency of premature ventricular beats, handgrip strength, and serum cholesterol were measured. These characteristics were correlated with the duration of exercise using the Bruce protocol. Univariate analysis indicated that treadmill performance was significantly and positively correlated with leisure-time activity and reports of sweating and dyspnea occurring regularly during such physical activity. Performance was negatively correlated with age, body mass index, resting heart rate, cigarette smoking, and consumption of caffeine-containing beverages. A total correlation of 0.75 was found between treadmill performance and 11 of the variables previously mentioned, and it increased to 0.81 by adding heart rate during submaximal exercise.

TABLE 13-9. Epidemiologic studies of exercise capacity assessed by exercise testing as it relates to mortality

Investigator	Year	Mean follow-up	Assessment	Subjects	Conclusions
Peters	1983	4.8 years	Bicycle ergometry	2779 healthy middle-aged men	Adjusted RR of 2.2 for low exercise capacity if other risk factors also present
Lie	1985	7.0 years	Bicycle ergometry	149 middle-aged elite athletes; 2014 healthy men	Higher quintiles of physical fitness associated with decreased coronary disease and mortality
Ekelund	1988	8.5 years	Bruce TM	4276 males	RR of 2.7 for cardiovascular death in men with low exercise capacity
Blair	1989	8 years	USAFSAM TM	10,224 males, 3120 females	Physical fitness inversely related to all-cause mortality
Blair	1995	5.1 years	USAFSAM TM	9777 men	Improvement in fitness between two tests (5 years apart) reduces mortality 44%
Snader	1997	2 years	Bruce TM	3400 patients referred for clinical reasons	Exercise capacity stronger predictor of death than Tl-201 defects; RR 4.4 for poor versus good exercise capacity
Erikssen	1998		Bicycle ergometry	1756 men	Graded, inverse relation between change in fitness in fitness on two exercise tests (7 to 10 years apart) and mortality, irrespective of initial fitness level
Myers	2002	6.2 years	Ramp TM	6213 patients referred for clinical reasons	Exercise capacity strongest predictor of mortality among clinical, risk factor and exercise test variables; each 1 MET increase conferred 12% improved survival
Mora	2003	20 years	Bruce TM	2994 asymptomatic women	Exercise capacity stronger predictor of mortality than ischemic criteria; Each 1 MET increase conferred 20% improved survival
Gulati	2003	8 years	Bruce TM	5721 asymptomatic women	17% better survival per MET achieved
Balady	2004	18 years	Bruce TM	1431 men, 1612 women without CHD at baseline	In high risk men, each 1 MET increase conferred 13% reduction in CHD risk

CHD, coronary heart disease; RR, relative risk; Tl-201, Thallium SPECT imaging; TM, treadmill; USAFSAM, United States Air Force School of Aerospace Medicine.

A prospective study by Peters et al[147] suggested that poor physical work capacity, as measured by bicycle ergometry in apparently healthy Los Angeles County workers, was related to subsequent MI. This was one of the first follow-up studies to measure exercise capacity directly, rather than to estimate activity level. An adjusted relative risk of 2.2 was found only in men with certain other risk factors present, namely above-median cholesterol, smoking, above-median systolic blood pressure, or a combination of these.

An impressive body of data has been published from the Aerobics Center in Dallas, using treadmill performance to associate physical fitness with health. In a cross-sectional study of 753 men, treadmill performance was found to be inversely related to body weight, percentage of body fat, lipids, glucose, and systolic blood pressure.[148] In a subsequent longitudinal study, men who were treadmill tested both before and after an exercise program were analyzed to determine if their performance had improved. Those men who reached the upper quartile of improved aerobic fitness exhibited decreases in lipids, diastolic blood pressure, serum glucose, uric acid, and weight. Regular exercise resulting in increased aerobic capacity was associated with decreased risk factors. In addition, they found that, in a study of 420 men who were divided into groups of former athletes and nonathletes, prior athleticism had no significant effect on cardiovascular risk factors, physical fitness, and exercise habits.[149]

This group also subsequently studied 10,244 men and 3120 women (99% of whom were white) who all were able to achieve 85% of age-predicted heart rate.[139] They divided physical fitness levels into quintiles by estimating VO_2 max from a baseline treadmill test. During an average follow-up of 8 years, they demonstrated by multivariate analysis adjusted for age, other known cardiac risk factors, and length of follow-up that all-cause mortality was inversely related to physical fitness. The relative risk in men and women in the highest quintile of fitness was 0.29 and 0.22, respectively. Simply changing from the lowest quintile of fitness to the second-lowest quintile cut the mortality in half for women (relative risk, 0.52) and by 60% in men (relative risk, 0.40). These results are presented in Table 13-10. This study was quite important at the time of publication, being one of the only analyses to prospectively study fitness in women, to include such a large sample size, and to document that gradations in physical fitness led to significant reductions in mortality.

The Lipid Research Clinics (LRC) Mortality Follow-up Study also used a baseline treadmill test as its estimate of physical fitness in its study of 3106 men followed-up for an average of 8.5 years.[140] This study reported a relative risk of cardiovascular death of 2.7 (95%; confidence interval 1.4 to 5.1, $P = 0.003$) for the less physically fit men, none of whom had evidence of cardiac disease at entry. An interesting study by Lie et al[150] in Norway prospectively followed groups of men with no known cardiac disease at entry for 7 years. One group of 149 middle-aged elite athletes (Nordic skiers) had an extremely low incidence of death (1%) after 7 years. The other group was composed of 2014 middle-aged healthy men who were further subdivided into physical fitness quartiles based on their performance on a bicycle ergometry test on entry. This quartile grouping was also consistent with the subject's level of leisure activity determined by questionnaire. The most fit quartile in this group had a 7-year mortality rate similar to that of the Nordic skiers, and a highly significant difference was found in survival between each of the quartiles. Physical fitness and leisure-time physical activity in this study were found to be significantly inversely related to mortality.

The LRC recently addressed this issue in women.[144] Among 2994 asymptomatic women followed-up over a period of 20 years, low exercise capacity, low heart rate recovery, and the inability to achieve target heart rate were independent predictors of mortality. After age-adjustment, there was a 20% reduction in mortality for every MET achieved on the treadmill. Women who were below the median values for both exercise capacity and heart rate recovery had a 3.5-fold increased risk

TABLE 13-10. Rates and relative risks of death* among 10,244 men and 3120 women in an 8-year follow-up, by gradients of physical fitness

Quintiles of fitness[†]	Men			Women		
	Number of deaths	Death per 100,000 man-years	Relative risk of death[‡]	Number of deaths	Deaths per 100,000 woman-years	Relative risk of death[‡]
1 (low)	75	64.0	1.00	18	39.5	1.00
2	40	25.5	0.40	11	20.5	0.52
3	47	27.1	0.42	6	12.2	0.31
4	43	21.7	0.34	4	6.5	0.15
5 (high)	35	18.6	0.29	4	8.5	0.22

*Age-adjusted.
[†]Quintiles of fitness determined by maximal exercise testing.
[‡]p for trend <0.05.
From Blair SN, Kohl HW, Paffenbarger RS, et al: Physical fitness and all-cause mortality. JAMA 1989;262:2395-2401.

of cardiovascular death. Importantly, although exercise capacity was a powerful predictor of risk, ST-segment depression was not associated with risk in these women. Similar observations were made from the St. James Women Take Heart Project, in which 5721 asymptomatic women (mean age 52 years) underwent exercise testing and were followed for a mean of 8.4 years.[111] After adjustment for Framingham risk score, there was a decrease in mortality of 17% for every MET increase in exercise capacity. These two studies are important in that they included large cohorts of women, as opposed to the vast majority of previous studies performed in men. They suggest that exercise capacity may be an even more powerful predictor of risk (17% to 20% risk reduction per MET) than that observed in men. In addition, they confirm that the prognostic value of the exercise test in women is associated with fitness-related variables (exercise capacity and heart rate recovery) more so than ischemic responses.

More recently, this issue has been addressed in clinical populations, for example, patients referred for exercise testing for clinical reasons.[50,141-143,145] In a recent study performed among U.S. Veterans, 6213 men underwent maximal exercise testing for clinical reasons and were followed for a mean of 6.2 years.[50] The subjects were classified into five categories by gradients of fitness. After adjustment for age, the researchers observed that the largest gains in terms of mortality were achieved between the lowest fitness group and the next lowest fitness group. Figure 13-1 illustrates the age-adjusted relative risks associated with the different categories of fitness. Among both normal subjects and

those with cardiovascular disease, the least fit individuals had more than four times the risk of all-cause mortality compared with the most fit. Importantly, an individual's fitness level was a stronger predictor of mortality than established risk factors such as smoking, high blood pressure, high cholesterol, and diabetes. Over the last few years, other cohorts, such as those from the Cleveland Clinic[143] and the Mayo Clinic[141,142] have documented the importance of exercise capacity as a predictor of mortality among clinically referred populations. These clinically based studies confirm the observations of Blair et al,[139] Framingham,[48] and the LRC Trial[140] among asymptomatic populations, underscoring the fact that fitness level has a strong influence on the incidence of cardiovascular and all-cause morbidity and mortality.

Studies Assessing Both Physical Activity Pattern and Fitness Level

Is *physical fitness* or *activity* necessary to achieve protection from CAD? This controversy is still debated in the literature[151-154] and some have argued that it is as much a rhetorical question as it is a scientific one. VO_2 max correlates with the level of physical activity, and for epidemiologic studies, estimated METs have been used as a reasonable expression of cardiovascular fitness.[50,139,141-143,145] Fitness level achieved on an exercise test is no doubt a more objective and reliable method of assessing a person's cardiovascular health than physical activity as reported by questionnaire. There has

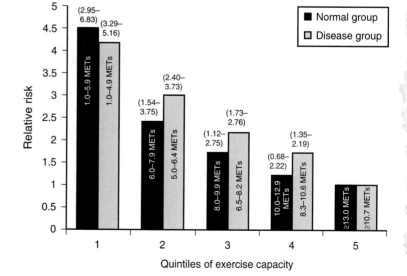

■ FIGURE 13-1

Age-adjusted relative risks of mortality by quintiles of exercise capacity among normal subjects and patients with cardiovascular disease. *(From Myers et al: Exercise capacity and mortality among men referred for exercise testing. New Engl J Med 2002;346:793-801).*

been some recent debate as to whether daily physical activity patterns largely determine one's fitness level, and therefore health risk, or whether fitness level predicts mortality independently from activity pattern.

Despite the abundance of reports related to fitness or activity and health outcomes, few studies have addressed both fitness and physical activity in the same population multivariately with other clinical and risk factor data. The available studies generally suggest that fitness level more strongly predicts outcomes than physical activity patterns.[151-153] There may be several reasons why this is the case. First, the quantification of physical fitness is more objective than physical activity. Fitness is generally determined directly from symptom or sign-limited exercise testing, whereas activity level is dependent upon subject recollection, the judiciousness with which subjects respond, and other limitations associated with questionnaires. In addition, the strength of exercise capacity relative to other clinical and exercise data in stratifying risk, while only recently appreciated,[137,138] is increasingly being recognized in the literature among both healthy[111,139,140,144] and clinically referred subjects.[50,141-143,145]

In the Copenhagen Male Study, the joint effects of fitness and leisure-time activity were analyzed in 4999 men aged 40 to 59 years.[155] The men were classified according to level of physical fitness by estimated maximal oxygen uptake, physical activity was determined by interview, and mortality and CHD incidence was recorded over a 17-year period. In sedentary men, fitness was not a predictor of future risk of CHD. In moderate or highly active men, however, fitness was a strong predictor of risk. The least fit (two least fit quintiles) physically active men had a higher CHD mortality rate; after adjustment for age, social class, and smoking in a multiple logistic regression equation, there was a 67% higher mortality risk for the lower fitness groups. These investigators concluded that: (1) being fit provides no protection against CHD—nor all-cause mortality—in sedentary men and (2) unfit, sedentary men have a higher risk of CHD than unfit, active men, that is, those performing light physical activity for at least 4 hours per week.

In an effort to further clarify this issue, we studied 6213 men referred for exercise testing between 1987 and 2000, and a subgroup of 842 who underwent an assessment of adulthood activity patterns.[153] The predictive power of exercise capacity and activity patterns, along with clinical and exercise test data, were assessed for all-cause mortality during a mean follow-up period of 5.5 ± 2 years.

Expressing the data by age-adjusted quartiles, exercise capacity was a stronger predictor of mortality than activity pattern (hazard ratio 0.56, $P < 0.001$). In a multivariate analysis, including clinical, risk factor, exercise test data, and activity patterns, exercise capacity and energy expenditure from adulthood recreational activity were the only significant predictors of mortality (hazard ratio for exercise capacity = 0.62, $P < 0.001$ and hazard ratio for activity = 0.72, $P = 0.002$ per quartile); these two variables were stronger predictors of mortality than established risk factors such as smoking, hypertension, obesity, and diabetes. Age-adjusted hazard ratios for exercise capacity per quartile were 1.0, 0.59, 0.46, and 0.28 ($P < 0.001$); age-adjusted hazard ratios for physical activity were 1.0, 0.63, 0.42, and 0.38 ($P < 0.001$). A 1000-kcal per week increase in activity was approximately similar to a 1-MET increase in fitness; both conferred a 20% mortality benefit. This analysis suggests that although exercise capacity determined from exercise testing and energy expenditure from weekly activity are *both* strong predictors of mortality, exercise capacity outperforms activity pattern in predicting risk. Importantly, however, both are stronger predictors of risk than other clinical and exercise test variables.

Meta-Analyses of Physical Activity and Health Outcomes

The large volume of data published over several decades has provided the opportunity to combine results in order to better define the association between physical activity and various outcomes. In 1987 Powell et al[157] performed an extensive review of 43 such studies and concluded that an inverse relationship between physical activity and the incidence of CHD was observed in over two thirds. Moreover, the relationship was strongest in those studies that best measured physical activity (Fig. 13-2).

In a recent meta-analysis, Williams[152] compared the dose-response relationships between leisure-time physical activity and fitness from published reports and their association with cardiovascular disease endpoints. The analysis included a remarkable 1,325,000 person-years follow-up. The results of the Williams meta-analysis[151] are summarized in Figure 13-3. Relative risks are plotted as a function of the cumulative percentages of the samples when ranked from least fit or active to most fit or active. In combining study

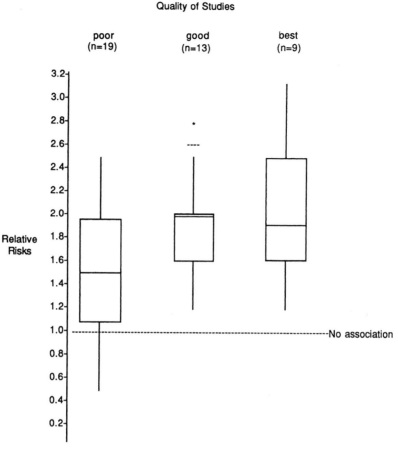

Quality of Studies

■ **FIGURE 13-2**

Box plot illustrating the relative risk of physical inactivity according to the scientific quality of the available studies. *(From Powell KE, Thompson PD, Caspersen CJ, Kendrick JS: Physical activity and the incidence of coronary heart disease. Am Rev Public Health 1987;8:253–287).*

results, a weighted average of the relative risks from the physical activity and fitness cohorts was computed at every 5th percentile between 5% and 100%. As illustrated in Figure 13-3, the risks of CHD decrease linearly with increasing percentiles of physical activity. This is contrasted by the fitness cohorts, in which a sharp drop in risk occurs before the 25th percentile of the fitness distribution. This suggests that the largest benefits in terms of CHD morbidity occur by the most unfit becoming moderately fit, confirming the observations in the Blair et al,[139] the Veterans Administration,[50] and other[106,107] studies. Perhaps more importantly, the precipitous drop in risk before the 25th percentile of the fitness distribution results in fitness being a more powerful predictor of CHD risk than physical activity. In other words, at all percentiles greater than the 25th, the

relative risk reduction is greater for fitness than physical activity. Williams[151] interpreted these findings to mean that formulating activity recommendations on the basis of fitness studies may inappropriately demote the status of cardiorespiratory fitness as a risk factor, while exaggerating the public health benefits of moderate amounts of physical activity.

This recent debate aside, it should be noted that dozens of studies over the last 4 decades have reported that *both* higher physical fitness levels *and* greater amounts of physical activity have an inverse association with the incidence of cardiovascular disease and all-cause mortality. Answering the question regarding whether fitness or activity more strongly predicts outcomes is a difficult undertaking, complicated by the fact that the two measures are related (with correlation

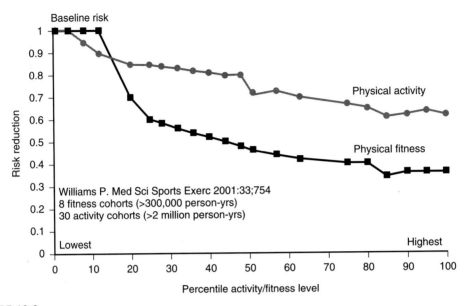

FIGURE 13-3

Degree of risk reduction in coronary heart disease or other cardiovascular diseases from 8 physical fitness and 30 physical activity cohorts. *(From Williams PT: Physical fitness and activity as separate heart disease risk factors: A meta-analysis. Med Sci Sports Exerc 2001:33;754–761).*

coefficients ranging in the order of 0.30 to 0.60), and because fitness also has a strong genetic component, in addition to the fact that fitness may be influenced by subclinical disease and other factors. Even with large, prospective analyses addressing both fitness and activity measures in the same population, a complete answer to this issue will remain elusive. Physical activity develops physical fitness, although the magnitude of the response to an exercise stimulus is likely genetically determined. Nevertheless, activity is likely required to develop and maintain a fitness level that is consistent with good health. This scientific question should not be a distraction from the important public health message that sedentary individuals should become more physically active.

Changes in Physical Fitness or Activity and Health Risk

Several groups of investigators have also studied *changes* in physical fitness (as assessed by serial treadmill testing) and its association with mortality risk. Blair et al[112] conducted two exercise evaluations, performed a mean of 4.9 years apart, to evaluate change or lack of change in fitness, and

mortality was determined over a 5-year follow-up. Age-adjusted all-cause mortality was highest in men who were physically unfit at both examinations (122/10,000 person-years), and the lowest death rate was observed in men who were physically fit at both examinations (39.6/10,000 person-years). Men who improved from unfit to fit between tests had a reduction in mortality risk of 44% relative to men who were unfit at both examinations. For each minute of increase in maximal treadmill time between tests, there was a corresponding 7.9% decrease in risk of all-cause mortality. The results were similar for cardiovascular mortality. Erikssen et al[113] made similar observations in Sweden; a graded inverse relationship was observed between change in fitness on two exercise tests (performed 7 to 10 years apart) and both cardiovascular and all-cause mortality, irrespective of initial fitness level.

In the Corpus Christi Heart Project, Steffen-Batey et al,[157] studied the association between change in level of physical activity and risk of death or reinfarction was studied in 406 patients who survived a first MI. Patients were interviewed at baseline and annually thereafter about physical activity, medical history, and risk factors for CHD. Change in level of activity after the infarction was categorized as: (1) sedentary, no change (referent group); (2) decreased activity; (3) increased activity; and (4) active, no change. Over a 7-year period, the relative risks of death were as follows: 0.21 for the active, no change group; 0.11 for the increased activity group; and 0.49 for the decreased activity group. The relative risks of reinfarction were as follows: 0.40 for the active, no change group; 0.22 for the increased activity group; and 0.93 for the decreased activity group. These findings are consistent with those observed among asymptomatic populations and suggest a beneficial role of increasing physical activity in men and women who survive a first MI.

RECOMMENDATIONS ON PHYSICAL ACTIVITY

Previous position statements published by the AHA,[115,158] the ACSM,[32] and the National Institutes of Health (NIH)[159] on the recommended quality and quantity of exercise were extended in 1996 with the publication of the Surgeon General's Report on Physical Activity and Health.[107] This document was the strongest policy statement ever made by the U.S. government concerning physical activity. It represented a historical turning point redefining exercise as a key component for health promotion and disease prevention. The federal government mounted a multiyear educational campaign based on this report. In this report, the epidemiologic evidence supporting physical activity in the prevention of CHD morbidity and mortality was reviewed in detail. The document also outlines how much exercise is necessary to achieve these benefits. It is suggested that each individual perform a moderate amount of activity daily, with the amount of activity emphasized rather than the intensity, for 30 minutes or more on most, and preferably on all days of the week. These activities can take the form of brisk walking, yard work or other household chores, jogging, or a wide variety of recreational activities. Repeated intermittent or shorter bouts of activity (at least 10 minutes), including occupational, nonoccupational, or tasks of daily living, have similar cardiovascular and health benefits if performed at a level of moderate intensity (such as brisk walking, cycling, swimming, home repair, and yard work) with an accumulated duration of at least 30 minutes per day. People who already meet these standards will receive additional benefits from increasing this to more vigorous activity.

The 30-minutes per day recommendation parallels an energy expenditure in the order of 1000 kcal per week, and comes from the observation that this degree of energy expenditure is achievable by most individuals, and is associated with 20% to 40% reductions in cardiovascular and all-cause morbidity and mortality. Despite the fact that this relatively small investment in physical activity yields a major benefit in health outcomes, studies have shown that few physicians discuss exercise with their patients.[160] Despite major educational efforts made by governmental agencies, the vast majority of adults in Western societies remain effectively sedentary,[106,107] in part due to the fact that physical activity is not currently integrated into the healthcare paradigm. Physicians need to be more proactive in educating and preparing previously sedentary individuals to become more physically active.

"Health" versus "Fitness" Benefits of Exercise

A noteworthy theme that is consistent in each of the recent documents described above is that considerable health benefits are derived from moderate levels of activity; it is generally not necessary to engage in vigorous activity to derive many of these benefits. In past decades, an exercise program was thought to be effective only if an improvement in some measure of cardiopulmonary function was observed. In recent years, however, the philosophy on recommending exercise as a means to this end ("fitness" measured by exercise capacity) has changed significantly. It is now appreciated that substantial health benefits can be achieved through modest amounts of regular exercise, irrespective of whether exercise results in a measurable improvement in exercise capacity. Epidemiologic studies have shown that death rates from cardiovascular causes are considerably lower even among individuals who engage in relatively small amounts of exercise, less than the threshold that was generally thought needed to increase exercise capacity.[32,106,107,115,153,158,159] Although this issue has also been debated, it is difficult to argue with the wealth of evidence demonstrating that modest amounts of activity are associated with considerable health benefits. As health professionals, it is important to be aware of the distinction between "health" and "fitness" when making activity recommendations to patients with cardiovascular disease, those at high risk for its development, and healthy adults.

DANGERS OF EXERCISE

Sudden death has been defined relative to the onset of symptoms, for example, instantaneous versus within 1, 6, or 24 hours. Autopsy findings in people dying instantaneously and those dying after 24 hours are different. Deaths occurring within 6 hours of onset of symptoms include all electrical deaths and are best defined as "sudden," because no anatomic change usually can be demonstrated. Most sudden deaths that occur during exertion do so within minutes of the onset of symptoms. Sudden cardiac death is herein defined as "death occurring unexpectedly within 6 hours of onset of symptoms in a previously healthy person." "Sudden" death, when defined this way, is the most frequent mode of death. The incidence of sudden death in the general population is high (15% to 30%) with the majority (80% to 90%) due to cardiovascular causes.

The mechanism of sudden cardiac death and acute MI in previously healthy adults is most often a rupture of an atherosclerotic plaque and acute coronary thrombosis. This has been confirmed by a number of autopsy studies in recent years, and has engendered the concept of the "vulnerable plaque" syndrome. Studies suggest that roughly 70% of MIs are caused by inflammation leading to "soft" or vulnerable plaque in the arterial wall. Exercise could induce disruption of a vulnerable plaque by the dynamic vasodilation and vasoconstriction that occurs with exercise, a "twisting" motion of the artery, or the abnormal vasoconstriction that occurs in atherosclerotic segments of a coronary artery during exercise.[1] In the following, some of the major studies on the incidence and causes of sudden death during exercise are reviewed.

Coronary Atherosclerosis in Joggers and Marathon Runners

Interest in causes of death in joggers and marathon runners was stimulated in the 1970s when claims were made that "marathon running provides complete immunity from CAD."[161] Since then, numerous cases of death in joggers and marathon runners have been reported. The most common cause of death has been coronary atherosclerosis (75%). The most common non-cardiovascular death in runners results from automobile accidents. Rare cardiovascular causes of death have been reported to include amyloidosis and tunnel coronary artery (2% each), myocarditis, congenital hypoplastic coronary arteries, heat stroke, prolapsed mitral valve, hypertrophic cardiomyopathy (HCM), and gastrointestinal hemorrhage (1% each). In about 10% of cases, the cause of death is unknown.

Siscovik et al[162] studied individuals who were reported by the paramedical immediate response system in Seattle to have had sudden death. They were compared with a matched sample that was randomly chosen by a special telephone-dialing device. To examine the risk of primary cardiac arrest during vigorous exercise, they interviewed the wives of 133 men who had died suddenly of heart disease that had not been previously diagnosed. The deceased were classified according to their time of cardiac arrest and the amount of their habitual vigorous activity. Among men with low levels of habitual activity, the relative risk of cardiac arrest during exercise compared with that at other times was 56. The risk during exercise among men at the highest activity level was also elevated, but only fivefold, and their overall risk of cardiac arrest at any time was only 40% that of sedentary men. This was the first study to clearly document that, although the risk of primary cardiac arrest is transiently increased during vigorous exercise, regular exercise markedly decreases the risk.

Waller and Roberts[163] reported on the autopsies of five conditioned runners aged 40 years and older, all of whom had severe coronary atherosclerosis. A series by Thompson et al[164] described 18 joggers, with five "exercising regularly" for at least 1 year and nine exercising for 3 or more years. Fifteen of 18 died suddenly while jogging, and of those, 13 had CHD. Waller[165] described 10 patients over 30 years of age who ran 1 to 55 miles per week for 1 to 12 years. All had at least one artery severely narrowed by an atherosclerotic plaque and six had MIs. As a sequel to their study of jogging deaths in California, Thompson et al[166] assessed the incidence of sudden death during jogging in Rhode Island. From 1975 through 1980, 12 men died during jogging, and the cause of death in 11 was CHD. From a telephone survey, they found that 7.4% of adult male Rhode Islanders jogged at least twice a week. The incidence of death from jogging was one death per year for every 7620 joggers and only one death per 396,000 man-hours of jogging. This rate is seven times the estimated death rate from CHD during more sedentary activities in Rhode Island. Vander et al[167] conducted a 5-year retrospective survey of fatal and nonfatal cardiovascular events that occurred in community recreation centers. Fifty-eight facilities reported 30 nonfatal and 38 fatal events. There was one nonfatal and one fatal event every 1,124,200 and 887,526 hours of participation, respectively.

What is the expected level of cardiovascular deaths among runners while running if one considers chance alone? This is an important question because it is often assumed that exercise is the cause when a person dies of cardiovascular causes during recreational running. Koplan[168] used data from the National Center of Health Statistics and found that approximately 100 cardiovascular deaths per year in runners in the United States can be predicted on a purely temporal basis. This is certainly higher than the number of deaths reported. Morales et al[169] described three healthy individuals—two males aged 34 and 54 years and one female 17 years of age—who died suddenly during strenuous exercise and were found to have a triad of pathologic findings. The pathologic triad was muscle bridging of the left anterior descending coronary artery, poor circulation to the posterior surface of the heart, and septal fibrosis. The angiographic finding of a coronary artery that passes underneath a band of myocardium is not that unusual and it has been debated whether or not it has functional significance. Some studies of coronary blood flow have suggested that the constriction of a coronary artery by this myocardial band during systole results in decreased flow; however, most coronary flow takes place during diastole. In regard to the second finding, there is great variability in the coronary artery distribution on the posterior surface of the heart around the crux and the posterior margin of the septum. In the most common situation, the right coronary artery branches into a posterior descending artery, which passes down the septum, giving off septal perforators. Often there are normal variations where the left circumflex provides this branch or there are only small arteries in the area. Lastly, septal fibrosis could be due to chronic ischemia. These anatomic findings could also be purely coincidental.

Noakes et al[170] presented four marathon runners with autopsy-proven coronary atherosclerosis. The first individual was a 44-year-old male who, after 14 months of training, had completed seven marathons in less than 4 hours each. He suddenly dropped dead half-way through a marathon. At autopsy he was found to have an old anteroseptal MI and 90% lesions of his left anterior descending and circumflex coronary arteries. The second was a 41-year-old man who, after 2 years of running, had a symptomatic MI. After release from the hospital, he returned to training and ran in five marathons. He was later hospitalized again with unstable angina and coronary angiography was performed. He was found to have severe triple vessel

CAD; while waiting for surgery, he died suddenly. The last two cases were 36- and 27-year-old athletes who had completed multiple marathons and were killed accidentally. Both had left anterior descending coronary artery lesions at autopsy; the younger had a 50% and the older had a 90% lesion.

An interesting review of this topic was later published by Noakes[171] in which the deaths of 36 marathon runners previously reported in the medical literature were described. This group had a mean age of 43.8 years (range, 18 to 70 years) and 75% had a cardiovascular cause of death. Seventy-one percent of these runners with coronary disease had forewarning symptoms that they tended to ignore and continued training. Of the 26 runners from whom data were available, 50% died within 24 hours of a competitive running event. Thus, unlike what was thought for many years, it is clear that high levels of aerobic performance do not exclude the presence of significant coronary disease, and symptoms in such patients should be taken seriously.

Virmani and McAllister[172] reported findings in 30 joggers or marathon runners who died from nontraumatic causes. Twenty-two men died with severe atherosclerosis; their ages ranged from 18 to 54 years (mean 36 years). The history of jogging was well documented in 18 patients who ran 7 to 105 miles per week (mean 33 miles) and had been running 1 to 28 years (mean, 10 years). Three were marathon runners and the others had been jogging for at least 6 months. Review of records revealed a family history of heart disease in nine, systemic hypertension in nine, and total cholesterol greater than 200 mg/dl in seven. None were diabetic and smoking history was uncertain. A history of CHD was present in eight (27%); of these, five were from a retrospective review of medical records. Nineteen died suddenly and three had a history of prolonged chest pain. In six patients, death occurred soon after jogging, and two were found dead in bed. At autopsy, the heart weight ranged from 345 to 600 g (mean, 432 g). In 16 patients, the heart weight was increased beyond the normal range. Of the four major arteries examined for severe atherosclerosis, only one artery was involved in nine patients (41%), two coronary arteries in nine (41%), and three and four coronary arteries in one each. Thrombi were noted in six (27%) patients. The most common single artery involved was the left anterior descending, and the most common combination was the left anterior descending and right coronary arteries. Of a total of 70 coronary arteries examined in 20 joggers,

34 (49%) were severely narrowed, and the average number of coronary arteries greater than 75% narrowed was 1.65 per jogger. Those with a history of CHD had a similar extent of coronary atherosclerosis as those without such histories (1.7 versus 1.6 coronary arteries narrowed per patient). In six of the 22 with severe coronary atherosclerosis, isolated healed MI was present; acute MI with or without healed MI was present in eight. A total of 14 (64%) of 22 who died of severe coronary atherosclerosis had MI.

Virmani and Robinowitz[173] studied another 11 male joggers with a mean age of 41 years (range, 19 to 59 years). Sudden death occurred while jogging in 9 of 11 men. Available risk factor history was as follows: two had hypercholesterolemia, one had systemic hypertension, and one had a family history of premature CHD. Only two had a history of prior cardiac disease: one had angina, and one had undergone left ventricular aneurysmectomy with coronary bypass surgery. A 43-year-old man had been jogging 50 miles per week for 5 to 6 years and had participated in several marathons. His heart weighed 600 g, an acute MI was found, and there was a greater than 75% cross-sectional area luminal narrowing of the three major coronary arteries, with thrombus in the left circumflex. Seven had at least two vessels severely narrowed, one had one-vessel disease, and the other two had been described as having severe coronary atherosclerosis. Acute or healed MIs were present in six of 10.

Causes of Death During or Soon After Exercise Other Than Jogging or Marathon Running.

Opie[174] reported the causes of sudden death in 21 athletes, 13 of whom took part in rugby or soccer. Eighteen were thought to be caused by CHD. The Squash Rackets Association has estimated that there may be 2.5 million people in the United Kingdom playing squash once or more a month. The circumstances surrounding 60 sudden deaths associated with squash playing were described by Northcote et al[175] in Glasgow. The mean age of those who died was 46 years (range, 22 to 66 years). They were able to collate a series of 89 sudden deaths associated with squash that occurred between October 1976 and February 1984 by examining press reports and by a prospective mail survey of sports centers and squash clubs throughout the United Kingdom.

Corrado et al[176] from Italy also found that sudden death in athletes occurs most often during or immediately after vigorous activity. Their postmortem studies of 22 young athletes (mean age, 23 years) showed arrhythmic cardiac arrest to be the most common cause of death (17 cases) and right ventricular dysplasia and atherosclerotic CAD were the most frequent underlying cardiovascular diseases (six and four cases, respectively). Of note, many of the athletes had experienced premonitory signs or had abnormal baseline ECGs.

A community-based participation screening examination appeared to prevent sudden death due to HCM in a 17-year prospective study of young people in Italy.[177] Of the 33,735 young athletes (mean age, 19 years) screened, 3016 were referred for echocardiography and 22 of them were excluded from competition due to HCM. Sudden death occurred in 269 of the total 2,009,600 subjects under the age of 35 years in the geographic area. Athletes accounted for 49 deaths and nonathletes for 220, resulting in rates of 1.6 versus 0.75 deaths per 100,000 persons, respectively (relative risk for nonathletes versus athletes = 2.1). The most common cause of death was right ventricular cardiomyopathy (22.4% of deaths). This study confirms the extremely low incidence of athletic sudden deaths, but points out potentially important ethnic differences; HCM may be more common in the United States, whereas right ventricular cardiomyopathy may be more common in Italy.

Maron et al[178] reported sudden unexpected death in 29 highly conditioned, competitive athletes aged 13 to 30 years (mean age, 19 years) drawn from news media reports, the registry of the cardiovascular division of the Armed Forces Institute of Pathology, and the pathology branch of the NIH. All had been active, highly conditioned members of an organized athletic team for at least 2 years. The type of sport varied, but basketball and football were most common. In 28 of the 29 athletes, death occurred suddenly without warning and was virtually instantaneous, occurring on the playing field in 13. One athlete survived 12 hours after collapse. In 22 athletes, death occurred during or soon after severe exertion, in two after mild exertion, and in five during sedentary activities. Structural cardiovascular abnormalities were found in 28 athletes and were the cause of sudden death in 22. Of these, the most common anatomic abnormality was HCM, which was present in 14. HCM was defined as asymmetric septal hypertrophy, with marked ventricular septal disorganization in another two. Four athletes had anomalous origin of the left coronary artery from the right sinus of Valsalva, including one patient with HCM. Four athletes had concentric left ventricular hypertrophy, two with and two without disorganization. Three athletes (24 to 28 years of age) had severe coronary atherosclerosis. Two died of aortic rupture; both had evidence of cystic medial necrosis, and one had Marfan's syndrome.

In six athletes, the cardiovascular abnormality was considered probable evidence of cardiovascular disease: five had hypertrophied hearts (420 to 530 g), one had mild prolapse of anterior and posterior mitral leaflets, and one had normal heart weight with a hypoplastic right coronary artery. Several died of coronary atherosclerosis, one after running a pass pattern in a professional football game. In this individual, they hypothesized that a blow to the chest while being tackled caused a hemorrhage into a plaque in the left anterior descending coronary artery. Several others had congenital anomalies of the coronary arteries. Virmani and Robinowitz[173] reviewed records of 32 individuals who died suddenly while engaging in either military training (six) or in other sports activity: basketball (six), running (eight), racquetball (two), volleyball (two), tennis (two), swimming, (two), football (two), and one each in gymnastics and bowling. Their ages ranged from 14 to 60 years, with a mean age of 28 years; 31 were males and one was female. The anatomic abnormalities were varied: coronary disease in eight, idiopathic myocarditis in four, congenital coronary abnormalities in three, HCM in two, tunnel coronary artery in two, abnormal mitral valve in two, intramural coronary thickening in two, and one each with rheumatic heart disease and aortic dissection. Four had left ventricular hypertrophy of unknown cause (420- to 600-g hearts) and were 17, 20, 21, and 32 years old. All died during exertion. Three who died while running had sickle cell trait and were only 17, 20, and 22 years old.

Maron et al[179] more recently quantified deaths during competitive sports among high school athletes over a 12-year period using an insurance database in Minnesota. During this period, there were 1,453,280 sports participations in 27 different sports, and there were 12 deaths due to cardiovascular disease. The risk of sudden death was 1 per 217,400 participants per year (or 0.46/100,000 annually); the risk was slightly higher in male athletes. The rare incidence of sudden death in this and other studies points out the practical and cost limitations associated with broad screening programs for young athletes.

The causes of death in Virmani and McAllister's[172] subjects were markedly different from those of Maron et al[179], probably because symptomatic individuals are excluded from military service and none was highly trained, whereas Maron's population included only trained athletes. Virmani's subjects had a wide age range, with only 25 being 30 years old or younger, whereas Maron's athletes were 13 to 30 years old, with a mean of 19 years. Prevalence of CHD is directly related to age. This has been confirmed in other studies of runners older than 40 years of age: CHD is the most common cause of death and they usually have had symptoms of CHD prior to the event. Moreover, all of these events are extremely unusual and it would be difficult to screen for them. It is known that athletes frequently have abnormal ECGs and even echocardiographic hypertrophy. In addition, they have a higher prevalence of false-positive exercise tests. However, screening for lipid abnormalities would be a wise public health measure regardless of a lack of specificity, and it would be advisable to get an echocardiogram on an athlete with symptoms or signs of HCM.

Van Camp et al[180] examined 136 deaths that occurred during or within 1 hour of sports participation over 10 years among high school or college athletes. Cardiac conditions were responsible for 100 of the cases, including HCM (56% of the cases), coronary artery anomalies (13%), myocarditis (7%), aortic stenosis (6%), and dilated cardiomyopathy (6%). Together, the studies performed among younger individuals (i.e., <30 years) demonstrate that CAD is a rare cause of exercise-related death in younger individuals. Among high school and college athletes, only about 30% of deaths associated with exercise are also associated with CAD. Rather, exercise-related deaths in young subjects are usually caused by either congenital cardiac abnormalities or nonatherosclerotic acquired cardiovascular diseases.

In a study that has been widely cited since the mid-1990s as evidence that regular exercise offers protection against triggering MI, Mittleman et al[181] conducted interviews among 1228 patients who had sustained an MI an average of 4 days earlier. Information was gathered regarding their usual annual frequency and intensity of physical exertion, along with their physical activity in the 26 hours prior to their MI. The estimated relative risk of MI in the hour after heavy physical exertion, as compared with less strenuous physical exertion or no physical exertion whatsoever, was 5.9. Comparing subjects who regularly participated in physical activity (equaling or more than five times per week) to those who participated in physical activity less than once a week the reactive risk for the less active was 107. Stated differently, while a bout of exercise transiently increases the risk of MI by six-fold, being habitually sedentary increased the risk of MI during exertion by 107 times. In a similar study from Germany, interviews were conducted among 1194 acute MI patients.[182] The adjusted relative risk of the infarction being associated with strenuous physical activity was 2.1. However, the risk of infarction among subjects who were regularly active (equal to or more than versus less than four times per week) was 5.3 times lower than those who were less active.

Effect of Environment

An important factor in sudden death among athletes and joggers is the climate in which exercise is being performed. Serious thermal injuries are preventable, and the ACSM recommends that long-distance races should not be conducted in temperatures that exceed 28°C (82.4°F). The amount of heat generated is directly related to the intensity of exercise. The body is only 25% efficient in converting calories generated into external work, and the remaining 75% of energy is converted into heat. Therefore, a large amount of heat must be lost by the body to prevent raising the core temperature.

If the body does not lose any heat, the core temperature would increase by 1°C every 5 minutes. It is the efficient mechanisms of thermoregulation of the body that prevent hyperthermia. These mechanisms include sweating and heat loss by radiation and by conversion. The factors that prevent heat loss are high ambient temperature, high humidity, dehydration (which prevents cutaneous vasodilation), extremes of age, debilitation, excessive clothing, and drugs that may impair thermoregulation. The spectrum of heat injury includes three well-recognized syndromes: (1) heat cramps; (2) heat exhaustion; and (3) heat stroke. Heat cramps are painful spasms in the muscles, whereas heat exhaustion is characterized by fatigue, hyperventilation, headache, lightheadedness, nausea, and muscle cramps. Patients with heat exhaustion sweat and have chills despite the core temperature being high. Heat stroke, the most serious of thermal injuries, is characterized by an altered state of consciousness that may progress rapidly to unconsciousness and seizure activity. The heat stroke patient is hot, flushed, and has dry skin because sweating has stopped. Dehydration and circulatory collapse soon follow. Body temperature is usually above 41°C (106°F) and laboratory tests show hemoconcentration, leukocytosis, azotemia, acidosis, abnormal liver function tests, and abnormal muscle enzymes. Treatment includes submersion in ice water and intravenous heparin to stop fibrinolysis. At autopsy, the findings usually are nonspecific and consist of petechial hemorrhages in the skin, mucous membranes, brain, lung, and heart. The hemorrhages in the heart are most pronounced in the epicardial and endocardial region, especially on the left side of the ventricular septum. Damage to myocardial filaments and intercalated discs have been described by electron microscopy in patients with malignant hyperthermia induced by anesthetic agents.

Summary of Exercise-Related Death in the Athlete

Although exercise contributes to sudden death in susceptible persons, numerous studies have demonstrated that the risk of exercise is extremely small and suggests that routine screening is not justified. Cardiovascular diseases responsible for sudden unexpected death in highly conditioned athletes are largely related to the age of the patient. In most young, competitive athletes (<35 years of age), sudden death is due to congenital cardiovascular disease. HCM appears to be the most common cause of such deaths, accounting for about half of the sudden deaths in young athletes. Other cardiovascular abnormalities that appear to be less frequent in young athletes include congenital coronary artery anomalies, ruptured aorta (due to cystic medial necrosis), idiopathic left ventricular hypertrophy, and coronary atherosclerosis. Very uncommon causes of sudden death include myocarditis, mitral valve prolapse, aortic valve stenosis, and sarcoidosis. The recent data from Italy implicating right ventricular dysplasia and hypertrophy as a major cause of sudden death in young athletes requires further study, because these findings have not been confirmed in other populations.

Cardiovascular disease in young athletes usually is unsuspected during life, and most athletes who die suddenly have experienced no cardiac symptoms. In only about 25% of the competitive athletes who die suddenly is underlying cardiovascular disease detected or suspected before participation, and rarely is the correct clinical diagnosis made. In contrast, in older athletes (≥35 years of age), sudden death is usually due to CAD. Noninvasive screening procedures currently are available that can detect many subjects at risk of sudden death, but with an uncertain specificity. However, although some potentially lethal diseases can be excluded by a relatively simple screening program, other diseases require expensive procedures, such as echocardiography, exercise testing, and cardiac catheterization. This means that the sensitivity of detecting diseases leading to sudden death increases in proportion to the financial resources that can be applied to the screening program. Thus, when a screening program designed to identify all cardiac diseases that have the potential to cause sudden death is planned by a community, school, or nonprofessional athletic team, the costs will be prohibitive. The practicality of applying a community or school screening program can be questioned because of the very low incidence of sudden unexpected death in young healthy individuals. Comprehensive screening programs are confined to individuals or organizations with adequate financial resources. Less expensive, limited screening can be undertaken by individuals or groups to identify some subjects at risk of sudden death during athletic competition. An important consideration is the education of the team physician. Symptoms and family history of sudden death or syncope should not be overlooked. However, due to high vagal tone, fainting can occur in young athletes. In addition, ECG abnormalities, S3 waves, and systolic murmurs are common.

The normal heart, even when subjected to vigorous forms of stress, is protected from lethal arrhythmias except in unusual conditions such as profound electrolyte derangement, thermal stress, or adverse drug reactions. Victims of sudden death almost always have underlying heart disease. CAD is found in about 80% of victims of sudden cardiac death, whereas other abnormalities, such as cardiomyopathy, valvular heart disease, or primary arrhythmic disorders, also may cause unexpected cardiac arrest. Although exertion-related death appears to be confined to patients with structural heart disease, a third of these individuals may be asymptomatic. Mechanisms underlying sudden death in cardiac patients include ventricular fibrillation and myocardial ischemia. Ventricular fibrillation is the arrhythmia usually underlying the sudden cardiac death syndrome, particularly in exertion-related events. In the follow-up of patients resuscitated from out-of-hospital ventricular fibrillation, Cobb and Weaver[183] recognized three major clinical settings in which ventricular fibrillation occurs: (1) as a complication of typical acute MI; (2) as a manifestation of transient myocardial ischemia, especially during or after exertion; and (3) as an event unassociated with ischemia and occurring while sedentary. In the latter setting, ventricular fibrillation most often occurs in patients with prior MI and left ventricular dysfunction.

Transient ischemia is a plausible cause for most episodes of exertion-related cardiac arrest in patients with coronary disease. In assessing resuscitated patients who collapsed during or after exertion, Cobb and Weaver[183] found that, compared with persons with non-exertion-related cardiac arrest, these patients had fewer limitations and more often had no recognized preceding heart disease. In addition, warning symptoms were noted in only about 25%, and less than one third had new Q waves. These patients have few episodes of ventricular arrhythmia during ambulatory monitoring. Although there has been no large, prospective assessment of the role of exertion in precipitating cardiac arrest, some relevant information is available. In patients treated by the paramedic system in Seattle, 36 (11%) of 316 consecutive victims had collapsed during or immediately after exertion or stress. This incidence is similar to that of the 26 of 150 (17%) patients reported in Miami. In autopsy registries, the incidence of exertion-related cardiac arrest was reported to be 10% to 30% of all sudden deaths. In studies of unexpected sudden death in younger persons, cardiac arrest commonly was associated with physical activity.

In a prospective 5-year survey by Hinkle et al[184] involving approximately 270,000 men, 42% of the sudden coronary deaths occurred in persons without previously recognized coronary disease. About one third of these deaths occurred within minutes of engaging in activities known to be associated with myocardial ischemia or in the setting of suspected sympathetic nervous system stimulation. As reported by the Cooper Clinic, in a predominantly normal population of middle-aged persons, one cardiac arrest occurred per 375,000 person hours of exercise. In the Framingham Study, there was a significant association between the mode of death and activity; sudden death occurred more often in the setting of physical activity. Cobb and Weaver[183] reported that in 133 men who experienced cardiac arrest in Seattle, the incidence of cardiac arrest was 5 to 56 times greater during high-intensity exercise than at other times. The persons considered in that study were aged 25 to 75 years and were without previously recognized cardiovascular disease. The estimated incidence of cardiac arrest during vigorous activity ranged from one case per 137,000 hours to one per 4.7 million hours at risk.

These studies serve to point out that physical exertion may precipitate cardiac arrest in the normal population and that prior recognition of susceptible individuals has not been possible. Exercise-induced cardiac arrest is a rare but real phenomenon, particularly in patients with known heart disease. However, the majority of sudden deaths are temporally associated with routine activities of daily life and not with exercise. Therefore, the number of deaths due to strenuous physical exertion is relatively modest. Exertion-related cardiac arrest usually is due to ventricular fibrillation or tachycardia, and studies show that exercise transiently increases this risk. Importantly, however, sudden death or MI during exercise is far less common among individuals who are regularly active versus those who are not, by a factor of 5 to 100 times.

Complications Other than Death

There are numerous risks for amateur and professional athletes. Heat stroke can be avoided by taking precautions for humid, hot environments, including adequate oral replacement of dilute electrolyte solutions. There is no place for fluid restriction in order to limit sweating. Runners can have heat stroke and still be actively sweating, although it was once taught that heat stroke was always preceded by cessation of sweating. Hematuria after a run can be due to bladder trauma and proteinuria can even be normal. Diarrhea and other gastrointestinal complaints are fairly common in runners during and after events. Numerous episodes of anaphylaxis thought to be exercise-induced have been reported. Diagnosis by the findings of bronchospasm and urticaria is important because treatment with epinephrine and antihistamines can be lifesaving.

Orthopedic Injuries. The greater public awareness and participation in physical activity is responsible for both general practitioners and sports medicine specialists noticing an increase in sports-related injuries among weekend and after-work athletes. Basketball and soccer leagues, ski vacations, evening runs, dance classes, and tennis cause injuries once found chiefly among professional and college athletes.

The Center for Sports Medicine in San Francisco compiled statistics on over 10,000 injuries treated at the center. They found that nine activities— basketball, dance, football, gymnastics, running, skiing, tennis, soccer, and figure skating— accounted for nearly three fourths of the injuries. More than two thirds of the injuries were caused by overuse—problems such as shin splints and tendonitis that develop from a repetitive trauma to muscle and bone. Tennis, aerobic dance, and running frequently cause such problems. The remaining injuries were acute ones—incidents that happened instantly—such as a sprained ankle. These tend to occur in skiing, football, basketball, and soccer. Injuries to the knee caused the most visits and skiers have the most knee problems. Aerobic dance causes more fractures than any other recreational activity. Many problems stem from acute injuries that occurred in the past. Unlike football injuries, most of the basketball injuries occur in participants older than 25 years of age.

Is the recommended physical activity safe? De Loes and Goldie[185] reported the incidence of injury from physical exercise as recorded by physician visits over the course of an entire year in a Swedish town with 31,620 inhabitants. They found that injuries from sports or physical exercise comprised 17% of all clinic visits for accidents. This compared with 26% home-related injuries and 19% work-related injuries. It should be noted that, whereas the Swedes play a great deal of ice hockey (the sport they found causing the greatest incidence of injury), they do not play football.

Education regarding how recreational injuries happen and how to treat them is an important step in prevention. Treatment may include weight lifting for rehabilitation, shoe inserts to correct irregularities in stride or foot strike, ultrasound and electrical stimulation for muscle tears and stiffness, and compression and icing to control swelling. Rest, ice, compression, and elevation are still the best treatment for most acute injuries. There has been a trend toward active rehabilitation. For instance, to treat a sprained ankle, a program that focuses on muscle strengthening is used because if ligaments do not heal well, a tear may become a persistent problem. Prolonged rest can cause a decrease in muscle mass around the ankle, resulting in a loss of strength. The muscles lose their ability to move quickly and stabilize the ankle. Instead, strengthening surrounding muscles will avoid atrophy. In many cases, the strengthened muscles will compensate for the deficient ligaments, making the joint stable for further activities.

Knochel[186] reported that "white collar rhabdomyolysis" (weekend competitive running in middle-aged, moderately conditioned people leading to rhabdomyolysis) is much more common than currently thought. Rhabdomyolysis refers to breakdown of muscle fibers and the release of myoglobin and other intracellular contents into the plasma. This syndrome can be avoided by ensuring gradual conditioning and reasonable competition.

SUMMARY

Animal studies have provided substantial evidence of the cardiovascular benefits of regular physical activity. Improved coronary circulation has been demonstrated in exercise-trained animals through increases in coronary artery size, capillary density, and collateral development in response to hypoxia. Studies utilizing various animal models have reported improvements in cardiac function secondary to exercise training. Improved intrinsic contractility, faster relaxation, enzymatic alterations, calcium availability, and enhanced autonomic and hormonal control of function all have been suggested as reasons for these findings.

These animal studies demonstrate that there are morphologic and metabolic changes that make the cardiovascular system better able to withstand stress, possibly even that imposed by atherosclerosis. The study by Kramsch et al[31] provides the strongest evidence for the favorable impact of exercise and diet on the primary prevention of coronary disease. However, although exercise lessened ischemic manifestations, only diet stopped the progression of coronary atherosclerosis. Although myocardial ischemia seems to be a necessary stimulus for the development of collateral vessels, exercise appears to enhance their development. Exercise probably does not affect the atherosclerotic process, but instead enlarges coronary arteries to provide protection via increased flow. Precisely how these observations made among animals relate to the human heart is unknown, particularly because many of the changes are age-related.

Echocardiographic studies have shown endurance training in young subjects to result in increased ventricular mass, wall thickness, volume, and function, but not all results have been conclusive, probably because of problems with measurement reproducibility. These increases in left ventricular mass may not occur in younger subjects unless higher levels of exercise are used and may never occur in older subjects. In cardiac patients, an exercise program may not lessen exercise-induced ischemia (as assessed by ST-segment depression), but multidisciplinary secondary prevention programs have recently been shown to retard the progression of, and even regress, angiographic CAD.

It is difficult to separate the association between physical inactivity, the atherosclerotic process, and other factors such as abnormal lipids, cigarette smoking, and hypertension. An inverse association between the level of activity and regression of atherosclerosis was reported by Hambrecht et al.[56]

Although regression of atherosclerosis has been repeatedly demonstrated in the 1990s with the use of statins, only a few of these studies have incorporated physical activity; thus, it is not possible at present to determine the independent contribution of physical activity to retarding or regressing the atherosclerotic process. Nevertheless, although physical inactivity does not necessarily precede the atherosclerotic process, its relationship to cardiac events is certainly strong. The level of exercise necessary to lessen the risk of cardiovascular death differs from that required to obtain the hemodynamic and morphologic benefits of more rigorous training. The latter requires careful attention to training intensity, duration, frequency, and mode. The prescription for good health, however, can be less demanding. Moderate or vigorous walking for a minimum of 30 minutes, five to seven times per week, is sufficient to obtain many of the health benefits from exercise.

Interestingly, activity surveys have demonstrated that more than 50% of the American population exercises less than 20 minutes three times a week. This makes inactivity a very prevalent risk factor and increases the population-attributable risk of inactivity in modern society far above that of other risk factors. Recent studies of primary prevention support a lifestyle of regular physical activity to decrease one's risk for CHD. Such physical activity helps to decrease other risk factors as well.[47,115,187,188] Regular, moderate exercise can improve one's quality of life by lessening fatigue and by increasing physical performance.

Although athletic deaths generate a great deal of interest in the public and the press, they are extremely rare. The guidelines on screening athletes suggest that all of the available screening techniques can cause more harm than good because of their high false-positive rates. Knowledge of the causes of such deaths, however, can help focus our attention appropriately. Unfortunately, even an exercise test is not effective for predicting exercise-related deaths in asymptomatic populations. The public health prescription of physical activity rather than the higher levels of exercise needed for physical fitness carries minimal risk.

Thus, both animal and human studies have shown beneficial effects on the heart from regular, sustained exercise. Large epidemiologic studies have shown significant benefits from improvements in physical fitness/activity, especially with regard to decreasing cardiac mortality. Specific recommendations have been put forth by various medical societies; these detail the precise extent and duration of exercise needed to improve both quantity and quality of life. The challenge ahead is to convince two thirds of the American public to step out of the ranks of the sedentary. They need not become Olympic athletes, but they must engage in at least moderate activity.

REFERENCES

1. Gordon JB, Ganz P, Nabel EG, et al: Atherosclerosis influences the vasomotor response of epicardial coronary arteries to exercise. J Clin Invest 1989;83:1946–1952.
2. Hambrecht R, Wolf A, Gielen S, et al: Effect of exercise on coronary endothelial function in patients with coronary artery disease. N Engl J Med 2000;342:454–460.
3. Moyna NM, Thompson PD: The effect of physical activity on endothelial function in man. Acta Physiol Scand 2004;180: 113–123.
4. Dunn AL, Trivedi MH, O'Neal HA: Physical activity dose-response effects on outcomes of depression and anxiety. Med Sci Sports Exerc 2001;33(suppl):S587–S597.
5. Bouchard C, Shephard RJ, Stephens T: Exercise, Fitness and Health. International Proceedings and Consensus Statement. Champaign, Ill., Human Kinetics, 1994.
6. Leon AS: Exercise following myocardial infarction. Current recommendations. Sports Med 2000;29:301–311.
7. Taylor RS, Brown A, Ebrahim S, et al. Exercise-based rehabilitation for patients with coronary heart disease: Systematic review and meta-analysis of randomized controlled trials. Am J Med 2004;116:682–692.
8. Thompson PC, Buchner D, Pina IL, et al. Exercise and physical activity in the prevention and treatment of atherosclerotic cardiovascular disease: A statement from the Council on Clinical Cardiology (Subcommittee on Exercise, Rehabilitation, and Prevention) and the Council on Nutrition, Physical Activity, and Metabolism (Subcommittee on Physical Activity). Circulation 2003;107:3109–3116.
9. Agency for Health Care Policy and Research: Guidelines for Cardiac Rehabilitation. US Dept. of Health and Human Services, 1995.
10. Poupa O, Rakusan K, Ostadal B: The effect of physical activity upon the heart of vertebrates. Physical activity and aging. Med Sports 1970;4:202–203.
11. Thmanek RJ, Tounton CA, Liskop KS: Relationship between age, chronic exercise, and connective tissue of the heart. J Gerontol 1972;27:33–38.
12. Ljungqvist A, Unge G: Capillary proliferation activity in myocardium and skeletal muscle of exercised rats. J Appl Physiol 1978;43:306–312.
13. Tepperman J, Pearlman D: Effects of exercise and anemia on coronary arteries of small animals as revealed by the corrosion-cast technique. Circ Res 1961;9:576–584.
14. Eckstein RW: Effect of exercise and coronary artery narrowing on coronary collateral circulation. Circ Res 1957;5:230–235.
15. Spear KL, Koerner JE, Terjung RL: Coronary blood flow in physically trained rats. Cardiovasc Res 1978;12:135–143.
16. Bloor CM, White FC, Sanders TM: Effects of exercise on collateral development in myocardial ischemia in pigs. J Appl Physiol 1984;56:656–665.
17. Heaton WH, Marr KC, Capurro NL, et al: Beneficial effects of physical training on blood flow to myocardium perfused by chronic collaterals in the exercising dog. Circulation 1978;57:575–581.
18. Cohen MV, Yipinstoi T, Scheuer J: Coronary collateral stimulation by exercise in dogs with stenotic coronary arteries. J Appl Physiol 1982;52:664–668.
19. Wang J, Wolin MS, Hintze TH: Chronic exercise enhances endothelium-mediated dilation of epicardial coronary artery in conscious dogs. Circ Res 1993;73:829–838.
20. Muller JM, Myers PR, Laughlin MH: Vasodilator responses of coronary resistance arteries of exercise-trained pigs. Circulation 1994;89: 2308–2314.
21. Billman GE, Schwartz PJ, Stone HL: The effects of daily exercise on susceptibility to sudden cardiac death. Circulation 1984;69: 1182–1189.
22. Posel D, Noakes T, Kantor P, et al: Exercise training after experimental myocardial infarction increases the ventricular fibrillation threshold before and after the onset of reinfarction in the isolated rat heart. Circulation 1989;80:138–145.
23. Hull SS Jr, Vanoli E, Adamson PB, et al: Exercise training confers anticipatory protection from sudden death during acute myocardial ischemia. Circulation 1994;89:548–552.
24. O'Conner GT, Buring JE, Yusaf S, et al: An overview of randomized trials of rehabilitation with exercise after myocardial infarction. Circulation 1989;80:234–244.
25. Oldridge NB, Guyatt GH, Fischer ME, et al: Cardiac rehabilitation with exercise after myocardial infarction. JAMA 1988;260:945–950.
26. Smart N, Marwick TH: Exercise training for patients with heart failure: A systematic review of factors that improve mortality and morbidity. Am J Med 2004;116:693–706.
27. Piepoli MF, Davos C, Francis DP, et al: Exercise training meta-analysis of trials in patients with chronic heart failure. BMJ 2004;328:189–195.
28. Holloszy JO: Minireview. Exercise and longevity: Studies on rats. J Gerontol 1988; 43:149–151.
29. Lundeberg T, Kohler R, Bucinskaite V, et al: Physical exercise increases survival after an experimental myocardial infarction in rates. Cardiology 1998;90:28–31.
30. Powers SK, Quindry J, Hamilton K: Aging, exercise, and cardioprotection. Ann NY Acad Sci 2004;1019:462–470.
31. Kramsch DM, Aspen AJ, Abramowitz BM, et al: Reduction of coronary atherosclerosis by moderate conditioning exercise in monkeys on an atherogenic diet. N Engl J Med 1981;305:1483–1489.
32. American College of Sports Medicine: Position stand on the recommended quantity and quality of exercise for developing and maintaining cardiorespiratory and muscular fitness in healthy adults. Med Sci Sports Exerc 1998;30:975–991.
33. Myers J, Froelicher VF: Exercise testing and prescription. Phys Med Rehabil Clin N Am 1995;6:117–151.
34. American Association of Cardiovascular and Pulmonary Rehabilitation: Guidelines for Cardiac Rehabilitation programs, 4th ed. Champaign, Ill., Human Kinetics, 2003.
35. Verrill DE, Ribisl PM: Resistive exercise training in cardiac rehabilitation: A review. Sports Med 1996;21:347–383.
36. Ehsani AA, Hagberg JM, Hickson RC: Rapid changes in left ventricular dimensions and mass in response to physical conditioning and deconditioning. Am J Cardiol 1978;42:52–56.
37. DeMaria AN, Neumann A, Lee G, et al: Alterations in ventricular mass and performance induced by exercise training in man evaluated by echocardiography. Circulation 1978;57:237–244.
38. Stein RA, Michielli D, Fox EL, et al: Continuous ventricular dimensions in man during supine exercise and recovery. Am J Cardiol 1978;41:655–660.
39. Parrault H, Peronnet F, Cleroux J, et al: Electro– and echocardiographic assessment of left ventricle before and after training in man. Can J Appl Sports Sci 1978;3:180–186.
40. Wolfe LA, Martin RP, Watson DD, et al: Chronic exercise and left ventricular structure and function in healthy human subjects. J Appl Physiol 1985;58:409–415.
41. Adams TD, Yanowitz FG, Fischer AG, et al: Noninvasive evaluation of exercise training in college-age men. Circulation 1981;64: 958–965.
42. Landry F, Bouchard C, Dumesnil J: Cardiac dimension changes with endurance training. JAMA 1985;254:77–80.
43. Ehsani AA, Heath GW, Haberg JM, et al: Effects of 12 months of intense exercise training on myocardial ST-segment depression in patients with coronary artery disease. Circulation 1981;64:1116–1124.
44. Ditchey RV, Watkins J, McKirnan MD, et al: Effects of exercise training on left ventricular mass in patients with ischemic heart disease. Am Heart J 1981;101:701–706.
45. Giannuzzi P, Temporelli PL, Corra U, et al: Antiremodeling effect of long-term exercise training in patients with stable chronic heart failure. Results of the exercise in left ventricular dysfunction and chronic heart failure trial. Circulation 2003;108:554–559.
46. Myers J, Ahnve S, Froelicher V, et al: A randomized trial of the effects of 1 year of exercise training on computer-measured ST segment displacement in patients with coronary artery disease. J Am Coll Cardiol 1984;4:1094–1102.
47. Haskell WL, Alderman EL, Fair JM, et al: Effects of intensive multiple risk factor reduction on coronary atherosclerosis and clinical

cardiac events in men and women with coronary artery disease: The Stanford Coronary Risk Intervention Project (SCRIP). Circulation 1994;89:975–990.

48. Kannel WB, Wilson P, Blair SN: Epidemiological assessment of the role of physical activity and fitness in development of cardiovascular disease. Am Heart J 1985;109:876–885.

49. Paffenbarger RS, Hyde RT, Wing AL, et al: The association of changes in physical-activity level and other lifestyle characteristics with mortality among men. N Engl J Med 1993;328:538–545.

50. Myers JN, Prakash M, Froelicher VF, et al: Exercise capacity and mortality among men referred for exercise testing. N Engl J Med 2002;346:793–801.

51. Blair SN, Kohl HW, Barlow CE, et al: Changes in physical fitness and all-cause mortality. A prospective study of health and unhealthy men. JAMA 1995;273:1093–1098.

52. Tanasescu M, Leitzmann MF, Rimm EB, et al: Exercise type and intensity in relation to coronary heart disease in men. JAMA 2002;288:1994–2000.

53. Vermeulen A, Lie K, Durrer D: Effects of cardiac rehabilitation after myocardial infarction: Changes in coronary risk factors and long-term prognosis. Am Heart J 1983;105:789–801.

54. Schuler G, Hambrecht R, Schlierf G, et al: Regular physical exercise and low-fat diet: Effects of progression of coronary artery disease. Circulation 1992;86:1–11.

55. DeBusk RF, Houston Miller N, Superko HR, et al: A case-management system for coronary risk factor modification after acute myocardial infarction. Ann Intern Med 1994;120:721–729.

56. Hambrecht R, Niebauer J, Marburger C, et al: Various intensities of leisure time physical activity in patients with coronary artery disease: Effects on cardiorespiratory fitness and progression of coronary atherosclerotic lesions. J Am Coll Cardiol 1993;22:468–477.

57. Fletcher BJ, Dunbar SB, Felner JM, et al: Exercise testing and training in physically disabled men with clinical evidence of coronary artery disease. Am J Cardiol 1994;73:170–174.

58. Nikolaus T, Schlierf G, Vogel G, et al: Treatment of coronary heart disease with diet and exercise-problems of compliance. Ann Nutr Metab 1991;85:1–7.

59. Kinsey GM, Fletcher BJ, Rice CR, et al: Coronary risk factor modification followed by home-monitored exercise in coronary bypass surgery patients: A four-year follow-up study. J Cardiopulm Rehabil 1989;9:207–212.

60. Cannistra LB, Balady GJ, O'Malley CJ, et al: Comparison of the clinical profile and outcome of women and men in cardiac rehabilitation. Am J Cardiol 1992;69:1274–1279.

61. Milani RV, Lavie CJ, Mehra MR: Reduction in C-reactive protein through cardiac rehabilitation and exercise training. J Am Coll Cardiol 2004;43:1056–1061.

62. Mattusch F, Dufaux B, Heine O, et al: Reduction of the plasma concentration of C-reactive protein following nine months of endurance training. Int J Sports Med 2000;21:21–24.

63. Vincent KR, Braith RW, Bottiglieri T, et al: Homocysteine and lipoprotein levels following resistance training in older adults. Prev Cardiol 2003;6:197–203.

64. Ali A, Mehra MR, Lavie CJ, et al: Modulatory impact of cardiac rehabilitation on hyperhomocysteinemia in patients with coronary artery disaese and "normal" lipid levels. Am J Cardial 1998;82:1543–1545.

65. Engblom E, Ronnemaa T, Hamaleinen H, et al: Coronary heart disease risk factors before and after bypass surgery: Results of a controlled trial on multifactorial rehabilitation. Eur Heart J 1992;13:232–237.

66. Kallio V, Hamaleinen H, Hakkila J, Luurila OJ: Reduction in sudden deaths by a multifactorial intervention programme after acute myocardial infarction. Lancet 1979;2:1091–1094.

67. Hamaleinen H, Luurila OJ, Kallio V, et al: Long-term reduction in sudden deaths after a multifactorial intervention programme in patients with myocardial infarction: 10-year results of a controlled investigation. Eur Heart J 1989;10:55–62.

68. Taylor CB, Miller NH: Principles of health behavior change: In ACSM Resource Manual for Exercise Testing and Prescription, 4th ed. Baltimore, Lippincott Williams & Wilkins, 2001, pp 556–561.

69. Ornish D, Brown SE, Scherwitz LW, et al: Can lifestyle changes reverse coronary heart disease? The Lifestyle Heart Trial. Lancet 1990; 336:129–133.

70. Savage PD, Lee M, Harvey-Berino J, et al: Weight reduction in the cardiac rehabilitation setting. J Cardiopulm Rehabil 2002;22:154–160.

71. Despres JP: Physical activity and adipose tissue: In Bouchard C, Shepard RJ, Stephens RJ (eds): Physical Activity, Fitness and Health. Champaign, Ill., Human Kinetics, 1994, pp 358–368.

72. Glenny AM, O'Meara S, Melville A, et al: The treatment and prevention of obesity: A systematic review of the literature. Int J Obes Relat Metab Disord 1997; 21:715–737.

73. Atkinson RL, Walberg-Rankin J: Physical activity, fitness, and severe obesity. In Bouchard C, Shepard RJ, Stephens T (eds): Physical Activity, Fitness and Health. Champaign, Ill., Human Kinetics, 1994, pp 696–711.

74. Avenell A, Brown TJ, McGee MA, et al: What interventions should we add to weight reducing diets in adults with obesity? A systematic review of randomized controlled trials of adding drug therapy, exercise, behaviour therapy or combinations of these interventions. J Hum Nutr Diet 2004;17:293–316.

75. Fagard RH: Physical activity, fitness, and hypertension. In Bouchard C, Shepard RJ, Stephens T (eds): Physical Activity, Fitness and Health. Champaign, Ill, Human Kinetics, 1994, pp 633–655.

76. Criqui MH, Mebane I, Wallace RB, et al: Multivariate correlates of adult blood pressures in nine North American populations: The lipid research clinics prevalence study. Prev Med 1982;11:391–402.

77. Pescatello LS, Franklin BA, Fagard R, et al: American College of Sports Medicine position stand. Exercise and hypertension. Med Sci Sports Exerc 2004;36:533–553.

78. Reaven PD, Barret-Connor E, Edelstein S: Relation between leisure-time physical activity and blood pressure in older women. Circulation 1991;83:559–565.

79. Carroll S, Cooke CB, Butterly RJ: Metabolic clustering, physical activity and fitness in nonsmoking middle-aged men. Med Sci Sports Exerc 2000;32:2079–2086.

80. Cooper KH, Pollock ML, Martin RP, et al: Physical fitness levels vs selected coronary risk factors: A cross-sectional study. JAMA 1976;236:166–169.

81. Hartung GH, Kohl HW, Blair SN, et al: Exercise tolerance and alcohol intake: Blood pressure relation. Hypertension 1990;16:501–507.

82. Gibbons LW, Blair SN, Cooper KH, Smith M: Association between coronary heart disease risk factors and physical fitness in healthy adult women. Circulation 1983;67:977–983.

83. Carnethon MR, Gidding SS, Nehgme R, et al: Cardiorespiratory fitness in young adulthood and the development of cardiovascular disease risk factors. JAMA 2003;290:3092–3100.

84. Aronson D, Sella R, Sheikh-Ahmad M, et al: The association between cardiorespiratory fitness and C-reactive protein in subjects with the metabolic syndrome. J Am Coll Cardiol 2004;44: 2003–2007.

85. Church TS, Barlow CE, Earnest CP, et al: Associations between cardiorespiratory fitness and C-reactive protein in men. Arterioscler Thromb Vasc Biol 2002;21:1869–1876.

86. Herrmann M, Wilkinson J, Schorr H, et al: Comparison of the influence of volume-oriented training and high-intensity interval training on serum homocysteine and its cofactors in young, healthy swimmers. Clin Chem Lab Med 2003;41:1525–1531.

87. Duncan GE, Perri MG, Anton SD, et al: Effects of exercise on emerging and traditional cardiovascular risk factors. Prev Med 2004;39:894–902.

88. Hahn RA, Teutsh SM, Rothenberg RB, Marks JS: Excess deaths from nine chronic diseases in the United States. JAMA 1986;264:2654–2659.

89. McGinnis JM, Foege WH: Actual causes of death in the United States. JAMA 1993;270:2207–2212.

90. Booth FW, Gordon SE, Carlson CJ, et al: Waging war on modern chronic disease: Primary prevention through exercise biology. J Appl Physiol 2000;88:774–787.

91. Haskell WL, Leon AS, Caspersen CJ, et al: Cardiovascular benefits and, assessment of physical activity and physical fitness in adults. Med Sci Sports Exerc 1992;24:S201–S220.

92. Manson JE, Greenland P, LaCroix AZ, et al: Walking compared with vigorous exercise for the prevention of cardiovascular events in women. N Engl J Med 2002;347:716–725.

93. Myers J, Atwood JE, Froelicher VF: Active lifestyle and diabetes. Circulation 2003;107:2392–2394.

94. Tanasescu M, Leitzmann MF, Rimm EB, et al: Physical activity in relation to cardiovascular disease and total mortality among men with type 2 diabetes. Circulation 2003;107;2435–2439.

95. Hu FB, Sigal RJ, Rich-Edwards JW, et al: Walking compared with vigorous physical activity and risk of type 2 diabetes in women: A prospective study. JAMA 1999;282:1433–1439.

96. Hu FB, Stampfer MJ, Solomon C, et al: Physical activity and risk for cardiovascular events in diabetic women. Ann Intern Med 2001;134:96–105.

97. Helmrich SP, Ragland DR, Leung RW, Paffenbarger RS: Physical activity and reduced occurrence of non-insulin dependent diabetes mellitus. N Engl J Med 1991;325:147–152.

98. Manson JE, Nathan DM, Kroleski AS, et al: A prospective study of exercise and incidence of diabetes among U.S. male physicians. JAMA 1992;268:63–67.

99. Manson JE, Rimm EB, Stampfer MJ, et al: Physical activity and incidence of non-insulin dependent diabetes mellitus in women. Lancet 1991;338:774–775.

100. Hagberg JM: Exercise, fitness, and hypertension. In Bouchard TC, Shepard RJ, Stephens T, et al. (eds): Exercise, Fitness, and Health. Champaign, Ill., Human Kinetics, 1994, pp 455–566.

101. Krousel-Wood MA, Muntner P, He J, et al: Primary prevention of essential hypertension. Med Clin North Am 2004;88:223–238.

102. Marcus R: Drinkwater B, Dalsky G, et al: Osteoporosis and exercise in women. Med Sci Sports Exerc 1992;24:S301–S307.

103. Murphy NM, Carroll P: The effect of physical activity and its interaction with nutrition and bone health. Proc Nutr Soc 2003; 62:829–839.

104. Lee I, Paffenbarger RS, Hsieh C: Physical activity and risk of developing colorectal cancer among college alumni. J Natl Cancer Inst 1991;83:1324–1329.

105. Thune I, Furberg AS: Physical activity and cancer risk; dose-response and cancer, all sites and site-specific. Med Sci Sports Exerc 2001;33(suppl):S530–S550.

106. Pate RR, Pratt MP, Blair SN, et al: Physical activity and public health. A recommendation from the Centers for Disease Control and Prevention and the American College of Sports Medicine. JAMA 1995;273:402–407.

107. U.S. Public Health Service, Office of the Surgeon General: Physical Activity and Health: A Report of the Surgeon General. Atlanta, U.S. Department of Health and Human Services, Centers for Disease Control and Prevention, National Center for Chronic Disease Prevention and Health Promotion, 1996.

108. Paffenbarger RS, Hyde RT, Wing AL, et al: Some interrelations of physical activity, physiological fitness, health, and longevity. In Bouchard C, Shephard RJ, Stephens T (eds): Physical Activity, Fitness, and Health, pp 119–133. Champaign, Ill., Human Kinetics, 1994.

109. Kohl HW: Physical activity and cardiovascular disease: Evidence for a dose response. Med Sci Sports Exerc 2001;33(suppl): S472–S483.

110. Lee IM, Paffenbarger RS: Do physical activity and physical fitness avert premature mortality? Exerc Sport Sci Rev 1996;24: 135–172.

111. Gulati M, Pandey DK, Arnsdorf MF, et al: Exercise capacity and the risk of death in women. The St James Women Take Heart Project. Circulation 2003;108:1554–1559.

112. Blair S, Kohl H III, Barlow C, et al: Changes in physical fitness and all-cause mortality: A prospective study of healthy and unhealthy men. JAMA 1995;273:1093–1098.

113. Erikssen G, Liestol K, Bjornholt J, et al: Changes in physical fitness and changes in mortality. Lancet 1998;352:759–762.

114. American College of Sports Medicine Position Stand: The recommended quantity and quality of exercise for developing and maintaining cardiorespiratory and muscular fitness, and flexibility in healthy adults. Med Sci Sports Exerc 1998;30:975–991.

115. Thompson PC, Buchner D, Pina IL, et al. Exercise and physical activity in the prevention and treatment of atherosclerotic cardiovascular disease: A statement from the American Heart Association Council on Clinical Cardiology (Subcommittee on Exercise, Rehabilitation, and Prevention) and the Council on Nutrition, Physical Activity, and Metabolism (Subcommittee on Physical Activity). Circulation 2003;107:3109–3116.

116. Centers for Disease Control and Prevention. Prevalence of sedentary lifestyle behavioral risk factor surveillance system, United States 1991. MMWR Morb Mortal Wkly Rep 1993;42:576–579.

117. Morris JN, Crawford MD: Coronary heart disease and physical activity. BMJ 1958;2:1485–1496.

118. Morris JN: Uses of Epidemiology. London, Churchill Livingstone, 1975.

119. Oliver RM: Physique and serum lipids of young London busmen in relation to ischemic heart disease. Br J Ind Med 1967;24: 181–187.

120. Stamler J, Kjelsberg M, Hall Y: Epidemiologic studies on cardiovascular-renal diseases: Analysis of mortality by age-race-sex-occupation. J Chronic Dis 1960;12:440–445.

121. Blackburn H, Taylor HL, Keys A: Coronary heart disease in seven countries. Circulation 1970;41:I154–I161.

122. Epstein L, Miller GJ, Stitt FW, et al: Vigorous exercise in leisure time, coronary risk factors, and resting electrocardiogram in middle-aged male civil servants. Br Heart J 1976;38:403–409.

123. Costas R, Garcia-Palmieri MR, Nazario E, et al: Relation of lipids, weight and physical activity to incidence of coronary heart disease. Am J Cardiol 1978;42:653–660.

124. Paffenbarger RS, Laughlin ME, Gima AS, et al: Work activity of longshoremen as related to death from coronary heart disease and stroke. N Engl J Med 1970;282:1109–1114.

125. Paffenbarger RS, Wing AL, Hyde RT: Physical activity as an index of heart attack risk in college alumni. Am J Epidemiol 1978;108: 161–167.

126. Paffenbarger RS, Wing AL, Hyde RT: Chronic disease in former college students: Physical activity as an index of heart attack risk in college alumni. Am J Epidemiol 1981;108:161–175.

127. Lee IM, Sesso HD, Oguma Y, et al: Relative intensity of physical activity and risk of coronary heart disease. Circulation 2003;107: 1110–1116.

128. Sesso HD, Paffenbarger RS, Lee IM: Physical activity and coronary heart disease in men: The Harvard Alumni Health Study. Circulation 2000;102:975–980.

129. Lakka TA, Venalainen JM, Rauramaa R, et al: Relation of leisure-time physical activity and cardiorespiratory fitness to the risk of acute myocardial infarction in men. N Engl J Med 1994;330:1549–1954.

130. Shaper AG, Wannamethee G: Physical activity and ischaemic heart disease in middle-aged British men. Br Heart J 1991;66: 384–394.

131. Slattery ML, Jacobs DR, Nichaman MZ: Leisure time physical activity and coronary heart disease death. The US Railroad Study. Circulation 1989;79:304–311.

132. Lee IM, Sesso HD, Paffenbarger RS: Physical activity and coronary heart disease risk in men. Does the duration of exercise episodes predict risk? Circulation 2000;102:981–986.

133. Kannel WB, Belanger A, D'Agostino R, et al: Physical activity and physical demand on the job and risk of CV disease and death: The Framingham study. Am Heart J 1986;112:820–825.

134. Leon AS, Connett J, Jacobs DR, Rauramaa R: Leisure-time physical activity levels and risk of coronary heart disease and death. JAMA 1987;258:2388–2395.

135. Morris CK, Ueshima K, Kawaguchi T, et al: The prognostic value of exercise capacity: A review of the literature. Am Heart J 1991;122:1423–1431.

136. Myers J, Gullestad L: The role of exercise testing and gas exchange measurement in the prognostic assessment of patients with heart failure. Curr Opin Cardiol 1998;13:145–155.

137. Mark DB, Lauer MS: The prognostic variable that doesn't get enough respect. Circulation 2003;108:1534–1536.

138. Myers J: Beyond ST-segment displacement: Newer diagnostic and prognostic markers from the exercise test. Am J Med Sports 2003;5:332–336.

139. Blair SN, Kohl HW III, Paffenbarger RS, et al: Physical fitness and all-cause mortality: A prospective study of healthy men and women. JAMA 1989;262:2395–2401.

140. Ekelund LG, Haskell WL, Johnson JL, et al: Physical fitness as a predictor of cardiovascular mortality in asymptomatic North American men. The Lipid Research Clinics Mortality Follow-up. N Engl J Med 1988;319:1379–1389.

141. Roger VL, Jacobsen SJ, Pellikka PA, et al: Prognostic value of treadmill exercise testing: A population-based study in Olmsted County, Minnesota. Circulation 1998;98:2836–2841.

142. Goraya TY, Jacobsen SJ, Pellikka PA, et al: Prognostic value of treadmill exercise testing in elderly persons. Ann Intern Med 2000;132:862–870.

143. Snader CE, Marwick TH, Pashkow FJ, et al: Importance of estimated functional capacity as a predictor of all-cause mortality

among patients referred for exercise thallium single-photon emission computed tomography: Report of 3,400 patients from a single center. J Am Coll Cardiol 1997;30:641–648.

144. Mora S, Redberg RF, Cui Y, et al: Ability of exercise testing to predict cardiovascular and all-cause death in asymptomatic women. A 20-year follow-up of the Lipid Research Clinics Prevalence Study. JAMA 2003;290:1600–1607.

145. Balady GJ, Larson MG, Vasan RS, et al: Usefulness of exercise testing in the prediction of coronary disease risk among asymptomatic persons as a function of the Framingham risk score. Circulation 2004;110:1920–1925.

146. Leon AS, Jacobs DR, DeBacker G, et al: Relationship of physical characteristics of life habits to treadmill exercise capacity. Am J Epidemiol 1981;113:653–660.

147. Peters RK, Cady LD, Bischoff DP, et al: Physical fitness and subsequent myocardial infarction in healthy workers. JAMA 1983;249: 3052–3056.

148. Blair SN, Cooper KH, Gibbons LW, et al: Changes in coronary heart disease risk factors associated with increased treadmill time in 753 men. Am J Epidemiol 1983;118:352–359.

149. Brill PB, Burkhalter HE, Kohl HW, et al: The impact of previous athleticism on exercise habits, physical fitness, and coronary heart disease risk factors in middle-aged men. Res Q Exerc Sport 1989;60:202–215.

150. Lie H, Mundal R, Erikssen J: Coronary risk factors and incidence of coronary death in relation to physical fitness. Seven year follow-up study of middle-aged and elderly men. Eur Heart J 1985;6:147–157.

151. Williams PT: Physical fitness and activity as separate heart disease risk factors: A meta-analysis. Med Sci Sports Exerc 2001;33: 754–761.

152. Blair SN, Jackson AS: Physical fitness and activity as separate heart disease risk factors: A meta-analysis. Med Sci Sports Exerc 2001;33:754–761.

153. Myers J, Kaykha A, George S, et al: Fitness versus physical activity patterns in predicting mortality in men. Am J Med 2005;117:912–918.

154. Blackburn H, Jacobs DR: Physical activity and the risk of coronary heart disease. N Engl J Med 1988;319:1217–1219.

155. Hein HO, Suadicani P, Gyntelberg F: Physical fitness or physical activity as a predictor of ischaemic heart disease? A 17-year follow-up in the Copenhagen Male Study. J Int Med 1992;232: 471–479.

156. Powell KE, Thompson PD, Caspersen CJ, Kendrick JS: Physical activity and the incidence of coronary heart disease. Annu Rev Public Health 1987;8:253–287.

157. Steffen-Batey L, Nichaman MZ, Goff DC, et al: Change in level of physical activity and risk of all-cause mortality or reinfarction. The Corpus Christi Heart Project. Circulation 2000;102: 2204–2209.

158. Fletcher GF, Blair SN, Blumenthal J, et al: Statement on exercise. Benefits and recommendations for physical activity programs for all Americans. A statement for health professionals by the committee on exercise and cardiac rehabilitation of the council on clinical cardiology. Circulation 1996;94:857–862.

159. National Institutes of Health: Consensus development conference statement on physical activity and cardiovascular health. Bethesda, Md, 1995.

160. Damush TM, Stewart AL, Mills KM, et al: Prevalence and correlates of physician recommendations to exercise among older adults. J Gerontol A Biol Sci Med Sci 1999;54:M423–M427.

161. Bassler TJ: Marathon running and immunity to atherosclerosis. Ann NY Acad Sci 1977;301:579–592.

162. Siscovik DS, Weiss NS, Fletcher RH, Lasky T: The incidence of primary cardiac arrest during vigorous exercise. N Engl J Med 1984;311:874–877.

163. Waller BF, Roberts WC: Sudden death while running in conditioned runners aged 40 years or over. Am J Cardiol 1980;45: 1291–1300.

164. Thompson PD, Stern MP, Williams P, et al: Death during jogging or running (in California). JAMA 1979;242:1265–1267.

165. Waller BF: Exercise-related sudden death in young (≤30 years) and old (>30 years) conditioned subjects. Cardiovasc Clin 1985;15:9–73.

166. Thompson PD, Funk EJ, Carleton RA, Sturner WQ: Incidence of death during jogging in Rhode Island from 1975 through 1980. JAMA 1982;247:2535–2538.

167. Vander L, Franklin B, Rubenfire M: Cardiovascular complications of recreational physical activity. Physician Sports Med 1982; 10:89–98.

168. Koplan JP: Cardiovascular deaths while running. JAMA 1979;242:2578–2579.

169. Morales AR, Romanelli R, Boucek RJ: The mural left anterior descending coronary artery, strenuous exercise and sudden death. Circulation 1980;62:230–237.

170. Noakes TD, Opie LH, Rose AG, et al: Autopsy-proved coronary atherosclerosis in marathon runners. N Engl J Med 1979;301:86–89.

171. Noakes TD: Heart disease in marathon runners: A review. Med Sci Sports Exerc 1987;19:187–194.

172. Virmani R, McAllister HA: Coronary heart disease at young age: A report of 187 autopsy patients who died of severe coronary atherosclerosis. Cardiovasc Rev Rep 1984;5:799–809.

173. Virmani R, Robinowitz M: Cardiac pathology and sports medicine. Hum Pathol 1987;18:493–501.

174. Opie LH: Sudden death and sport. Lancet 1975;306:263–266.

175. Northcote RJ, Evans ADB, Ballantyne D: Sudden death in squash players. Lancet 1984;323:148–151.

176. Corrado D, Thiene G, Nava A, et al: Sudden death in young competitive athletes: Clinicopathologic correlations in 22 cases. Am J Med 1990;89:588–595.

177. Corrado D, Basso C, Schiavon M, Thiene G: Screening for hypertrophic cardiomyopathy in young athletes. N Engl J Med 1998;339:364–369.

178. Maron BJ, Epstein SE, Roberts WC: Causes of sudden death in competitive athletes. J Am Coll Cardiol 1986;7:204–214.

179. Maron BJ, Shirani J, Poliac LC, et al: Sudden death in young competitive athletes. Clinical, demographic, and pathological profiles. JAMA 1996;276:199–204.

180. Van Camp SP, Bloor CM, Mueller FO, et al: Nontraumatic sports death in high school and college athletes. Med Sci Sports Exerc 1995;27:641–647.

181. Mittleman MA, Maclure M, Tofler GH, et al: Triggering of acute myocardial infarction by heavy physical exertion. Protection against triggering by regular exertion. N Engl J Med 1993;329: 1677–1683.

182. Willich SN, Lewis M, Lowel H, et al: Physical exertion as a trigger of acute myocardial infarction. N Engl J Med 1993;329: 1684–1690.

183. Cobb LA, Weaver D: Exercise: A risk for sudden death in patients with coronary artery disease. J Am Coll Cardiol 1986;7:215–219.

184. Hinkle LE, Whitney JA, Lehman EW, et al: Occupation, education, and coronary heart disease. Science 1968;161:238–246.

185. De Loes M, Goldie I: Incidence rate of injuries during sport activity and physical exercise in a rural Swedish municipality: Incidence rates in 17 sports. Int J Sports Med 1988;9:461–467.

186. Knochel JP: Catastrophic medical events with exhaustive exercise: "White collar rhabdomyolysis." Kidney Int 1990;38:709–719.

187. Leon AS: Physiological interactions between diet and exercise in the etiology and prevention of ischaemic heart disease. Ann Clin Res 1988;20:114–120.

188. Myers J: Exercise and cardiovascular health. Circulation 2003;107:e2–e5.

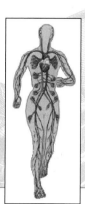

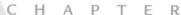

fourteen

Cardiac Rehabilitation

INTRODUCTION

Cardiac rehabilitation developed in the 1960s as a treatment for patients who had sustained a myocardial infarction (MI). Before the 1970s, the patient who had an MI was almost completely immobilized for 6 weeks or more and was even washed, shaved, and fed by others in order to keep the work of the heart to a minimum (Table 14-1). It was thought that this approach provided the heart with the opportunity to form a firm scar. The patient was also told not to expect to be able to return to a normal life. These were incorrect beliefs, particularly with an uncomplicated MI. Prolonged immobilization not only did not speed healing but exposed the patient to the additional risks of venous thrombosis, pulmonary embolism, muscle atrophy, lung infection, and deconditioning. Equally serious was the psychological result of such an approach, which often led to psychological impairment.

Today, the physician's approach to the patient with acute MI has changed dramatically.[1] The infarct is often interrupted by thrombolysis and/or coronary interventions that leave the heart relatively undamaged and able to withstand future ischemic stresses. When the infarct completes because of delay in treatment or confounding illnesses, a relatively brief period of time monitored by the advanced technology in the coronary care unit is followed by early mobilization, sitting at the bedside, graduated exercise and, in the uncomplicated case, discharge of the patient from the hospital in less than a week. This policy has been shown by randomized trials to be safe from the point of view of cardiac complications. In-patient rehabilitation is brief, but interaction with healthcare professionals, educational videos, and pamphlets can begin the patient's education. Iatrogenic deconditioning is no longer a problem, because there are no medical concerns about beginning a walking program very early. Psychological rehabilitation takes place in the doctor's office, along with prescribing exercise and education. Certainly all patients do not need all rehabilitative interventions, but exercise programs, educational sessions, group therapy, and psychological and vocational counseling are available in most communities, and nearly all patients benefit in some way from the various components of comprehensive rehabilitation.

Hospital admission for an acute MI or an intervention to avoid its progression is a stressful experience, one with a powerful impact. But it must be remembered that hospital discharge, although less dramatic, can be equally stressful after the patient has relied on the highly protective hospital support systems. Discharge into an uncertain future and to home and work, where one is considered disabled, can be as harmful to one's self-esteem as the acute event itself. The healthcare system is faced with the difficult task not only of supervising the physical recovery of the patient, but also of maintaining morale, providing education, helping the family cope and provide support, and facilitating the return to a gratifying lifestyle. Cardiac rehabilitation can be considered as the conservation of human life. Its goal is to restore the patient to optimal physiologic, psychological, and vocational status.

Though the death rate for coronary heart disease (CHD) has been decreasing steadily since the mid-1960s, it still remains the leading cause of

TABLE 14–1. Previous recommendations for bed rest following acute myocardial infarction from major cardiology textbooks

Lewis T (Diseases of the Heart. New York, Macmillan, 1937)	8 wk of bed rest
White PD (Heart Disease, 3rd ed. New York, Macmillan, 1945)	4 wk of bed rest
Wood P (Diseases of the Heart and Circulation, 2nd ed. London, Eyre and Spottiswoode, 1960)	3–6 wk of bed rest
Friedberg CK (Diseases of the Heart, 3rd ed. Philadelphia, W.B. Saunders, 1996)	2–3 wk of minimum bed rest
Wood P (Diseases of the Heart and Circulation, 3rd ed. London, Eyre and Spottiswoode, 1968)	2 wk of bed rest

death in the United States.[2] Four deaths in every 10 are due to cardiac disorders and of these, 90% can be attributed to CHD. The four distinct clinical manifestations of CHD are primary cardiac arrest, stable angina pectoris, acute coronary syndromes (ACS),[1] and acute MI. The resting ECG is critical to guiding therapy with ST elevation indicating the prompt application of thrombolysis or percutaneous coronary interventions (PCI) and ST depression requiring antiplatelet drugs (see Fig. 9-1).

Each year 900,000 people in the United States experience an acute MI. Of these, roughly 225,000 die, including 125,000 who die before obtaining medical care. The fatality rate in MI patients is temporally related to onset. The risk of death is highest within the first 24 hours of onset of signs and/or symptoms and declines throughout the following year. Following the onset of a first-time MI in middle-aged males, 30% to 50% die within 30 days and 85% of these deaths occur within the first 24 hours. Those patients with a first-time MI who actually reach a hospital alive have a 10% to 18% risk of dying before discharge. The mortality thereafter falls from an annualized rate of 9% over months 2 through 6, to 4% for months 7 through 30, to 3% over the next 3 years. Other studies have suggested a mortality rate of 11% in the first 3 months after hospital discharge and lower rates thereafter. In comparison to standard medical therapy, thrombolytic therapy is associated with a highly significant 20% reduction in 35-day mortality among patients with acute MI and ST elevation, corresponding to an overall reduction of 21 deaths per 1000 patients treated. All of these statistics are less meaningful than in the past due to two changes in healthcare: (1) the use of troponin to define MI[3] and ACS and (2) data supporting emergency PCI as superior to thrombolysis.[4] Temporal comparison studies have suggested a contemporary reduction in mortality due to modern therapies and prevention.[2,5] The impact of the 30% reduction in mortality with implantable defibrillators in patients with history of MI with LV dysfunction has not even been factored in yet.

Disability Due to MI

Cardiovascular diseases, largely atherosclerotic, are also the leading cause of activity limitation and disabled worker benefits in the United States and are the fourth leading cause of days lost from work. In fact, coronary artery disease (CAD) alone is responsible for almost one out of five disability allowances paid by the Social Security Administration. However, the total economic impact of disability related to cardiovascular diseases results from the combination of Social Security benefits, welfare support, disability insurance income, unemployment compensation, loss of taxable revenue, and reduced worker productivity related to these diseases. From a purely economic standpoint, it is essential that patients with CAD be rehabilitated as quickly and efficiently as possible in order to enable their return to remunerative employment. Just as important, however, is the psychosocial impact of heart disease, which cannot be measured in dollars lost. Clearly, improved quality of life, including lessened depression and an expedient return to preillness social roles within the family and community, should be another important goal in the effective rehabilitation of patients with heart disease.

With the addition of thrombolysis and acute catheter interventions to MI treatment, disability incurred by an MI has decreased. Today's standard practice is that 85% or more of MI patients undergo cardiac catheterization. Because of the functional benefits observed in cardiac rehabilitation, physicians have extended rehabilitation services to other groups of patients. These patients include those who have undergone PCI, coronary artery bypass grafting (CABG), pacemakers for cardiac resynchronization, transplantation, and valve surgery. Other patients for consideration include those limited by angina or heart failure or whose heart disease is complicated by additional illnesses, particularly diabetes, the metabolic syndrome, and renal insufficiency. We begin this chapter by reviewing the pathophysiology of MI as it relates to rehabilitation.

PATHOPHYSIOLOGY OF AN ACUTE MYOCARDIAL INFARCTION

Infarct Severity

MIs basically are divided into two groups: those that evolve Q waves and result in larger area/transmural myocardial cell death, and those that do not evolve Q waves and only result in smaller area/subendocardial cell death.[6] Subendocardial MI cannot be localized, whereas transmural MI can be roughly localized by the Q-wave pattern. Attempts have been made to judge the size or severity of an MI electrocardiographically by Q-wave and R-wave scores, and body surface mapping has even been used, but these methods only provide rough estimates. In general, the greater the number of areas with Q waves and the greater the R-wave loss, the larger the MI. Non-Q-wave MIs are not often associated with complications such as congestive heart failure (CHF) or shock; however, they can be complicated, particularly when a prior MI has occurred or the patient has diabetes. With an uncomplicated MI, prognosis is particularly good if the patient does not have a prior MI or a decreased ejection fraction. Because more myocardium has survived, patients with non-Q-wave MIs are more likely to suffer ischemic events. Anterior Q-wave MIs usually are larger than inferior infarcts and are more likely to be associated with CHF and cardiogenic shock. Anterior infarcts are also more likely to cause aneurysms and a greater decrease in ejection fraction. Surprisingly, however, in follow-up studies, anterior Q-wave MIs have a similar or only slightly poorer prognosis than inferior Q-wave MIs.[7] Fifteen percent of patients with Q-wave MIs lose their Q waves over the following year but still have the same prognosis as those who do not lose their Q waves.

Using magnetic resonance imaging (MRI) to determine the pathologic basis of Q-wave and non-Q-wave MI, a total of 100 consecutive patients with documented previous MIs were recently studied.[8] Subendocardial damage was associated with Q waves about a third of the time, while transmural damage was associated with Q waves only about two thirds of the time. As MI size and number of transmural segments increased by MRI, the probability of Q waves on the ECG increased. These findings did not hold for lateral MI. In a multivariate model, the transmural extent of MI was not an independent predictor of Q waves when total size of MI was removed. The Q-wave/non-Q-wave distinction can be useful, but it is determined by the total size rather than transmural extent of underlying MI.

Risk Prediction

The pathophysiologic determinates of prognosis are: (1) the amount of viable myocardium and (2) the amount of myocardium in jeopardy. Inferences can be made regarding these two factors clinically if a patient has had CHF, or cardiogenic shock, and continued chest pain, or ischemia. Cardiac catheterization assesses this by ejection fraction and the number of vessels occluded. The clinical findings manifested by abnormalities related to these two factors are the basis for several indices that have been used to predict risk. These apply when the infarction damage has not been averted by an intervention. Clinical data remain very useful in triaging patients with regard to the necessary length of stay in the hospital. Patients without these criteria, that is, those with uncomplicated MIs, can be discharged within 3 to 5 days, while those with these criteria require longer hospitalization and closer observation. If the infarction has been averted, the completeness of the revascularization of the intervention determines the outcome.

Healthcare professionals must be able to advise post-MI patients as to what they should or should not do to improve their prognosis. One strategy has been to identify high-risk patients by using various clinical markers and test results.[9,10] Clinical markers that have indicated high risk include: prior MI, CHF, cardiogenic shock, tachycardia, continued chest pain, older age, stroke or transient ischemic attack (TIA), and complicating illnesses. Procedures used to determine risk, with some success, have included the chest x-ray, routine ECG, ambulatory monitoring, radionuclide cardiac tests, exercise testing, and most recently, cardiac biomarkers.[11] The assumption has been that patients at high risk should be considered for intervention; these interventions are CABG and PCI. Because of easy access to these procedures, nearly all patients with history of MI undergo cardiac catheterization prior to discharge, particularly because PCI is currently superseding thrombolysis.[12] Exercise testing is now less often used to decide who needs cardiac catheterization, because catheterization is the clinical norm. In addition, success of PCI is being promoted as superior to exercise testing and clinical risk status for providing criteria for early discharge after MI.

Morbidity and mortality in postinfarction patients who have complicated courses are much higher than in those with uncomplicated MIs. Diabetes doubles the mortality with any type of MI. The criteria for a complicated MI are listed in Table 14-2. The progressive ambulation program should be delayed until such individuals reach an uncomplicated status, and even then progressive ambulation should be slower.

CARDIAC REHABILITATION

Early Ambulation

Prior to 1960, patients with acute MI were thought to require prolonged restriction of physical activity. Patients were often kept at strict bed rest for 2 months with all activities performed by nursing personnel. The concern was that physical activity could lead to complications such as ventricular aneurysm formation, cardiac rupture, heart failure, dysrhythmias, reinfarction, or sudden death. Hospitalization could last for 3 to 4 months with limitations of activities for at least 1 year. Table 14-1 summarizes the recommendations for bed rest in some of the major cardiology textbooks in this century. This approach was based on pathologic studies that indicated that at least 6 weeks were required for necrotic myocardium to form a firm scar, and on the increased prevalence of cardiac rupture reported among patients who infarcted in mental hospitals, where bed rest could not be enforced.

TABLE 14–2. The presence of any one or more of the following criteria classify a myocardial infarction as complicated

Prior myocardial infarction
Continued cardiac ischemia (pain, late enzyme rise)
Left ventricular failure (congestive heart failure, new murmurs, chest x-ray changes)
Shock (blood pressure drop, pallor, oliguria)
Important cardiac dysrhythmias (PVCs greater than 6/min, atrial fibrillation)
Conduction disturbances (bundle branch block, AV block, hemiblock)
Severe pleurisy or pericarditis
Complicating illnesses
Marked creatine kinase rise without a noncardiac explanation
Age >75 yr
Stroke or transient ischemic attack

Animal Experiments of Training Early After Infarction

Hammerman et al[13] designed a study to evaluate the effects of early exercise on late scar formation in a rat model. After occlusion of the proximal left coronary artery, infarct extent was assessed 24 hours later by ECG criteria. The rats were divided into two groups: eight were subjected to daily graded swimming for up to 45 minutes a day for a week, followed by 2 weeks of no swimming; seven served as a control group. Twenty-two days after coronary occlusion, the hearts of both groups were excised and wall thickness determined histologically. A ratio for transmural infarcts was obtained from multiple measurements by dividing scar thickness by noninfarcted septal wall thickness. In the exercise group, there was marked scar thinning. Infarct extent was similar in both groups. They concluded that short-term swimming during the first week after an MI had effects on scar formation when assessed 2 weeks later. A study by Kloner and Kloner,[14] with rats forced to swim 7 days post-MI, reported similar results. Studies performed more recently by Gaudron et al[15] and Oh et al[16] demonstrated that training groups of rats, shortly after experimentally induced infarctions, showed evidence of abnormal ventricular remodeling, including dilation, shape distortion, and scar thinning. Hochman and Healy[17] performed similar experiments and found no signs in their rats of myocardial thinning or aneurysm formation. However, the relevance of rats forced to swim in this manner to the clinical situation is uncertain.

The many animal studies of the 1950s and 1960s were followed by controlled clinical studies of early mobilization, and a greater incidence of death or other complications was not observed among patients mobilized early in the period following an MI compared to those who remained longer in bed rest. In fact, it has been widely recognized for over 30 years that bed rest is associated with many negative physiologic consequences (see in the following sections). The promising results of these studies led to recommendations of gradual mobilization during the early stages following an MI. In many patients, the major cause of decreased exercise capacity is enforced bed rest. The exercise prescription for MI patients in the coronary care unit can avoid iatrogenically induced deconditioning.

Chair Treatment

A revolutionary approach to treatment occurred in the 1940s, when Levine and Lown[18] recommended "chair treatment" for the patient that had experienced an MI. This emphasized the benefits of the sitting versus the supine position for increasing peripheral venous pooling and reducing preload on the myocardium. Levine and Lown theorized correctly that such a reduction would lead to a decrease in resting left ventricular wall tension and to a decrease in myocardial oxygen demand, in addition to decreasing the risk of thrombosis and pulmonary embolism.

Physiologic studies performed since then have documented the hemodynamic alterations caused by bed rest and deconditioning. After prolonged bed rest, tachycardia and hypotension are common upon standing. They are most likely caused by alterations in the baromotor reflexes and by the hypovolemia that occurs with bed rest. Clearly, the disability secondary to most MIs is due both to bed rest and to myocardial dysfunction. The spontaneous hemodynamic improvement usually seen is due both to improving function (scar formation and possibly compensatory hypertrophy) and to a return to normal activities.

Bed Rest: Lack of Activity versus Effects of Gravity

There are now well-defined hemodynamic alterations due to deconditioning from bed rest. These are outlined in Table 14-3. The classic 1968 study by Saltin et al[19] demonstrated that young men maintained at bed rest for 3 weeks demonstrated a 20% to 25% decrease in maximal oxygen uptake. Other than decreased functional capacity, prolonged bed rest can result in orthostatic hypotension and

TABLE 14–3. Physiologic consequences of prolonged bed rest

Loss of muscle mass, strength, and endurance
Decreased plasma and blood volume
Decreased ventricular volume
Increased hematocrit and hemoglobin
Diuresis and natriuresis
Venous stasis
Bone demineralization
Increased heart rate at rest and submaximal levels of activity
Decreased resting and maximum stroke volume
Decreased maximum cardiac output
Decreased maximal oxygen uptake
Increased venous compliance
Increased risk of venous thrombosis and thromboembolism
Decreased orthostatic tolerance
Increased risk of atelectasis, pulmonary emboli

venous thrombosis through a loss of blood volume, in which plasma loss exceeds red blood cell mass loss. Pulmonary function is decreased, and the patient can be in negative nitrogen and calcium balance.

The question has been raised as to whether the deleterious hemodynamic effects of bed rest, including decreased exercise capacity, are due to inactivity or to the loss of the upright exposure to gravity. There are at least four reasons supporting the concept that much of these alterations are caused simply by the latter: (1) supine exercise does not prevent the deconditioning effects of being in bed; (2) there is both a less dramatic and a slower decline in maximal oxygen uptake with chair rest than with bed rest; (3) there is a greater decrease in maximal oxygen uptake after a period of bed rest measured during upright exercise versus supine exercise, and (4) a lower body positive-pressure device decreases the deconditioning effects of bed rest. Clearly, intermittent exposure to gravitational stress during the bed rest stage of hospital convalescence from surgery or MI obviates much of the deterioration in cardiovascular performance that can follow these events. Previous efforts to limit the decrease in functional capacity after an acute MI or surgery have emphasized low-level activities, but studies suggest that simple exposure to gravitational stress substantially accomplishes this.[20]

Progressive Activity

A consideration often forgotten when dealing with older patients or those with complicating illnesses is the level of activity that they maintained prior to their MI. If a patient was physically limited prior to their event, then the plan for progressive ambulation must be modified. It is generally not practical to expect a patient to be more physically active after an MI than before—unless the patient was previously limited by angina that disappeared later. It is important to assess the exercise capacity and activity level that existed prior to the MI.

In addition to the oxygen cost and the heart rate achieved during activity, the duration of the activity must be considered. The effect of prolonged exercise on myocardial scar formation in the acute recovery phase has not been carefully studied, but it is known that during prolonged steady-state dynamic exercise, heart rate increases, myocardial contractility declines, and left ventricular volume increases. It is apparent then, that even though certain work levels can be achieved by a patient, prolonged exercise should be avoided in the acute recovery phase. Probably the safest recommendation is to tell patients not to fatigue themselves and to limit the duration of exercise by their fatigue level and perceived exertion.

Postdischarge activity recommendations have had little basis for their enforcement. Activities involving a return to work, to driving, and/or to sexual activity have been based on clinical judgments rather than physiologic assessments. Because of this, physicians have left much of this up to their patients—allowing them to see how they respond in terms of symptoms—rather than the traditional, very conservative approach, which can foster invalidism. These decisions should be made considering the consequence of the coronary event (ischemia or symptoms of congestive failure, or dysrhythmias) and the nature of the activities (manual labor versus deskwork, light driving versus congested freeway driving, and sex with an established partner versus other relationships).

The impetus for mobilizing patients who had an MI or underwent surgery evolved from clinical studies assessing the physiologic effects of activity in these patients in the 1960s and 1970s. In 1961, Cain et al[21] reported on the use of a progressive activity program for acute MI patients. They had difficulty getting this report accepted for publication because the approach was considered dangerous. They reported 335 patients with an uncomplicated MI who were at least 15 days postinfarction. The patients previously had been restricted to bed, chair, and commode. The ECG was monitored after the patient performed activities such as climbing stairs and walking up a grade. In 1964, Torkelson[22] reported results in 10 patients with an uncomplicated MI. On the sixth week of the in-hospital rehabilitation program, a low-level treadmill test was performed using 1.7 mph at a 10% grade. He concluded that the treadmill test was a valuable procedure for the documentation of the specific exercise response of patients recovering from an acute MI.

Later publications did not include ECG monitoring as part of progressive ambulation. Instead, generalized statements as to the activities on each post-infarct day were made for all patients, rather than individualized activity progression. Sivarajan et al[23] described 12 patients with an acute MI whose symptoms, signs, and hemodynamic and ECG responses during and after three activities (sitting upright, walking to the toilet, and walking on a treadmill) were assessed. Studies of these activities were done at 3, 6, and 10 days after infarction. They concluded that successful performance of these three activities provided useful criteria for discharge.

Hayes et al[24] studied 189 patients with an uncomplicated MI selected at random for early or late mobilization and discharge from the hospital. Patients were admitted to the study once they had spent more than 48 hours in a coronary care unit, if they were free of pain, and if they showed no evidence of heart failure or significant dysrhythmias. One group of patients was mobilized immediately and discharged home after a total of 9 days in the hospital, and the second group was mobilized on the 9th day and discharged on the 16th day. Outpatient assessment was carried out 6 weeks after admission. No significant differences were observed between the groups in terms of morbidity or mortality.

In a randomized study, Bloch et al[25] studied the effects of early mobilization after uncomplicated MI. For the study, 154 patients younger than 70 years of age who were hospitalized for an acute MI and had no complications on day 1 or day 2 were randomly assigned to two treatment groups. In the early mobilization group, patients were treated by a physical therapist with a progressive activity program that began on day 2 or day 3 after infarction. In the control group, the patients underwent the traditional hospital regimen of strict bed rest for 3 or more weeks. The mean duration of hospitalization was 21 days for active patients and 33 days for the control group. The follow-up period ranged from 6 to 20 months, with an average of 11 months. There were no significant differences between the two groups with regard to hospital or follow-up mortality; rates of reinfarction, dysrhythmias, heart failure, angina pectoris, or ventricular aneurysm; or on the results of an exercise test. On follow-up examination, there was greater disability in the control group than in the active group.

Sivarajan et al[26] have reported on the effects of early initiation of supervised exercises in preventing deconditioning after an acute MI. Eighty-four patients were randomized to a control group and 174 to an exercise group. The exercise program began an average of 4.5 days after admission. The mean discharge was 10 days after admission for both groups. There were no differences between the two groups in the clinical, hemodynamic, or ECG responses to a low-level treadmill test performed on the day before hospital discharge. In addition, there were no significant differences between the two groups in the incidence of cardiovascular complications or death. By the time this well-designed study was funded, the standard of community medical care in Seattle included early ambulation and discharge. Therefore, the control group received treatment that was hardly different from the exercise group. In addition, for safety reasons, the sicker patients who most needed rehabilitation were excluded from this study. Six patients needed cardiac surgery prior to discharge in the exercise group, but none required it in the control group, which can be explained by chance distribution (failure of randomization) rather than by the mild exercises employed. These three randomized studies of patients with uncomplicated infarctions have provided strong evidence that the risks of early ambulation are minimal and that progressive mobilization during the early stages of an acute MI should be recommended.

Exercise Testing Before Hospital Discharge

The low-level exercise test early after an acute MI (from 3 days to 3 weeks) has been shown to be safe. Today, it is a standard part of the treatment for MI patients in many hospitals. This test has many benefits, including clarification of the response to exercise and work capacity, determination of an exercise prescription, and recognition of the need for additional medical therapy or surgery. It appears to have prognostic value, can have a beneficial psychological impact on recovery, and is an effective part of rehabilitation. The applications and interpretation of exercise testing early after an acute MI are detailed in Chapter 9.

EXERCISE PRESCRIPTION

Exercise training can be an important part of cardiac rehabilitation for returning a patient to his or her formerly active lifestyle, or as functional of a lifestyle as possible, after an acute cardiac event. An early definition of cardiac rehabilitation was provided by the World Health Organization (WHO)[27] as "the sum of activities required to ensure them the best possible physical, mental, and social conditions so that they may, by their own efforts, resume as normal a place as possible in the life of the community... and that...rehabilitation cannot be regarded as an isolated form of therapy, but must be integrated into the whole treatment of which it constitutes only one facet." The explicit principles of exercise prescription, including frequency, intensity, duration and exercise mode, absolute and relative contraindications to exercise, and guidelines for terminating exercise, as outlined by the American College of Sports Medicine (ACSM)[28] and the American Association of Cardiovascular and Pulmonary Rehabilitation (AACVPR),[29] were described in Chapter 13, and should be specifically tailored to each individual patient.

When prescribing exercise, two basic physiologic principles should be considered. Myocardial oxygen consumption is the amount of oxygen required by the heart to maintain itself and to do the work of pumping blood to the other organs. It cannot be measured directly without catheters but can be estimated by the product of systolic blood pressure (SBP) and heart rate (double product). The higher the double product, the higher the myocardial oxygen consumption, and vice versa. Patients usually experience their angina at the same double product, unless affected by other factors such as catecholamine level, left ventricular end-diastolic volume, oxyhemoglobin dissociation as affected by acid-base balance, and coronary artery spasm.

The second principle concerns ventilatory oxygen uptake (VO_2), which is the amount of oxygen taken in from inspired air by the body to maintain itself and to do the work of muscular activity. Measuring VO_2 requires the collection of expired air, gas analyzers, and a skilled technician (these techniques are detailed in Chapter 3). However, VO_2 can be estimated from knowing the workload on a treadmill or cycle ergometer. Because the body's mechanical efficiency is relatively constant, estimates of the oxygen cost of various activities without using gas analysis can be applied between individuals. There are many tables giving the approximate oxygen cost of different activities. Because oxygen uptake is equal to arteriovenous oxygen difference (a-VO_2 difference) multiplied by the cardiac output, and a-VO_2 difference widens by roughly the same amount between individuals at maximal exercise, maximal oxygen uptake is sometimes considered an approximation of maximal cardiac output. However, patients with diseased hearts often have a lower cardiac output, a wider a-VO_2 difference, and a lower VO_2 than normal subjects performing the same submaximal workload.

Another important physiologic concept, which is an important consideration for exercise prescription, is the type of work performed. *Dynamic* work (bicycling, running, jogging) requires the movement of large muscle groups and requires a high blood flow and increased cardiac output. This movement is rhythmic, offers little resistance to flow, and provides a "pumping" action from alternating contraction and relaxation that helps return blood to the heart. The converse type of muscular work is *isometric,* which involves a relatively constant muscular contraction and thus limits the increase in blood flow. Activities such as lifting a weight or squeezing a ball are relatively isometric. For this type of exercise, blood pressure must be increased in order to force blood into the active, contracting muscles. Pressure work demands much more oxygen supply to the heart than flow work, and because coronary artery blood flow depends upon cardiac output, the myocardial oxygen supply can become inadequate. In addition, dynamic exercise is more easily controlled or graded, so that myocardial oxygen demand can be gradually increased, whereas isometric exercise can increase myocardial oxygen demands very quickly. Thus, appropriate contraindications must be considered before patients with cardiovascular disease are initiated into a resistance-exercise training program.

However, nearly all forms of exercise require a combination of dynamic and isometric contractions to one extent or another. When performed properly, resistance exercise enhances muscular strength and endurance, and has been shown to provide not only cardiovascular benefits, but favorable metabolic adaptations and benefits to bone health as well. Thus, appropriately guided resistance exercise is widely used today as a complement to aerobic exercise in rehabilitation programs.

Circuit Training

Kelemen et al[30] performed a prospective, randomized evaluation of the safety and efficacy of 10 weeks of circuit weight training in coronary disease patients aged 35 to 70 years. Circuit weight training consisted of a series of weight-lifting exercises using a moderate load with frequent repetitions. Patients had participated in a supervised cardiac rehabilitation program for a minimum of 3 months before the study. Control patients ($n = 20$) continued with their regular exercise, consisting of a walk/jog and volleyball program, whereas the experimental group ($n = 20$) substituted circuit weight training for volleyball. No sustained arrhythmias or cardiovascular problems occurred. The experimental group significantly increased exercise tolerance by 12%, whereas there was no change in the control patients. Circuit weight training was safe and resulted in significant increases in aerobic endurance and musculoskeletal strength compared with traditional exercise used in cardiac rehabilitation programs. Sparling et al[31] have also demonstrated the safety and efficacy of circuit weight training in patients with cardiovascular disease. In a 6-month study of 16 men, there was a 22% gain in strength, without an increase in

blood pressure. As with more traditional aerobic training programs, circuit weight training programs have been shown to have musculoskeletal and metabolic benefits, including improved insulin sensitivity in diabetics.[32] Numerous other investigators have recently made similar observations. The AACVPR guidelines[29] have even outlined recommendations on weight training for low-risk patients, an activity once thought to be far too dangerous for this population.

INTERVENTION STUDIES

There have been hundreds of studies published documenting the benefits of cardiac rehabilitation in patients recovering from an MI. Landmark studies performed in the late 1970s helped to define cardiac rehabilitation as a standard of care and provided important data not only on the physiologic effects of exercise training, but also data on the effects of exercise on cardiovascular mortality and reinfarction. These studies are summarized in Table 14-4. A few of the major studies are reviewed in the following.

Kallio et al[33] were part of a WHO-coordinated project to assess the effects of a comprehensive rehabilitation and secondary prevention program on morbidity, mortality, return to work, and various clinical, medical, and psychosocial factors after an MI. The study included 375 consecutive patients younger than 65 years of age treated for acute MI from two urban areas in Finland between 1973 and 1975. General advice on rehabilitation and secondary preventive measures was given to all patients who were discharged from the hospital. On discharge, the patients were randomly allocated to an intervention or to a control group, both of which were followed-up for 3 years. Patients in the control group were followed by their own doctors and were seen by the study team only once a year during the 3-year follow-up. The program for the intervention group was started 2 weeks after hospital discharge. An exercise prescription was determined from a bicycle test, and for most patients the program was supervised.

After the 3-year follow-up, the cumulative coronary mortality was significantly smaller in the intervention group than in the controls (18.6% versus 29.4%). This difference was mainly due to a reduction of sudden deaths in the intervention group (5.8% versus 14.4%). The reduction was greatest during the first 6 months after infarction. Total mortality was 21.8% in the intervention group and 29.9% in the control group. Although this was

TABLE 14-4. Summary of the early randomized trials of cardiac rehabilitation assessing cardiac events, mortality, or both in patients with coronary disease

Investigator	Population randomized												Percent mortality							
	Total	Cntrls	Ex	Exclusions (>Yr)	% women	Mean no. Mo entry after ml	Mean age	Yr follow-up	Dropouts		Return to work		Re-ml		Sudden		Cardiac		Total	
									Cntrl	Ex	Cntrl	Ex	Cntrl	Ex	Cntrl	Ex	Cntrl	Ex	Cntrl	Ex
Kentala 1972	158	81	77	>65	0	1.75	53	2			5%	8%	5%	8%			12%	10%	14%	14%
Wilhelmsen 1975	315	157	158	>57	11	3	51	4		46%			21%	18%			18%	16%	22%	18%
Palatsi 1976	380	200	180	>65	19	2.5	52	2.5		35%	33%	36%	15%	12%	3%	6%	14%	10%	14%	10%
Kallio 1979	357	187	188	>65	19	3	55	3					11%	18%	14%	6%	29%	19%	30%	22%
Mayou 1981	129	42	44	>60	0	1	51	1.5	25%	25%	30%	57%								
NEHDP 1981	651	328	323		0	14	52	3	31%	23%			7%	5%			6%	4%	7%	5%
Carson 1982	303	152	151	>70	0	1.5	52	2.1	45%	46%			7%	8%					14%	8%
Ontario 1982	761	371	390	>54	0	6	48	3.3	13%	15%			10%	9%			4%	4%	7%	10%
Sivarajan 1982	172	84	88	>70	20	0.13	56	0.50									2%	4%		
Bengtsson 1983	171	90	81	>65	0	1.5	56	1	6%	17%	73%	75%	4%	2%					7%	10%
Carson 1983	303	152	151	>70	0	1.5	51	3.5	4%	4%	81%	81%	7%	7%					14%	8%
Roman 1983	193	100	93		10	2	55	9					23%	17%	7%	4%	17%	10%	24%	14%
Vermeulen 1983	98	51	47	>55	0	1.75	49	5	14%	17%			18%	9%			10%	4%	10%	4%
Froelicher 1984	146	74	76	>65	0	4	53	1	7%	9%			1%	1%					0%	1%
Hung 1984	53	23	30	>70	0	0.75	55	0.5		45%	59%	66%	7%	9%	0%	0%	3%	0%	3%	0%
Hedback 1985	297	154	143	>65	15	1.5	57	1					16%	5%			8%	8%	8%	9%
Marra 1985	167	83	84	>65		2	57	4.5					11%	6%			5%	6%	6%	7%
Hamalainen 1989	375	187	188	>65	20	<1		10					19%	26%	23%	13%	47%	35%	52%	44%
DeBusk 1994	585	292	293	>70	21	0.10	57	1	12%	15%			7%	3%			3%	4%	3%	4%

Cntrl, controls; Ex, exercise; MI, myocardial infarction.

a landmark study, two weak points were (1) that more patients in the intervention group than in the control group took antihypertensive medications and beta-blockers and (2) that exercise capacity measured at 1, 2, and 3 years after acute infarction was similar in both groups.

Kentala[34] studied 298 consecutive men less than 65 years of age admitted to the University of Helsinki Hospital in 1969 with a diagnosis of acute MI. They were divided by the year of birth: controls were from odd number years ($n = 146$) and exercisers were from even number years ($n = 152$). The average age of patients in both groups was 53 years. Exclusions for controls included 10 with uncertain diagnosis, 24 who died in the hospital, five who refused or were not informed, four who had other severe disease, and 22 who lived too far away. Exclusions for the exercise group included 12 with uncertain diagnosis; 21 who died in the hospital; three who were not informed; three with other severe diseases, and 36 who lived too far away. Eighty-one controls and 77 exercisers were accepted for the study. Of the 81 controls, four died, three were hospitalized, and one refused to particpate, leaving 73 at 1-year follow-up. Of the 77 randomized to exercise, five died, three were hospitalized, and one refused to participate, leaving 69 at 1-year follow-up. Unless contraindicated, patients were kept on anticoagulation; beta-blockers were avoided. Both groups made their own decisions on tobacco smoking, and diet information was given. The training group also was urged to increase home activities in addition to the exercise program, especially walking.

There were two training sessions weekly for the exercise group, for the exercise group, later increasing to three per week, with 20 minutes of warm-up, 20 minutes of exertion (bicycle, rowing, stairs), followed by a cool-down phase. The exercise heart rate was targeted to 10 beats less than the maximal heart rate from exercise testing. There was no difference in morbidity or mortality between the groups after 1 year. Both groups showed clear decreases in heart rate for given workloads, and both groups showed improved maximal workload, especially in those patients with greater than 70% attendance. Return to work was not influenced by training; 68% who worked before their MI returned to work after 1 year.

Palatsi[35] performed a nonrandomized trial of 380 patients who were younger than 65 years old, and recovering from MI. Patients were excluded if they had locomotive limitations, psychological problems, or CHF. The first 100 patients were allocated to an exercise program and the second 100 were the controls. The next 50 patients entered the

exercise group, and then 50 entered the control group. The final total included 180 patients for exercise, including 37 women, and 200 controls, including 34 women. Patients with non-Q-wave MIs were treated with bed rest for 3 days, were allowed to sit for 1 week, were allowed to walk on the 10th day, and were discharged on the 12th day. Q-wave MI patients had bed rest for 7 days, were sitting after 1 week, were allowed to walk on the 14th day, and were discharged on the 16th day.

Exercise training began 10 weeks after the MI and included breathing and relaxation exercises, calisthenics, and walking that progressed to running in place. Heart rate was at least 70% of the maximal rate during daily 30-minute sessions performed at home. Once a month, the patients returned for revision of their exercise program. No effort was made to change smoking habits. The authors concluded that home training was not as effective as continual supervised programs, but nevertheless accelerated recovery of aerobic capacity. Rehabilitation was associated with slightly lower total mortality versus controls (14% versus 10%) (NS). However, there were no between-group differences in symptoms, smoking habits, serum cholesterol, or return to work.

Wilhelmsen et al[36] studied patients who were born in 1913 or later and who were hospitalized for an MI between 1968 and 1970 in Goteborg, Sweden. Patients were randomized to a control group ($n = 157$) or an exercise group ($n = 158$). Fifteen of the controls and 20 of the exercisers were women. The only criterion was an age of 60 years or older, but 27% of patients were excluded for cardiac complications. The two groups were comparable for prevalence of hypertension, diabetes mellitus, treatment with digoxin, smoking status, CHF, and previous MI. The exercise group trained three times a week for 30 minutes per session. Calisthenics, cycling, and running were performed at 80% of the maximal age-predicted heart rate. All follow-up treatments were the same except for the exercise program. After 1 year, the exercise group showed increased work capacity and lower blood pressure, but no difference in blood lipids. At 1 year, only 39% continued to come to the hospital to exercise, whereas 21% trained elsewhere. Initially, compliance to the exercise sessions was 18%, but it decreased to 63% at 1 year. Smoking after MI was found to be a significant predictor of fatal recurrent MI. There was also an association between smoking cessation and attending the exercise program. No significant differences were seen with respect to cause, type, or place of death.

Wilhelmsen et al concluded that antismoking advice and treatment with beta-blockers deserve higher priority than exercise training in the secondary prevention of MI.

The National Exercise and Heart Disease Project (NEHDP) included 651 men post-MI enrolled in five centers in the United States.[37] It was a randomized 3-year clinical trial reporting the effects of a prescribed supervised exercise program starting 2 to 36 months after MI (80% were more than 8 months' post-infarction). In this study, 323 randomly selected patients performed exercise three times a week that was designed to increase their heart rate to 85% of that achieved during treadmill testing, and 328 patients served as controls. This study was carefully designed by experts who took 2 years to complete the protocol. An initial low-level exercise session in both groups, to exclude the faint of heart who would not comply with an exercise program, was surprisingly effective in improving patient performance.

The 3-year mortality rate was 7.3% (24 deaths) in the control group versus 4.6% (15 deaths) in the exercise group. Deaths from all cardiovascular causes (acute MI, sudden death, arrhythmias, CHF, cardiogenic shock, and stroke) for the 3-year follow-up were 6.1% (20 deaths) in the control group versus 4.3% (14 deaths) in the exercise group. Neither difference was statistically significant. However, when deaths due to acute MI were considered as a separate category, the exercise group had a significantly lower rate: one acute fatal MI per 3 years (0.3%) in the exercise group versus eight fatal MIs (2.4%) in the control group ($P < 0.05$). The rate of all recurrent MI per 3 years, fatal and nonfatal, did not differ significantly between groups— 23 cases (7.0%) in the control versus 17 cases (5.3%) in the exercise group. The number of rehospitalizations for reasons other than MI was also similar in the two groups (27.4% versus 28.5% over 3 years). The need for bypass surgery was also similar in both groups—16 controls and 17 exercisers underwent surgery during the 3-year period. This study suggests a beneficial effect of cardiac rehabilitation on morbidity and mortality, but a definitive conclusion was not reached as there were insufficient participants due to financial limitations and dropouts.

Despite the fact that the exercise group demonstrated 37% and 24% reductions in mortality and reinfarction rates, respectively, this study was not definitive from a statistical standpoint. However, it did demonstrate the feasibility of resolving this important issue. It is unfortunate that it was discontinued, especially because the results were so encouraging: 1400 patients (more than twice the actual sample size) would have been required to demonstrate a statistically significant reduction in mortality rate in the exercise group if the reported trend persisted. The patients in the exercise group who suffered a reinfarction had a lower mortality rate, suggesting that an exercise program increases an individual's ability to survive an MI.

The Ontario Study included seven Canadian centers that collaborated in a randomized prospective trial.[38] The study involved 733 men with prior history of MI who underwent random stratified allocation to either a high- or low-intensity exercise group. Patients were excluded for cardiac failure, insulin-dependent or uncontrolled diabetes, diastolic hypertension, orthopedic problems, or severe lung disease. The two groups were comparable for initial MI, angina, hypertension, type A personality, smokers, ex-smokers, and cholesterol level. Stratifying variables included: (1) the presence or absence of hypertension, (2) blue versus white collar employment, (3) presence or absence of angina, and (4) type A and B personality. The high-intensity group trained by walking or jogging at 65% to 85% of their maximal oxygen uptake for 1 hour twice a week. This continued for 8 weeks, after which they trained four times a week on their own. The low-intensity group trained once a week with relaxation exercises, volleyball, bowling, or swimming for 1 hour. They attempted to keep their heart rate at less than 50% of maximal oxygen uptake. Both groups were encouraged to stop smoking and control their weight. Less than 5% of the low-intensity group regularly exercised vigorously. The dropout rate was 47%. The rate of reinfarction in the high-intensity group was 14% versus 13% in the low-intensity group. They found that the high-intensity exercise program had similar results to one designed to produce a minimal training effect and did not reduce the risk of reinfarction.

Bengtsson[39] reported on 171 MI patients younger than 65 years of age who were randomized to a control and exercise group. Patients were excluded for CHF, aortic insufficiency, hepatitis, polio, diabetes, new MI, thyroid disorders, stroke, or psychological problems. The rehabilitation program consisted of an outpatient examination, counseling, and supervised exercise (large muscle group interval training by use of bicycles, calisthenics, and jogging for 30 minutes twice a week for 3 months at 90% of maximal heart rate). There were no reported differences between groups for age, sex, number of infarcts, highest enzyme level, heart size, number of days in the hospital, number of admissions, angina, CHF, arrhythmias, or depression or hypochondriasis on the Minnesota Multiphasic Personality Inventory. The authors reported 100% compliance to the program. The exercisers showed lower mean systolic blood pressure (SBP) at rest and lower diastolic blood pressure at high workloads than controls. Equal percentages of the exercise group and the controls (74%) returned to work. The exercisers performed 31% heavier work at the end of training and 63% at the end of follow-up. It was concluded that at 1 year, all patients were less physically and socially active than they were before their MI. They were more dependent on their relatives than before and they had a poor understanding of their illness. The rehabilitation program—including exercise, education, counseling, and social measures during the first 5 months after an acute MI— did not change outcome 8 to 19 months after the MI compared to controls when considering physical fitness, return to work, psychological factors, and an understanding of their illness.

Carson et al[40] performed their 3½ year study in a population of 1311 male MI patients. Of these, 12.5% died in the hospital, 4% died after discharge but prior to follow-up, and 4.8% failed to attend follow-up appointments. Thus, 70% of the original admissions remained. Patient exclusions included being older than 70 years of age or having CHF, cardiac enlargement, lung disease, hypertension, insulin, angina, orthopedic or medical problems, or personality disorders. After these exclusions, 442 patients were considered suitable and 139 of these declined, leaving 303. These patients were accepted into the study and were randomized to either a control or exercise group. There was no group difference with regard to site of MI, number of MIs, highest enzyme level, smoking habits, known diabetes, previous angina or MI, cholesterol levels, family history, left ventricular failure, or occupation. The exercise group trained in a gym twice a week for 12 weeks at 85% of the exercise test-determined maximal heart rate or until symptoms of angina, shortness of breath, or a poor SBP response occurred. Isometric exercise was avoided. The dropout rate was 17% in the exercise group and 6% in the controls. Mean age at death was significantly different in the two groups: 50 years in the exercise group and 57 years in the control group. Return to work was 81% in both groups, and both groups showed a similar decrease in smoking after their MI. They concluded that the difference in fitness between the exercise and control patients after completion of the study was highly significant. There was no significant decrease in mortality for the exercise group except for those with an inferior wall MI.

Vermeulen et al[41] described a prospective randomized trial with a 5-year follow-up. Approximately 1 month after MI, patients underwent a symptom-limited exercise test. There was no total population description, no training description, no dropout rate reported, and no return to work described. Both the control and exercise groups received the same dietary advice. They found that rehabilitation did not influence smoking habits but lowered serum cholesterol. The 6-week rehabilitation program was associated with a 50% decrease in progression of CAD compared to the control group. The incidence of progression of CAD was significantly decreased in patients smoking less than 20 cigarettes a day. They concluded that cardiac rehabilitation is safe and greatly benefits patients with history of MI due to direct effects on myocardial perfusion and lowering of cholesterol levels.

Roman[42] studied 139 patients, including 19 women, who entered into a cardiac rehabilitation program. The control and exercise groups were comparable for age, sex, and MI location. The exercise group trained 30 minutes three times a week at 70% of maximum heart rate for an average of 42 months. At the 9-year follow-up, the control group had 24 cardiac deaths, including 15 acute MIs, seven sudden deaths, and two with CHF. The trained group had 13 deaths, which included seven acute MIs, four sudden deaths, and two patients with CHF. The mortality rate was 5.2% for the control group and 2.9% for the rehabilitation group. There were 23 recurrent MIs in the control group (4.9% per year) and 16 recurrent MIs in the rehabilitation group (3.6% per year). There was no difference in the incidence of myocardial ischemia, severe arrhythmias, or cerebrovascular events between the two groups. There was a significant decrease in angina in the exercise group. The overall attendance was 76%, and the dropout rate was 4.1% in the exercise group and 3.9% among controls.

Mayou[43] studied 129 men, 60 years of age or younger, admitted to the hospital with an MI. They were sequentially allocated to normal treatment, exercise training, or counseling groups. The control group received standard in-patient care, advice booklets, and one to two regular clinic visits as outpatients. They had no other education, walking program, or instructions for exercise. The exercise group received the normal treatment plus eight sessions (twice a week) of circuit training in groups, written reminders, and reviews of their results. The counseling group received normal treatment plus discussion groups, they kept a daily-activity diary, had couples therapy, and had three to four follow-up sessions. The three groups were comparable socially, medically, and psychologically. Patients excluded were 13 who died and one with a stroke. Evaluation was performed after 12 weeks using exercise testing and standard tests of psychological state and social adjustment. There were no differences among the groups in psychological outcome, physical activity, or satisfaction with leisure or work. The exercise patients were more enthusiastic about their treatment and achieved higher workloads on exercise testing. At 18 months, the significant findings included a better outcome in terms of overall satisfaction, hours of work, and frequency of sexual intercourse for the counseled group. The dropout rate was 25% overall. There was no difference in exercise capacity at 6 weeks, but at 12 weeks there was a nonsignificant increase in the exercise group. The groups were similar in terms of return to work, activities, sexual activity, and ratings of quality of life. There were no group differences in compliance to advice on smoking, diet, or exercise. They concluded that exercise training increased confidence during exercise in the early stages of convalescence, but that the exercise program had little value with regard to cardiac performance, daily function, or emotional state.

Hedback et al[44] performed a retrospective study in Sweden with a control group of 154 patients and an intervention group of 143 patients; 23 of the controls and 22 of the exercisers were women. There was no group difference regarding age, sex, risk factors for MI, rate of employment, income level, MI location or size, arrhythmias, medications, or heart size on discharge chest x-ray. Exclusions for the training group included severe CHF, arthritis, and stroke. Thirty-one declined to enter the program. Of the 84 patients who began the training program, 79 completed it. Both groups were treated the same during their acute hospitalization. Training began 6 weeks after MI, following a bicycle test. Training was performed on a bicycle to a maximal heart rate of 5 beats below maximal heart rate as determined during the exercise test. If symptoms or signs occurred, heart rate was limited to 15 beats below maximal heart rate. Sessions were 25 to 30 minutes long. This was done for 4 weeks and then replaced by calisthenics and jogging plus a home program. Patients with a cholesterol level of 8 mmol/L were referred to a dietician. Beta-blockers were administered to 60% of the patients.

One year following the MI, there was no group difference in mortality, but the exercise group had a significantly lower rate of nonfatal reinfarction, fewer uncontrolled hypertensives, and fewer smokers.

Meta-Analysis

The overall benefits of cardiac rehabilitation are now widely accepted. Comprehensive reviews confirming these benefits are available.[45,46] Because of the time and expense involved in conducting controlled studies with large numbers of patients, few such trials have been performed. We are left with numerous studies showing significant benefits in exercise capacity, and often psychosocial benefits, but frequently only trends toward improved morbidity and mortality. Meta-analysis has gained popularity in recent years as a method of combining separate but similar studies, and this approach has recently yielded some very important information on the efficacy of cardiac rehabilitation. May et al[47] presented the first such summary of the long-term trials in secondary prevention after MI (Table 14-5). Trials reported prior to November 1981 were considered in which both intervention and follow-up were carried out beyond the time of hospital discharge. Random assignment and at least a total sample size of 100 patients were required. Total mortality was used whenever possible, in order to minimize bias. All patients randomized were included in the mortality estimates to reduce the bias of differential withdrawal. Effectiveness was calculated by considering the percent reduction in deaths that would have occurred if the intervention had been applied to the control group. Although few of the interventions resulted in a significant difference, all of them, except for antiarrhythmic therapy, showed a trend toward efficacy. The 19% reduction in death rate from exercise training suggests that exercise is as safe and effective as other available means of secondary prevention.

To circumvent the problem of inadequate sample sizes, O'Connor et al[48] performed a meta-analysis of 22 randomized trials of cardiac rehabilitation involving 4554 patients. They found a 20% reduction of risk for total mortality, a 22% reduction for cardiovascular mortality, and a 25% reduction in the risk for fatal reinfarction. Oldridge et al[49] performed a similar meta-analysis with 10 randomized trials including 4347 patients and found a similar reduction for all-cause death and cardiovascular death in the patients undergoing

TABLE 14-5. Mortality associated with randomized intervention trials after myocardial infarction considered epidemiologically valid

Intervention	Number of studies (with significant difference)	Number of patients randomized	Length of follow-up (range of means)	% Mortality controls	% Mortality intervention	Effectiveness (% reduction, in deaths)
Antidysrhythmics	6 (0)	1675	4 mo–2 yr	10.3	10.8	–4.6
Lipid-lowering agents	9 (1)	19,834	21 mo–11 yr	23.6	19.4	17.8
Anticoagulants	5 (0)	2327	2–6 yr	17.7	13.7	22.6
Platelet-active drugs	7 (0)	13,298	1–3 yr	10.5	9.7	7.6
Beta-blockers	11 (4)	11,325	9 mo–2 yr	11.5	8.8	23.5
Exercise	6 (1)	2752	1–4.5 yr	14.7	11.9	19

From May GS, Eberlein KA, Furberg CD, et al: Secondary prevention after myocardial infarction: A review of long-term trials. Prog Cardiovasc Dis 1982;24:331–352.

cardiac rehabilitation. A summary of the Oldridge results are presented in Table 14-6, in which the pooled odds ratios for the combined studies suggest 24% and 25% reductions in all-cause and cardiovascular deaths, respectively, among the exercise groups. Criticisms of these analyses are that each of the pooled studies was not uniform in its treatment of patients, and a non-exercise intervention done in the different trials may have biased the results. Nevertheless, these two meta-analyses have been widely cited and have been highly influential in support of cardiac rehabilitation.

Recently, Taylor et al[50] performed an updated meta-analysis of rehabilitation trials among patients with CHD. While the aforementioned studies focused on research performed during the 1970s and 1980s, the latter study included trials performed through 2003. A total of 48 trials met the inclusion criteria, including 8940 patients. Compared to usual care, cardiac rehabilitation was associated with reduced all-cause mortality (odds ratio [OR] = 0.80) and cardiac mortality (OR = 0.74). In addition, participation in cardiac rehabilitation was associated with greater reductions in cholesterol, triglycerides, and SBP. However, there were no differences between rehabilitation and usual care groups in nonfatal reinfarctions or revascularization rates. Importantly, the effect of

rehabilitation on mortality was independent of chronic heart failure diagnosis, type of rehabilitation, dose of exercise intervention, length of follow-up, trial quality, or trial publication data.

Although the mortality effects of exercise-based rehabilitation on outcomes in patients with prior history of MI have been known for some time (i.e., since the 1980s), meta-analyses among patients with heart failure (HF) have only recently been performed. Until the late 1980s, activity was generally restricted in patients with HF, due largely to concerns over safety and unknown effects on the myocardial remodeling process. During the 1990s, numerous trials demonstrated that exercise training is safe in these patients, and several landmark trials were published that employed highly technological imaging techniques that allayed concerns over the effects of training on left ventricular remodeling. This is addressed in more detail later in this chapter (see Table 14–11).

A collaborative study of European centers that performed exercise training trials in patients with HF during the 1990s was recently completed (termed the ExtraMATCH study).[51] This meta-analysis involved controlled exercise trials in HF, and was designed to provide estimates of treatment benefits on mortality and hospital admission. Nine trials met the study inclusion criteria,

TABLE 14-6. Meta-analysis of controlled exercise trials in patients following myocardial infarction

	No. of events/no. of patients			
	% Treatment	Control	Pooled odds ratio (95% CI)	P
All-cause death	236/1823 (12.9)	289/1791 (16.1)	0.76 (0.63–0.92)	0.004
Cardiovascular death	204/2051 (9.9)	252/1993 (12.6)	0.75 (0.62–0.93)	0.006

From Oldridge NB, Guyatt GH, Fischer ME, Rimm AA: Cardiac rehabilitation after myocardial infarction. Combined experience of randomized clinical trials. JAMA 1988;260:945–950.

comprising a total of 395 exercise intervention patients and 406 controls. After a mean follow-up period of 705 days, it was found that exercise training reduced mortality in the order of 35%. Using death or hospital admission as an endpoint, exercise was associated with a 28% reduction in mortality. Moreover, there was no evidence that any subgroup (elderly, severely reduced exercise capacity or ventricular function, type of HF, duration of training, or gender) would be less likely to benefit from training.

Smart and Marwick[52] performed a similar but less restrictive analysis, including a search of the medical literature on exercise training in HF between 1966 and 2003. A total of 81 studies were included in the analysis, which included aerobic training studies, strength training, inspiratory muscle training, and combinations of these approaches. There were no reports of deaths associated with more than 60,000 patient-hours of exercise. No significant differences were observed between the exercise and control groups in total adverse events. However, the mortality rate was lower among subjects who participated in an exercise program versus those randomized to a control group (OR = 0.71, $P = 0.06$).

These meta-analyses have provided strong support for the application of cardiac rehabilitation in clinical practice. They demonstrate the mortality benefits associated with exercise training, and have led many to suggest that regular physical activity can provide a powerful protective effect against recurrent MI and death that should be additive to the current standardized interventions (PCI, beta-blockade, statins, bypass surgery). This evidence has sustained the growth of cardiac rehabilitation as an important component of healthcare around the world. However, the meta-analyses have limitations, and the issue is often raised that none of the single-center studies alone have been sufficiently powered to adequately document changes in mortality. In the absence of such data directly testing the hypothesis that exercise training reduces subsequent MI and mortality, scientific and popular perceptions regarding the benefits of exercise will support it as a treatment modality for cardiovascular disease.

Mechanism for Reduced Mortality with Exercise Training

The precise mechanism as to why an exercise program may reduce mortality is unknown. Aside from the physiologic benefits of training and its favorable effect on cardiovascular risk factors (discussed later in this chapter), other mechanisms may include a reduction in the incidence of ventricular fibrillation and its effect on ischemic preconditioning. A reduction in ventricular fibrillation might help explain the reduction in sudden death demonstrated in the meta-analyses,[47-52] and has been suggested by the observations of an increased fibrillation threshold after training in animal studies, which is associated with heightened vagal tone.[53-55] The reduction in sudden death in subjects randomized to exercise programs may also be partly explained by the availability of defibrillators and trained personnel to resuscitate victims of exercise-related fibrillation. Alternatively, it has been suggested that training represents a form of *ischemic preconditioning*, which refers to the observation that brief periods of ischemia before coronary occlusion can reduce subsequent infarct size.[56-58] Ischemic preconditioning has been suggested to help lessen the effects of subsequent ischemia, through any of several mechanisms. These include enhancing thrombolysis by the release of adenosine and its effect on platelet aggregation, enhanced collateral blood flow (with chronic ischemia), or through a complex series of second messenger pathways in the heart.[59]

Newer Concepts Regarding Physiologic Benefits of Exercise Training

A longstanding and attractive hypothesis is the concept that exercise training can reverse or retard the progression of atherosclerosis. The observation that regression of atherosclerosis occurred in animal studies dating back to the 1950s continues to stimulate interest in the effects of exercise on the coronary vasculature in humans. While this idea was largely rejected during the 1970s and 1980s, several notable studies were performed during the 1990s indicating that exercise training, when combined with multidisciplinary risk management, can improve myocardial perfusion.[60-62] This has been demonstrated indirectly using nuclear imaging[60] and directly by angiography.[61,62] Because most of these studies involved multidisciplinary risk reduction (e.g., diet, smoking cessation, stress management, and pharmacologic management of risk factors, including statin therapy) in addition to exercise training, it is not possible to determine the independent effects of exercise training.

There is also debate regarding the mechanism by which the apparent improvement in myocardial perfusion might occur following training. It is generally considered unlikely that changes in coronary blood flow during exercise in animals would apply to humans. Three mechanisms could potentially explain an improvement in perfusion after training: (1) direct regression of atherosclerotic lesions, (2) formation of collateral vessels, or (3) a change in the dynamics of epicardial flow via flow-mediated or endogenous stimuli of the vessel. Although there has been evidence of small but significant improvements in lumen diameter after intensive exercise and risk reduction programs in patients with CAD, no evidence exists that collateral vessel formation occurs after training in humans. Interestingly, although changes in lumen diameter following these intervention programs are quite small, they are associated with considerable reductions in hospital admissions for cardiac reasons.[62] This suggests that patients in the intervention groups may achieve greater plaque stability, without large changes in the coronary artery lumen.

In terms of the third mechanism, that is, changes in epicardial flow dynamics after training, a significant amount of recent research has demonstrated that training improves endothelial dysfunction, thus permitting enhanced peripheral and coronary blood flow in response to exercise. This represents a paradigm shift in the pathophysiology of CAD. The last decade has brought an awareness that the luminal diameter of epicardial vessels changes rapidly in response to mechanical (flow-related) and endogenous or pharmacological stimuli. Hambrecht et al[63] studied the effects of exercise training in patients with reduced ventricular function and reported that leg blood flow during acetylcholine infusion was enhanced compared to controls. The improvement after training was attributed to an increase in endothelium-dependent vasodilation with an increase in basal nitric oxide formation. In a subsequent study, these investigators demonstrated an improvement in endothelium-dependent vasodilation in epicardial vessels as well as resistance vessels in patients with CAD. After 4 weeks of exercise training, there was a 29% increase in coronary artery flow reserve in comparison to the nonexercise control group.[64]

These findings have been confirmed by other groups,[65-67] and suggest an important role of endothelial dysfunction contributing to inadequate blood flow in patients with cardiovascular disease. Exercise training appears to have a profound effect on the vasodilatory properties of the vasculature. Further exploration into the effects of exercise training on the dynamic behavior of the endothelium is an important target area for future research in both patients with and without existing cardiovascular disease.

RISK OF EXERCISE TESTING AND TRAINING IN CARDIAC REHABILITATION

Risk of Exercise Testing

There is a small but definite incidence of cardiac arrest associated with exercise testing of cardiac patients, particularly in the early minutes of recovery from the exercise test. The first study to address this was a large multicenter survey of complications by Rochmis and Blackburn,[68] which showed a combined mortality and morbidity rate of four events per 10,000 tests. In a retrospective review by Irving and Bruce[69] of 10,751 symptom-limited exercise tests, five cardiac arrests were reported. All occurred in the first 4 minutes of recovery, and all five patients survived after defibrillation (one arrest per 2000 tests). Based on these results, the relative risk of developing cardiac arrest with exercise testing (lasting 15 minutes) can be estimated to be one arrest per 538 hours of treadmill exercise, or 160 times greater than what might be expected to occur spontaneously (one death per 88,000 hours, assuming a 10% yearly rate of sudden death).

Perhaps due to expanded knowledge concerning indications, contraindications, and endpoints, maximal exercise testing appears safer today than 30 years go. Gibbons et al[70] reported the safety of exercise testing in 71,914 tests conducted over a 16-year period. The complication rate was 0.8 per 10,000 tests. This is markedly lower than earlier studies, but it was conducted in a population that was generally healthier. The authors also suggested that the low complication rate might be due to the use of a cool-down walk, which may make the recovery period safer. However, we have found that out of 3351 tests in our laboratory, no cardiac arrests occurred, and sustained ventricular tachycardia occurred in only five patients.[71] In general, our population is a higher risk group, and all patients are placed supine immediately after the test for diagnostic purposes. In 1997, Franklin et al[72] reported their experience from 8 years of exercise testing (more than 58,000 tests) using nonphysician healthcare providers. Their very low morbidity (2.1 per 10,000) and mortality (0.3 per 10,000) rates underscore the recent debate as to whether physician supervision is always necessary for exercise testing. More recently, we conducted a survey of 72 exercise laboratories in the VA Health Care System.[73] Among a total of 75,828 exercise tests, an event rate (defined as an event serious enough to require hospitalization) of 1.2 per 10,000 tests was reported (three MIs, one sustained ventricular tachycardia). Thus, the recent studies are consistent in the observation that the rate of events during exercise testing is low (≈1 per 10,000); this appears to be true for both clinical and asymptomatic populations. The overall complication rates from exercise testing of studies in the literature are summarized in Table 14-7.

Risk of Complications during Exercise Training

Haskell[74] surveyed 30 cardiac rehabilitation programs in North America using a questionnaire to assess major cardiovascular complications. This survey included approximately 14,000 patients including 1.6 million exercise-hours.

Of 50 cardiopulmonary resuscitations (CPR), eight resulted in death, and of seven MIs, two resulted in death. Exercise programs resulted in four other fatalities occurring after hospitalization. Thus, there was one nonfatal event per 35,000 patient-hours and one fatal event per 160,000 patient-hours. The complication rates were lower in ECG-monitored programs. These programs reported a 4% annual mortality rate during exercise, which is a rate not different from that expected for such patients. Other programs have reported rates of CPR ranging from 1 in 6000 to 1 in 25,000 man-hours of exercise. Such events are difficult to predict, can occur in patients with mild as well as more severe forms of disease, and can occur at any time after being in a program.

A Seattle cardiac rehabilitation program (CAPRI) reported a comparatively high rate of one CPR in 6000 exercise-hours.[75] Of 15 patients requiring defibrillation, the CAPRI group successfully

TABLE 14–7. Complication rates of exercise testing from previous studies

Investigator	No. of tests	Morbidity rate (per 10,000)	Mortality rate (per 10,000)	Total complications (per 10,000)	Physician supervised?
Rochmis & Blackburn (JAMA 1971;217:1061–1065)	170,000	2.4	1.0	3.4	Yes*
Stuart & Ellestad (Chest 1980;77:94–97)	518,448	8.4	0.5	8.9	Yes*
Scherer & Kaltenbach (Disch Med Wochenschr 1979;33:1161–1165)	353,638†	0	0	0	Yes*
	712,285‡	1.4	0.2	1.6	Yes*
Young et al (Circulation 1984;70:184–191)	1,377§	232	0	232	Yes*
Atterhog et al (Am Heart J 1979;98:572–579)	50,000	5.2	0.4	5.6	Yes*
Cahalin et al/Blessey (Exercise Standards and Malpractice Reporter 1989;3:69–74)	18,707	3.8	0.9	4.7	No
DeBusk (Exercise Standards and Malpractice Reporter 1988;2:65–70)	>12,000	—	2.5	—	No
Gibbons et al (Circulation 1989;80:846–850)	71,914	0.7	0.1	0.8	Yes*
Lem et al (Heart Lung 1985;14:280–284)	4,050	0.3	0	0.3	No
Yang et al (Arch Intern Med 1991;151:349–353)	3,351	14.9‖	0	14.9	Yes*
Knight et al (Am J Cardiol 1995;75:390–391)	28,133	3.2	0	0.3	No
Franklin et al (Circulation 1995;92(suppl I):737.)	58,047	2.1	0.3	2.4	No
Myers et al (J Cardiopulm Rehabil 2000;20:251–258)	75,828	1.2	0	4.0	Yes¶

*>85% of these tests were directly supervised by physicians; †Athletes; ‡Coronary patients; §Patients with a history of malignant ventricular arrhythmias; ‖Sustained ventricular tachycardia only; ¶73% supervised directly by physicians.

resuscitated all of them. Eleven had angiography, which showed single-vessel disease in four patients and multivessel disease in seven. Subsequently, the CAPRI record improved and they reported defibrillating two patients simultaneously; on another occasion, a physician monitoring an exercise class was defibrillated. Of 2464 patients observed during a 13-year period, 25 cardiac arrests occurred during 375,000 hours of supervised exercise, a rate of one arrest per 15,000 hours. Similar incidence rates were reported in Toronto and in Atlanta, where five arrests occurred in 75,000 hours of exercise, and a similar rate of one arrest per 12,000 hours (total of 36,000 gymnasium-hours) was reported in Connecticut. In CAPRI, 12 of the 25 victims had been enrolled for 12 or more months. Fibrillation was recorded in 23 cases and ventricular tachycardia in two. Prompt defibrillation was carried out and all patients survived. Each cardiac arrest was a "primary" arrhythmic event, and none was associated with acute MI. Eighteen of the 25 patients had ST-segment depression and five had developed hypotension with prior exercise testing.

Fletcher et al[76] reported that five coronary disease patients were resuscitated after ventricular fibrillation in an exercise program. Multivessel coronary disease that could be treated with bypass surgery was present in four of the patients. Resuscitation was required unexpectedly and at unpredictable times, occurring 2 to 48 months after being in the exercise program.

In the largest of these studies, Van Camp and Peterson[77] obtained statistics from 167 randomly selected outpatient cardiac rehabilitation programs and found that the incidence rate for cardiac arrest was 8.9 per million patient-hours. Of these cardiac arrests, 86% were successfully resuscitated, giving an incidence rate for death of 1.3 per million patient-hours. This compares favorably with the estimated fatality rate for unselected joggers at 2.5 per million person-hours of jogging.[78] There also was no significant difference in the cardiac event rate between rehabilitation programs with or without ECG monitoring. These data have been widely cited to document that the risk of exercise training is quite small.[79]

The incidence of exertion-related cardiac arrest in cardiac rehabilitation programs is low, and because of the availability of rapid defibrillation, death rarely occurs. The 2005 AHA Scientific Statement on Cardiac Rehabilitation and Secondary Prevention of Coronary Heart Disease[80] lists the occurrence of major cardiac events during supervised exercise in contemporary programs ranging from 1 per 50,000 to 1 per 120,000 patient-hours of exercise. It is noteworthy that studies have shown that in fact, the majority of sudden deaths are temporally associated with routine activities of daily life and not with exercise. Moreover, cardiac events during exercise are more likely to occur among habitually sedentary individuals, by a rate of 20 to 30 times.[81]

SPONTANEOUS IMPROVEMENT POSTMYOCARDIAL INFARCTION

Clearly, the natural course of healing after an MI is associated with some improvement in function, irrespective of engaging in a formal exercise program. Several groups have tried to quantify this. To document spontaneous improvement in aerobic capacity, the Stanford group measured VO_2 max within the first 3 months after an uncomplicated MI.[82] Forty-six men underwent symptom-limited maximal treadmill tests at 3 and 11 weeks after an MI. There was a significant increase between the two periods in heart rate, rate pressure product, and oxygen uptake during exercise. The mean maximal heart rate increased from 137 to 150; VO_2 max increased from 21 to 27 mL/kg/min; and maximal SBP, double product, and oxygen pulse also increased.

To evaluate hemodynamic changes after MI, Kelbaek et al[83] measured VO_2 max and performed invasive studies at rest and during two submaximal exercise levels. Thirty men were studied 2, 5, and 8 months after an uncomplicated MI. Fourteen patients participated in an exercise program during the first 3 months of the study, whereas the other 16 patients attended the training during the second 3-month period. An increase in VO_2 max occurred at the fifth month in both groups, 16% and 11%, respectively, along with an increase in cardiac index at the same relative submaximal workload. Later in the study, only slight increments in VO_2 max and no changes in hemodynamics were recorded within or between the two groups. They concluded that poor medical advice and pensions appeared to be the major factors responsible for unnecessary unemployment after an acute MI.

In a comprehensive review, Greenland and Chu[84] analyzed eight controlled studies of supervised exercise programs and their effects on physical work capacity. In all the studies reviewed, exercise capacity improved after the intervention, whether the patients were in a control or active intervention group. This suggests that either a patient's exercise capacity is artificially limited by the patient himself or herself or by the physicians caring for them (e.g., a low-level predischarge exercise test), or there is a spontaneous improvement in exercise capacity as time passes following infarction. However, the exercise groups always had a greater exercise capacity than the control groups after the interventions—on the order of 20% to 25% better. Studies that failed to show any benefit might have been limited by exercise programs of inadequate duration, as it probably takes longer than 3 months for at least some of the cardiac adaptations to occur, and also by compliance with the exercise program or prescription.

To study the extent to which spontaneous improvement may occur in patients with reduced ventricular function after an MI, bypass surgery, or both, Goebbels et al[85] studied 67 consecutive patients referred to a residential rehabilitation program in Switzerland. A month after their myocardial event, 42 patients had normal ventricular function (ejection fraction >50%) and were randomized to an exercise or control group. Twenty-five other patients had reduced ventricular function after their myocardial event and were also randomized to exercise and control groups. After 8 weeks of training, peak VO_2 increased only in the group with reduced ventricular function; the exercise group with normal ventricular function did not change significantly. Conversely, control patients with normal ventricular function increased peak VO_2 spontaneously (by 19%), whereas control patients with reduced ventricular function did not improve peak VO_2. The authors suggested that patients with depressed ventricular function strongly benefit from rehabilitation, whereas most patients with preserved ventricular function following an MI or CABG tend to improve spontaneously after the event.

CARDIAC CHANGES IN CORONARY HEART DISEASE PATIENTS

Many favorable physiologic changes have been documented in patients with CHD who have undertaken an aerobic exercise program. These include lower submaximal and resting heart rate, decreased symptoms, and increased maximal oxygen uptake. Peripheral adaptations are thought to be mostly responsible for these changes, and controversy has existed for many years as to the effects of chronic exercise on the heart itself. In a review of the effects of exercise training on myocardial vascularity and perfusion, Scheuer[86] concluded that, in the normal animal heart, there is strong evidence

that chronic training promotes myocardial capillary growth and enlargement of extramural vessels. However, it is unclear if these changes actually increase perfusion or protect the heart during ischemia. Controversy remains as to whether or not exercise training can promote coronary collaterals in the animal model subjected to chronic ischemia, even though the landmark study using ischemic pigs performed by Bloor et al[87] supports this contention.

There have been a number of attempts to demonstrate the effects of exercise training on the hearts of patients with CHD. Ferguson et al[88] performed coronary angiography on 14 patients before and after 13 months of exercise. Despite a 25% increase in maximal oxygen uptake, collateral vessels were observed in only two coronary arteries, and four of 14 patients demonstrated progression of disease. Nolewajka et al[89] studied 10 male patients before and after 7 months of exercise training. Neither the exercisers nor the 10 control patients showed any changes in coronary angiograms, myocardial perfusion as assessed by intracoronary injection of radionuclides, or ejection fraction. Sim and Neill[90] also failed to demonstrate cardiac changes in trained angina patients, including assessment of myocardial blood flow and oxygen consumption. Whether these negative findings can be explained by limitations in the techniques, patient selection, inadequate intensity, or length of training is uncertain. In the 1990s, evidence demonstrating angiographic regression of coronary disease in humans became available for the first time. However, it is unclear whether these changes are due strictly to intensive therapy with the newer lipid-lowering drugs, or to diet and/or exercise. This issue is reviewed in more detail in the following sections.

Assessment of Cardiac Changes Using Radionuclides

With the advent of radionuclide techniques in the late 1970s and 1980s, numerous efforts were made to assess the effects of exercise training on myocardial perfusion and function in both normal subjects and patients with cardiovascular disease. Verani et al[91] used radionuclide ventriculography and thallium scintigraphy to evaluate 16 coronary patients before and after 12 weeks of exercise training. Thirty patients entered the study, but only 16 completed it. Ten patients had a documented MI at least 2 months prior, and all but one of the others had angiographic documentation of coronary disease. Nine patients received pro-pranolol throughout the exercise period. Both post-training exercise studies were performed at the same double product as in the pretraining studies. For the ventriculography, a multicrystal camera was used and scintigraphy accomplished within 10 seconds of completion of exercise. After the training program, 15 of the 16 patients had improved exercise tolerance. Resting mean left ventricular ejection fraction increased from 52% to 57%, but no change was noted in exercise ejec-tion fraction or regional wall motion abnormali-ties. The thallium studies also were unchanged.

The Duke group reported the effects of 6 months of exercise training on treadmill and radionuclide ventriculography performance in 15 patients, all less than 6 months post-MI.[92] A training effect was demonstrated by a lower heart rate at a submaximal workload and longer treadmill time in spite of a wide variation in resting ventricular function (ejec-tion fractions ranging from 17% to 67%). The mean ejection fraction, end-diastolic volume, and wall motion abnormalities during rest and at matched workloads and heart rates were not significantly different after training. DeBusk and Hung[93] ran-domized 11 CHD patients to a home exercise pro-gram and 10 to a control group 3 weeks post-MI. There was no significant difference in resting or exercise ejection fraction or thallium perfusion images between the two groups after 8 weeks. Todd et al[94] from Scotland reported improvement in thallium scores among 40 male patients with stable angina after 1 year of following the Canadian Air Force plan for physical fitness.

A group from Heidelberg, Germany, performed a series of studies on the effects of exercise and a low-fat diet on myocardial perfusion in patients with CAD using radionuclide techniques.[95-97] In the first of these studies, 18 patients with stable angina and mild hypercholesterolemia (mean 242 ± 32 mg/dL) underwent a combined regimen of low-fat/low-cholesterol diet and supervised high-intensity training for one year. After the study period, serum cholesterol had decreased to 202 ± 31 mg/dL and low-density lipoprotein (LDL), very low-density lipoprotein were lowered to normal levels, and work capacity increased by 21%. Stress-induced myocardial ischemia by thallium[201] scintigraphy was reduced by 54% in the exercise group, whereas no changes were observed in blood lipids or measures of ischemia among controls. In a second, larger study, 56 patients were randomized to a similar diet and exercise regimen and com-pared with a control group at 1 year. The interven-tion group demonstrated significant decreases in body weight, total cholesterol, and triglycerides. Exercise capacity increased by 23%, whereas there were no changes in these variables in the control group. Exercise-induced myocardial ischemia by thallium[201] scintigraphy decreased by 13% ($P < 0.05$). In addition, significantly more patients demonstrated angiographic regression of coronary lesions in the exercise group, whereas significantly more control patients demonstrated angiographic progression. In a third study by this group, a reduction in radionuclide evidence of myocardial ischemia in patients who exercised was not limited to those exhibiting regression of coronary arteriosclerotic lesions, suggesting that regular exercise and a low-fat diet may retard pro-gression of coronary disease, independent from regression of stenotic lesions.

Perfext

Our group at the University of California, San Diego (UCSD) performed a study called PERFEXT (PERFusion, PERFormance, EXercise Trial).[98] The San Diego community was informed about the recruitment of male CHD patients between the ages of 35 and 65 years for a free exercise program. The responding volunteers were a select group of highly motivated patients who were encouraged to accept randomization by being promised that if they were originally assigned to the control group, they could join the exercise classes after the 1-year study was completed. Potential subjects were screened to determine if they: (1) had CHD, (2) were willing to be randomized and comply with either a low-level home walking program or a medically supervised exercise program at UCSD Hospital, (3) could discontinue their medications for testing, (4) had no complicating illnesses or locomotive limitations, (5) had not recently been in an exercise program, and (6) had the approval of their physician. The patients were classified by the following criteria: (1) history of MI, (2) stable exertional angina pectoris, or (3) CABS. Disease stability was assured by careful history taking and by not allowing the patient to enter the study until at least 4 months after a cardiac event, a change in symptoms, or surgery.

Of all the men interested in participating, 161 patients were interviewed, signed consent forms, and agreed to randomization. The patients were then scheduled for three entry exercise tests done on separate days, usually within a 2-week period. A thallium treadmill test was done first, for famil-iarization, followed by a maximal oxygen uptake

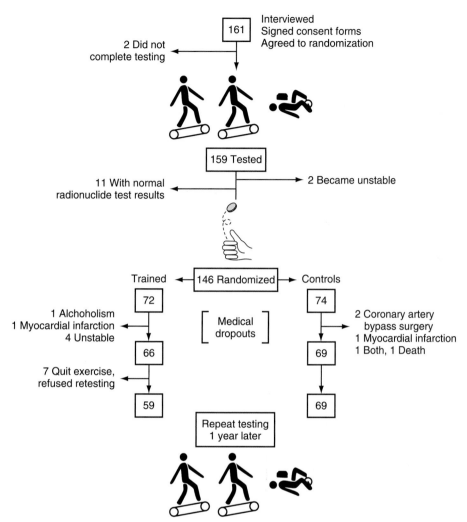

FIGURE 14–1

Patient distribution and flow in the PERFEXT study. From Froelicher VF, Jensen D, Genter F, et al: A randomized trial of exercise training in patients with coronary heart disease. *(From JAMA 1984; 252:1291–1297. Copyright 1984, American Medical Association).*

treadmill test and a supine bicycle radionuclide study. Of the 161 patients who enrolled in the study, 15 were excluded; 2 did not complete baseline testing, 2 became unstable, and 11 had normal radionuclide test results. Of 146 patients who were randomized, 72 were in the training group and 74 were in the control group. Patients randomized to the exercise group underwent 1 year of supervised exercise sessions; the exercise intensity progressed in standard fashion throughout the year. The study design is outlined in Figure 14-1.

Significant training effects in the intervention group were evidenced by a decrease in resting and submaximal heart rates, as well as significant increases in measured and estimated maximal oxygen uptake (Table 14-8). The control group showed a significant decrease in exercise capacity; this was partially because of the lower maximal heart rate obtained at 1 year. There was also a small but significant decline in the submaximal heart rate and rate pressure product in the control group, probably due to habituation. No changes were observed in maximal perceived exertion, respiratory exchange ratio, or SBP between the two groups initially or at 1 year, or between the initial and 1-year tests. Analysis of variance confirmed that the training effect, including an increase in peak VO_2, occurred in subgroups of the exercise intervention patients relative to controls. These subgroups included

TABLE 14–8. Initial and 1-year measurements from maximal treadmill testing in perfext[98]

Test	Control (n = 69)	Exercise intervention group (n = 59)
Heart rate, beats/min		
Supine		
Initial	66 (9)	69 (12)
1 year	69 (11)	65 (11)
Mean difference	2.2 (10)	−3.8 (10)
Submaximal, 3.3 mph/5%		
Initial	125 (15)	126 (16)
1 year	121 (160)	118 (15)
Mean difference	−3.1 (11)*	−9.3 (12)†
Maximal		
Initial	154 (19)	156 (22)
1 year	149 (23)	154 (22)
Mean difference	−5.2 (13)*	−2.2 (11)
Rate pressure product		
Submaximal, 3.3 mph/5%		
Initial	209 (44)	215 (47)
1 year	199 (49)	196 (42)
Mean difference	−8 (35)†	−19 (34)*
Maximal		
Initial	279 (57)	286 (59)
1 year	273 (60)	289 (67)
Mean difference	−6 (46)	3 (50)
Maximal oxygen uptake		
Estimated, mL/kg/min		
Initial	33 (8)	33 (9)
1 year	32 (8)	37 (9)
Mean difference	1.3 (5)	4.7 (6)†
% change	−3 (18)	18 (24)†
Measured, L/min		
Initial	2.1 (.5)	2.2 (.6)
1 year	2.0 (.5)	2.3 (.6)
Mean difference	−0.1 (.3)*	0.1 (.3)†
% change	−4 (17)*	8.5 (17)†

*Significant change from initial within group; †Significant change between groups.

those with and without the following features: a history of a Q-wave MI, treadmill test-induced angina, ejection fraction less than 0.40, abnormal exercise test-induced ST-segment depression, beta-blocker administration, or a dropping ejection fraction response.

Radionuclide ventriculography demonstrated a baseline increase in both end-systolic and end-diastolic volume in response to supine exercise. We examined the effect of training relative to controls on the following variables: heart rate, ejection fraction, end-diastolic and end-systolic volumes, stroke volume, and cardiac output. Each of these variable was tested at rest and at each of the three stages, and the percentage of change from rest to each of the three stages was calculated for each variable. There were no significant differences at rest, during the three stages of exercise, or the percentage of change from rest to exercise between the control and trained group at 1 year in ejection fraction, end-diastolic volume, stroke volume, or cardiac output. However, the intervention group, relative to controls, had significantly lower percentage changes in end-systolic volume at all three workloads. The data suggested that the magnitude of the intervention effect differed in the MI and non-MI groups, although this was not statistically significant; the intervention effect appeared consistently stronger in the non-MI than in the MI group.

The exercise intervention group also demonstrated a significant improvement in the exercise thallium images after 1 year, using the Atwood scoring system[99] as well as computer techniques.[100] However, comparing thallium scans side-by-side, which has been done effectively to evaluate surgical intervention, was not successful in the clinical assessment of changes in myocardial perfusion following the exercise program. Disappointingly, the ST-segment changes did not show an improvement, nor did they agree with the thallium changes.[101]

One of the only changes in ventricular function or volume of a consistent nature was the significantly lower percentage of change in end-systolic volume in the exercise intervention patients, which could not be explained as being due to a decreased afterload because there were no significant differences in blood pressure at any stage of bicycle exercise. It would appear that the trained heart calls on the Frank-Starling mechanism to a lesser extent than the untrained heart, probably due to lessened ischemia or improved contractility. This response may not have been seen had the patients' legs been elevated during supine exercise testing (Table 14-9).

TABLE 14–9. Estimated changes in stroke volume and cardiac output during supine bicycle exercise after 1 year[98]

	Exercise-intervention group		
Measurement	With angina (n = 20)	Without angina (n = 39)	P value
Resting supine stroke volume	−9.9 mL	7 mL	0.06
Stroke volume, stage 2	−14.9 mL	11.9 mL	0.02
Maximal stroke volume	−10.9 mL	10.3 mL	0.03
Maximal cardiac output	−1.0 L/min	1.3 L/min	0.05

The other significant change was the effect of the intervention on stroke volume and maximal cardiac output. Training is known to increase both, but the differential effect due to angina was surprising. The decrease in stroke volume and cardiac output in the angina patients was accompanied by a lessening of ischemia and an increase in end-systolic volume in response to supine exercise. This suggests that absolute volume changes had to occur that could not be detected because of the variability of the volume technique. Future studies need to address the mechanism of this response.

In routine clinical practice, cardiac rehabilitation is begun as soon as possible after a cardiac event. However, given our study design and sample size limitation, we chose only to study patients with stable CHD. Studying patients more acutely post-MI is complicated by the degrees of severity and by the variable rate of spontaneous improvement. Our results may not be applicable to the cardiac population immediately postevent.

One point of criticism might be that our patients did not exercise hard enough and that if they had, more definite improvements might have been possible. However, even if we chose those patients who trained the most intensely or who had the highest exercise class attendance, we did not find greater changes. Surprisingly, there was a poor correlation between the intensity or attendance and radionuclide or aerobic capacity changes. In fact, there was a poor correlation between the change in aerobic capacity and changes in the radionuclide tests. A paradox related to this developed during the 1980s; Ehsani et al[102] reported impressive cardiac changes in a highly selected group of cardiac patients with asymptomatic ST-segment depression exercised at very high levels. Hossack and Hartwick[103] also have reported an increased risk for exercise-induced events in similar patients. The question remains whether the usual cardiac patient can be exercised safely at higher levels than usually accepted and, if so, whether more definite cardiac changes can be demonstrated.

Care must be taken in interpreting many of the studies evaluating the effect of chronic exercise in cardiac patients. Often initial testing is submaximal, whereas follow-up tests are on a higher level because of increased patient and technician confidence and enthusiasm. This should be suspected when there are large increases in maximal heart rate, blood pressure, respiratory exchange ratio, or perceived exertion. Our study did not show significant changes in these parameters because we took care to encourage patients to perform a maximal effort in their initial test. In addition, if oxygen uptake is estimated from treadmill time rather than measured, the changes are usually very much exaggerated.

THE EFFECT OF AN EXERCISE PROGRAM ON THE VENTILATORY THRESHOLD

The noninvasive measurement of the ventilatory or lactate threshold has been considered in numerous exercise-training trials to document the benefits of chronic exercise during submaximal levels. Some investigators have suggested that the ventilatory threshold may even represent a more clinically relevant point than maximal exercise, because most activities of daily living are performed below the ventilatory threshold. Thus, it has been an important index of cardiopulmonary function. It is also often suggested that the intensity of exercise training must occur at intensities near or above the ventilatory threshold to ensure increases in cardiorespiratory variables such as peak VO_2, VO_2 at the ventilatory threshold, or improvements in markers of ventilatory efficiency. Many studies have demonstrated that this point can be changed with programs of exercise training. Increases in the ventilatory threshold, expressed either as an absolute value (VO_2 in mL/min), or as a relative percentage of peak VO_2, typically parallel the changes observed in peak VO_2 after training. Although the reason the ventilatory or lactate threshold improves after training has been the source of some debate, the most likely explanation is a greater rate of lactate removal from the blood during exercise.[104,105]

CHANGES IN THE EXERCISE ECG WITH EXERCISE TRAINING

It is attractive to think that myocardial perfusion could be evaluated noninvasively during exercise by the exercise ECG; there have been a number of efforts to address this. Previous studies in this area have had mixed results; these are reviewed in the preceding chapter (see Table 13-6). As part of PERFEXT, 48 patients who exercised and 59 control patients had computerized exercise ECGs performed initially and 1 year later.[101] ST-segment displacement was analyzed 60 msec after the end of the QRS complex in the three-dimensional X, Y, and Z leads and utilizing the spatial amplitude derived from them. There were no significant differences between the groups except for less ST-segment displacement at a matched workload, but this could be explained by a lowered heart rate. It is unlikely that myocardial perfusion could be changed after training to an extent that is great enough to cause differences in ST-segment displacement. It is also unlikely that the ST segment is sensitive enough to detect such changes.

THE EFFECT OF BETA-BLOCKERS ON EXERCISE TRAINING

There is evidence that a functioning sympathetic nervous system may be necessary to achieve the beneficial hemodynamic alterations of training. In addition, the limitation in cardiac output due to beta-blockade may result in fatigue and reduce the intensity of training or compliance to exercise. Moreover, if ischemia (theoretically the major stimulus for collateral development) is lessened by beta-blockade, this potential benefit of training also could be impeded. Beta-adrenergic blockade is now used widely to treat patients both with CHD and heart failure. However, one of the beneficial hemodynamic effects of both regular exercise and beta-blockade is that heart rate at rest and submaximal workloads is decreased. If beta-adrenergic stimulation is needed for the effects of exercise training to occur or if beta-blockade lessens the ischemia necessary to promote collateralization, then beta-blockade might be expected to interfere with the beneficial results of exercise. Beta-blockade also could increase perceived exertion and fatigue, thus lessening the tolerance for higher exercise levels and adherence to an exercise program. Therefore, a pharmacologically imposed limitation in heart rate and cardiac output during exercise may prohibit obtaining an optimal training effect.

The mechanisms by which hemodynamic changes occur secondary to regular exercise are poorly understood. High levels of sympathetic stimulation are present during aerobic exercise. It has been shown that regular intermittent infusions of dobutamine in dogs result in cardiovascular changes similar to those induced by an exercise program. However, the dogs did not get a true "training" effect. Other support for the importance of sympathetic stimulation for achieving the changes induced by exercise is that prolonged infusion of epinephrine has enhanced myocardial contractility and induced hypertrophy in dogs. Likewise, it has been discovered that sympathectomy abolishes the increase in the heart/body weight ratio produced by exercise in rats. Hossack et al[106] reported ventilatory changes during exercise in response to a single 40-mg oral dose of propranolol. They hypothesized that the changes

were due to inhibited glucose metabolism that could impede the training effect, but this has not been substantiated. These observations suggest that repeated, sustained sympathetic stimulation might be an important factor in exercise training. If beta-adrenergic sympathetic stimulation is needed for an exercise effect to occur, then beta-blockade might be expected to interfere with this process.

In 1974, Malmborg et al[107] first reported that a training effect could not be obtained in coronary patients with angina on beta-blockers. However, their exercise program was only held for 18 minutes twice a week. Obma et al[108] later reported a conflicting result. Their patients were limited by angina but demonstrated a significant increase in peak estimated oxygen uptake after an 8-week, 30- to 60-minute, 5 to 7 days per week exercise program. Pratt et al[109] retrospectively studied 35 patients with CHD who underwent a 3-month walk-jog-cycle training program. Fourteen patients had received no beta-blockers, 14 received 30 to 80 mg of propranolol per day, and seven patients received 120 to 240 mg of propranolol per day at the discretion of their physicians. Training consisted of three 1-hour periods per week at 70% to 85% of maximal pre-training heart rate. Each group's estimated peak oxygen uptake, assessed while on medications, increased after training: by 27% in those not taking beta-blockers, by 30% in those on a low dose, and by 46% in those on a high dose.

Vanhees et al[110] compared two groups of patients with past history of MI but without angina pectoris; 15 were receiving beta-blockers and 15 were not receiving them. Propranolol and metoprolol were the beta-blockers most commonly used, at daily doses ranging from 30 to 120 and 75 to 200 mg, respectively. Exercise training was performed between 60% and 80% of their maximal capacity for 3 months. Both groups showed lower heart rates, SBP, and rate pressure products after training, both at rest and during submaximal exercise. Testing was done while on beta-blockers, but surprisingly the maximal heart rate was only about 13 beats per minute higher in the group not on beta-blockers. Heart rate decreases were significantly less in the group on beta-blockade, whereas SBP decreases were less pronounced in the other group. Peak measured oxygen uptake increased an average of about 35% in both groups, but maximal heart rate and rate pressure product were also higher in both groups.

Pavia et al[111] studied 27 patients enrolled in a cardiac rehabilitation program after an uncomplicated MI. Fourteen patients were taking metoprolol as prescribed by their referring physician, and 13 patients were on an individually prescribed medical regimen not including a beta-blocker. Both groups underwent a training program lasting 3 months using a training intensity designed to approximate the ventilatory threshold. After the rehabilitation program, the groups increased peak VO_2 similarly (33% increase in the beta-blocker group and 27% increase in the placebo group, $P < 0.01$). Marked increases were also observed in VO_2 at the ventilatory threshold (28% and 39% increases in the beta-blocker and placebo groups, respectively).

Because both exercise training and beta-blockade have only become widely accepted therapies for patients with heart failure as of late, this issue has only recently been addressed in this population. Two recent studies from France[112,113] reported that exercise-training responses were similar between heart failure patients receiving beta-blockade therapy and those not receiving beta-blockade therapy. Although data in this group are limited, it appears that beta-blockers do not impair functional adaptations to an exercise program in heart failure.

Controversy even exists among normal subjects and the effects of beta-blockade. Ewy et al[114] studied 27 healthy male adults (mean age, 24 years) who first underwent two maximal treadmill tests. They were then randomly assigned to either a placebo group or to sotalol 320 mg per day. A third maximal treadmill test was performed 1 week after the administration of the agents. Subjects then participated in a 13-week training program in which they exercised 45 minutes five times a week at a training heart rate equivalent to 75% of measured maximal oxygen uptake. A fourth maximal treadmill test was performed at the conclusion of the training program while taking the agent; 7 days after cessation of medication, a fifth maximal treadmill test was performed. Measured VO_2 max was increased following training in both groups; however, in the beta-blocked group this was demonstrated only off beta-blockers. These findings suggest that stroke volume had attained its maximal physiologic capacity during beta-adrenergic blockade, and the reduction in maximal heart rate with beta-blockade prevented cardiac output to increase optimally following training. These observations are supported by Tesch and Kaiser,[115] who observed markedly reduced VO_2 max values in highly trained athletes after acute administration of propranolol.

Sable et al[116] studied normal young men before and after 5 weeks of aerobic training. In double-blind fashion, eight received placebo and nine received propranolol throughout the period, while training at the same intensities. Maximal exercise tests were performed before starting the drug regimen and training, and were then repeated 3 to 5 days after completing the exercise program, when beta-blockade was withdrawn. The subjects who received propranolol had no increase in measured VO_2 max, whereas the placebo group changed from a mean of 44 to 53 mL/kg/min. Maximal heart rate was unchanged in both groups. High levels of propranolol had been maintained by monitoring plasma levels, with daily doses ranging from 160 to 640 mg. This contradicts the findings reported in other studies, possibly because of the high levels of beta-blockade achieved. However, when these investigators repeated the same protocol in the subjects using low doses of beta-blockers, a similar attenuation of changes in VO_2 max was observed.

Similarly, Marsh et al[117] studied 12 normal individuals before and after a 6-week intensive exercise program. Six subjects were randomized to low-dose propranolol, and six were randomized to placebo and trained at similar intensities. All testing was performed off beta-blockade. Maximal oxygen uptake increased significantly in the placebo group, but was unchanged in those receiving propranolol. These authors concluded that high levels of sympathetic stimulation during training were necessary for the conditioning process to occur.

The work of Gordon et al[118] at Stanford, who randomized normal subjects to drug or placebo and then trained them, has shown particularly interesting results. Beta-blockade eliminated the echocardiographic changes in left ventricular posterior wall and septal thickening that was found in the placebo group who underwent training. Other investigators who have done studies of cardiac patients have not randomized the patients to beta-blockade, but have instead taken patients selected by their physicians to be on or off beta-blockade. Naturally, this can bias the findings. Other possible explanations for the different results obtained in studies of the effects of beta-blockers on training include: (1) inadequate total time in training, (2) high initial levels of training or fitness, (3) differences in the suppression of maximal heart rate by beta-blockade, and (4) successful blinding of subjects as to drug treatment in some studies.

We performed an analysis of patients in PERFEXT who exercised for 1 year versus controls, in which patients were placed on beta-blockers at the prerogative of their physicians.[119] The patients' medical records were reviewed to see who had taken beta-blockers, as prescribed by their physicians, during the year of training for the exercise group and the year of observation for the controls. This information was then used to separate them into four groups: (1) controls on beta-blockers, (2) controls not taking beta-blockers, (3) trained subjects on beta-blockers, and (4) trained subjects not taking beta-blockers. All testing was performed after beta-blocker withdrawal. More patients in the exercise group who were on beta-blockers had exercise test-induced angina than those who were not on beta-blockers (64% versus 16%, $P < 0.01$), and they tended to have more ST-segment depression and higher thallium ischemia scores. There was a trend for a higher prevalence of prior bypass surgery in those not on beta-blockers. These differences are probably due to exercise training making limitations due to angina more obvious and leading to beta-blocker administration. The average exercise intensity in the beta-blocker group for the year was 77% $\pm$ 14% of measured oxygen uptake, and average calories expended per session was 323 $\pm$ 104 (ranging from 130 to 719). There were no significant differences in these values between those on or off beta-blockers. Attendance at exercise sessions was a mean of 76% $\pm$ 18% (ranging from 23% to 97%) with no difference between those on or off beta-blockers (73% versus 78% for those on and off beta-blockers, respectively).

Two-way analysis of variance revealed highly significant changes in the treadmill parameters due to the exercise intervention. No interaction was detected due to beta-blocker status during the year. There was no correlation between beta-blocker dosage and the change in measured oxygen uptake in the exercise group. No other changes in treadmill parameters, including maximal heart rate, blood pressure, perceived exertion, or respiratory exchange ratio were detected. The changes in submaximal heart rate were significant despite the rebound effect of beta-blocker withdrawal.

Considering the clinical classifications of angina, prior MI, and CABS revealed significant ($P < 0.01$) improvement only in the thallium scintigrams of the patients in the exercise program with exercise test-induced angina. Therefore, three-way analysis of variance for angina, beta-blockers, and intervention was performed. Although there was a trend for this improvement to be concentrated in angina patients not taking beta-blockers, this did not reach statistical significance.

By design, patients were selected by their physicians to be on or off beta-blockers, and beneficial effects of exercise training were demonstrated. This clinical study is different from that studying the effects of beta-blockers on exercise training in normal subjects. Conflicting results exist as to the effects of being randomized to beta-blockade in normal subjects as compared with studies among patients with CHD engaged in exercise training. In coronary patients selected for beta-blockade treatment by their physicians, the answer regarding the beneficial effects of exercise is more definitive. From previous studies it has been demonstrated that expected changes in oxygen uptake, submaximal heart rate, and exercise duration usually occur in patients who engage in exercise training. Our study supports this, but also demonstrates no preferential difference between those patients trained on or off beta-blockers. In addition, PERFEXT demonstrated an increase in myocardial perfusion, implied by improved thallium scintigrams in angina patients in an exercise program. These findings and those summarized above support the beneficial effects of exercise training in coronary patients taking beta-blocker medications. A summary of the studies that have addressed this issue is presented in Table 14-10.

COMPLIANCE

The success and benefit of any exercise training program obviously are directly related to the amount of exercise actually performed by the patient—in other words, their compliance with the exercise prescription. Kentala[120] reported that only 13% of his patients carried out their assigned exercise prescription at least 70% of the time. As time progressed, compliance fell. At 3 months, compliance was 80%; 1 year later, compliance was only 45% to 60%; and at 4 years it was only 30% to 55%. These findings are similar to those from the U.S. National Exercise and Heart Disease Project,[121] in which compliance to exercise participation dropped from 80% after 2 months of supervised training to only 13% after 3 years. These and other studies clearly show that adherence to physical activity is often unsatisfactory in the absence of some form of continued follow-up or supervision.

Several options are available to improve compliance behavior: reduce the waiting time for enrollment; expert supervision; tailoring of the exercise prescription to avoid physical discomfort or frustration; use of variable activities, including games; incorporation of social events; recalling absent patients; involving the patient's family or spouse in the program; case management; and involving the patients in monitoring themselves and their progress.

TABLE 14-10. Summary of studies evaluating the effects of beta-blockade on exercise training

Investigator	Population	Duration	Drug(s)	Findings
Lester 1978	Normals ($n = 6$)	6 wk	Propranolol	Peak VO_2 increase 24%
	Normals ($n = 6$)		No beta-blocker	Peak VO_2 increase 25%
Pratt 1981	CAD ($n = 14$)	12 wk	Propranolol (30-80 mg/day)	Peak VO_2 increase 30%
				Peak VO_2 increase 46%
	CAD ($n = 7$)		Propranolol (120–240 mg/day)	Peak VO_2 increase 27%
	CAD ($n = 14$)		No beta-blocker	
Sable 1982	Normals ($n = 9$)	5 wk	Propranolol	No change in peak VO_2
	Normals ($n = 8$)		No beta-blocker	Peak VO_2 increase 21%
Laslett 1983	CAD ($n = 11$)	12 wk	Propranolol	METs increase 17%
	CAD ($n = 25$)		No beta-blocker	METs increase 12%
Vanhees 1984	CAD ($n = 15$)	12 wk	Atenolol, metoprolol, propranolol	Peak VO_2 increase 37%
	CAD ($n = 14$)		No beta-blocker	Peak VO_2 increase 34%
Ehsani 1985	CAD ($n = 13$)	48 wk	Propranolol, nadolol, timolol	Peak VO_2 increase 36%
	CAD ($n = 13$)		No beta-blocker	Peak VO_2 increase 35%
Fletcher 1985	CAD ($n = 50$)	12 wk	Various	Exercise time increase 32%
Savin 1985	Normals ($n = 13$)	6 wk	Atenolol	Peak VO_2 increase 17%
	Normals ($n = 11$)		Propranolol	Peak VO_2 increase 17%
	Normals ($n = 15$)		No beta-blocker	Peak VO_2 increase 19%
Wilmore 1985	Normals ($n = 47$)	15 wk	Atenolol	Peak VO_2 increase 18%
			Propranolol	Peak VO_2 increase 17%
			No beta-blocker	Peak VO_2 increase 17%
Ciske 1986	CAD ($n = 24$)	4 wk	Propranol, atenolol, metoprolol, timolol	Peak VO_2 increase 16%
	CAD ($n = 15$)		No beta-blocker	Peak VO_2 increase 21%
Madden 1988	CAD ($n = 9$)	12 wk	Propranolol	Peak VO_2 increase 11%
	CAD ($n = 7$)		Atenolol	Peak VO_2 increase 22%
	CAD ($n = 8$)		No beta-blocker	Peak VO_2 increase 12%
Ades 1990	CAD ($n = 10$)	10 wk	Metoprolol	Peak VO_2 increase 24%
	CAD ($n = 10$)		Propranolol	Peak VO_2 increase 8%
	CAD ($n = 10$)		No beta-blocker	No change in peak VO_2
Pavia 1995	CAD ($n = 14$)	12 wk	Metoprolol	Peak VO_2 increase 33%
	CAD ($n = 13$)		No beta-blocker	Peak VO_2 increase 27%
Malfatto 1998	CAD ($n = 20$)	48 wk	Atenolol, metoprolol	Exercise capacity increase 23%
	CAD ($n = 19$)		No beta-blocker	Exercise capacity increase 22%
Forissier 2001	CHF ($n = 24$)	4 wk	Carvedilol	Peak VO_2 increase 16.6%

CAD, coronary artery disease; CHF, chronic heart failure.

PATIENTS WITH LEFT VENTRICULAR DYSFUNCTION

Prior to the 1990s, patients with left ventricular dysfunction were thought to be poor candidates for exercise programs. This was out of concern for safety and the general thinking that they were unable to benefit from training. Safety concerns have been dispelled, however, by numerous studies that have been published since the late 1980s. Today it is recognized that patients with CHF derive considerable benefits from cardiac rehabilitation. With improvements in therapy (e.g., thrombolytics, ACE inhibitors, beta-blockade), survival among patients with CHF has improved considerably, and more of these patients are available as candidates for rehabilitation. The incidence of CHF is currently about 500,000 per year in the United States, and these improvements in therapy mean that this number will continue to increase. Recent studies suggest that the major physiologic benefit from training in CHF occurs in the skeletal muscle rather than in the heart itself.[122-126] A summary of the major randomized studies in heart failure is presented in Table 14-11. Extensive studies have been performed on the effects of training on central hemodynamics, peripheral blood flow, myocardial remodeling after an MI using echocardiographic and MRI techniques, and skeletal muscle metabolism.[122-134] These studies are nearly universal in their demonstration that training has beneficial effects on these systems. In addition, the rather

TABLE 14–11. Trials of exercise training in humans with impaired left ventricular function

Randomized controlled studies	Number subjects	Mean lvef(%)	Etiology	Program duration	Adaptions due to training
Coats et al (Lancet 1990;335:63–66)	17	20	CAD	8 wk	↑ Peak VO_2 2.4 mL/kg/min, ↑ exercise time 2 min, ↓ HRrest ↑QoL ↓ Ventilation, ↓ Symp, ↑ vagal tone
Meyer et al (J Intern Med 1991;230:407–413)	12	23	CAD	8 wk	↑ Peak VO_2 1.6 mL/kg/min, ↑ exercise time 1.4 Min
Jette et al (Circulation 1991;84:151–157)	7 versus 8	23	>10 wk post-MI	4 wk	↑ Peak VO_2 3.6 mL/kg/min, ↑ peak work rate 13 W, ↑ PWP 9 mmHg
Adamopoulos et al (Am J Cardiol 1993;21:1101–1106)	12	23	Stable CAD	8 wk	↑ Peak VO_2 1.9 mL/kg/min, ↑ exercise time 3 min, ↓ PCr use, ↑ ADP recovery
Kostis et al (Chest 1994;106:996–1001)	7 versus 13	35	>12 wk post-MI	12 wk	↑ Exercise time 1 min, ↑ QoL
Kayanakis et al (Presse Med 1994;23:121–126)	24 versus 24	30	DCM-CAD	3 wk	↑ Peak VO_2 0.1 mL/kg/min, ↑ vascular resistance
Barlow et al (Circulation 1994;89:1144–1152)	5 versus 5	23	CAD	8 wk	↑ Peak VO_2 1.3 mL/kg/min, ↑ peak work rate 16%, ↓ [K+]a, ↓ lactate
Belardinelli et al (Circulation 1995;91:2775–2784)	36 versus 19	26	DCM-CAD	8 wk	↑ Peak VO_2 1.2 mL/kg/min, ↓ lactate, ↑ diastolic function, ↑ a-VO2
Kilavouri et al (Eur Heart J 1995;16: 490–495)	12 versus 8	24	DCM-CAD	3 mo	↑ Peak VO_2 3.2 mL/kg/min, ↑ exercise time, ↑ vagal tone, ↓ symp
Hambrecht et al (J Am Coll Cardiol 1995;25:1239–1249)	12 versus 10	26	DCM-CAD	6 mo	↑ Peak VO_2 5.8 mL/kg/min, ↓ NYHA, ↑ mitochondria, ↑ peak leg VO2 ↑ max cardiac output
Keteyian et al (Ann Intern Med 1996; 124:1051–1057)	21 versus 19	21	DCM-CAD	24 wk	↑ Peak VO_2 2.4 mL/kg/min, ↑ exercise time 2.8 min, ↑ peak work rate
Dubach et al (J Am Coll Cardiol 1997;29:1591–1598; Circulation 1997;95:2060–2067)	12 versus 13	32	CAD	2 mo	↑ Peak VO_2 4.5 mL/kg/min, ↑ max cardiac output, ↑ peak work rate 36%
Meyer et al (Am J Cardiol 1997;80:56–60; Am Heart J 1997;133:447–453)	18	21	DCM-CAD	3 wk	↑ Peak VO_2 2.4 mL/kg/min, ↑ 6-min walk test, ↓ VE/VCO$_2$
Demopoulos et al (Circulation 1997;95:1764–1767)	8 versus 8	23	DCM-CAD	12 wk	↑ Peak VO_2 3.1 mL/kg/min, ↑ calf blood flow
Hambrecht et al (Circulation 1998;98:2709–2715)	10 versus 10	23	DCM-CAD	26 wk	↑ Peak VO_2 26%, marked improvement in endothelial dysfunction
Myers et al (Med Sci Sports Exerc 1999;31:929–937)	12 versus 13	32	CAD	8 wk	29% ↑ in peak VO_2, 39% ↑ in VO_2 AT, ↓ in lactate at matched work rates, ↓ VE/VCO$_2$ slope, improved ventilatory efficiency
Bellardinelli et al (Circulation 1999;99:1173–1182)	50 versus 49	28	DCM-CAD	52 wk	↑ Peak VO_2 18%, ↑ thallium ischemia scores, ↑ QoL, ↓ mortality (RR = 0.37), ↓ hospital readmission (RR = 0.29)

TABLE 14–11. Trials of exercise training in humans with impaired left ventricular function—*cont'd*

Randomized controlled studies	Number subjects	Mean lvef(%)	Etiology	Program duration	Adaptions due to training
Hambrecht et al (JAMA 2000; 283:3095–3101)	36 versus 37	27	DCM-CAD	26 wk	↑ Peak VO$_2$ 4.8 mL/kg/min, ↑ exercise time 4 min, ↑ LVEF, ↓ peak exercise TPR, ↑ stroke volume
Myers et al (Am Heart J 2000;139:252–261)	12 versus 13	32	CAD	8 wk, 1 year follow-up	27% ↑ peak VO$_2$, no change in LVEF, LV volumes, or wall thickness by MRI
Linke et al (J Amer Coll Cardiol 2001;37:392–397)	11 versus 11	25	DCM-CAD	4 wk	↑ Peak VO$_2$ 21%, ↑ VO$_2$ AT 19%, improved endothelium-dependent vasodilation
Erbs et al (Eur J Cardiovasc Prev Rehab 2003;10: 336–344)	36 versus 37	17	DCM-CAD	26 wk	↑ Peak VO$_2$ 32%, ↑ VO$_2$ AT 49%, ↑ resting and peak exercise, stroke volume
Giannuzzi et al (Circulation 2003;108:554–559)	45 versus 45	25	DCM-CAD	26 wk	↑ Peak VO$_2$ 17%, ↓ LV volumes, 4% ↑ in LVEF, ↑ 6-min walk distance, ↑ QoL
Single Limb Training					
Minotti et al (J Clin Invest 1990;86: 751–758)	5	27	CAD-DCM	4 wk	↑ Peak VO$_2$ 0.9 mL/kg/min, ↑ exercise time, ↓ PCr use
Koch et al (Chest 1992;101:231S–235S)	13 versus 12	26	CAD-DCM	3 mo	↑ Exercise time 3 min, ↑ QoL, ↑ strength
Stratton et al (J Appl Physiol 1994;76:1575–1582)	10	na	CAD-DCM	1 mo	↑ Exercise time 10 min, ↑ pH, ↑ PCr, ATP resynthesis
Piepoli et al (Am J Physiol 1995;269:H1428–H1436)	9	26	CAD	6 wk	↑ Peak VO$_2$ 0.7 mL/kg/min, ↑ exercise time 3.2 min, ↓ ergo-reflex activity
Magnusson et al (Eur Heart J 1996;17:1048–1055)	11	21	CAD-DCM	2 mo	↑ Peak VO$_2$ 0.8 mL/kg/min, ↑ peak work rate, ↑ cross-sectional area
Gordon et al (Clin Cardiol 1996;19: 568–574)	14 versus 7	28	CAD-DCM	8 wk	↑ Peak VO$_2$ 0.1 mL/kg/min, ↑ capillary, ↑ oxidative enzyme activity, ↑ peak work rate, ↑ strength, ↑ muscle citrate synthase
Hambrecht et al (Circulation 1998;98:2709–2715.)	10 versus 10	24	CAD-CHF	6 mo	↑ Peak VO$_2$ 3.7 mL/kg/min, ↑ endothelium-dependent vasodilation
Nonrandomized or Uncontrolled Studies					
Lee et al (Circulation 1979;60:1519–1526.)	18	18	>6 post-MI	18 mo (12–42)	↑ Exercise time 1.1 Min
Conn et al 1982	10	20	>3 mo post-MI	12 mo (4–37)	↑ Peak work rate 1.5 METS
Arvan et al 1998	25	29	>12 wk post-MI	12 wk	↑ Peak VO$_2$ 7 mL/kg/min, ↑ exercise time 4 min
Sullivan et al (Circulation 1998;78:506–515.)	12	9–33	CAD-DCM	16–24 wk	↑ Peak VO$_2$ 3.8 mL/kg/min, leg a-VO$_2$ diff, ↑ leg flow, ↓ lactate production
Jugdutt et al (J Am Coll Cardiol 1988;12:367–372.)	7	43	6–32 wk post-MI	12 wk	↑ Total work, ↓ LVEF 13%
Scalvini et al (Cardiology 1992;80:417–423.)	6	32	>6 mo post-MI	5 wk	↑ Peak work rate 9 W, ↓ peak VO$_2$ mL/kg/min

Continued

TABLE 14–11. Trials of exercise training in humans with impaired left ventricular function—*cont'd*

Randomized controlled studies	Number subjects	Mean Ivef(%)	Etiology	Program duration	Adaptions due to training
Belardinelli et al (J Amer Coll Cardiol 1995;26:975–982)	27	30	CAD-DCM	8 wk	↑ Peak VO₂ 2.8 mL/kg/min, ↑ peak work rate 21%, ↓ HRrest, ↑ lactate threshold 20%, ↑ skeletal muscle mitochondria
Kavanagh et al (Heart 1996;76:42–49)	30	22	CAD-DCM	52 wk	↑ Peak VO₂ 2.6 mL/kg/min, ↑ LVEF 5.8%, ↓ symptoms, ↓ HRrest
Wilson et al (Circulation 1996;94:1567–1572)	32	23	CAD-DCM	3 mo	↑ Peak VO₂ 1.2 mL/kg/min, ↑ exercise time 1.5 min
Demopoulos et al (J Am Coll Cardiol 1997;29:597–603)	16	21	CAD-DCM	12 wk	↑ Peak VO₂ 3.5 mL/kg/min, ↑ leg blood flow, ↓ VE/VCO₂, ↑ lactate threshold
Single Limb Training					
Kellerman et al (Cardiology 1990;77:130–138)	11	30	>6 mo post-MI or CABG	36 mo	↑ Work rate achieved, ↑ LVEF
Hertzeanu et al (Am J Cardiol 1993;71: 24–27)	11	31	>2 yr post-MI	60 mo	↓ NA, ↓ ventricular arrhythmias, ↑ work rate achieved, ↑ QoL
Horning et al (Circulation 1996;93:210–214)	12	21	CAD-DCM	4 wk	↑ Endothelial function
Respiratory Muscle Training					
Mancini et al (Circulation 1995;91:320–329)	14	22	CAD-DCM	3 mo	↑ Peak VO₂ 1.8 mL/kg/min, ↑ 6-min walk 320 ft, ↓ Borg score

ADP/ATP, adrenaline diphosphate/triphosphate; a-v, arteriovenous; CAD, coronary artery disease; DCM, dilated cardiomyopathy; HEART RATE, heart rate; [K⁺]a, arterial potassium concentration; LVEF, left ventricular ejection fraction (%); MI, myocardial infarction; mo, months; NA, noradrenaline; PCᵣ, phosphocreatinine; QoL, quality of life; RR, relative risk; Symp, sympathetic activity; TRP, total peripheral resistance; Vagal, vagal activity; VO₂, peak oxygen consumption (mL, min⁻¹. kg⁻¹); wk, weeks.

extensive experience with training in CHF patients now available in the literature has not been associated with increased morbidity or mortality. As mentioned earlier, two recent meta-analyses have demonstrated improved survival among heart failure patients participating in exercise programs.[51,52] Numerous studies have demonstrated improvements in symptoms, and some of the studies have documented improvements in quality of life.[125,134,135]

EFFECTS OF TRAINING ON POSTINFARCT REMODELING

Myocardial remodeling is a term that has been used to describe the adaptations of the heart during the months following an MI. These adaptations may include myocardial wall thinning, aneurysm formation, expansion of the infarct area, and ventricular dilatation. These responses are clearly precursors to the development of heart failure and are important prognostic markers after an infarction.

The concerns regarding the effects of training on the hearts of patients with reduced ventricular function after an infarction were reignited in 1988 with the publication of a study from a Canadian group. Judgutt et al[136] studied 13 patients with anterior Q-wave MIs using echocardiography before and after supervised low-level exercise training. They found that patients with evidence of greater left ventricular asynergy (akinesis or dykinesis) at baseline had more detrimental ventricular shape distortion, with expansion and thinning of their left ventricle after exercise training. This was thought to be secondary to remodeling of an incompletely healed infarct zone.

The provocative observations of Judgutt et al[136] were supported by several animal studies published in the early 1990s, some of which demonstrated severe global left ventricular dilation, left ventricular shape distortion, and scar thinning after periods of training.[15,16,137] However, subsequent controlled trials among humans did not confirm these findings.[125,127,129,132,138-140] Giannuzzi et al[138] completed a multicentric controlled trial of exercise training in Italy. After 1 year, patients in both the trained and control groups whose ejection fractions were equal to or less than 40% demonstrated some degree of additional global and regional dilation. Importantly, however, training had no effect on this response, and there was no effect in either group among patients with ejection fractions more than 40%. These investigators also completed a larger randomized trial in patients with left ventricular dysfunction after an MI.[137] After 6 months, patients in the control group demonstrated increases in both end-systolic and end-diastolic volumes, and a worsening in both wall motion abnormalities and regional dilation relative to patients in the exercise group. The latter study was the first to suggest that an exercise program may actually attenuate abnormal remodeling in patients with reduced ventricular function.

Data from Switzerland using MRI confirm that exercise training in patients with reduced left ventricular function following an MI is effective in improving exercise capacity,[124,127,132] and supports the recent Agency for Health Care Policy and Research recommendations[141] that this modality is a useful adjunct to medical therapy in these patients. Training did not cause further myocardial damage (i.e., wall thinning, infarct expansion, changes in ejection fraction, or increase in ventricular volume),[124,132] nor were there any long-term changes (1-year follow-up) in these measures assessed using MRI.[127] The application of MRI to assess the remodeling process by this group represents a significant advance in precision over previous studies.

Most recently, Giannuzzi et al[129] randomized 90 patients with heart failure into a 6-month exercise program or a control group. Detailed echocardiographic measures of left ventricular size and function revealed that patients in the trained group actually attenuated abnormal remodeling. Left ventricular volumes increased in the control group, but trained subjects showed reductions in left ventricular volumes, and an improvement in ejection fraction. In addition, trained subjects demonstrated significant improvements in peak VO_2, 6-minute walk performance, and quality of life, and fewer hospital admissions for heart failure. This trial provided the most definitive evidence that training in

heart failure does not cause further damage to the left ventricle.

EXERCISE TRAINING IN POST-TRANSPLANT PATIENTS

There are increasing numbers of patients who have undergone cardiac transplantation for end-stage heart failure, and today more than three quarters of these patients remain alive after 5 years.[142] The question has been raised as to whether these patients also can benefit from exercise training. Because the transplant patient's heart is denervated, some intriguing hemodynamic responses to exercise are observed. The heart is not responsive to the normal actions of the parasympathetic and sympathetic systems. The absence of vagal tone explains the high resting heart rate in these patients (100 to 110 beats per minute) and the relatively slow adaptation of the heart to a given amount of submaximal work.[143-145] This slows the delivery of oxygen to the working tissue, contributing to an earlier-than-normal metabolic acidosis and hyperventilation during exercise. Maximal heart rate is lower in transplant patients than in normal persons, which contributes to a reduction in cardiac output and exercise capacity. Only a few reports in the literature discuss the effects of training after cardiac transplantation. These results are encouraging, and suggest that post-transplant patients do indeed respond favorably to training. These studies have demonstrated increases in peak oxygen uptake, reductions in resting and submaximal heart rates, and improved ventilatory responses to exercise.[146,147] Whether the major physiologic adaptation to training is improved cardiac function, changes in skeletal muscle metabolism, or simply an improvement in strength remains to be determined.[146] Psychosocial studies of rehabilitation in transplant patients are lacking, as are the effects of regular exercise on survival.

ELDERLY PATIENTS

The prevalence of coronary disease increases as the population ages; roughly 25% of individuals equal to or older than 65 years of age have significant coronary disease. Older coronary patients are at particularly high risk for disability. There has been an emphasis on research funding for preventing disability in the elderly, and along with this has come an interest in the effects of cardiac rehabilitation on physical functioning in elderly patients. Williams et al[148] studied 361 patients grouped according to age with 76 patients who were 65 years of age or older, all of whom were post-acute MI or post-CABG and enrolled in a 12-week exercise program. They found that the improvement in physical capacity by the elderly group was the same as for the younger groups, and that benefits from cardiac rehabilitation were unrelated to age. Ades et al[149] performed a comprehensive evaluation of exercise training in elderly (mean, 69 ± 6 years) coronary patients. Forty-five patients who had sustained a recent cardiac event (MI or CABS) participated in a 12-week, 3 hours per week, outpatient program. Exercise time to exhaustion on a submaximal endurance treadmill protocol was increased more than 40%, with associated decreases in serum lactate, perceived exertion, respiratory exchange ratio, minute ventilation, heart rate, and SBP. The 40% increase in submaximal exercise capacity was contrasted by a far more modest 16% increase in peak VO_2. In a comprehensive study by Lavie and Milani,[150] a formal cardiac rehabilitation program in 268 consecutive patients older than 65 years was reported. In addition to a marked increase in exercise capacity (34%), improvements were observed in BMI, lipids, and quality of life scores. Demonstrable improvements were also reported in anxiety, depression, hostility scores, and somatization. Similar observations were made by this group of investigators among very elderly (≥75 years) patients.[151] The findings from these studies are very important because, as was mentioned earlier, the majority of MIs occur in this age group, and this will increasingly be the case as the population ages.

EXERCISE PROGRAMS FOR PATIENTS POST-BYPASS SURGERY

Coronary artery bypass surgery has been shown to prolong life and relieve angina in selected groups of patients with CAD. Advances in operative techniques, including cardioplegia, the use of the internal mammary artery, and more complete revascularization have improved operative results. Postoperative exercise programs are one means of optimizing the surgical result and helping those with inadequate revascularization. Because of the large number of patients undergoing coronary artery bypass and their potential for rehabilitation, some of these patients have been included in exercise rehabilitation programs. The number of studies that have been reported assessing the

effects of exercise rehabilitation on exercise capacity, return to work, or quality of life in patients who have undergone bypass surgery is now considerable.[152-171]

These studies differ considerably in terms of design (many were retrospective), study entry (some used preoperative exercise tolerance as the baseline, others used postoperative exercise capacity as the baseline), and duration of follow-up. Most previous studies only considered patients with successful surgery that alleviated angina, whereas our study group included approximately one third with signs or symptoms of ischemia.

A summary of studies evaluating the effects of cardiac rehabilitation after bypass surgery is presented in Table 14-12. The evidence would suggest that patients who have recently undergone bypass surgery respond to exercise training much the same was as patients with history of MI (mean increase in exercise tolerance 30%, with a range of 7% to 73%). Several observations among these studies are noteworthy. Fletcher et al[157] reported that patients who participated in a rehabilitation program had greater exercise capacity, smoked less, were less often rehospitalized, and were more often fully employed compared to patients who dropped out of their program. Similarly, Perk et al[159] demonstrated less medication use and fewer hospitalizations in patients with history of CABG who participated in an exercise program. Nakai et al[158] reported an improved graft patency rate at 7 weeks post-CABG among patients who exercised (98% patency in the exercise group versus 80% patency in the control group), as documented by coronary angiography. In two randomized studies, Dubach et al[164,165] observed that among patients who were randomized 1 month after surgery, control patients improved their exercise capacity to a similar extent as patients who participated in the 1-month concentrated residential programs typical of central Europe. This finding may reflect something unique about the spontaneous time course of healing after bypass surgery, or that 1 month does not provide an adequate training stimulus, or both.

In the PERFEXT study,[171] CABG patients represented a third of the total study group. Among 53 CABG patients who were randomized, 28 were in the exercise-intervention group and 25 in the control group. This was a unique opportunity to evaluate the effects of CABG in rehabilitation because the numbers were fairly high, radionuclide changes were assessed, and, unlike many studies, it was a controlled trial. The mean time from surgery until entry into the study was 2 years, with a

TABLE 14–12.   Summary of studies evaluating the effects of cardiac rehabilitation after bypass surgery

Investigator	Study design	No. of subjects	Study entry	Duration	% Change in exercise capacity
Oldridge 1978	Prospective	21	1 week postsurgery	32 mo	Exercise: 28% Control: 3%
Gohlke 1982	Retrospective	467	postsurgery	5 yr	Exercise: 37%
Waites 1983	Retrospective	22	9 mo postsurgery	6 mo	Exercise: 25%
Kappagoda 1983	Randomized, prospective	30	1–2 days postsurgery	9 mo	Exercise: 73% Control: 29.6%
Stevens 1984	Retrospective	204	44 days postsurgery	4 mo	Supervised: 19% Unsupervised: 18%
Froelicher 1985	Randomized, prospective	53	Mean 2 yr postsurgery	1 year	Exercise: 7.1% Control: 2.9%
Maresh 1985	Retrospective	54	30 days postsurgery	12 wk	Exercise: 56%
Ben-Ari 1986	Prospective	96	10–14 days postsurgery	1 year	Exercise: 81 watts Control: 61 watts
Hedback 1990	Randomized, retrospective	147	6 wk postsurgery	1 year	Exercise: 32% Control: 23%
Dubach 1993	Randomized, crossover	28	1 mo postsurgery	3 mo	Exercise: 16% Control: 19%
Dubach 1995	Randomized, prospective	42	25 days postsurgery	4 wk	Exercise: 11% Control: 14%
Goodman 1999	Prospective	31	8–10 wk postsurgery	12 wk	Exercise:13%
Adachi 2001	Prospective	57	2 wk postsurgery	2 wk	Exercise: 42% Control: 4%
Kodis 2001	Retrospective	1042	6–8 wk postsurgery	6 mo	Exercise: 21%

standard deviation of 2 years and a range of 6 months to 9 years. This time period was rather long and exercise training likely has a greater effect if applied sooner. Favorable training effects were observed, however, which were similar to the larger group, but radionuclide changes were not found to be significant.

The effects of revascularization vary, but many patients are presently 10 to 20 years or more post-CABG; there is a recurrence rate of angina of 5% or less 1 year postsurgery. Randomized trials of aspirin and statins have demonstrated improved graft patency, and so efficacy could be improved even further. The available studies, although limited by methodology, patient numbers, and highly variable details of the rehabilitation programs employed, demonstrate that exercise programs improve exercise capacity and the ability to return to work in patients who have undergone CABG.

REHABILITATION AFTER PERCUTANEOUS CORONARY INTERVENTION

The exponential growth in percutaneous transluminal coronary angioplasty (PTCA) since its first clinical application in 1977 by Andreas Gruentzig

has been dramatic. Today, more than one million coronary angioplasty and stent implantation procedures are performed annually. Despite improvements in equipment and techniques, late vessel restenosis occurs frequently within 3 to 6 months of the procedure. Depending on the types of patients studied and the definition of restenosis, it occurs in 12% to 48% of patients.[172] Because an average of 30% of patients will experience restenosis, this constitutes a significant number of patients who are destined to have recurrence of symptoms associated with ischemia. Currently, the annual risk of a major cardiac event following PCI is 5% to 7%. Cardiac rehabilitation can assist these patients symptomatically as well as physically and mentally in coping with their coronary disease. Fitzgerald et al[173] have shown that despite the minimal invasiveness of PTCA and lack of any physical contraindications, some patients have found it difficult to return to work because of low self-confidence; only 81% of PTCA patients actually return to work.[174] It would therefore seem practical to offer cardiac rehabilitation to these patients so that they, too, can benefit from an improvement in exercise capacity.

Ben-Ari et al[175] studied the effects of cardiac rehabilitation in patients with history of PTCA and compared them to a group of matched patients who received usual care post-PTCA without rehabilitation. They found a higher physical work capacity and ejection fraction in the rehabilitation group compared to controls, and lower total cholesterol, lower LDL, and higher HDL as well. There was no difference in the rate of restenosis at 5.5 months of follow-up. Further work by this group documented a higher return to work after their program.[176] In Japan, Kubo et al[177] recently evaluated the effects of exercise training on the development of restenosis after PTCA. Single photon emission computed tomography (SPECT) imaging was performed 1 and 13 weeks after PTCA in 18 patients who underwent exercise training and 20 controls. After the study period, the restenosis rate was 17% in the exercise group versus 40% among controls. Patients in the exercise group demonstrated improvements in exercise capacity and significantly improved SPECT redistribution images, whereas these variables remained unchanged among controls.

The results of the PCI versus Exercise Training (PET) study were recently published.[178] This was a unique trial performed in Germany which will likely have an important impact for some time. The PET study was a randomized trial designed to compare the effects of exercise training versus standard PCI with stenting on clinical symptoms, angina-free exercise capacity, myocardial perfusion, cost-effectiveness, and frequency of a combined clinical endpoint (cardiovascular death, stroke, bypass surgery, angioplasty, acute MI, and worsening angina with objective evidence resulting in hospitalization). A total of 101 male patients younger than or equal to 70 years of age were recruited after routine coronary angiography and randomized to 12 months of exercise training (20 minutes of bicycle ergometry per day) or to PCI. Cost-efficiency was calculated as the average expense (in U.S. dollars) needed to improve the Canadian Cardiovascular Society class by 1 class. The results demonstrated that exercise training was associated with a higher event-free survival (88% versus 70% in the PCI group) and increased maximal oxygen uptake (+16%). To gain 1 Canadian Cardiovascular Society class, $6956 was spent in the PCI group versus $3429 in the training group. Compared with PCI, the 12-month program of regular physical exercise resulted in superior event-free survival and exercise capacity at lower costs, notably owing to reduced rehospitalizations and fewer repeat revascularizations. This landmark trial was the first to directly compare cardiac rehabilitation with an invasive intervention in a randomized

fashion, and suggests that, at least in some patients with stable CAD, lifestyle intervention can be an alternative approach to an interventional strategy. As a minimum, PCI should be combined with aggressive lifestyle intervention, including exercise.

RETURN TO WORK

The presumed inability to resume gainful employment can contribute greatly to a patient's loss of self-esteem and perceived economic impotence. A concerted effort by the medical/rehabilitation team must be directed to allay these concerns.[179] A symptom-limited exercise test, if normal, can do much to encourage and reinstill confidence in patients to resume their job-related activities. Conversely, an exercise test showing a lower exercise capacity can be used to guide a patient's level of activity at work.

Occupational evaluation and counseling was shown to be of benefit by Dennis et al,[180] who decreased the time interval between infarction and return to work by an average of 32% by counseling low-risk patients. Cost-benefit analysis of these same patients revealed that total medical costs per patient during the 6 months post-MI were lower by $502, and their occupational income generated during this same time period was $2102 greater.[181] The fact that people are working longer into their later years, and 80% of patients younger than 65 years of age eventually return to work after their MIs underscores the fact that many patients with history of MI can benefit from this type of counseling. Engblom et al[182] assessed the effects of a rehabilitation program 5 years after CABS in Finland. The patients who were randomized to an exercise program after their surgery demonstrated better physical function scores (Nottingham Health Profile), better perception of health, and better perception of quality of life compared to controls. However, a greater proportion of these patients were working only at the 3-year evaluation (not at 4 or 5 years). The Agency for Health Care Policy and Research Guidelines on Cardiac Rehabilitation[141] summarized the results of 28 studies, and the results of the effects of rehabilitation on return to work were mixed. Return to work is a complex issue that is influenced by social and political factors, economic incentives or disincentives to resume working, employer attitudes, and preillness employment status of the patient.[141] Few of these factors have been considered in studies on the effects of rehabilitation on return to work, and this remains an area in need of further study.

RISK-FACTOR MODIFICATION

Given the recurrence rate of reinfarction and overall cardiovascular mortality in survivors of MI, theoretical benefits of risk factor modification in this high-risk population could be very significant.[183] There have been numerous efforts to assess the effects of controlled, multifactorial risk-factor reduction programs on cardiovascular risk. Exercise training programs alone have inconsistent effects on smoking cessation, lipids, and body weight.[141] However, multifactorial programs including exercise, lipid-lowering therapy, dietary education and counseling, and other interventions have been demonstrated to be effective (Fig. 14-2). As part of a WHO study, Kallio et al[33] performed a multifactorial intervention combined with cardiac rehabilitation in patients with history of MI

beginning 2 weeks after their event. They found a decrease in blood pressure, lower body weight, and improved serum cholesterol and triglycerides in the treated group; however, smoking decreased by 50% in both the treated and control groups. The National Exercise and Heart Disease Project[184] showed a reduction in LDL fractions. An analysis of 10-year mortality from cardiovascular disease in relation to cholesterol level by Pekkanen et al[185] demonstrated the importance of serum cholesterol in men with pre-existing cardiovascular disease. Hamalainen et al[186] noted a reduction in sudden deaths by almost 50% in patients enrolled in an aggressive, multifactorial intervention program for 10 years post-MI. Their interventions included control of smoking, hypertension, and lipids, and the use of antiarrhythmic agents in addition to beta-blockers.

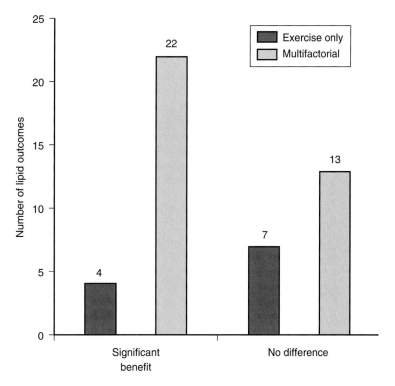

■ **FIGURE 14–2**

Changes in lipid levels in 18 randomized controlled trials of cardiac rehabilitation by intervention strategy-exercise only versus multifactorial intervention. *(From Agency for Health Care Policy and Research, Guidelines for Cardiac Rehabilitation, 1995).*

Note: Effects of types of cardiac rehabilitation interventions on lipid levels in randomized controlled trials (significant reductions in total cholesterol, LDL cholesterol, and triglyceride levels, and significant increases in HDL cholesterol levels). Multifactorial rehabilitation interventions appear more likely to effect a beneficial change in lipid levels than does exercise training alone. All trials compared rehabilitation versus control patients. Some studies reported more than one lipid result.

Previously, it was argued that when atheromas are well established and cause symptoms, alterations in serum cholesterol would have little effect. In recent years, it has been demonstrated repeatedly that this is not the case. Evidence that the progression of coronary atherosclerosis may be arrested and actually reversed with aggressive dietary and medical therapy is accumulating.[187,188] Meta-analysis of lipid-lowering trials using digital coronary angiography now consistently confirm that this is the case. The recent multidisciplinary risk reduction trials that have included exercise training as a component and their effect on the atherosclerotic process are summarized in Table 14-13. The data presented in Table 14-13 are noteworthy in several respects. Atherosclerotic regression, when it occurs, is demonstrated much more often in patients who receive lipid-lowering agents, dietary, or other interventions compared with controls. It also should be noted that the percentage reductions in coronary arterial lumen diameter are small, and they do not occur in all patients in the treatment groups. Lastly, although exercise training has been included as a component of multifactorial intervention, it is difficult at present to determine the effects of diet, drugs, exercise, or other interventions independently.

Nevertheless, the recent observation that the atherosclerotic process can be reversed has had a major effect on clinical practice. Current recommendations suggest that all individuals with existing heart disease should have aggressive management to lower their LDL cholesterol to below 100.[189] The interaction of triglycerides with gene site activity, typing of apo-B, ultracentrifugation of LDL, and other new findings are leading to an exciting new hope that atherosclerosis can be treated more effectively. These studies are promising and emphasize the medical rehabilitation team's responsibility to encourage patients to alter lifestyles that could be deleterious to their health and institute medical therapy as necessary to control cardiac risk factors.

PREDICTING OUTCOME IN CARDIAC REHABILITATION PATIENTS

Cardiac rehabilitation programs can be expensive and may be difficult to provide to some patients due to financial reasons, lack of insurance, distance to the hospital or rehabilitation facility, comorbidities, or other reasons. If a patient's likelihood of improving work capacity could be predicted on the basis of initial data, much time and money could be saved and rehabilitation services could be directed to patients who would benefit the most. Several groups have made efforts to address this, and most have been rather disappointing. Pierson et al[190] recently studied 60 patients who participated in an outpatient rehabilitation program for 5 to 9 months. The best predictor of a training response was low baseline fitness level; there was no association between the increase in exercise tolerance during rehabilitation and age, revascularization status, or markers of ischemia.

In the PERFEXT study, peak VO_2 and other markers of a training effect were considered and the following questions were addressed[191]: (1) Can clinical features prior to training predict whether or not beneficial changes occur with training?, (2) do initial treadmill or radionuclide measurements contribute information to improve this prediction?, and (3) does the intensity of training over the year predict beneficial changes? Our major finding was that a patient's success or failure in improving aerobic capacity following a 1-year aerobic exercise program was poorly predicted on the basis of initial clinical, treadmill, or radionuclide data. Correlations between initial parameters and outcome were poor. Training intensity had little to do with outcome. Those with ischemic markers (exercise test-induced angina, ST depression, or dropping ejection fraction) did not have a different response to training than patients without ischemia; neither did those with markers of myocardial damage. History of CABS or MI had no bearing on whether a patient's work capacity would improve following the training period. Multivariate analyses did not greatly improve the ability to predict outcome. Previous studies have found that those with the lowest initial measured oxygen uptake often have the largest improvement with an exercise program, but this was not the case in PERFEXT.

Thus, a very detailed initial evaluation did not allow accurate prediction of who would benefit from training and who would not. Even those patients whose characteristics suggested they had the most ischemia or largest scar showed as much improvement from training as patients without such characteristics. Therefore, it would appear that using angina, a low resting ejection fraction, ST-segment depression, or a dropping ejection fraction with exercise as contraindications to an exercise program is unjustified. Because many of the benefits obtained from an exercise program are intangible, it seems inappropriate to eliminate any patient from an exercise program on the basis

TABLE 14-13. Human coronary regression studies using exercise as an intervention

Study	Study population	Length	Intervention	Result (% of sample)
Exercise Therapy Heidelberg Hambrecht 1993	62 (No LM CAD, no bypass, no hypercholesterolemia)	1 yr	Low-fat diet, exercise	Progression-intervention (10%) Control (45%) No change-intervention (62%) Control (49%) Regression-intervention (28%) Control (6%)
Heidelberg Schuler 1992	36 (CAD, stable symptoms)	1 yr	Low-fat diet, intensive exercise >3 hours/wk	Progression-intervention (28%) Control (33%) No change-intervention (33%) Control (61%) Regression-intervention (39%) Control (6%)
Lifestyle Heart Trial Ornish et al 1990	41 (35–75, no lipid-lowering drugs, no CAD, no recent MI, 5 females)	1 yr	Diet (low-fat, vegetarian) smoking cessation, stress management training, exercise	Progression-intervention (18%) Control (53%) No change-intervention (0%) Control (5.3%) Regression-intervention (82%) Control (42.7%)
Lifestyle Heart Trial Ornish et al 1998	35 (moderate to severe CHD, 20 intervention and 20 control)	1 yr and 5 yr	Diet (low-fat, vegetarian) smoking cessation, stress management training exercise	1 yr (relative change) Progression-intervention (5.4%) Control (0%) Regression-intervention (0%) Control (4.5%) 5 yr (relative change) Progression-intervention (27.7%) Control (0%) Regression-intervention (0%) Control (7.9%)
Schuler et al 1992	36 (stable angina pectoris, 18 intervention, 18 control)	1 yr	Low-fat and cholesterol exercise >3 hr/week	Regression-intervention (38.9%) Control (5.6%) No change-intervention (33%) Control (61%) Progression-intervention (27.8%) Control (33%)
Schuler et al 1992	113 (stable angina pectoris)	1 yr	Low-fat diet, exercise	Progression-intervention (23%) Control (43%) Regression-intervention (32%) Control (17%) No change-intervention (45%) Control (35%) New lesions-intervention (15%) Control (14%) New occlusions-intervention (10%) Control (14%)
SCRIP Haskell 1994	300 (angiographically detectable atherosclerosis, 41 females)	4 yr	Low-fat and cholesterol diet, exercise, weight loss, smoking less/cessation, niacin, lovastatin, gemfibrozil, probucol	Progression-intervention (50.4%) Control (49.6%) Regression-intervention (21%) Control (10%)
Bellardinelli 2001	118 randomized to exercise or control	6 mo	Exercise training	Restenosis rate 29% exercise, 33% control; Residual diameter stenosis 30% lower in exercise group
Hambrecht 2004	101 randomized to PCI or intervention	1 year	Exercise training	Exercise 32% progression; PCI 45% progression; Better event-free survival in exercise group

of clinical, treadmill, or radionuclide data. Van Dixhoorn et al[192] added psychosocial variables and were better able to predict "failure" to improve than success. Data from the major exercise trials in chronic heart failure were recently combined, and there were no variables at baseline that were found to be significant predictors of success.[193] Mixed results have been observed by other investigators on this issue,[194] and more studies are needed that include hemodynamic, exercise, clinical, and psychosocial variables.

NEW MODELS OF CARDIAC REHABILITATION

Changes in reimbursement patterns over the last 15 years, along with the demonstration that clinical outcomes can be improved by multidisciplinary risk factor intervention,[195,196] have led to the development of new models of cardiac rehabilitation. The need for new approaches has also been fueled by the recent observation that a wider spectrum of patients can benefit from cardiac rehabilitation (e.g., valvular surgery, heart failure, transplantation, peripheral vascular disease, and the elderly). Moreover, innovative strategies have been proposed in order to increase the proportion of eligible patients who receive cardiac rehabilitation services despite reductions in reimbursement. In addition, physicians have not been particularly effective in assisting patients in achieving defined risk factor goals,[197-202] and strategies have been suggested to facilitate a greater proportion of patients meeting evidence-based treatment guidelines.

Models that have been developed to meet these needs include the transformation of rehabilitation centers into "secondary prevention centers",[196] the "inclusive chronic disease model",[203] the implementation of affordable, evidence-based, comprehensive risk reduction in primary and secondary prevention settings,[195,204] home exercise programs,[205,206] and case-management systems.[207-210] The concept that cardiac rehabilitation should be the primary medium to implement comprehensive cardiovascular risk reduction has been embraced by the American Heart Association (AHA),[196] the Agency for Health Care Policy and Research Clinical Practice Guidelines,[141] and the AACVPR.[29] The recent AHA consensus statement on "Core Components of Rehabilitation/Secondary Prevention Programs"[193] defines specific evidence-based risk factor goals for management of lipids, blood pressure, weight, smoking cessation, diabetes management, and physical activity (Table 14-14).

This model provides an integrated system that includes appropriate triage, education, counseling on lifestyle interventions, and long-term follow-up.

Several studies have demonstrated the efficacy of comprehensive risk factor management using a *case management* approach. In each of these studies, a nurse or exercise physiologist, as case manager, functions as the coordinator and the point of contact who identifies, triages, provides surveillance on safety and efficacy, performs follow-up, and in many instances, quantifies patient outcomes. Case management has been the cornerstone of recent multidisciplinary efforts to reduce cardiovascular risk. In addition, it has provided a framework for comprehensive management of existing disease, particularly for patients with heart failure.[62,207-210] This approach involves the coordination of risk reduction strategies for targeted groups of patients by a single individual, most commonly a nurse or exercise physiologist, with appropriate medical supervision. The case management concept is based on the idea that risk factors are strongly interrelated, and an individualized, integrated approach to management will optimize care such that clinical outcomes will be improved and costs will be saved. The case management approach has been applied in various settings over the last decade and has been successful in reducing risk markers for CAD and improving outcomes in patients with existing disease. Some of the more prominent studies performed during the 1990s using case management approaches are described in the following.

The Butterworth Heath System in Michigan reorganized their cardiac rehabilitation program to focus on improvement in long-term outcomes using a case-management model.[208] The model included the use of referral pathways, education sessions, and intervention by social workers as necessary. In addition, they added regular phone call follow-up to assess the effectiveness of the risk-reduction interventions. One year after initiating the program, 77% of patients were on appropriate lipid-lowering therapy, 78% reported exercising at least 3 days a week, and 66% of prior smokers reported smoking cessation.

The MULTIFIT program of DeBusk et al[207] has been a model for other case management programs, and its success led to it being adopted by the Kaiser Permanente Health Care System. MULTIFIT is a case-managed program for patients hospitalized with acute MI in Northern California. Patients were randomized to either special risk reduction intervention by a nurse case manager or to usual care. The intervention patients received

TABLE 14–14.   Core components for cardiac rehabilitation/secondary prevention programs

Lipid Management
- Short-term: Assessment and modification of interventions until LDL < 100 mg/dL.
- Long-term: LDL < 100 mg/dL. Secondary goals include HDL > 40 mg/dL and triglycerides < 200 mg/dL.

Hypertension Management
- Short-term: Assessment and modification of interventions until BP < 140 mmHg systolic and < 90 mmHg diastolic; in patients with heart failure, diabetes, and renal failure BP < 130 mmHg systolic and < 85 mmHg diastolic.
- Long-term: BP < 140 mmHg systolic and < 90 mmHg diastolic; in patients with heart failure, diabetes, and renal failure, BP < 130 mmHg systolic and < 85 mmHg diastolic.

Smoking Cessation
- Short-term: Patient will demonstrate readiness to change by initially expressing decision to quit (contemplation) and selecting a quit date (preparation). Subsequently the patient will quit smoking and use of all tobacco products (action); adhere to pharmacotherapy, if prescribed; practice strategies as recommended; and resume cessation plan as quickly as possible when relapse occurs.
- Long-term: complete abstinence from smoking and use of all tobacco products at 12 mo from quit date.

Weight Management
- In patients with BMI > 25 kg/m2 and/or waist > 40 inches in men (102 cm) and > 35 inches (88 cm) in women: Establish reasonable short- and long-term weight goals individualized to patient and associated risk factors (e.g., reduce body weight by at least 10% at a rate of 1–2 lbs/wk over a period of time up to 6 mo).
- Short-term: Continued assessment and modification of interventions until progressive weight loss is achieved. Have patient participate in on-site weight loss program or provide referral to specialized nutrition weight loss programs such that weight goals are achieved.
- Long-term: Adherence to diet and exercise program aimed toward attainment of established weight goal.

Diabetes Management
- In patients with diabetes:
  - Short-term: Develop a regimen of dietary adherence and weight control which includes: exercise, oral hypoglycemic agents, insulin therapy, and optimal control of other risk factors. Drug therapy should be provided and/or monitored in concert with primary healthcare provider.
  - Long-term: Normalization of fasting plasma glucose (80–110 mg/dL or HbA$_1$c < 7.0), minimization of diabetic complications, control of associated obesity, hypertension (<130/85 mmHg), and hyperlipidemia.
- Refer patients without known diabetes whose fasting glucose is >110 mg/dL to their primary healthcare provider for further evaluation and treatment.

Physical Activity Counseling
- Increased physical activity, which includes 20–30 min per day of moderate physical activity on ≥5 days/wk, and increased activity in usual routines; e.g., parking farther away from entrances, walking two or more flights of stairs, walking 15 min during lunch break.
- Increased participation in domestic, occupational, and recreational activities.
- Improved psychosocial well-being, reduction in stress, facilitation of functional independence, prevention of disability, and enhancement of opportunities for independent self-care to achieve recommended goals.

BMI, body mass index; BP, blood pressure; HBA$_1$C, glycosylated hemoglobin; HDL, high-density lipoprotein; LDL, low-density lipoprotein. From the AHA and AACVPR: Scientific Statement on Core Components of Cardiac Rehabilitation/Secondary Prevention Programs. Circulation 2000;102:1069–1073.

education and counseling regarding smoking cessation, regular physical activity, and nutrition. Medical management, such as lipid-lowering therapy, was instituted as indicated for risk factors not controlled by lifestyle change. Much of the intervention was mediated by phone and mail contact. The intervention group showed greater improvement at 6 months and 1 year in functional capacity, rate of smoking cessation, and changes in LDL-C compared with the usual care group, and subsequent analyses have shown MULTIFIT to be cost-effective.[210]

The recently completed Cardiac Hospital Atherosclerosis Management Program (CHAMP)[209] compared outcomes among 302 patients enrolled in a case-managed risk reduction intervention and compared them with 256 control patients. All were discharged from UCLA Medical Center with a diagnosis of CAD or other vascular disease. The case managed approach emphasized close adherence to appropriate use of aspirin, beta-blockers, ACE inhibitors, and lipid-lowering agents, combined with outpatient exercise, nutrition, and smoking cessation counseling. After the study period, there was greater use of appropriate medications, an increase in the percentage of patients achieving an LDL-C level less than 100 mg/dl, a reduction in recurrent MI, and a lower 1-year mortality.

At Stanford, a randomized, controlled trial funded by the NIH was performed to evaluate the efficacy of case-managed, physician-directed multirisk factor intervention (the SCRIP Study).[62] Case managers coordinated care along with a team of nutritionists, psychologists, and physicians to provide clinical and lifestyle interventions, attempting to achieve nationally recognized goals for risk factor reduction. Three hundred subjects were randomized to intervention or usual care groups. After the 4-year study period, the intervention group demonstrated an increase in exercise participation; reductions in dietary fat and cholesterol intake; reductions in SBP, body mass index and blood lipids; an improvement in glucose tolerance; and a 27% reduction in Framingham Risk Score. These changes were associated with reductions in hospitalizations and coronary events. Angiographic results included both a decreased progression of CAD and greater stabilization of plaque in the intervention group.

The home-based model of rehabilitation, validated at Stanford University in the 1980s,[205] has been used in many centers over the last 15 years. This approach uses home exercise that is either unmonitored or monitored via telephone or computer. Some programs feature regular feedback via telephone or home visits, and recent approaches have used exercise monitoring devices such as pedometers, accelerometers, and heart rate recording devices to encourage and document compliance with prescribed exercise. Safety and efficacy of these home programs have been shown to be similar to those of more conventional programs.[205,206]

FUTURE DIRECTIONS FOR CARDIAC REHABILITATION

Cardiac rehabilitation professionals must continue to develop innovative means to deliver their services and to document what they are doing by using outcome assessment and cost control. They must gather evidence on consequences of care—not just at completion of formal treatment, but much later—and with assessment tools that are sensitive to lifestyle factors associated with disease risk and progression, as well as quality of life. Their services must have a focus that is population-based, with a primary responsibility to manage capitated enrollees. Rather than respond to hospital directors, they must relate to executives responsible for managing primary care. Re-engineering is critical. Cardiac rehabilitation professionals must start asking, "Do we really need this particular aspect of rehabilitation?," "Is there a better and cheaper way to deliver this service?," and "Which patients really need and benefit from a particular component?" No longer can each hospital or clinic have a program simply to be competitive. One or two centers will be sufficient for each community. The following

sections describe suggestions for the survival of cardiac rehabilitation.

As suggested by Ribisl et al,[203,211] a new era requires a new model. The old model of a standard, fixed 36-session program in which every patient receives the same intervention, regardless of specific needs or characteristics, is outmoded and a disservice to patients. Part of the reason for adhering to the old model was failure to interact with third-party payers in the design of appropriate programs that met patient needs. The security of a safe and reliable means of obtaining reimbursement was the driving force behind this approach—and programs have been reluctant to make any change because of fear that revenues would be lost. Some observations or suggestions follow in subsequent sections, as well as recommendations of several models for consideration that are based on impressions of current trends and opportunities that exist today.

Initiate Patient Contact Early

Too many patients are leaving the in-patient setting without being contacted by the cardiac rehabilitation specialists. Efforts must be intensified to ensure an early contact during the in-patient setting. The cardiac rehabilitation team must be integrated into the clinical pathway to work with these patients at this ideal time. Waiting until well after discharge has proven to be ineffective. The current trend is to reduce the length of both the hospital stay and the follow-up period as a method of cost saving. Thus, it becomes even more important that these patients be provided with an opportunity to interact with rehabilitation specialists who can assist them in their recovery. Practitioners must be more active in educating primary care physicians, managed care administrators, and consumers about the value of rehabilitation. Under a capitated system, they must be convinced that low-technology alternatives are in place to minimize costs. They also must be able to readily access services so admissions occur at acceptable rates when appropriate cases arise. With cardiac rehabilitation care serving approximately 15% to 20% of eligible patients today, utilization is low.

Reach a More Diverse Pool of Patients

The treatment plan for patients with cardiovascular disease is really limited to a single diagnosis. It is unusual to find an older patient who is free of other diagnoses of chronic disease. It is likely that many patients with cardiac disease have one or more additional diseases such as obesity, diabetes, chronic obstructive pulmonary disease,[212] arthritis, or other complications that must be taken into account in the intervention plan. Yet few programs market their services to patients with these other diagnoses and thereby lose a key opportunity to serve the widest client base with a common set of interventional strategies applicable to the treatment of multiple disease. For instance, weight control is an important intervention in the treatment of those chronic diseases that are aggravated by obesity. Dietary modification, including a reduction of fat and cholesterol intake, and an increase in complex carbohydrates in the form of whole grains, fresh fruits, and vegetables, is not only essential in clinical efforts to slow the progress of atherosclerotic lesions, but also helps the diabetic, arthritic, and the obese. The *benefits of exercise* to each of these chronic disease groups are well documented, as are the use of relaxation and cognitive strategies in *behavior change*. Cardiac rehabilitation needs to consider a new and broader identity and expand its scope of practice to include all chronic disease—especially as the aged segment of our patient population continues to grow, requiring the most costly services available in the healthcare system.

Increase Physician Awareness

There is a clear lack of awareness among those in the medical profession who are responsible for making decisions regarding the treatment options available to their patients in the community. It is a well-recognized fact that physicians infrequently counsel their patients regarding healthy habits, even though most authorities would agree to the benefits. Whether it is a lack of awareness of the availability of these services or whether it is simply negligence, ignorance, or skepticism—the fact remains that few patients are being referred to rehabilitative programs. The critical step in any effort to change this pattern rests with the primary care physician, who now serves as a "gatekeeper" to these potential services. Primary care physicians must become an integral part of the treatment plan for their patients who are most likely to benefit from cardiac rehabilitation. They must become educated about the short- and long-term benefits; otherwise, without this collaborative treatment planning and consequent increase in clientele, it is unlikely that these programs can survive in the future. Because training in preventive strategies has never been an integral part of medical education, efforts must be made to convince current practitioners and medical students about the benefits to patients.

Include Underserved Populations

The misconception that cardiovascular disease predominantly afflicts men is a major deterrent to referrals of women to rehabilitative programs. Cardiovascular disease is still the major cause of death in women and mortality rates are comparable between the sexes. Other groups, who are underserved, due to reasons of economics as well as misconception, are the elderly, the poor or uneducated, and minorities. The population being served in most programs across the nation remains relatively young, white, professional, and male.

Expand Utilization

Although less than 20% of all eligible cardiac patients are referred to cardiac rehabilitation programs, 100% of all eligible patients could benefit from some form of cardiac rehabilitation. One reason for this discrepancy may be a physician belief system that fails to incorporate secondary prevention (e.g., cardiac rehabilitation) into the patient's treatment plan. Physicians should become more familiar with alternatives to their current practice and utilize other healthcare professionals to efficiently and economically extend their capacity to treat their patients. Ideally, specialists who would determine their needs and individualize a program would see every patient at a rehabilitation center. All of the modalities of rehabilitation would be considered (home-based to monitored groups) without outside pressures to enter patients into expensive approaches. In addition, eligibility should be expanded to the elderly, patients with CHF, and those patients in need of post-surgical intervention. In some circumstances, all the rehabilitation needed or available might be counseling by a primary care physician. Patients who are more successful in changing their lifestyle behaviors report that the physician's recommendation had a strong influence on their willingness to change. Physicians who are confident and have good counseling skills are often effective in changing the behavior of their patients. Physicians with good personal health habits and positive health beliefs are also more likely to have a positive influence on their patients' lifestyles. It has even been suggested that the traditional physical examination in apparently healthy persons is a waste of physician and patient time—time that could better be spent on counseling to encourage better lifestyle habits.

Highlight Potential Reduction in Mortality

Cardiac rehabilitation is successful, as demonstrated by several independent meta-analyses described earlier in this chapter; these rigorous analyses have demonstrated 25% reductions in cardiovascular mortality. This mortality benefit was recently extended to patients with heart failure[51,52] In fact, these latter analyses demonstrated that the mortality benefit may even be slightly greater in patients with heart failure. Numerous studies have documented the benefits of lowering serum cholesterol using drugs. Angiographic studies have consistently shown regression or slowing of progression, whereas one recent follow-up study found a 25% and 42% reduction in mortality and CABS, respectively. Because recent studies indicating regression of coronary disease and decrease in events with cholesterol-lowering statins underscore the benefits of rehabilitation, the control of lipid abnormalities must be a key part of any rehabilitation program.

Document Cost-Efficacy

Like all clinical interventions today, cardiac rehabilitation programs must demonstrate to hospital administrators that they are cost effective. Although such documentation is likely to exist for many, if not most, programs, few have made the effort to publish such data. There has been a proliferation of research methodologies in recent years that consider alternative ways of conducting economic evaluation of healthcare.[213] Although this has added some uncertainty of approach, standardization is coming and decision makers are beginning to consider these findings as they reformulate the scope of their health insurance coverage. Importantly, recent studies clearly demonstrate that cardiac rehabilitation is cost-effective. Oldridge et al[214] performed an economic evaluation of patients 1 year after randomization to either an 8-week rehabilitation intervention or usual care and revealed that cardiac rehabilitation is an efficient use of healthcare resources. Ades et al[215] presented the results of a 3-year economic evaluation of patients undergoing 12 weeks of rehabilitation, which revealed that per capita

hospitalization charges for rehabilitation participants were $739 lower than for nonparticipants. Bondestam et al[216] described the effects of early rehabilitation that relied totally upon the primary healthcare system on consumption of medical care resources during the first year after acute MI in patients 65 years of age or older. Patients from one primary healthcare district were assigned to a rehabilitation program, whereas patients from a neighboring district constituted a control group. The rehabilitation measures were initiated very early after the infarction with individual counseling in the home of the patient and later in the local health center, where 21% of the patients also joined a low-intensity exercise group. During the first 3 months there was a significantly lower incidence of rehospitalization in the intervention group, expressed both in terms of percentage of patients and days of rehospitalization. Visits to the emergency department without rehospitalization also were significantly lower in the intervention group. After 12 months the differences still remained, with the exception of no intergroup difference in follow-up relative to days of rehospitalization. In the matched groups the same result was seen. Although readmissions and emergency department visits generally were well justified in the intervention group, vague symptoms dominated among the controls. Levin et al[217] presented the results of an economic evaluation of patients followed-up for 5 years after rehabilitation intervention or usual care that demonstrated that mean patient costs were $8800 lower in the rehabilitation group. These cost-savings associated with rehabilitation compare favorably to the cost-effectiveness of other preventive measures, with the exception of smoking cessation.[218]

SUMMARY

Cardiac rehabilitation has been going through the same dramatic changes as the entire healthcare system. However, its principles have become part of good medical practice. The outcome for nearly all clinical interventions carried out for cardiovascular disease can be improved by lifestyle intervention, and cardiac rehabilitation has been an important medium for these lifestyle changes. A major challenge that remains is providing rehabilitation services to a greater proportion of eligible patients. The emphasis on the health benefits of physical activity, rather than physical fitness and the reduction of iatrogenic deconditioning, have decreased the emphasis on exercise prescription and the phased approach. Cardiac rehabilitation is appropriately evolving from simple exercise programs toward comprehensive secondary prevention. As studies continue to demonstrate physiologic benefits, improved mortality, and cost efficacy, rehabilitation and secondary prevention will become a standard of care for patients with cardiovascular disease.

REFERENCES

1. Braunwald E, Antman EM, Beasley JW, et al: ACC/AHA 2002 guideline update for the management of patients with unstable angina and non-ST segment elevation myocardial infarction—summary article: A report of the American College of Cardiology/American Heart Association task force on practice guidelines (Committee on the Management of Patients With Unstable Angina). J Am Coll Cardiol 2002;40:1366–1374.
2. Arciero TJ, Jacobsen SJ, Reeder GS, et al: Temporal trends in the incidence of coronary disease. Am J Med 2004;117:228–233.
3. Dargie H: Myocardial infarction: Redefined or reinvented? Heart 2002;88:1–3.
4. Dalby M, Bouzamondo A, Lechat P, Montalescot G: Transfer for primary angioplasty versus immediate thrombolysis in acute myocardial infarction: A meta-analysis. Circulation 2003;108:1809–1814.
5. Goldman L, Phillips KA, Coxson P, et al: The effect of risk factor reductions between 1981 and 1990 on coronary heart disease incidence, prevalence, mortality and cost. J Am Coll Cardiol 2001;38:1012–1017.
6. Maisel AS, Ahnve S, Gilpin E, et al: Prognosis after extension of myocardial infarct: The role of Q-wave or non-Q-wave infarction. Circulation 1985;71:211–217.
7. Maisel AS, Gilpin E, Hoit B, et al: Survival after hospital discharge in matched populations with inferior or anterior myocardial infarction. J Am Coll Cardiol 1985;6:731–736.
8. Moon JC, De Arenaza DP, Elkington AG, et al: The pathologic basis of Q-wave and non-Q-wave myocardial infarction: A cardiovascular magnetic resonance study. J Am Coll Cardio. 2004;44:554–560.
9. Guidelines for Risk Stratification after Myocardial Infarction. American College of Physicians. Ann Intern Med 1997;126:556–560.
10. Eagle KA, Lim MJ, Dabbous OH, et al: A validated prediction model for all forms of acute coronary syndrome: Estimating the risk of 6-month postdischarge death in an international registry. JAMA 2004;291:2727–2733.
11. Plebani M, Zaninotto M: Cardiac markers: Present and future. Int J Clin Lab Res 1999;29:56–63.
12. Cucherat M, Bonnefoy E, Tremeau G: Primary angioplasty versus intravenous thrombolysis for acute myocardial infarction. Cochrane Database Syst Rev 2003;3:CD001560.
13. Hammerman H, Schoen FJ, Kloner RA: Short-term exercise has a prolonged effect on scar formation after experimental acute myocardial infarction. J Am Coll Cardiol 1983;2:979–982.
14. Kloner RA, Kloner JA: The effect of early exercise on myocardial infarct scar formation. Am Heart J 1983;106:1009–1014.
15. Gaudron P, Hu K, Schamberger R, et al: Effect of endurance training early or late after coronary artery occulusion on left ventricular remodeling, hemodynamics, and survival in rats with chronic transmural myocardial infarction. Circulation 1994;89:402–412.
16. Oh BH, Ono S, Rockman HA, Ross J: Myocardial hypertrophy in the ischemic zone induced by exercise in rats after coronary reperfusion. Circulation 1993;87:598–607.
17. Hochman JS, Healy B: Effect of exercise on acute myocardial infarction in rats. J Am Coll Cardiol 1986;7:126–132.
18. Levine SA, Lown B: The "chair" treatment of acute coronary thrombosis. Trans Assoc Am Physicians 1951;64:316–319.
19. Saltin B, Blomquist G, Mitchell JH, et al: Response to exercise after bed rest and after training. Circulation 1968;1(suppl VII):37–38.
20. Convertino VA: Effect of orthostatic stress on exercise performance after bed rest: Relation to in-hospital rehabilitation. J Cardiopulm Rehabil 1983;3:660–663.
21. Cain HD, Frasher WG, Stivelman R: Graded activity program for safe return to self-care after myocardial infarction. JAMA 1961;177:111–120.
22. Torkelson LO: Rehabilitation of the patient with acute myocardial infarction. J Chronic Dis 1964;17:685–704.
23. Sivarajan ES, Snydsman A, Smith B, et al: Low-level treadmill testing of 41 patients with acute myocardial infarction prior to discharge from the hospital. Heart Lung 1977;6:975–980.
24. Hayes MJ, Morris GK, Hampton JR: Comparison of mobilization after two and nine days in uncomplicated myocardial infarction. BMJ 1974;3:10–13.
25. Bloch A, Maeder J, Haissly J, et al: Early mobilization after myocardial infarction: A controlled study. Am J Cardiol 1974;34:152–157.
26. Sivarajan E, Bruce RA, Almes MJ, et al: A randomized study of cardiac rehabilitation. N Engl J Med 1981;305:357–362.
27. World Health Organization (WHO) Report of Expert Committee: Rehabilitation of patients with cardiovascular diseases. Technical report no. 270. Geneva, WHO, 1964.
28. American College of Sports Medicine: Guidelines for Exercise Testing and Prescription, 6th ed. Baltimore, Lippincott Williams & Wilkins, 2000.
29. American Association of Cardiovascular and Pulmonary Rehabilitation: Guidelines for Cardiac Rehabilitation Programs, 4th ed. Champaign, Ill, Human Kinetics, 2003.
30. Kelemen MH, Stewart KJ, Gillilan RE, et al: Circuit weight training in cardiac patients. J Am Coll Cardiol 1986;7:38–42.
31. Sparling PB, Cantwell JD, Dolan CM, Niederman RK: Strength training in a cardiac rehabilitation program: A six-month follow-up. Arch Phys Med Rehabil 1990;71:148.
32. Sanchez OA, Leon A: Resistance exercise for patients with diabetes mellitus. In Graves JE, Franklin BA (eds): Resistance Training for Health and Rehabilitation. Champaign Ill, Human Kinetics, 2001, pp 295–318.
33. Kallio V, Hamalainen H, Hakkila J, Luurila OJ: Reduction in sudden deaths by a multifactorial intervention programme after acute myocardial infarction. Lancet 1979;2:1091–1094.
34. Kentala E: Physical fitness and feasibility of physical rehabilitation after myocardial infarction in men of working age. Ann Clin Res 1972;4:1–25.
35. Palatsi I: Feasibility of physical training after myocardial infarction and its effect on return to work, morbidity, and mortality. Acta Med Scand Suppl 1976;599:1–100.
36. Wilhelmsen L, Sanne H, Elmfeldt D, et al: A controlled trial of physical training after myocardial infarction. Prev Med 1975;4:491–508.
37. Shaw LW: Effects of a prescribed supervised exercise program on mortality and cardiovascular mortality in patients after a myocardial infarction. Am J Cardiol 1981;48:39–46.
38. Shepard RJ: Exercise regimens after myocardial infarction: Rationale and results. Cardiovasc Clin 1985;14:145–157.
39. Bengtsson K: Rehabilitation after myocardial infarction. Scand J Rehabil Med 1983;15:1–9.
40. Carson P, Phillips R, Lloyd M, et al: Exercise after myocardial infarction: A controlled trial. J R Coll Physicians Lond 1982;16:147–151.
41. Vermeulen A, Liew KI, Durrer D: Effects of cardiac rehabilitation after myocardial infarction: Changes in coronary risk factors and long-term prognosis. Am Heart J 1983;105:798–801.
42. Roman O: Do randomized trials support the use of cardiac rehabilitation? J Cardiopulm Rehabil 1985;5:93–96.
43. Mayou RA: A controlled trial of early rehabilitation after myocardial infarction. J Cardiopulm Rehabil 1983;3:397–402.
44. Hedback B, Perk J, Perski A: Effect of a post-myocardial infarction rehabilitation program on mortality, morbidity, and risk factors. J Cardiopulm Rehabil 1985;5:576–583.
45. Agency for Health Care Policy and Research. Guidelines for Cardiac Rehabilitation, 1995.
46. Ades PA: Cardiac rehabilitation and secondary prevention of coronary heart disease. N Engl J Med 2001;345:892–902.
47. May GS, Eberlein KA, Furberg CD, et al: Secondary prevention after myocardial infarction: A review of long-term trials. Prog Cardiovasc Dis 1982;24:331–352.
48. O'Connor GT, Buring JE, Yusuf S, et al: An overview of randomized trials of rehabilitation with exercise after myocardial infarction. Circulation 1989;80:234–244.

49. Oldridge NB, Guyatt GH, Fischer ME, Rimm AA: Cardiac rehabilitation after myocardial infarction. Combined experience of randomized clinical trials. JAMA 1988;260:945–950.

50. Taylor RS, Brown A, Ebrahim S, et al: Exercise-based rehabilitation for patients with coronary heart disease: Systematic review and meta-analysis of randomized controlled trails. Am J Med 2004;16:682–692.

51. Piepoli MF, Davos C, Francis DP, Coats AJ: Exercise training meta-analysis of trials in patients with chronic heart failure. BMJ 2004;328:189.

52. Smart N, Marwick TH: Exercise training for heart failure patients: A systemic review of factors that improve patient mortality and morbidity. Am J Med 2004;116:693–706.

53. Kent KM, Smith ER, Redwood DR, et al: Electrical stability of acutely ischemic myocardium. Circulation 1973;47:291–298.

54. Billman GE, Schwartz PJ, Stone HL: The effects of daily exercise on susceptibility to sudden cardiac death. Circulation 1984;69:1182–1189.

55. Hull SS, Vanoli E, Adamson PB, et al: Exercise training confers anticipatory protection from sudden death during acute myocardial ischemia. Circulation 1994;89:548–552.

56. Kloner RA, Bolli R, Marban E, et al: Participants, medical and cellular implications of stunning, hibernation, and preconditioning: An NHLBI workshop. Circulation 1998;97:1847–1867.

57. Abete P, Ferrara N. Cacciatore F, et al: Angina-induced protection against myocardial infarction in adult and elderly patients: A loss of preconditioning mechanism in the aging heart? J Am Coll Cardiol 1997;30:947–954.

58. Maybaum S, Ilan M, Mogilevsky J, et al: Improvement in ischemic parameters during repeated exercise testing: A possible model for myocardial preconditioning. Am J Cardiol 1996;78:1087–1091.

59. Kloner RA: Preinfarct angina and exercise: Yet another reason to stay physically active. J Am Coll Cardiol 2001;38:1366–1368.

60. Schuler G, Hambrecht R, Schlierf G, et al: Myocardial perfusion and regression of coronary artery disease in patients on a regimen of intensive physical exercise and low fat diet. J Am Coll Cardiol 1992;19:34–42.

61. Hambrecht R, Niebauer J, Marburger C, et al: Various intensities of leisure time physical activity in patients with coronary artery disease: Effects on cardiorespiratory fitness and progression of coronary atherosclerotic lesions. J Am Coll Cardiol 1993;22:468–477.

62. Haskell WL, Alderman EL, Fair JM, et al: Effects of intensive multiple risk factor reduction on coronary atherosclerosis and clinical cardiac events in men and women with coronary artery disease: The Stanford Coronary Risk Intervention project (SCRIP). Circulation 1994;89:975–990.

63. Hambrecht R, Wolf A, Gielen S, et al: Effect of exercise on coronary endothelial function in patients with coronary artery disease. N Engl J Med 2000;342:454–460.

64. Hambrecht R, Fiehen E, Weigl C, et al: Regular physical exercise corrects endothelial dysfunction and improves exercise capacity in patients with chronic heart failure. Circulation 1998;98:2709–2715.

65. Edwards DG, Schofield RS, Lennon SL, et al: Effect of exercise training on endothelial function in men with coronary artery disease. Am J Cardiol 2004;93:617–620.

66. Gokce N, Vita JA, Bader DS, et al: Effect of exercise on upper and lower extremity endothelial function in patients with coronary artery disease. Am J Cardiol 2002;90:124–127.

67. Moyna NM, Thompson PD: The effect of physical activity on endothelial function in man. Acta Physiol Scand 2004;180:113–123.

68. Rochmis P, Blackburn H: Exercise tests: A survey of procedures, safety and litigation experience in approximately 170,000 tests. JAMA 1971;217:1061–1066.

69. Irving JB, Bruce RA: Exertional hypotension and postexertional ventricular fibrillation in stress testing. Am J Cardiol 1977;39:849–851.

70. Gibbons L, Blair SN, Kohl HW, Cooper K: The safety of maximal exercise testing. Circulation 1980;80:846–852.

71. Yang JC, Wesley RC Jr, Froelicher VF: Ventricular tachycardia during routine treadmill testing. Arch Intern Med 1991;151:349–353.

72. Franklin BA, Gordon S, Timmis GC, O'Neill WW: Is direct physician supervision of exercise stress testing routinely necessary? Chest 1997;111:262–264.

73. Myers J, Voodi L, Umann T, Froelicher VF: A survey of exercise testing: Methods, utilization, interpretation, and safety in the VAHCS. J Cariopulm Rehabil 2000;20:251–258.

74. Haskell WL: Cardiovascular complications during exercise training of cardiac patients. Circulation 1978;57:920–924.

75. Hossack KF, Hartwig R: Cardiac arrest associated with supervised cardiac rehabilitation. J Cardiac Rehab 1982;2:402–408.

76. Fletcher G, Cantwell JD, Murray PM, Thomas RJ: Exercise and the heart: Current management of service exercise-related cardiac events. Chest 1988;93:1264–1269.

77. Van Camp SP, Peterson RA: Cardiovascular complications of outpatient cardiac rehabilitation programs. JAMA 1986;256:1160–1163.

78. Thompson PD, Funk EJ, Carleton RA, Sturner WQ: Incidence of death during jogging in Rhode Island from 1975 through 1980. JAMA 1982;247:2535–2538.

79. Thompson PD: The benefits and risks of exercise training in patients with chronic coronary artery disease. JAMA 1988;259:1537–1540.

80. Leon AS, Franklin BA, Costa F et al: Cardiac rehabilitation and secondary prevention of coronary heart disease. An American Heart Association Scientific Statement from the Council on Clinical Cardiology (Subcommittee on Exercise, Cardiac Rehabilitation, and Prevention (and the Council on Nutrition, Physical Activity, and Metabolism (subcommittee on Physical Activity), in collaboration with the American Association of Cardiovascular and Pulmonary Rehabilitation. Circulation 2005;111:369–376.

81. Giri S, Thompson PD, Kiernan FJ, et al: Clinical and angiographic characteristics of exertion-related acute myocardial infarction. JAMA 1999;282:1731–1736.

82. Miller NH, Haskell WL, Berra K, DeBusk RF: Home versus group exercise training for increasing functional capacity after myocardial infarction. Circulation 1984;70:645–649.

83. Kelbaek H, Eskildsen P, Hansen PF, Godtfredsen J: Spontaneous and/or training-induced hemodynamic changes after myocardial infarction. Int J Cardiol 1981;1:205–213.

84. Greenland P, Chu JS: Efficacy of cardiac rehabilitation services. With emphasis on patients after myocardial infarction. Ann Intern Med 1988;109:650–666.

85. Goebbels U, Myers J, Dziekan G, et al: A randomized comparison of exercise training in patients with normal vs. reduced ventricular function. Chest 1998;113:1387–1393.

86. Scheuer J: Effects of physical training on myocardial vascularity and perfusion. Circulation 1982;66:491–495.

87. Bloor CM, White F, Sanders T: Effects of exercise on collateral development in myocardial ischemia in pigs. J Appl Physiol 1984;56:656–665.

88. Ferguson RJ, Petitclerc R, Choquette G, et al: Effect of physical training on treadmill exercise capacity, collateral circulation and progression of coronary disease. Am J Cardiol 1974;34:764–772.

89. Nolewajka AJ, Kostuk WJ, Rechnitzer PA, et al: Exercise and human collateralization: An angiographic and scintigraphic assessment. Circulation 1979;60:114–122.

90. Sim DN, Neill WA: Investigation of the physiological basis for increased exercise threshold for angina pectoris after physical conditioning. J Clin Invest 1974;54:763–770.

91. Verani MS, Hartung GH, Harris-Hoepfel J, et al: Effects of exercise training on left ventricular performance and myocardial perfusion in patients with coronary artery disease. Am J Cardiol 1981;47:797–803.

92. Cobb FR, Williams RS, McEwan P, et al: Effects of exercise training on ventricular function in patients with recent myocardial infarction. Circulation 1982;66:100–108.

93. DeBusk RF, Hung J: Exercise conditioning soon after myocardial infarction: Effects on myocardial perfusion and ventricular function. Ann NY Acad Sci 1982;382:343–351.

94. Todd IC, Bradnam MS, Cooke MBD, Ballantyne D: Effects of daily high-intensity exercise on myocardial perfusion in angina pectoris. Am J Cardiol 1991;68:1593–1600.

95. Schuler G, Schlierf G, Wirth A, et al: Low-fat diet and regular, supervised physical exercise in patients with symptomatic coronary artery disease: Reduction of stress-induced myocardial ischemia. Circulation 1988;77:172–181.

96. Schuler G, Hambrecht R, Schlierf G, et al: Regular physical exercise and low-fat diet: Effects on progression of coronary artery disease. Circulation 1992;86:1–11.

97. Schuler G, Hambrecht R, Schlierf G, et al: Myocardial perfusion and regression of coronary artery disease in patients on a regimen of intensive physical exercise and low fat diet. J Am Coll Cardiol 1992;19:34–42.

98. Froelicher VF, Jensen D, Genter F, et al: A randomized trial of exercise training in patients with coronary heart disease. JAMA 1984;252:1291–1297.

99. Atwood JE, Jensen D, Froelicher VF, et al: Agreement in human interpretation of analog thallium myocardial perfusion images. Circulation 1981;64:601–609.

100. Sebrechts CP, Klein JL, Ahnve S, et al: Myocardial perfusion changes following 1 year of exercise training assessed by thallium-201 circumferential count profiles. Am Heart J 1986;112:1217–1226.

101. Myers J, Ahnve S, Froelicher V, et al: A randomized trial of the effects of 1 year of exercise training on computer-measured ST segment displacement in patients with coronary artery disease. J Am Coll Cardiol 1984;4:1094–1102.

102. Ehsani AA, Martin WH, Heath GW, Coyle EF: Cardiac effects of prolonged and intense exercise training in patients with coronary artery disease. Am J Cardiol 1982;50:246–254.

103. Hossack KF, Hartwick R: Cardiac arrest associated with supervised cardiac rehabilitation. J Cardiac Rehabil 1982;2:402–408.

104. Donovan CM, Brooks GA: Endurance training affects lactate clearance, not lactate production. Am J Physiol 1983;244:E83–E92.

105. Myers J, Ashley E: Dangerous curves—A perspective on exercise, lactate and the anaerobic threshold. Chest 1997;111:787–795.

106. Hossack KF, Bruce RA, Kusumi F: Altered exercise ventilatory responses by apparent propranolol-diminished glucose metabolism: Implications concerning impaired physical training benefit in coronary patients. Am Heart J 1981;102:378–382.

107. Malmborg R, Isaccson S, Kallivroussis G: The effect of beta-blockade and/or physical training in patients with angina pectoris. Curr Ther Res Clin Exp 1974;16:171–183.

108. Obma RT, Wilson PK, Goebel ME, Campbell DE: Effect of a conditioning program in patients taking propranolol for angina pectoris. Cardiology 1979;64:365–371.

109. Pratt CM, Welton DE, Squired WG, et al: Demonstration of training effect during chronic beta-adrenergic blockade in patients with coronary artery disease. Circulation 1981;64:1125–1129.

110. Vanhees L, Fagard R, Amery A: Influence of beta-adrenergic blockade on the hemodynamic effects of physical training in patients with ischemic heart disease. Am Heart J 1984;108:270–275.

111. Pavia L, Orlando G, Myers J, et al: The effect of beta-blockade therapy on the response to exercise training in postmyocardial infarction patients. Clin Cardiol 1995;18:716–720.

112. Forissier JF, Vernochet P, Bertrand P, Charbonnier B, et al: Influence of carvedilol on the benefits of physical training in patients with moderate chronic heart failure. Eur J Heart Fail 2001;3:335–342.

113. Currier D, Galinier M, Pathak A, et al: Rehabilitation of patients with congestive heart failure with or without beta-blockade therapy. J Card Fail 2001;7:241–248.

114. Ewy GA, Wilmore JH, Morton AR, et al: The effect of beta-adrenergic blockade on obtaining a trained exercise state. J Cardiac Rehabil 1983;3:25–29.

115. Tesch PA, Kaiser P: Effects of beta-adrenergic blockade on 02 uptake during submaximal and maximal exercise. J Appl Physiol 1983;54:901–905.

116. Sable DL, Brammell HL, Shehan MV, et al: Attenuation of exercise conditioning by beta-adrenergic blockade. Circulation 1982;65: 679–684.

117. Marsh RC, Hiatt WR, Brammel HL, Horowitz L: Attenuation of exercise conditioning by low dose beta-adrenergic receptor blockade. J Am Coll Cardiol 1983;2:551–556.

118. Gordon EP, Savin WM, Bristow MR, Haskell WL: Cathecholamines and cardiac hypertrophy in exercise training. Circulation 1983;68:III–376.

119. Froelicher VF, Sullivan M, Myers J, Jensen D: Can patients with coronary artery disease receiving beta blockers obtain a training effect? Am J Cardiol 1985;55:155D–161D.

120. Kentala E: Physical fitness and feasibility of physical rehabilitation after myocardial infarction in men of working age. Ann Clin Res 1972;4(suppl 9):1–84.

121. Dorn J, Naughton J, Imamura D, Trevisan M: Correlates of compliance in a randomized exercise trial in myocardial infarction patients. Med Sci Sports Exerc 2001;33:1081–1089.

122. Piepoli MF, Flather M, Coats AJ: Overview of studies of exercise training in chronic heart failure: The need for a prospective randomized multicenter European trial. Eur Heart J 1998;19: 830–841.

123. Hambrecht R, Niebauer J, Fiehn E, et al: Physical training in patients with stable chronic heart failure: Effects on cardiorespiratory fitness and ultrastructural abnormalities of leg muscles. J Am Coll Cardiol 1995;25:1239–1249.

124. Dubach P, Myers J, Dziekan G, et al: Effect of high intensity exercise training on central hemodynamic responses to exercise in men with reduced left ventricular function. J Am Coll Cardiol 1997; 29:1591–1598.

125. Pina IL, Apstein CS, Balady GJ, et al: Exercise and heart failure: A statement from the American Heart Association Committee on exercise, rehabilitation, and prevention. Circulation 2003;107: 1210–1225.

126. Stratton J, Dunn J, Adamopoulos S, et al: Training partially reverses skeletal muscle metabolic abnormalities during exercise in heart failure. J Appl Physiol 1994;76:1575–1582.

127. Myers J, Goebbels U, Dzeikan G, et al: Exercise training and myocardial remodeling in patients with reduced ventricular function: One-year follow-up with magnetic resonance imaging. Am Heart J 2000;139:252–261.

128. Hambrecht R, Gielen S, Linke, et al: Effects of exercise training on left ventricular function and peripheral resistance on patients with chronic heart failure. JAMA 2000;283:3095–3101.

129. Giannuzzi P, Temporelli PL, Corra U, Tavazzi L: Antiremodeling effect of long-term exercise training in patients with stable chronic heart failure: Results of the Exercise in Left Ventricular Dysfunction and Chronic Heart Failure (ELVD-CHF) Trial. Circulation 2003;108:554–559.

130. Sullivan MJ, Higginbotham MB, Cobb FR: Exercise training in patients with severe left ventricular dysfunction: Hemodynamic and metabolic effects. Circulation 1988;78:506–515.

131. Coats A, Adamopoulos S, Radaelli A, et al: Controlled trial of physical training in chronic heart failure. Circulation 1992; 85:2119–2131.

132. Dubach P, Myers J, Dzieken G, et al: Effect of exercise training on myocardial remodeling in patients with reduced left ventricular function after myocardial infarction: Application of magnetic resonance imaging. Circulation 1997;95:2060–2067.

133. Hambrecht R, Fiehn E, Weigl C, et al: Regular physical exercise corrects endothelial dysfunction and improves exercise capacity in patients with chronic heart failure. Circulation 1998;98: 2709–2715.

134. Coats AJS, Adamopoulos S, Meyer TE, et al: Effects of physical training in chronic heart failure. Lancet 1990;335:63–66.

135. Tyni-Lenne R, Gordon A, Sylven C: Improved quality of life in chronic heart failure patients following local endurance training with leg muscle. J Cardiac Failure 1996;2:111–117.

136. Judgutt BI, Michorowski BL, Kappagoda CT: Exercise training after anterior Q-wave myocardial infarction: Importance of regional left ventricular function and topography. J Am Coll Cardiol 1988; 12:363–372.

137. Oh BH, Ono S, Gilpin E, Ross J: Altered left ventricular remodeling with beta-adrenergic blockade and exercise after coronary reperfusion in rats. Circulation 1993;87:608–616.

138. Giannuzzi P, Tavazzi L, Temporelli PL, et al: Long-term physical training and left ventricular remodeling after anterior myocardial infarction. Results of exercise in anterior myocardial infarction (EAMI) trial. J Am Coll Cardiol 1993;22:1821–1829.

139. Giannuzzi P, Corra U, Gattone M, et al: Attenuation of unfavorable remodeling by exercise training in postinfarction patients with left ventricular dysfunction: Results of exercise in left ventricular dysfunction (ELVD) trial. Circulation 1997;96:1790–1797.

140. Cannistra LB, Davidoff R, Picard MH, Balady GJ: Effect of exercise training after myocardial infarction on left ventricular remodelling relative to infarct size. J Cardiopulm Rehabil 1999; 19:373–380.

141. Agency for Health Care Policy and Research Clinical Practice Guidelines: Cardiac Rehabilitation. Washington, D.C., U.S. Department of Health and Human Services, 1995.

142. Hosenpud JD, Bennett LE, Keck BM, et al: The Registry of the International Society for Heart and Lung Transplantation: Fifteenth official report. J Heart Lung Transplant 1998;17:656–668.

143 Stinson EB, Griepp RL, Schroeder IS, et al: Hemodynamic observations one and two years after cardiac transplantation in man. Circulation 1972;14:1181–1193.

144. Gullestad L, Myers J, Edvardsen T, et al: Predictors of exercise capacity and the impact of angiographic coronary artery disease in heart transplant recipients. Am Heart J 2004;147:49–54.

145. Borrelli E, Pogliaghi S, Molinello A, et al: Serial assessment of peak VO2 and VO2 kinetics early after heart transplantation. Med Sci Sports Exerc 2003;35:1798–1804.

146. Shephard RJ: Responses of the cardiac transplant patient to exercise and training. Exerc Sport Sci Rev 1992;20:297–320.

147. Marconi C, Marzorati M: Exercise after heart transplantation. Eur J Appl Physiol 2003;90:250–259.

148. Williams MA, Maresh CM, Esterbrooks DJ, et al: Early exercise training in patients older than age 65 years compared with that in younger patients after acute myocardial infarction or coronary artery bypass grafting. Am J Cardiol 1985;55:263–266.

149. Ades P, Waldmann M, Poehlman E, et al: Exercise conditioning in older coronary patients: Submaximal lactate response and endurance capacity. Circulation 1993;88:572–577.

150. Lavie CJ, Milani RV: Impact of aging on hostility in coronary patients and effects of cardiac rehabilitation and exercise training in elderly persons. Am J Geriatr Cardiol 2004;13:125–130.

151. Lavie CJ, Milani RV: Effects of cardiac rehabilitation programs in very elderly patients ≥75 years of age. Am J Cardiol 1995;76:177–179.

152. Oldridge NB, Nagle FJ, Balke B, et al: Aortocoronary bypass surgery: Effects of surgery and 32 months of physical conditioning on treadmill performance. Arch Phys Med Rehabil 1978;59:268–275.

153. Soloff PH: Medically and surgically treated coronary patients in cardiovascular rehabilitation: A comparative study. Int J Psychiatry Med 1980;9:93–106.

154. Horgan JH, Teo KK, Murren KM, et al: The response to exercise training and vocation counselling in post-myocardial infarction and coronary artery bypass surgery patients. Ir Med J 1980;74:463–469.

155. Hartung GH, Rangel R: Exercise training in post-myocardial infarction patients: Comparison of results with high risk coronary and post-bypass patients. Arch Phys Med Rehabil 1981;62:147–153.

156. Dornan J, Rolko AF, Greenfield C: Factors affecting rehabilitation following aortocoronary bypass procedures. Can J Surg 1982;25:677–680.

157. Fletcher BJ, Lloyd A, Fletcher GF: Outpatient rehabilitative training in patients with cardiovascular disease: Emphasis on training method. Heart Lung 1988;17:199–205.

158. Nakai Y, Kataoka Y, Bando M, et al: Effects of physical exercise training on cardiac function and graft patency after coronary artery bypass grafting. J Thorac Cardiovasc Surg 1987;93:65–72.

159. Perk B, Hedback E, Engvall G: Effects of cardiac rehabilitation after CABS on readmissions, return to work, and physical fitness. Scand J Soc Med 1990;18:45–53.

160. Robinson G, Froelicher VF, Utley JR: Rehabilitation of the coronary artery bypass graft surgery patient. J Cardiac Rehabil 1984;4:74–86.

161. Foster C: Exercise training following cardiovascular surgery. Exerc Sport Sci Rev 1986;14:303–323.

162. Gohlke H, Schnellbacher K, Samek L, et al: Long-term improvement of exercise tolerance and vocational rehabilitation after bypass surgery: A five-year follow-up. J Cardiac Rehabil 1982;2:531–540.

163. Ben-Ari E, Kellermann JJ, Fisman E, et al: Benefits of long-term physical training in patients after coronary artery bypass grafting–A 58 month follow-up and comparison with a non-trained group. J Cardiopulm Rehabil 1986;6:165–170.

164. Dubach P, Litscher K, Kuhn M, et al: Cardiac rehabilitation in Switzerland: Efficacy of the residential approach following bypass surgery. Chest 1993;103:611–615.

165. Dubach P, Myers J, Dziekan G, et al: Effect of residential cardiac rehabilitation following bypass surgery: Observations in Switzerland. Chest 1995;108:1434–1439.

166. Hedbach B, Perk J, Engvall J, Areskog N-H: Cardiac rehabilitation after coronary artery bypass grafting: Effects on exercise performance and risk factors. Arch Phys Med Rehabil 1990;71:1069–1073.

167. Maresh C, Harbrecht J, Flick B, Hartzler G: Comparison of rehabilitation benefits after percutaneous transluminal coronary angioplasty and coronary artery bypass graft surgery. J Cardiac Rehabil 1985;5:124–130.

168. Waites T, Watt E, Fletcher G: Comparative functional and physiologic status of active and dropout coronary bypass patients of a rehabilitation program. Am J Cardiol 1983;51:1087–1090.

169. Stevens R, Hanson P: Comparisons of supervised and unsupervised exercise training after coronary bypass surgery. Am J Cardiol 1984;53:1524–1528.

170. Kappagoda CT, Greenwood PV: Physical training with minimal hospital supervision of patients after coronary artery bypass surgery. Arch Phys Med Rehabil 1984;65:57–60.

171. Froelicher V, Jensen D, Sullivan M: A randomized trial of the effects of exercise training after coronary artery bypass surgery. Arch Intern Med 1985;145:689–692.

172. Holmes DR, Vliestra RE, Smith HC, et al: Restenosis after percutaneous transluminal coronary angioplasty (PTCA): A report from the PTCA registry of the National, Heart, Lung, and Blood Institute. Am J Cardiol 1989;53:77C–81A.

173. Fitzgerald ST, Becker DM, Celentano DP, et al: Return to work after percutaneous transluminal coronary angioplasty. Am J Cardiol 1989;64:1108–1112.

174. Meier B, Gruentzig AR: Return to work after coronary artery bypass surgery in comparison to coronary angioplasty. In PJ Walter (ed.): Return to Work After Coronary Bypass Surgery: Psychosocial and Economic Aspects. New York, Springer-Verlag, 1995, pp 171–176.

175. Ben-Ari E, Rothbaum DA, Linnmeir TJ, et al: Benefits of a monitored rehabilitation program versus physician care after percutaneous transluminal coronary angioplasty: Follow-up of risk factors and rate of restenosis. J Cardiopulm Rehabil 1992;7:281–285.

176. Ben-Ari E, Rothbaum DA, Linnmeier TA, et al: Return to work after successful coronary angioplasty: Comparison between a comprehensive rehabilitation program and patients receiving usual care. J Cardiopulm Rehabil 1992;12:20–24.

177. Kubo H, Yano K, Hirai H, et al: Preventive effect of exercise training on recurrent stenosis after percutaneous transluminal coronary angioplasty (PTCA). Jpn Circ J 1992;56:413–421.

178. Hambrecht R, Walther C, Mobius-Winkler S, et al: Percutaneous coronary angioplasty compared with exercise training in patients with stable coronary artery disease. A randomized trial. Circulation 2004;109:1371–1378.

179. Haskell WL: Restoration and maintenance of physical and psychosocial function in patients with ischemic heart disease. J Am Coll Cardiol 1988;12:1090–1121.

180. Dennis C, Houston-Miller N, Schwartz RG, et al: Early return to work after uncomplicated myocardial infarction: Results of a randomized trial. JAMA 1988;260:214–220.

181. Picard MH, Dennis C, Schwartz RG, et al: Cost-benefit analysis of early return to work after uncomplicated acute myocardial infarction. Am J Cardiol 1989;63:1308–1314.

182. Engblom E, Korpilahti K, Hamalainen H, et al: Quality of life and return to work 5 years after coronary artery bypass surgery. Long term results of cardiac rehabilitation. J Cardiovasc Rehabil 1997;17:29–36.

183. Siegel D, Grady P, Browner WS, Hulley SB: Risk factor modification after myocardial infarction. Ann Intern Med 1988;109:213–218.

184. LaRosa JC, Cleary P, Muesing RA, et al: Effect of long-term moderate physical exercise on plasma lipoproteins: The National Exercise and Heart Disease Project. Arch Intern Med 1982;142:2269–2274.

185. Pekkanen J, Linn S, Meiss G, et al: Ten year mortality from cardiovascular disease in relation to cholesterol level among men with and without preexisting cardiovascular disease. N Engl J Med 1990;332:1700–1707.

186. Hamalainen H, Luurila OJ, Kallio V, et al: Long-term reduction in sudden deaths after a multifactorial intervention programme in patients with myocardial infarction: 10-year results in a controlled investigation. Eur Heart J 1989;10:55–62.

187. Schell WD, Myers JN: Regression of atherosclerosis: A review. Prog Cardiovasc Dis 1997;39:483–496.

188. Feeman WE, Niebauer J: Prediction of angiographic stabilization/regression of coronary atherosclerosis by a risk factor graph. J Cardiovasc Risk 2000;7:415–423.

189. Third Report of the National Cholesterol Education Program (NCEP) Expert Panel on Detection, Evaluation and Treatment, High Blood Cholesterol in Adults (Adults Treatment Panel III) final report. Circulation 2002;106:3143–3421.

190. Pierson LM, Miller LE, Herbert WG: Predicting exercise training outcome from cardiac rehabilitation. J Cardiopulm Rehabil 2004;24:113–118.

191. Hammond KH, Kelly TL, Froelicher VF, Pewen W: Use of clinical data in predicting improvement in exercise capacity after cardiac rehabilitation. J Am Coll Cardiol 1985;6:19–26.

192. Van Dixhoorn E, Duivenvoorden H, Pool G: Success and failure of exercise training after myocardial infarction: Is the outcome predictable? J Am Coll Cardiol 1990;15:974–980.

193. European Heart Failure Training Group: Experience from controlled trials of physical training in chronic heart failure. Protocol and patient factors in effectiveness in the improvement in exercise tolerance. Eur Heart J 1998;19:466–475.

194. Myers J, Froelicher VF: Predicting outcome in cardiac rehabilitation. J Am Coll Cardiol 1990;15:983–985.

195. Ades PA, Balady GJ, Berra K: Transforming exercise-based cardiac rehabilitation programs into secondary prevention centers: A national imperative. J Cardiopulm Rehabil 2001;21:263–272.

196. Balady G, Ades P, Comoss P, et al: Core components of cardiac rehabilitation/secondary prevention programs: A statement for healthcare professions from the American Heart Association and the American Association of Cardiovascular and Pulmonary Rehabilitation Writing Group. Circulation 2000;102:1069–1073.

197. Wee CC, McCarthy EP, Davis, et al: Physician counseling about exercise. JAMA 1999;282:1583–1588.

198. Sherman SE, Hershman WY: Exercise counseling: How do general internists do? J Gen Intern Med 1993;8:243–248.

199. Damush TM, Stewart AL, Mills KM, et al: Prevalence and correlates of physician recommendations to exercise among older adults. J Gerontol A Biol Sci Med Sci 1999;54:M423–M427.

200. Sueta C, Chowdhury M, Boccussi S: Analysis of the degree of undertreatment of hyperlipidemia and congestive heart failure secondary to coronary artery disease. Am J Cardiol 1999;83:1303–1307.

201. Schrott H, Bittner V, Vittinghoff E, et al: Adherence to national cholesterol education program treatment goals in postmenopausal women with heart disease: The heart and estrogen/progestin replacement study (HERS). JAMA 1997;277:1281–1286.

202. Ribisl PM: Exercise: The unfilled prescription. Am J Med Sports 2001;3:13–21.

203. Ribisl PM: The inclusive chronic disease model: Reaching beyond cardiopulmonary patients. In Jobin J, Maltais F, Poirier P, Leblanc P, Simard C (eds): Advancing the Frontiers of Cardiopulmonary Rehabilitation. Champaign, Ill, Human Kinetics, 2002, pp 29–36.

204. Gordon NF, Salmon RD, Mitchell BS, et al: Innovative approaches to comprehensive cardiovascular disease risk reduction in clinical and community-based settings. Curr Atheroscler Rep 2001;3:498–506.

205. DeBusk RF, Haskell WL, Miller NH, et al: Medically directed at-home rehabilitation soon after clinically uncomplicated acute myocardial infarction: A new model for patient care. Am J Cardiol 1985;55:251–257.

206. Ades P, Pashkow F, Fletcher G, et al: A controlled trial of cardiac rehabilitation in the home setting using electrocardiographic and voice transtelephonic monitoring. Am Heart J 2000;139:543–548.

207. DeBusk RF, Houston-Miller N, Superko HR, et al: A case-management system for coronary risk factor modification after acute myocardial infarction. Ann Intern Med 1994;120:721–729.

208. Levknecht L, Schriefer J, Schriefer J, Maconis B: Combining case management, pathways, and report cards for secondary cardiac prevention. Jt Commun Qual Improv 1997;23:162–174.

209. Fonarow GC, Gawlinski A, Moughrabi S, Tillisch JH: Improved treatment of coronary heart disease by implementation of a Cardiac Hospitalization Atherosclerosis Management Program (CHAMP). Am J Cardiol 2001;87:819–822.

210. West JA, Miller NH, Parker K, et al: A comprehensive management system for heart failure improves clinical outcomes and reduces medical resource utilization. Am J Cardiol 1997;79:58–63.

211. Froelicher VF, Herbert W, Myers J, Ribisl P: How cardiac rehabilitation is being influenced by changes in healthcare delivery. J Cardiopulm Rehabil 1996;16:151–159.

212. Ries AL, Kaplan RM, Limberg TM, Prewitt LM: Effects of pulmonary rehabilitation on physiologic and psychosocial outcomes in patients with chronic obstructive pulmonary disease. Ann Intern Med 1995;122:823–832.

213. Drummond M, Brandt A, Luce B, Rovira J: Standardizing methodologies for economic evaluation in health care. Int J Technol Assess Health Care 1993;9:26–36.

214. Oldridge N, Furlong W, Feeny D, Guyatt GH: Economic evaluation of cardiac rehabilitation soon after acute myocardial infarction. Am J Cardiol 1993;72:154–161.

215. Ades PA, Huang D, Weaver SO: Cardiac rehabilitation participation predicts lower rehospitalization costs. Am Heart J 1992;123:916–921.

216. Bondestam E, Breikss A, Hartford M: Effects of early rehabilitation on consumption of medical care during the first year after acute myocardial infarction in patients 65 years of age or older. Am J Cardiol 1995;75:767–771.

217. Levin LA, Perk J, Hedback B: Cardiac rehabilitation: A cost analysis. J Intern Med 1991;230:427–434.

218. Ades PA, Pashkow FJ, Nestor JR: Cost effectiveness of cardiac rehabilitation after myocardial infarction. J Cardiopulm Rehabil 1997;17:222–231.

index

Note: Page numbers in *italics* refer to illustrations; page numbers followed by the letter t refer to tables.

N